Biomedical Imaging

Biomedical Imaging

Edited by **Thomas Jackson**

hayle
medical

New York

Published by Hayle Medical,
30 West, 37th Street, Suite 612,
New York, NY 10018, USA
www.haylemedical.com

Biomedical Imaging
Edited by Thomas Jackson

International Standard Book Number: 978-1-63241-405-2 (Hardback)

The publisher's policy is to use permanent paper from mills that operate a sustainable forestry policy. Furthermore, the publisher ensures that the text paper and cover boards used have met acceptable environmental accreditation standards.

Printed in the United States of America.

Contents

Preface   VII

Chapter 1   **Recovering 3D Shape with Absolute Size from Endoscope Images Using RBF
            Neural Network**   1
            Seiya Tsuda, Yuji Iwahori, M. K. Bhuyan, Robert J. Woodham and Kunio Kasugai

Chapter 2   **Closed Contour Specular Reflection Segmentation in Laparoscopic Images**   12
            Jan Marek Marcinczak and Rolf-Rainer Grigat

Chapter 3   **High Performance GPU-Based Fourier Volume Rendering**   18
            Marwan Abdellah, Ayman Eldeib and Amr Sharawi

Chapter 4   **Automatic Classification of Normal and Cancer Lung CT Images Using Multiscale
            AM-FM Features**   31
            Eman Magdy, Nourhan Zayed and Mahmoud Fakhr

Chapter 5   **Imaging Performance of Quantitative Transmission Ultrasound**   38
            Mark W. Lenox, James Wiskin, Matthew A. Lewis, Stephen Darrouzet, David Borup
            and Scott Hsieh

Chapter 6   **Incidence of Brain Abnormalities Detected on Preoperative Brain MR Imaging
            and their Effect on the Outcome of Cochlear Implantation in Children with
            Sensorineural Hearing Loss**   46
            Xiao-Quan Xu, Fei-Yun Wu, Hao Hu, Guo-Yi Su and Jie Shen

Chapter 7   **Learned Shrinkage Approach for Low-Dose Reconstruction in Computed
            Tomography**   52
            Joseph Shtok, Michael Elad and Michael Zibulevsky

Chapter 8   **Statistical Analysis of Haralick Texture Features to Discriminate Lung
            Abnormalities**   72
            Nourhan Zayed and Heba A. Elnemr

Chapter 9   **Automated Feature Extraction in Brain Tumor by Magnetic Resonance Imaging
            Using Gaussian Mixture Models**   79
            Ahmad Chaddad

Chapter 10 **Evaluation of Algebraic Iterative Image Reconstruction Methods for Tetrahedron
            Beam Computed Tomography Systems**   90
            Joshua Kim, Huaiqun Guan, David Gersten and Tiezhi Zhang

Chapter 11 **Lung Segmentation in 4D CT Volumes Based on Robust Active Shape
            Model Matching**   104
            Gurman Gill and Reinhard R. Beichel

Chapter 12   **Automated Classification of Glandular Tissue by Statistical Proximity Sampling**   113
Jimmy C. Azar, Martin Simonsson, Ewert Bengtsson and Anders Hast

Chapter 13   **Edge Detection in Digital Images Using Dispersive Phase Stretch Transform**   124
Mohammad H. Asghari and Bahram Jalali

Chapter 14   **Automated Diagnosis of Otitis Media: Vocabulary and Grammar**   130
Anupama Kuruvilla, Nader Shaikh, Alejandro Hoberman and Jelena Kovačević

Chapter 15   **Endoscopy-MR Image Fusion for Image Guided Procedures**   145
Anwar Abdalbari, Xishi Huang and Jing Ren

Chapter 16   **Classifying Dementia Using Local Binary Patterns from Different Regions in Magnetic Resonance Images**   155
Ketil Oppedal, Trygve Eftestøl, Kjersti Engan, Mona K. Beyer and Dag Aarsland

Chapter 17   **Automated Segmentation and Object Classification of CT Images: Application to *In Vivo* Molecular Imaging of Avian Embryos**   169
Alexander Heidrich, Jana Schmidt, Johannes Zimmermann and Hans Peter Saluz

Chapter 18   **Respiratory Motion Compensation Using Diaphragm Tracking for Cone-Beam C-Arm CT: A Simulation and a Phantom Study**   179
Marco Bögel, Hannes G. Hofmann, Joachim Hornegger, Rebecca Fahrig, Stefan Britzen and Andreas Maier

Chapter 19   **Insight into the Molecular Imaging of Alzheimer's Disease**   189
Abishek Arora and Neeta Bhagat

Chapter 20   **Clutter Mitigation in Echocardiography Using Sparse Signal Separation**   206
Javier S. Turek, Michael Elad and Irad Yavneh

Chapter 21   **Optic Disc Segmentation by Balloon Snake with Texture from Color Fundus Image**   224
Jinyang Sun, Fangjun Luan and Hanhui Wu

Chapter 22   **Skin Parameter Map Retrieval from a Dedicated Multispectral Imaging System Applied to Dermatology/Cosmetology**   238
Romuald Jolivot, Yannick Benezeth and Franck Marzani

Chapter 23   **Automatic Extraction of Blood Vessels in the Retinal Vascular Tree Using Multiscale Medialness**   253
Mariem Ben Abdallah, Jihene Malek, Ahmad Taher Azar, Philippe Montesinos, Hafedh Belmabrouk, Julio Esclarín Monreal and Karl Krissian

Permissions

List of Contributors

Preface

Biomedical Imaging is a fast growing field of medicine. Technological changes and constant demand for improved diagnosis led to the growth and advancement of this discipline. This area has acquired a completely different outlook over the years. It involves collection, analysis, and deduction of results with the use of techniques such as Magnetic resonance imaging (MRI), computed tomography (CT) scan, ultrasound, neutron imaging, digital radiography and tomosynthesis, Positron emission tomography (PET), etc. This book traces the progress of the field of biomedical imaging and serves as a complete source of knowledge on the present status of this important area. This book is a valuable compilation of topics, ranging from the basic to the most complex advancements in the field of biomedical imaging. It is an essential guide for both academicians and those who wish to pursue this discipline further.

The information shared in this book is based on empirical researches made by veterans in this field of study. The elaborative information provided in this book will help the readers further their scope of knowledge leading to advancements in this field.

Finally, I would like to thank my fellow researchers who gave constructive feedback and my family members who supported me at every step of my research.

Editor

Recovering 3D Shape with Absolute Size from Endoscope Images Using RBF Neural Network

Seiya Tsuda,[1] **Yuji Iwahori,**[1] **M. K. Bhuyan,**[2] **Robert J. Woodham,**[3] **and Kunio Kasugai**[4]

[1]*Department of Computer Science, Chubu University, 1200 Matsumotocho, Kasugai 487-8501, Japan*
[2]*Department of Electronics and Electrical Engineering, IIT Guwahati, Guwahati 781039, India*
[3]*Department of Computer Science, University of British Columbia, Vancouver, BC, Canada V6T 1Z4*
[4]*Department of Gastroenterology, Aichi Medical University, 1-1 Karimata, Yazako, Nagakute 480-1195, Japan*

Correspondence should be addressed to Seiya Tsuda; tuda_g@cvl.cs.chubu.ac.jp

Academic Editor: Richard H. Bayford

Medical diagnosis judges the status of polyp from the size and the 3D shape of the polyp from its medical endoscope image. However the medical doctor judges the status empirically from the endoscope image and more accurate 3D shape recovery from its 2D image has been demanded to support this judgment. As a method to recover 3D shape with high speed, VBW (Vogel-Breuß-Weickert) model is proposed to recover 3D shape under the condition of point light source illumination and perspective projection. However, VBW model recovers the relative shape but there is a problem that the shape cannot be recovered with the exact size. Here, shape modification is introduced to recover the exact shape with modification from that with VBW model. RBF-NN is introduced for the mapping between input and output. Input is given as the output of gradient parameters of VBW model for the generated sphere. Output is given as the true gradient parameters of true values of the generated sphere. Learning mapping with NN can modify the gradient and the depth can be recovered according to the modified gradient parameters. Performance of the proposed approach is confirmed via computer simulation and real experiment.

1. Introduction

Endoscopy allows medical practitioners to observe the interior of hollow organs and other body cavities in a minimally invasive way. Sometimes, diagnosis requires assessment of the 3D shape of the observed tissue. For example, the pathological condition of a polyp often is related to its geometrical shape. Medicine is an important area of application of computer vision technology. Specialized endoscopes with a laser light beam head [1] or with two cameras mounted in the head [2] have been developed. Many approaches are based on stereo vision [3]; however, the size of endoscope becomes large and this imposes a burden on the patient. Here, we consider a general purpose endoscope, of the sort still most widely used in medical practice.

Here, shape from endoscope image is considered. Shape from shading (SFS) [4] and Fast Marching Method [5] based SFS approach [6] are proposed. These approaches use orthographic projection, while an extension of FMM to the perspective projection is proposed in [7] or further extension of FMM to both point light source illumination and perspective projection is proposed in [8]. Recent extensions include generating Lambertian image from the original multiple color images [9, 10]. Application of FMM includes the solution [11] to the oblique light source problem using neural network learning [12].

Iwahori et al. [13] developed Radial Basis Function Neural Network (RBF-NN) photometric stereo, where RBF-NN is powerful to achieve the multiple dimensional nonparametric functional approximation between input and output mapping.

Recently, VBW model [14], which is based on solving the Hamilton-Jacobi equation, has been proposed to recover a shape from an image taken under the conditions of point light source illumination and perspective projection. However the result recovered by VBW model is relative and there is a problem that VBW gives much smaller values of surface gradient and height distribution than those of true values.

That is, it is impossible to apply the VBW model to obtain the exact shape and size.

This paper proposes a new approach to recover the 3D shape with absolute size from 2D image taken under the condition of both point light source illumination and perspective projection. While the VBW model approach can recover the relative shape with relative scale, the proposed approach obtains absolute depth by improving the gradient modification by RBF neural network. The final purpose of this approach is to support the medical diagnosis of the status of polyp if polyp is benign or malignant by recovering 3D shape with its absolute size.

The proposed approach generates a Lambertian sphere model. VBW model is applied for the generated sphere and shape is recovered. Here RBF-NN is used and learned with this sphere to improve the accuracy of recovered shape, where input and output of the neural network are the surface gradient parameters obtained via VBW model as input and the corresponding true values as output, respectively.

The proposed approach is evaluated and it is confirmed that the obtained shape is improved via computer simulation and real experiments.

2. VBW Model

VBW model [14] is proposed as a model to calculate the depth from the view point under the conditions of point light source illumination and perspective projection by solving the Hamilton-Jacobi equations [15] combined with the model of Faugeras and Prados models [16, 17]. Lambertian reflectance is assumed for a target object as another condition.

The following processing is applied for each point of the image. First, the initial value for the depth $Z_{default}$ is given using (1) as in [18]:

$$Z_{default} = -0.5 \log \left(I f^2 \right), \tag{1}$$

where I represents the normalized image intensity and f is the focal length of the lens.

Next, the combination of gradient parameters which gives the minimum gradient is selected from the difference of the depth for the neighboring points. The depth Z is calculated from (2) and the process is repeated until Z does not change for that at the previous stage. Here, (x, y) represent the image coordinates, Δt represents the width of time, (m, n) represent the minimum gradient for (x, y) directions, and $Q = f/\sqrt{x^2 + y^2 + f^2}$ represents the coefficient of the perspective projection, respectively:

$$
\begin{aligned}
&Z(x, y) \\
&= Z(x, y) + \Delta t \exp\left(-2Z(x, y)\right) \\
&\quad - \Delta t \\
&\quad \cdot \left(\frac{If^2}{Q} \sqrt{f^2 \left(m(x)^2 + n(y)^2\right) + \left(xm(x) + yn(y)\right)^2 + Q^2} \right).
\end{aligned}
\tag{2}
$$

Here, it is noted that the shape obtained via VBW model gives the relative scale, not absolute one. This means that obtained result gives the smaller values of surface gradients than those actual values.

3. Proposed Approach

3.1. NN Learning for Modification of Surface Gradient. When uniform Lambertian reflectance is assumed, the intensity depends on the dot product of surface normal vector and light source vector with the inverse square law for illuminance. The image intensity of the surface is determined as follows:

$$E = C \frac{(\mathbf{s} \cdot \mathbf{n})}{r^2}, \tag{3}$$

where E is image intensity, C is reflectance parameter, $\mathbf{s}$ is a unit vector towards a point light source, $\mathbf{n}$ is a unit surface normal vector, and r is the distance between a point light source and surface point.

The basic assumption is that both of point light source and center of lens are located at the origin of (X, Y, Z) coordinates and image projection is perspective projection. That is, the object is viewed and illuminated from the view point. Here, the actual endoscope image has the color textures and specular reflectance. Using the approach proposed in the paper [19] can convert the original input image into the uniform Lambertian gray scale image.

VBW model gives the relative result for the true size and shape. VBW model also assumes the condition that Lambertian image is used to recover the shape as a target. The result gives the small values of surface gradient and the depth. Here, the modification of surface gradient and improvement of the recovered shape are considered. First the surface gradient at each point is modified with neural network (NN), and then the depth is modified from modified surface gradient parameters $(p, q) = (\partial Z/\partial X, \partial Z/\partial Y)$. RBF-NN (Radial Basis Function Neural Network) [12] is used for the learning for modification of surface gradient of the result obtained by VBW model.

Expanding (3) with parameters (p, q, Z) derives the following:

$$E = C \frac{(-px - qy + f) f^2}{(x^2 + y^2 + f^2)^{3/2} Z^2 (p^2 + q^2 + 1)^{1/2}}, \tag{4}$$

where (x, y) are image coordinates, f is focal length of the lens, and Z is depth.

Sphere image is synthesized using (4) and VBW model is applied to this sphere image. Surface gradient parameters (p, q) are obtained using forward difference of Z obtained from VBW model. Calculated (p, q) and the corresponding true (p, q) for the synthesized sphere are given to the RBF-NN as input vector and output vector, respectively, and NN learning is applied. After NN learning, this NN can be used to modify the recovered shape for other images. Original endoscope image is shown in Figure 1(a) and generated Lambertian image using [19] is shown in Figure 1(b) as an example.

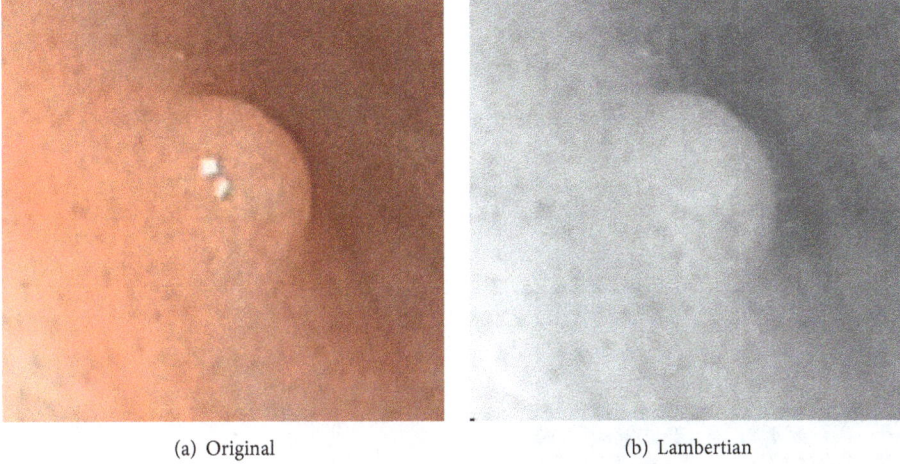

(a) Original   (b) Lambertian

FIGURE 1: Endoscope image and Lambertian image.

The synthesized sphere image used in NN is shown in Figure 2(a). Surface gradients obtained by VBW model are shown in Figures 2(b) and 2(c) and the corresponding true (p, q) of this sphere are shown in Figures 2(d) and 2(e), respectively. Various points are sampled from a sphere and NN learning is done except points with so large values of (p, q). Procedure of NN learning is shown in Figure 3.

3.2. NN Generalization and Modification of Z.
Learned NN is used for generalization for another test object. Modification of (p, q) using learned NN is applied to test object and depth Z is calculated and updated using modified (p, q). To apply this NN to endoscope image, specular component is removed and uniform Lambertian image is generated based on our previous preprocessing for endoscope image in [19]. This is because endoscope image includes color textures and specular reflectance components and it is necessary to generate a uniform Lambertian sphere with gray scale image.

Next, VBW model is applied to this Lambertian image and (p, q) are calculated from the obtained Z distribution. Calculated (p, q) are input to the learned NN and the modified (p, q) are obtained as output of NN. The depth Z is calculated and updated by (5) using modified (p, q), where (5) is also the original equation derived in [8]:

$$Z = \sqrt{\frac{CV(-px - qy + f)}{E(p^2 + q^2 + 1)^{1/2}}}, \quad (5)$$

where p, q, E, f, and C are the same parameters as those in (4), while $V = f^2 / (x^2 + y^2 + f^2)^{3/2}$.

The flow of processing described above is shown in Figure 4.

4. Experimental Results

4.1. NN Learning.
Sphere was synthesized with radius 5 mm whose center is located at $(0, 0, 15)$ with the focal length 10 mm of the lens and reflectance parameter set to 100.

The image size is 9 mm $\times$ 9 mm and pixel size is 256 $\times$ 256 pixels. This sphere was recovered by VBW model and the result gave the gradient parameters (p, q) as shown in Figures 2(b) and 2(c), respectively. These (p, q) are used as input of NN and the corresponding true (p, q) shown in Figures 2(d) and 2(e) are used as output of NN. Learning was done under the condition of the error goal $1.0e - 1$, the maximum number of learning epochs 500. The results of learning are shown in Figure 5.

As shown in Figure 5, NN learning was done with 500 epochs. Also, processing time for NN learning was around 70 seconds.

A sphere has a variety of surface gradients and it is used for the NN learning. After a sphere is used for NN learning, not only a sphere object but also another object with another shape including convex or concave surfaces is also applied in the generalization process. This is because surface gradient for each point is modified by NN and this modification does not depend on the shape of target object.

4.2. Computer Simulation.
Computer simulation is done to confirm the performance of NN generalization. The first experiment is done under the condition that the reflectance factor is 50 and the focal length is 10 mm for a sphere with radius 3 mm. The center of a sphere is set at $(0, 0, 15)$, as shown in Figure 6. The image size is 9 mm $\times$ 9 mm and the pixel size is 360 $\times$ 360 pixels. True depth is shown in Figure 7(a) and the result of VBW model is shown in Figure 7(b), while the improved result is shown in Figure 7(c). The mean error of gradient parameters and depth is shown in Table 1.

The mean errors of surface gradient and depth are shown in Table 1. In Table 1, the depth had improvement of the mean error from 1.84 to 0.03; that is, mean error became 0.02 times less in comparison with that by VBW model. Generalization of NN was quite good for the different condition of Z with another size and shape. It took 40 seconds in total. It is shown that the obtained result was improved from Figures 7(a), 7(b), and 7(c) and Table 1. These results suggest that error tends to increase at the points where the values of (p, q) become

(a) Sphere

(b) p by VBW

(c) q by VBW

(d) True p

(e) True q

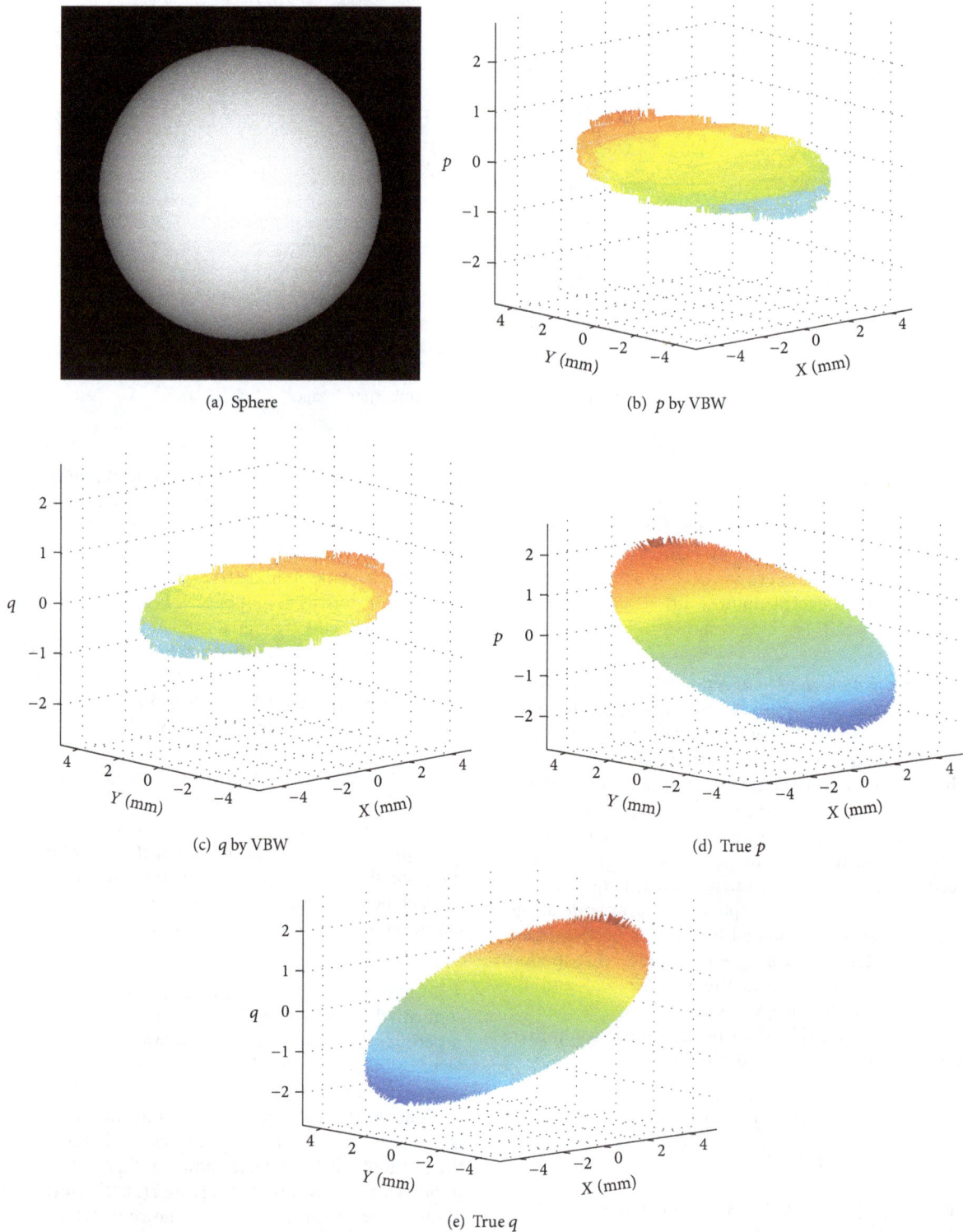

Figure 2: Synthesized sphere for NN learning.

large, because the number of sampled points with the larger values of (p, q) was smaller using every equal number of dot sampling.

Next, synthesized cosine curved surface was used, whose center is located at the coordinate (0, 0, 12). Here, the reflectance parameter C is 120, the focal length f is 10 mm,

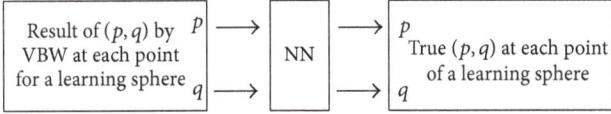

FIGURE 3: Learning flow.

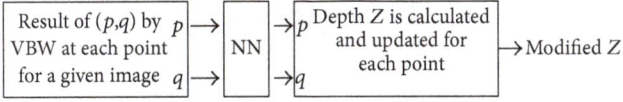

FIGURE 4: Flow of NN generalization.

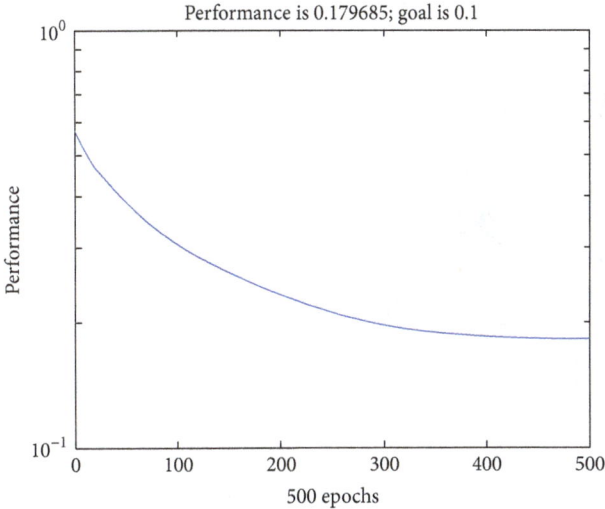

FIGURE 5: Learning result.

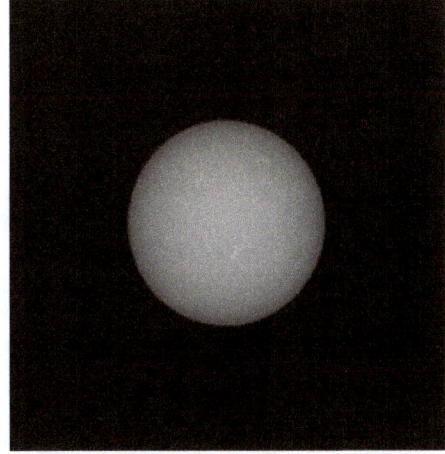

FIGURE 6: Sphere image.

TABLE 1: Mean error.

	p	q	Z [mm]
VBW	11.24	11.24	1.84
Proposed	0.41	0.41	0.03

TABLE 2: Mean error.

	p	q	Z [mm]
VBW	23.04	23.04	0.86
Proposed	0.33	0.33	0.26

waveform cycle is 4 mm, and ± amplitude is 1 mm. Synthesized image is shown in Figure 8.

Using the learned NN, (p, q) obtained from VBW were input and generalized. (p, q) were modified and Z was further updated using (5). The true depth is shown in Figure 9(a). Recovered result by VBW is shown in Figure 9(b) for Figure 8 and modified depth using NN and (5) is shown in Figure 9(c).

The mean errors of surface gradient and depth are shown in Table 2. In Table 2, the depth had improvement of the mean error from 0.86 to 0.26; that is, mean error became 0.3 times less in comparison with that by VBW model. Generalization of NN was quite good for the different condition of Z with another size and shape. It took 9 seconds to recover the shape while it took 61 seconds for NN learning with 428 learning epochs; that is, it took 70 seconds in total.

It is confirmed that the shape is improved with modification in the proposed approach from Figure 9. This means that NN modified (p, q) for each point and Z are modified correctly.

4.3. Real Image Experiments.

Real endoscope image is used in the experiments. First, NN was learned using a synthesized sphere as well. Then, VBW is applied to real endoscope image which is converted into uniform Lambertian image. Surface gradients (p, q) were modified with NN; then Z was calculated and updated for each point of endoscope image, where the focal length f, the image size, and camera movement ΔZ were assigned to the same known parameters as those in the computer simulation. Endoscope image is shown in Figure 10(a). Generated Lambertian image is shown in Figure 10(b). Result by VBW is shown in Figure 11(a) and modified result is shown in Figure 11(b).

In Figure 10(b), the specular reflection component was removed in comparison with Figure 10(a) of input image, and it is confirmed that the converted image has become a gray scale image with uniform reflectance. It is also confirmed that Figure 11(b) gives larger height than Figure 11(a), via modification. Except the cast shadow region, the processing was done correctly and improved the depth. The size of polyp was 1 cm and the processing time for shape modification was 9 seconds. It took 9 seconds to recover the shape while it took 117 seconds for NN learning with 540 learning epochs; that is, it took 126 seconds in total. Although the quantitative evaluation is difficult, medical doctors with experience of endoscope diagnosis evaluated the result and qualitatively correct evaluations have been obtained for the result. Thus, it was confirmed that the proposed approach is effective for the real endoscope image.

Another experiment is done for three cases of endoscopic image. Endoscope image of the first case is shown in Figure 12(a), and this Lambertian image generated is in

(a) True Z

(b) Z by VBW

(c) Modified Z

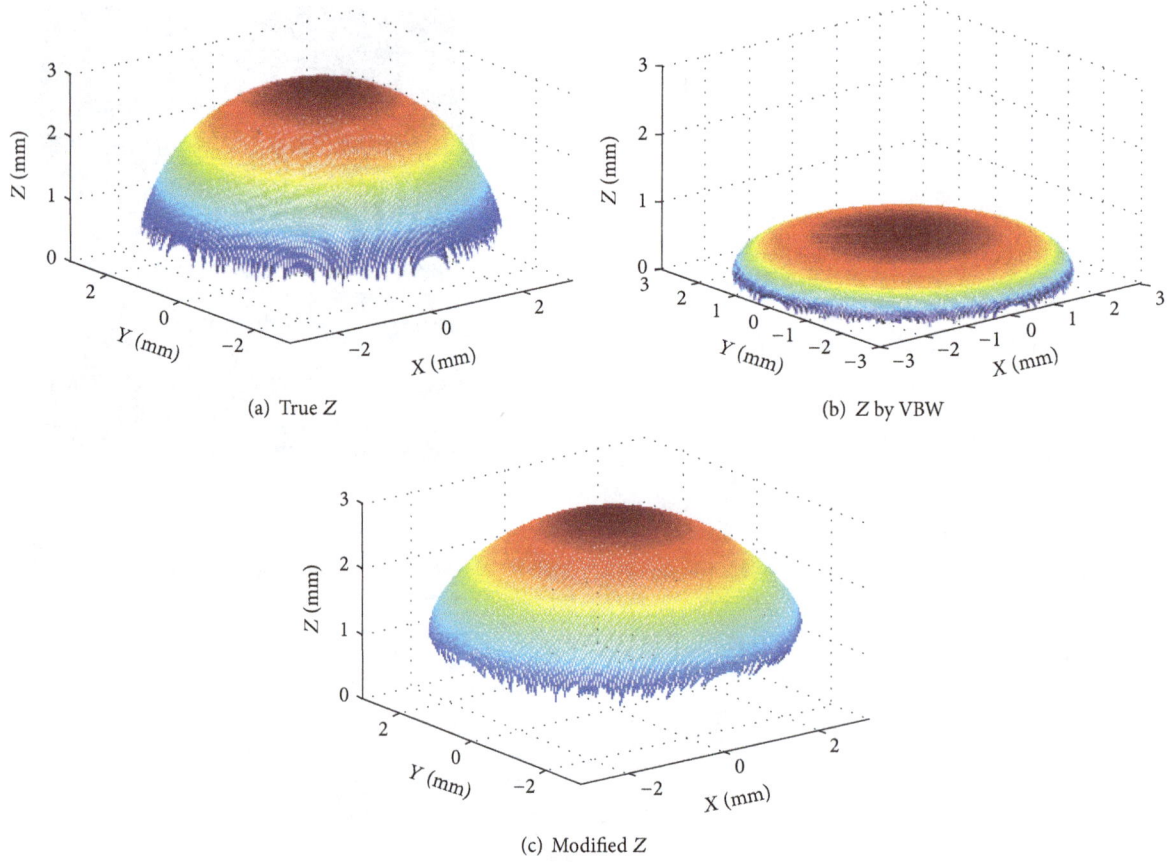

FIGURE 7: Results.

FIGURE 8: Cosine model.

Figure 12(b). The result for Figure 12(b) is shown in Figure 13(a), while that for the proposed approach is shown in Figure 13(b), respectively.

Endoscope image of second case is shown in Figure 14(a), and this Lambertian image generated is in Figure 14(b). The result for Figure 14(b) is shown in Figure 15(a), while that for the proposed approach is shown in Figure 15(b), respectively.

Endoscope image of third case is shown in Figure 16(a), and this Lambertian image generated is in Figure 16(b). The result for Figure 16(b) is shown in Figure 17(a), while that for the proposed approach is shown in Figure 17(b), respectively.

In Figure 13(b), the size of polyp was 2 mm. In Figures 12(b), 14(b), and 16(b), the specular reflection component was removed in comparison with Figures 12(a), 14(a), and 16(a) of input image, and it is confirmed that the converted images have become a gray scale images with uniform reflectance, recpectively. It is also confirmed that Figures 13(b), 15(b), and 17(b) give larger height than Figures 13(a), 15(a), and 17(a) via modification, respectively. Learning time in all examples is about 60 seconds, while it took about 10 seconds to recover the modified shape. In Figures 15(b) and 17(b), the proposed approach can recover the rough concave/convex shape. It was confirmed that the gradient modification is effective to other shapes except a sphere. The result by VBW model represents convex and concave shape with relative scale for whole examples. However the height result by VBW model gives very small height and does not represent actual height, which means the height obtained is relative. The advantage of the proposed approach is that it can recover 3D shape with absolute size of polyp by keeping the original convex and concave conditions to obtain the actual status of polyp.

(a) True Z

(b) Z by VBW

(c) Modified Z

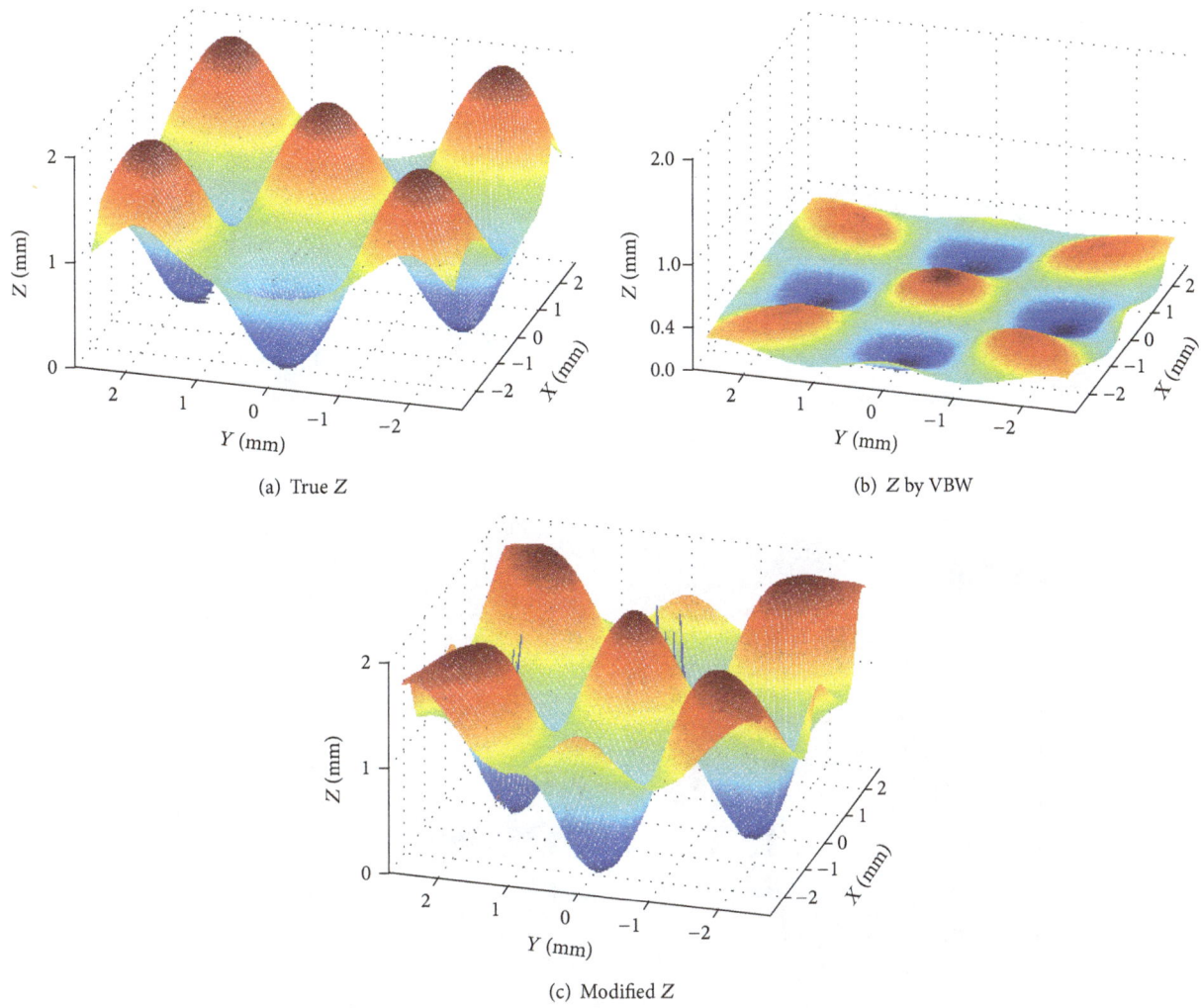

FIGURE 9: Results.

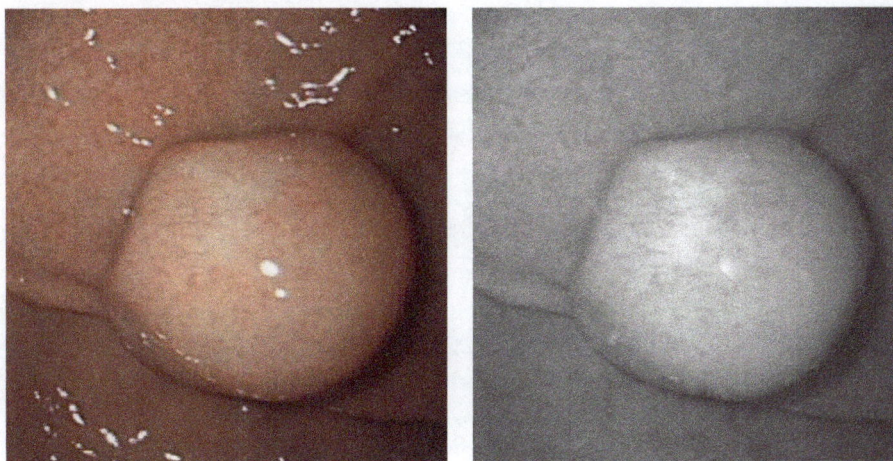

(a) Endoscope

(b) Lambertian

FIGURE 10: Endoscope image and generating Lambertian image.

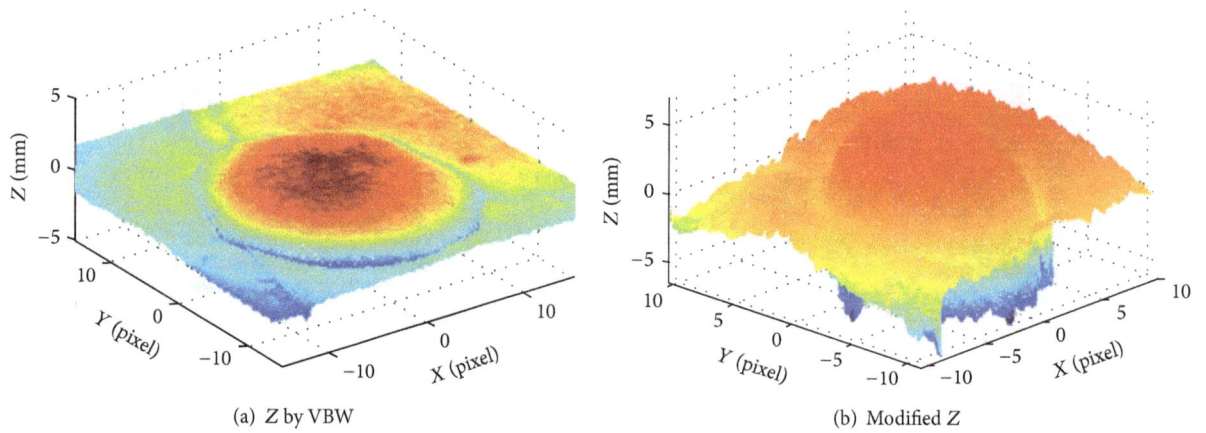

(a) Z by VBW

(b) Modified Z

FIGURE 11: Result for endoscope images.

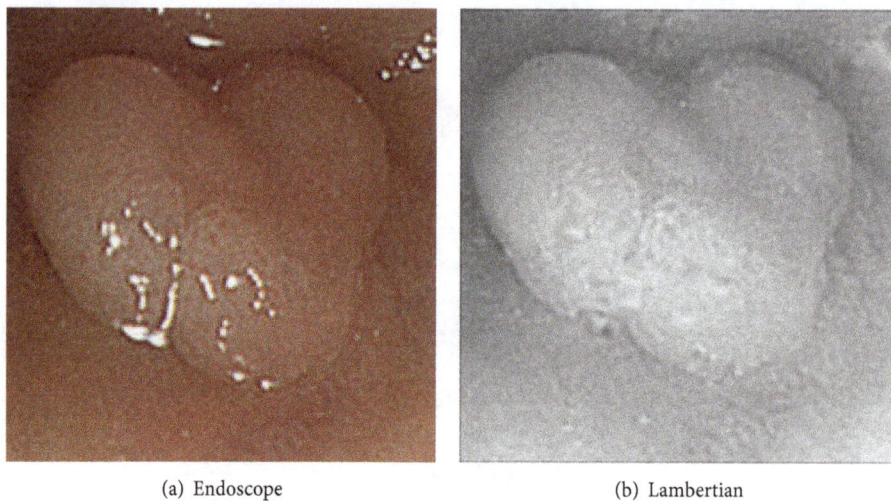

(a) Endoscope

(b) Lambertian

FIGURE 12: Endoscope image and generating Lambertian image.

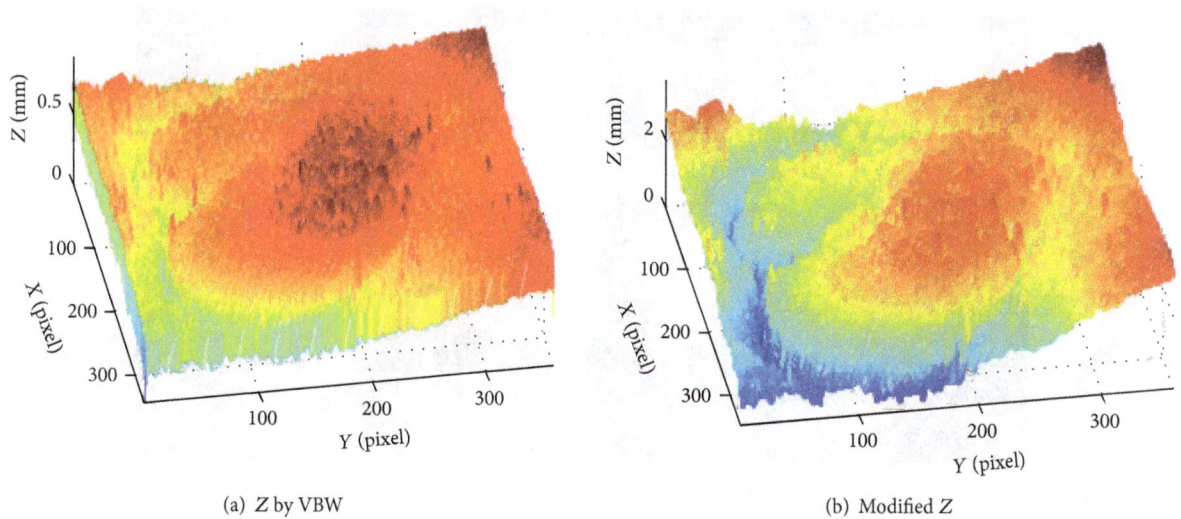

(a) Z by VBW

(b) Modified Z

FIGURE 13: Result for endoscope images.

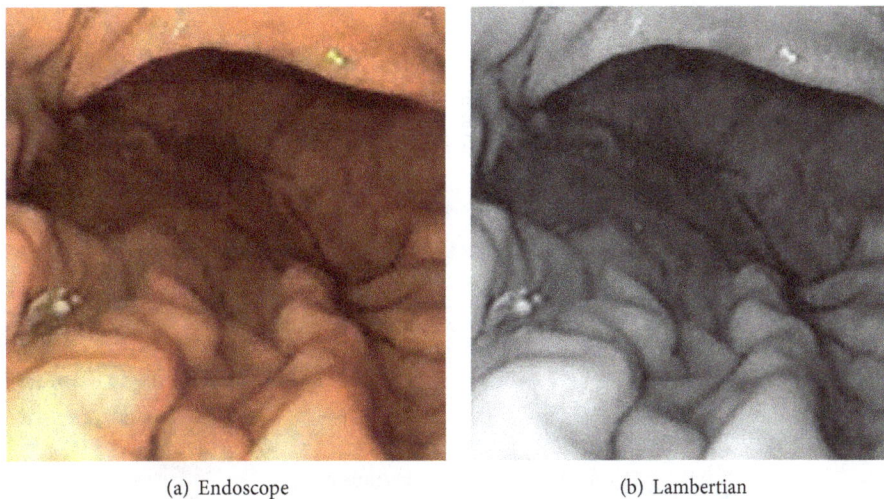

(a) Endoscope

(b) Lambertian

FIGURE 14: Endoscope image and generating Lambertian image.

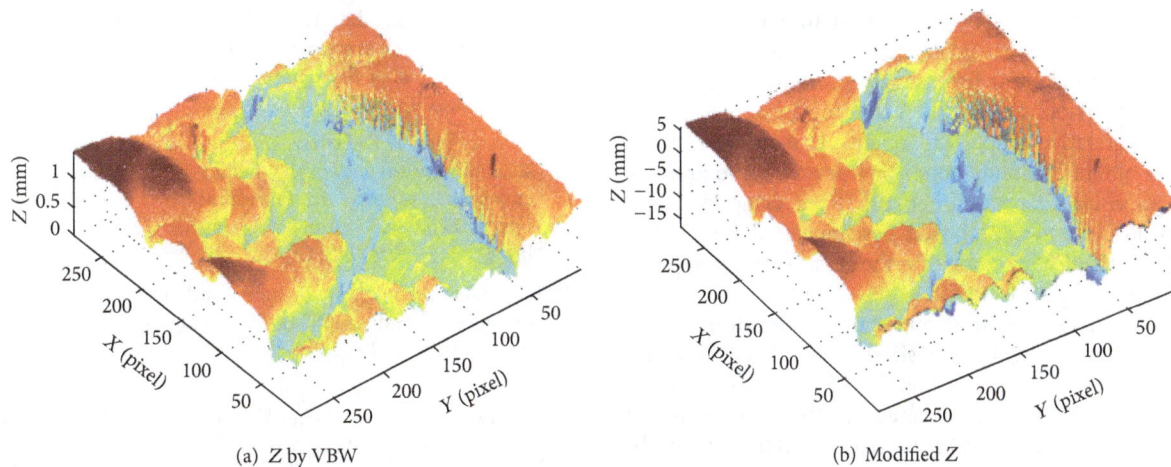

(a) Z by VBW

(b) Modified Z

FIGURE 15: Result for endoscope images.

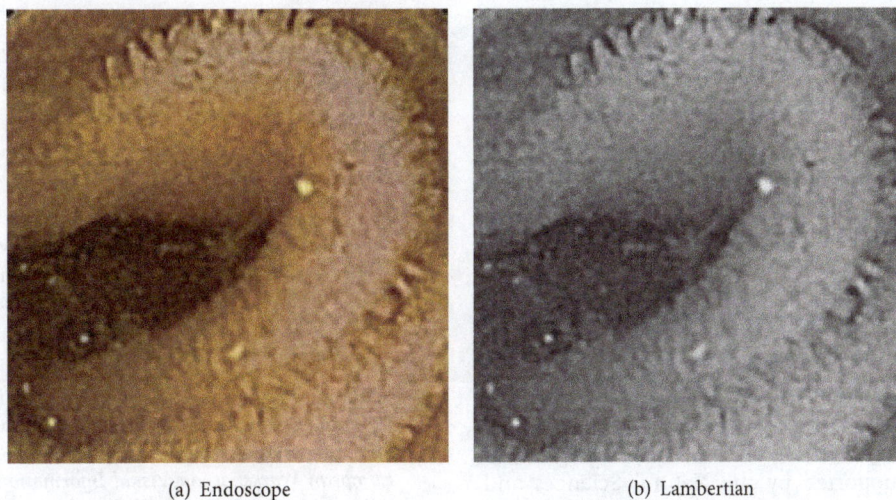

(a) Endoscope

(b) Lambertian

FIGURE 16: Endoscope image and generating Lambertian image.

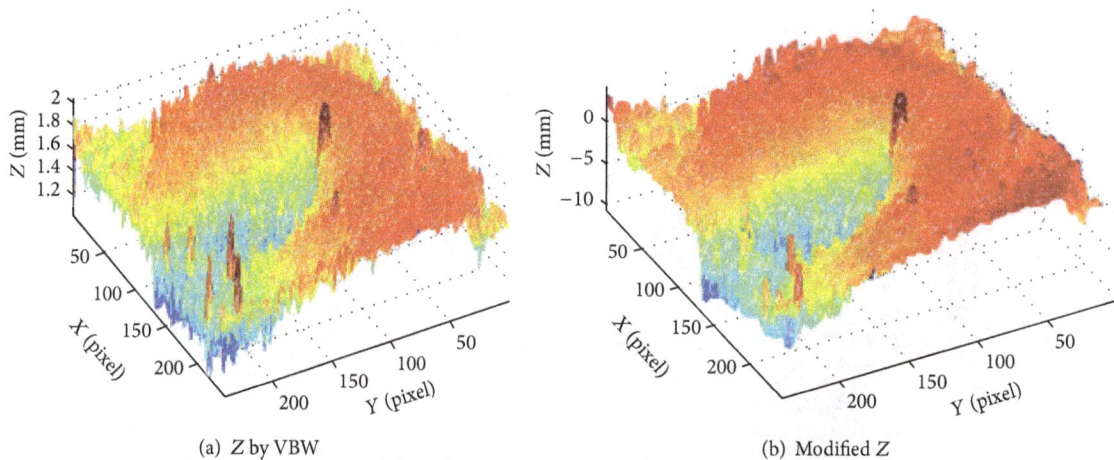

(a) Z by VBW

(b) Modified Z

FIGURE 17: Result for endoscope images.

5. Conclusion

This paper proposed a new approach to recover the 3D shape with absolute size from 2D image taken under the condition of both point light source illumination and perspective projection. While the VBW model approach can recover the relative shape with relative scale, the proposed approach obtains absolute depth by improving the gradient modification by RBF neural network. Recovering 3D shape with its absolute size proposed here makes it possible to support the medical diagnosis for the status of polyp if polyp is benign or malignant.

NN was introduced to demonstrate the modification of surface gradient using a synthesized sphere. VBW model is used to recover the original shape and further modification of accuracy of shape is performed via RBF-NN. Here, no parametric functional form has been assumed to improve the shape via NN. This has an important role in recovering the correct Z from the modified surface gradient. The approach is evaluated in computer simulation and real experiment using endoscope images. It was confirmed that the approach can improve the accuracy of recovered shape with acceptable error range. Other extensions of shape recovery algorithm or NN modification with whole camera parameters remain in the further subject.

Conflict of Interests

The authors declare that there is no conflict of interests regarding the publication of this paper.

Acknowledgments

Iwahori's research is supported by Japan Society for the Promotion of Science (JSPS) Grant-in-Aid for Scientific Research (C) (26330210) and Chubu University Grant. Woodham's research is supported by the Natural Sciences and Engineering Research Council (NSERC). The authors would like to thank the related lab member for useful discussions in this paper.

References

[1] H. Nakatani, K. Abe, A. Miyakawa, and S. Terakawa, "Three-dimensional measurement endoscope system with virtual rulers," *Journal of Biomedical Optics*, vol. 12, no. 5, Article ID 051803-1, 2007.

[2] F. Mourgues, F. Devemay, and E. Coste-Maniere, "3D reconstruction of the operating field for image overlay in 3D-endoscopic surgery," in *Proceedings of the IEEE and ACM International Symposium on Augmented Reality (ISAR '01)*, pp. 191–192, New York, NY, USA.

[3] T. Thormaehlen, H. Broszio, and P. N. Meier, "Three-dimensional endoscopy," in *Proceedings of the 2001 Falk Symposium*, pp. 199–212, 2001.

[4] B. K. P. Horn, "Obtaining shape from shading information," in *The Psychology of Computer Vision*, P. H. Winston, Ed., pp. 115–155, McGraw-Hill, 1975.

[5] J. A. Sethian, "A fast marching level set method for monotonically advancing fronts," *Proceedings of the National Academy of Sciences of the United States of America*, vol. 93, no. 4, pp. 1591–1595, 1996.

[6] R. Kimmel and J. A. Sethian, "Optimal algorithm for shape from shading and path planning," *Journal of Mathematical Imaging and Vision*, vol. 14, no. 3, pp. 237–244, 2001.

[7] S. Y. Yuen, Y. Y. Tsui, and C. K. Chow, "A fast marching formulation of perspective shape from shading under frontal illumination," *Pattern Recognition Letters*, vol. 28, no. 7, pp. 806–824, 2007.

[8] Y. Iwahori, K. Iwai, R. J. Woodham, H. Kawanaka, S. Fukui, and K. Kasugai, "Extending fast marching method under point light source illumination and perspective projection," in *Proceedings of the 20th International Conference on Pattern Recognition (ICPR '10)*, pp. 1650–1653, August 2010.

[9] Y. Ding, Y. Iwahori, T. Nakamura, L. He, R. J. Woodham, and H. Itoh, "Shape recovery of color textured object using fast marching method via self-calibration," in *Proceedings of the 2nd European Workshop on Visual Information Processing (EUVIP '10)*, pp. 92–96, Paris, France, July 2010.

[10] D. R. Neog, Y. Iwahori, M. K. Bhuyan, R. J. Woodham, and K. Kasugai, "Shape from an endoscope image using extended

Fast Marching Method," in *Proceedings of the 5th Indian International Conference on Artificial Intelligence (IICAI '11)*, pp. 1006–1015, December 2011.

[11] Y. Iwahori, K. Shibata, H. Kawanaka, K. Funahashi, R. J. Woodham, and Y. Adachi, "Shape from SEM image using fast marching method and intensity modification by neural network," in *Recent Advances in Knowledge-Based Paradigms and Applications*, vol. 234 of *Advances in Intelligent Systems and Computing*, chapter 5, pp. 73–86, Springer, 2014.

[12] Y. Ding, Y. Iwahori, T. Nakamura, R. J. Woodham, L. He, and H. Itoh, "Self-calibration and image rendering using RBF neural network," in *Knowledge-Based and Intelligent Information and Engineering Systems: 13th International Conference, KES 2009, Santiago, Chile, September 28–30, 2009, Proceedings, Part II*, vol. 5712 of *Lecture Notes in Computer Science*, pp. 705–712, Springer, Berlin, Germany, 2009.

[13] Y. Iwahori, R. J. Woodham, M. Ozaki, H. Tanaka, and N. Ishii, "Neural network based photometric stereo with a nearby rotational moving light source," *IEICE Transactions on Information and Systems*, vol. 80, no. 9, pp. 948–957, 1997.

[14] O. Vogel, M. Breuß, and J. Weickert, "A direct numerical approach to perspective shape-from-shading," in *Proceedings of the Vision, Modeling, and Visualization Conference (VMV '07)*, pp. 91–100, Saarbrücken, Germany, November 2007.

[15] S. H. Benton, *The Hamilton-Jacobi Equation: A Global Approach*, vol. 131, Academic Press, 1977.

[16] E. Prados and O. Faugeras, "A mathematical and algorithmic study of the Lambertian SFS problem for orthographic and pinhole cameras," Tech. Rep. 5005, INRIA, 2003.

[17] E. Prados and O. D. Faugeras, "Unifying approaches and removing unrealistic assumptions in Shape from Shading: mathematics can help," in *Proceedings of the 8th European Conference on Computer Vision (ECCV '04)*, Prague, Czech Republic, May 2004.

[18] E. Prados and O. Faugeras, "Shape from shading: a well-posed problem?" in *Proceedings of the IEEE Computer Society Conference on Computer Vision and Pattern Recognition (CVPR '05)*, vol. 2, pp. 870–877, June 2005.

[19] Y. Shimasaki, Y. Iwahori, D. R. Neog, R. J. Woodham, and M. K. Bhuyan, "Generating lambertian image with uniform reflectance for endoscope image," in *PRoceedings of the International Workshop on Advanced Image Technology (IWAIT '13)*, 1C-2 (Computer Vision 1), pp. 60–65, Nagoya, Japan, January 2013.

2

Closed Contour Specular Reflection Segmentation in Laparoscopic Images

Jan Marek Marcinczak and Rolf-Rainer Grigat

Hamburg University of Technology, Schlossstraße 20, 21079 Hamburg, Germany

Correspondence should be addressed to Jan Marek Marcinczak; jan.marcinczak@tu-harburg.de

Academic Editor: Tiange Zhuang

Segmentation of specular reflections is an essential step in endoscopic image analysis; it affects all further processing steps including segmentation, classification, and registration tasks. The dichromatic reflectance model, which is often used for specular reflection modeling, is made for dielectric materials and not for human tissue. Hence, most recent segmentation approaches rely on thresholding techniques. In this work, we first demonstrate the limited accuracy that can be achieved by thresholding techniques and propose a hybrid method which is based on closed contours and thresholding. The method has been evaluated on 269 specular reflections in 49 images which were taken from 27 real laparoscopic interventions. Our method improves the average sensitivity by 16% compared to the state-of-the-art thresholding methods.

1. Introduction

One major concern in laparoscopic image processing is specular reflections which are present in the majority of laparoscopic interventions and affect all following processing. Specular reflections are most pronounced if the surface normal bisects the angle between the incident light and the camera. They are caused by moist tissue and appear as white glare or light-colored glare in the images. Many different approaches to segment specular reflections have been proposed in the previous decades. Most of them are based on the dichromatic reflection model [1, 2]. Let i be the incident angle, e the exitance angle, g the phase angle, and λ the wavelength. The reflectance $L_s(\lambda, i, e, g)$ and $L_b(\lambda, i, e, g)$ model the surface reflection and the body reflection. The radiance $L(\lambda, i, e, g)$ reflected by a surface can be defined as

$$L(\lambda, i, e, g) = L_s(\lambda, i, e, g) + L_b(\lambda, i, e, g). \tag{1}$$

The dichromatic reflection model holds for dielectric surfaces and separates the spectral reflection from the geometric reflection [3–5]:

$$L(\lambda, i, e, g) = m_s(i, e, g)\, c_s(\lambda) + m_b(i, e, g)\, c_b(\lambda), \tag{2}$$

where $m_s(i, e, g)$ and $m_b(i, e, g)$ are geometric scaling factors and $c_s(\lambda)$ and $c_b(\lambda)$ are spectral power distributions. The body reflection (diffuse reflection) and the specular reflection form linear clusters in a color histogram [6]; fitting linear subspaces to these clusters can be used to detect specular reflections in images, and the diffuse color can be reconstructed by projection. However, in practice, surface roughness and the imaging geometry make the fitting of subspaces inaccurate [7]. Additionally, the assumption of dielectric surfaces is not fulfilled by human tissue. Nevertheless, several algorithms have been proposed that use the dichromatic model in an endoscopic environment [8, 9]. However, Vogt et al. show that simple S channel thresholding in the HSV color space achieves similar accuracy on endoscopic images [10]. Several adaptive thresholding techniques have been proposed that make use of nonlinear color transformations to separate the specular reflections from bright tissue in color space [9, 11]. Most of the specular reflection segmentation algorithms have in common that thresholding is used to segment the central part of the reflections, and the bright region surrounding the reflection is segmented in a second step. In the following, we will refer to this region where specular reflection is still strong, but body reflection increases as specular lobe. Commonly, this region is segmented by applying morphological operations to the thresholded image or using region growing [12]. As mentioned by several authors, single threshold techniques have limited accuracy [13, 14]. Bright parts of the tissue commonly intersect with weak specular reflections in color space. The approach of Oh et al. [14] is similar to our approach as they distinguish between weak and strong reflections using multiple thresholds. In our approach, specular reflections are classified as weak, intermediate, and strong reflections. We demonstrate that closed contours can be used to detect weak reflections which would be missed by thresholding techniques. The segmentation of weak, intermediate, and strong reflections is combined to obtain the final segmentation.

In here, Sections 2 and 3 discuss methods and results. First, thresholding techniques for specular reflection segmentation are detailed in Sections 2.1 and 2.2. These methods are applied in conjunction with the specular lobe segmentation described in Section 2.3. Section 2.4 defines our hybrid approach combining thresholding techniques with closed contour segmentation. The results of our approach are compared to the classical techniques in Section 3.

2. Methods

The most common techniques for specular reflection segmentation in endoscopic images are thresholding methods [9–11, 13, 14]. In the following sections, we detail the specular peak thresholding algorithm and outline a second thresholding method which we refer to as cone thresholding. In the evaluation, we compare these thresholding techniques to our hybrid approach which is explained in Section 2.4.

2.1. Specular Peak Thresholding. A common assumption for specular reflections is that they are located in the brightest peak in the histogram of an image. Stehle selects the brightest peak of the luminance channel of the YUV color space [15], while Saint-Pierre et al. perform a nonlinear transformation. Let $I : \Omega \rightarrow \mathbb{R}^3$ be an RGB image; the transformed image $I_t : \Omega \rightarrow \mathbb{R}^3$ is defined by

$$I_t(\mathbf{x}) = (1 - S(\mathbf{x})) I(\mathbf{x}), \tag{3}$$

where $S(\mathbf{x})$ is the saturation channel of $I(\mathbf{x})$ using the HSV color space [16]. This transformation decreases the color values depending on their distance to the gray-axis. The transformation is based on the assumption that most specular reflections will be located close to the gray-axis and have a low saturation. This transformation increases the gap between specular reflections and tissue in the histogram [11]. The threshold is selected by the following criterion. Let $h(t)$ be the histogram of the Y channel of I_t and $t = \{0, \ldots, 255\}$. The threshold t_{spec} is given by

$$t_{\text{spec}} = \max\left\{t \mid \bar{h}(t) - \bar{h}(t + 1) > 0\right\}, \tag{4}$$

with

$$\bar{h}(t) = \begin{cases} 1 & \text{if } h(t) - h(t + 1) > 0, \\ 0 & \text{if } h(t) - h(t + 1) \leq 0. \end{cases} \tag{5}$$

In [11], the threshold t_{spec} is directly used to detect specular reflections. However, in our experiments this segmentation was not robust; if no specular reflections are present in the image, the brightest parts of the tissue will be classified as specular reflections. Furthermore, different specular reflections might appear at different intensity levels and lead to several peaks in the high intensity range of the histogram $h(t_i)$. Therefore, we apply the two following steps to increase the robustness of the algorithm. First, we allow only thresholds $t_{\text{spec}} > t_{\text{min}}$. Second, we convolve $h(t_i)$ with a Gaussian kernel $\mathcal{N}(t_i, \sigma)$ to merge the peaks of $h(t_i)$ that are caused by different specular reflections. The set $\mathcal{S} \subseteq \Omega$ of specular reflections is given by $\mathcal{S} = \{\mathbf{x} \in \Omega \mid I_{\text{gray}}(\mathbf{x}) > t_{\text{spec}}\}$, where I_{gray} is the Y channel of I_t. This approach sets the threshold according to the brightest specular peak in $h(t_i) \star \mathcal{N}(t_i, \sigma)$.

2.2. Cone Thresholding. One drawback of the specular peak thresholding technique is the assumption that specular reflections are represented by a single peak in the histogram of an image. In practice, this is not always the case. Specular reflections appear at different intensity levels and can lead to several peaks in the histogram. Therefore, another technique which relies on defining a cone in the RGB color space as specular reflections can be used. The cone is located on the axis $\mathbf{n}_{r=g=b} = \begin{pmatrix} 1 & 1 & 1 \end{pmatrix}^{\text{T}}$ for which $r = g = b$, which implicitly assumes a perfect white balance. Let $\mathbf{I} : \Omega \rightarrow \mathbb{R}^3$ with $\Omega \subseteq \mathbb{R}^2$ be an RGB image. The projection of $\mathbf{I}(\mathbf{x})$ on $\mathbf{n}_{r=g=b}$ is given by

$$\mathbf{p}_{r=g=b}(\mathbf{x}) = \frac{\langle \mathbf{n}_{r=g=b}, \mathbf{I}(\mathbf{x}) \rangle}{|\mathbf{n}_{r=g=b}|} \mathbf{n}_{r=g=b}. \tag{6}$$

The set $\mathcal{S}_{\text{spec}}$ of specular reflections is then defined by

$$\mathcal{S}_{\text{spec}} = \left\{ \mathbf{x} \in \Omega \mid \left| \mathbf{I}(\mathbf{x}) - \mathbf{p}_{r=g=b}(\mathbf{x}) \right| \right.$$
$$\left. < a \left(\frac{\langle \mathbf{n}_{r=g=b}, \mathbf{I}(\mathbf{x}) \rangle}{|\mathbf{n}_{r=g=b}|} - x_0 \right) \right\}. \tag{7}$$

The parameters x_0 and a define the tip and the slope of the cone. This detection algorithm relies on the assumption that the specular reflections are close to the gray-axis of the RGB space. The advantage of this segmentation algorithm is that it does not suffer from multiple peaks in the histogram of the image. However, one should keep in mind that the RGB color space is a hardware-dependent color space. Therefore, the parameters x_0 and a need to be adjusted for different hardware.

2.3. Specular Lobe Segmentation. The thresholding techniques outlined in the previous sections segment the central part of the specular reflections. To obtain a segmentation of the entire specular reflection, specular lobe segmentation needs to be applied. We use a technique similar to [11] which is based on region growing [12]. Instead of using

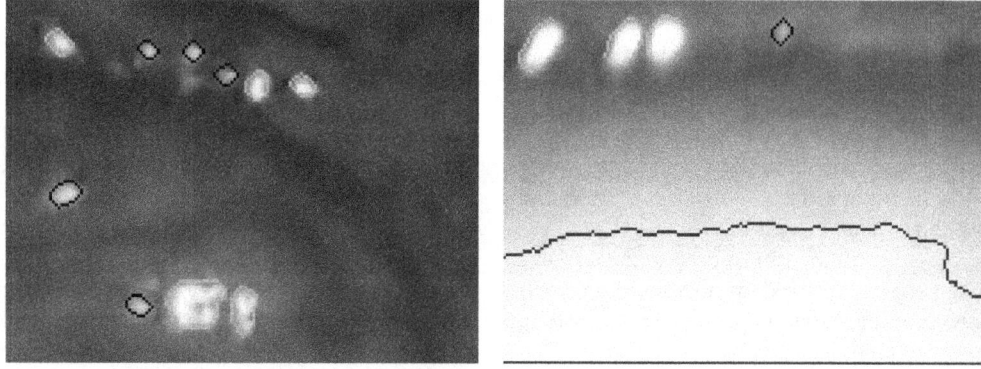

(a) The brighter specular reflections in this image are of
Type 2. The weak, small reflections are of Type 3 and are
segmented using closed contours

(b) In the lower part of the image, a large reflection of Type
1 can be observed. The three reflections in the upper left are
of Type 2. The small, weak reflection is of Type 3

FIGURE 1: Two regions of interest show reflections of Types 1, 2, and 3. Both images are taken from laparoscopic sequences of the liver.
Segmentation is performed using the hybrid contour thresholding algorithm.

a single threshold for the region growing, we compute thresholds based on the specular reflection intensities. For every connected component $\mathscr{S}_{cc,i} \subset \mathscr{S}_{spec}$, with $i = 1, \ldots, N$, where N is the number of connected components in $\mathscr{S}_{spec}$, the mean value of the connected component is estimated by

$$\mu_{cc,i} = \frac{1}{|\mathscr{S}_{cc,i}|} \sum_{j=1}^{|\mathscr{S}_{cc,i}|} I\left(\mathbf{x_j}\right), \quad \text{where } \mathbf{x_j} \in \mathscr{S}_{cc,i}. \quad (8)$$

The region growing algorithm adds a pixel $\mathbf{x}$ to the set $\mathscr{S}_{lobe}$ if

$$I\left(\mathbf{x}\right) > c\mu_{cc,i}, \quad (9)$$

where c is a scaling factor and $I(\mathbf{x})$ is the luminance channel of the YUV color image. The final segmentation is given by $\mathscr{S}_{spec} \cup \mathscr{S}_{lobe}$. The optimal parameter c for different thresholding algorithms is given in Figure 3. In the following evaluation, specular lobe segmentation is used together with the outlined thresholding algorithms.

2.4. Hybrid Closed Contour Thresholding. Single threshold segmentation techniques have an upper limit of accuracy which is often caused by bright tissue which is classified as specular reflection. An increase in precision can be achieved by using different models for specular reflections. In laparoscopic videos of the liver surface, different types of specular reflections appear. The first types of reflections are large specular reflections which occur in situations where the endoscope is located very close to the organ surface (Type 1). As the image intensities at specular reflections of Type 1 are very high and often clipped in the center part, thresholding can be used to segment this type of specular reflections. Another property of this type of reflection is the slowly, radial decreasing intensity. More difficult to detect are small, weak reflections located further apart from the endoscope. These reflections are caused by moist curved organ surfaces. The intensities of these small specular reflections can be low, depending on the surface geometry and the underlying

tissue. However, most of this type of reflections have a step-shaped border, which can be used for detection and precise segmentation. In the proposed segmentation algorithm, this type of specular reflections is split up into small reflections with high intensity (Type 2) and specular reflections that have low intensities even in the center (Type 3). All three types are illustrated in Figure 1. For Types 2 and 3, the contour is used to determine the segmentation boundary. For every connected component in the binary image that was created by cone thresholding, it is checked if the component is enclosed by a contour; this contour is used for segmentation. If no closed contour is found, the reflection is classified as Type 1. To detect reflections of Type 3, closed contours are used as seed points. An overview of this approach is given in Figure 2. In the following, $\mathscr{S}_{Type1}$ denotes the set of pixels segmented as specular reflections by thresholding. The Canny edge detector is used to compute a binary edge map $I_{Edge}(\mathbf{x})$ of the laparoscopic image $I(\mathbf{x})$ [17]. The liver surface is smooth and lacks edges or corners. Therefore, most of the strong filter responses are caused by the boundaries of specular reflections. A morphological closing operation is used to close small gaps in the contours. Let $\mathscr{S}_{cc,i}$ denote the set of pixels of the connected component i that is enclosed by the contours of $I_{Edge}(\mathbf{x})$. The set of Type 2 reflections $\mathscr{S}_{Type2}$ is obtained by the connected components that contain at least one pixel of $\mathscr{S}_{Type1}$. The weak Type 3 reflections are segmented using constraints on the connected components $\mathscr{S}_{cc}$ that are not elements of $\mathscr{S}_{Type2}$. The specular reflections $\mathscr{S}_{Type3}$ are given by the connected components $\mathscr{S}_{cc,i}$ that fulfill the following constraints:

$$E\left[I\left(\mathbf{x}\right)\right] > t_{av}, \quad \text{where } \mathbf{x} \in \mathscr{S}_{cc,i},$$

$$E\left[I\left(\mathbf{x}\right)\right] - E\left[I\left(\hat{\mathbf{x}}\right)\right] > t_{diff}, \quad \text{where } \mathbf{x} \in \mathscr{S}_{cc,i}, \ \hat{\mathbf{x}} \in \delta\mathscr{S}_{cc,i},$$

$$|\mathscr{S}_{cc,i}| > t_{cc,min},$$

$$|\mathscr{S}_{cc,i}| < t_{cc,max}. \quad (10)$$

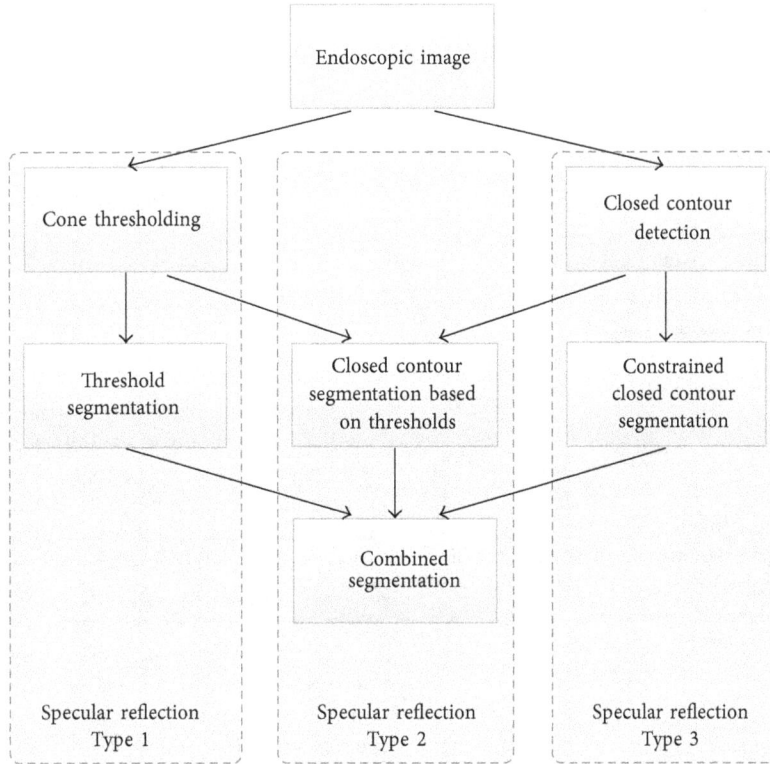

FIGURE 2: Overview of the hybrid closed contour thresholding algorithm. Three different process lines are used for the detection and are combined in a final segmentation. The contour-based segmentation is capable of segmenting even tiny specular reflections which cannot be detected by a single threshold. Furthermore, the closed contour supports reflections of Type 2, which have been detected by thresholding with a precise boundary. Reflections of Type 1 are large specular reflections with a smooth gradient and a bright central part.

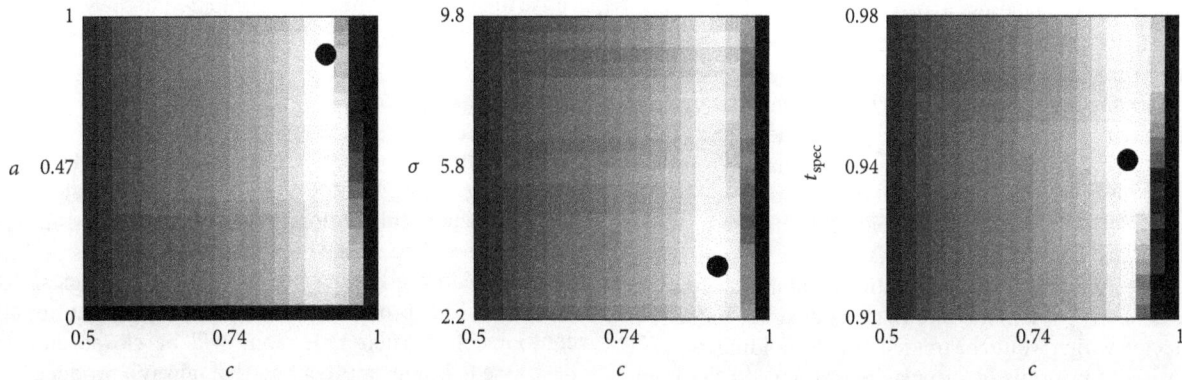

(a) Parameter space of the cone thresholding algorithm spanned by x_0 and a. For visualization, the 3-dimensional parameter spaces x_0, a, and c were reduced to the slice containing the optimal parameters $x_0 = 0.89$, $a = 0.89$, and $c = 0.92$

(b) Parameter space of the specular peak thresholding algorithm spanned by σ and c. The maximal Jaccard index is located at $\sigma = 3.4$ and $c = 0.92$

(c) Parameter space of gray-level thresholding spanned by t_{spec} and c. The maximum Jaccard index is labeled by the red dot. $t_{\text{spec}} = 0.94$ and $c = 0.92$

FIGURE 3: Parameter optimization using the Jaccard index. The dot labels the optimal parameter values. The optimal parameters are used in the evaluation.

The perimeter of $\mathscr{S}_{\text{cc},i}$ is denoted by $\delta\mathscr{S}_{\text{cc},i}$, and $E[I(\mathbf{x})]$ denotes the expectation value. The last two constraints assure that only closed contours of a specific size are considered to be specular reflections of Type 3. The first two constraints are based on the aspect that the average intensity of specular reflections is limited by a lower boundary and that there should be a high decrease in intensity close to the perimeter of the reflections. The final segmentation of specular reflections is then given by $\mathscr{S}_{\text{Type1}} \cup \mathscr{S}_{\text{Type2}} \cup \mathscr{S}_{\text{Type3}}$.

TABLE 1: The hybrid closed contour algorithm achieves the best results compared to thresholding techniques in terms of the Jaccard index and sensitivity. Note the high value for Q_1 and the sensitivity; this increase is caused by the reflections of Type 3 (T3) which are missed by the other algorithms.

Algorithm	$\overline{F}_{\text{Jaccard}}$	Q_1	Q_3	Sensitivity				PPV
				T1	T2	T3	Avg.	
Gray-level thresholding	0.55	0.26	0.80	1	0.96	0.10	0.74	0.96
Specular peak thresholding	0.60	0.38	**0.87**	1	0.81	0	0.61	**0.99**
Cone thresholding	0.60	0.37	0.81	1	0.91	0.10	0.70	**0.99**
Hybrid closed contour	**0.66**	**0.55**	0.82	1	**0.97**	**0.69**	**0.90**	0.96

The bold font highlights the best result for each category.

3. Results

In this section, we evaluate the specular reflection algorithms outlined in the previous sections. The evaluation is performed on a dataset of 49 laparoscopic images taken from 27 patients. The images contain 269 true specular reflections. Ground truth segmentation of specular reflection is given by manual segmentation of the specular reflections. The quality of the resulting segmentation is determined using the Jaccard index [18]:

$$F_{\text{Jacard}} = \frac{t_p}{t_p + f_p + f_n}, \tag{11}$$

where t_p, f_p, and f_n are the true positives, false positives, and false negatives. The Jaccard index is used to measure the overlap of a given segmentation with the ground truth segmentation. The advantage of this error metric is that the amount of true negatives is not considered; in laparoscopic images, the area of specular reflections is usually very small. Therefore, the specificity might be high although the segmented area is several times larger than the true specular reflection. The parameters for the thresholding technique were determined by maximizing the Jaccard index. Figure 3 shows the results of the parameter optimization. One of the main advantages of the hybrid segmentation is that it detects small reflections which would be missed by thresholding techniques. As the Jaccard index computes the overlap of the segmentation with the ground truth, small reflections will give only slight improvements. To demonstrate that many small reflections are detected which would be missed by thresholding, we state the sensitivity in terms of specular reflections. As the number of true negative reflections is unknown—we only have background and specular reflections—the specificity cannot be computed. Therefore, we use the positive prediction value (PPV) to consider the false positives:

$$\text{PPV} = \frac{t_p}{t_p + f_p}, \tag{12}$$

where t_p and f_p are the number of true and false reflections detected by the segmentation algorithms. Furthermore, we use the the average Jaccard index $\overline{F}_{\text{Jacard}}$ and the quartiles Q_1, Q_3 of the distribution of the Jaccard index to determine the robustness of the segmentation algorithms. The results are given in Table 1. The results demonstrate the limited accuracy that can be achieved by thresholding techniques for specular reflection segmentation; the cause for this upper limit is an overlap in the color space between specular reflections and the brightest part of the tissue. However, even the adaptive thresholding technique outlined in Section 2.1 just slightly improves accuracy. One reason for that is the assumption that the specular reflections are located in a single peak of the histogram. This assumption is not fulfilled if reflections of Type 1 and Type 3 are present in one image.

The hybrid approach using closed contours and thresholding achieves the highest sensitivity and the best segmentation results in terms of the Jaccard index. The sensitivity is increased by 16% and Q_1 by 0.17 compared to the best thresholding results. Small weak reflections are detected by their closed contours and give rise to this improvement. Furthermore, the closed contours increase the accuracy of the segmentation for specular reflections of Type 2 which explains the higher Jaccard index. However, there are some closed contours that are falsely classified as specular reflections and cause the PPV to drop slightly compared to the specular peak thresholding and the cone thresholding algorithm.

4. Conclusion

In this section, it was shown that using a hybrid approach combining closed contours and thresholding significantly improves the segmentation of specular reflection in laparoscopic videos. The closed contour computation is performed using the Canny edge detector and the morphological closing operation. This process has the disadvantage that not all the contours of specular reflections will be closed and might be missed. Using approaches that always produce closed contours such as polar transformations and shortest path computations [19, 20] could increase the sensitivity. However, many open contours are not caused by specular reflections; in a brief test, closing open contours using polar transformation increased the false positives in a large scale. Therefore, we apply morphological operations to obtain all contours that contain only small gaps. This leads to a tradeoff between a high sensitivity and an adequate PPV.

References

[1] S. A. Shafer, "UUsing color to separate reflection components," *Color Research and Application*, vol. 10, no. 4, pp. 210–218, 1985.

[2] T. Gevers and H. Stokman, "Classifying color edges in video into shadow-geometry, highlight, or material transitions,"

IEEE Transactions on Multimedia, vol. 5, no. 2, pp. 237–243, 2003.

[3] G. J. Klinker, S. A. Shafer, and T. Kanade, "The measurement of highlights in color images," *International Journal of Computer Vision*, vol. 2, no. 1, pp. 7–32, 1988.

[4] J. B. Park and A. C. Kak, "A truncated least squares approach to the detection of specular highlights in color images," in *Proceedings of the IEEE International Conference on Robotics and Automation (ICRA '03)*, vol. 1, pp. 1397–1403, Taiwan, September 2003.

[5] A. Artusi, F. Banterle, and D. Chetverikov, "A survey of specularity removal methods," *Computer Graphics Forum*, vol. 30, no. 8, pp. 2208–2230, 2011.

[6] C. L. Novak and S. A. Shafer, "Anatomy of a color histogram," in *Proceedings of the IEEE Computer Society Conference on Computer Vision and Pattern Recognition CVPR '92*, pp. 599–605, IEEE, 1992.

[7] P. Tan, S. Lin, L. Quan, and H.-S. Shum, "Highlight removal by illumination-constrained inpainting," in *Proceedings of the 9th IEEE International Conference on Computer Vision*, pp. 164–169, October 2003.

[8] D. Stoyanov and G. Z. Yang, "Removing specular reflection components for robotic assisted laparoscopic surgery," in *Proceedings of the IEEE International Conference on Image Processing (ICIP '05)*, pp. 632–635, September 2005.

[9] O. El Meslouhi, M. Kardouchi, H. Allali, T. Gadi, and Y. Benkaddour, "Automatic detection and inpainting of specular reflections for colposcopic images," *Central European Journal of Computer Science*, vol. 1, pp. 341–354, 2011.

[10] F. Vogt, D. Paulus, and H. Niemann, "Highlight substitution in light fields," in *Proceedings of the International Conference on Image Processing (ICIP '02)*, vol. 1, pp. 637–640, September 2002.

[11] C.-A. Saint-Pierre, J. Boisvert, G. Grimard, and F. Cheriet, "Detection and correction of specular reflections for automatic surgical tool segmentation in thoracoscopic images," *Machine Vision and Applications*, vol. 22, no. 1, pp. 171–180, 2011.

[12] C. R. Brice and C. L. Fennema, "Scene analysis using regions," *Artificial Intelligence*, vol. 1, no. 3-4, pp. 205–226, 1970.

[13] M. Arnold, A. Ghosh, S. Ameling, and G. Lacey, "Automatic segmentation and inpainting of specular highlights for endoscopic imaging," *Eurasip Journal on Image and Video Processing*, vol. 2010, article 9, Article ID 814319, 2010.

[14] J. Oh, S. Hwang, J. Lee, W. Tavanapong, J. Wong, and P. C. de Groen, "Informative frame classification for endoscopy video," *Medical Image Analysis*, vol. 11, no. 2, pp. 110–127, 2007.

[15] T. H. Stehle, "Specular reflection removal in endoscopic images," in *Proceedings of the 10th International Student Conference on Electrical Engineering*, Prague, Czech Republic, 2006.

[16] M. Ebner, *Color Constancy*, vol. 7, Wiley, New York, NY, USA, 2007.

[17] J. Canny, "A computational approach to edge detection," *IEEE Transactions on Pattern Analysis and Machine Intelligence*, vol. 8, no. 6, pp. 679–698, 1986.

[18] P. Jaccard, "Etude comparative de la distribution florale dans une portion des alpes et des jura," *Bulletin Del La Societe Vaudoise Des Sciences Naturelles*, vol. 37, pp. 547–579, 1901.

[19] A. Mishra, Y. Aloimonos, and C. L. Fah, "Active segmentation with fixation," in *Proceedings of the 12th International Conference on Computer Vision*, pp. 468–475, IEEE, 2009.

[20] S. J. Chiu, C. A. Toth, C. B. Rickman, J. A. Izatt, and S. Farsiu, "Automatic segmentation of closed-contour features in ophthalmic images using graph theory and dynamic programming," *Biomedical Optics Express*, vol. 3, no. 5, pp. 1127–1140, 2012.

3

High Performance GPU-Based Fourier Volume Rendering

Marwan Abdellah, Ayman Eldeib, and Amr Sharawi

Biomedical Engineering Department, Cairo University, Giza 12613, Egypt

Correspondence should be addressed to Marwan Abdellah; marwan.m.abdellah@ieee.org

Academic Editor: Tzung-Pei Hong

Fourier volume rendering (FVR) is a significant visualization technique that has been used widely in digital radiography. As a result of its $\mathcal{O}(N^2 \log N)$ time complexity, it provides a faster alternative to spatial domain volume rendering algorithms that are $\mathcal{O}(N^3)$ computationally complex. Relying on the *Fourier projection-slice theorem*, this technique operates on the spectral representation of a 3D volume instead of processing its spatial representation to generate attenuation-only projections that look like *X-ray radiographs*. Due to the rapid evolution of its underlying architecture, the graphics processing unit (GPU) became an attractive competent platform that can deliver giant computational raw power compared to the central processing unit (CPU) on a per-dollar-basis. The introduction of the compute unified device architecture (CUDA) technology enables embarrassingly-parallel algorithms to run efficiently on CUDA-capable GPU architectures. In this work, a high performance GPU-accelerated implementation of the FVR pipeline on CUDA-enabled GPUs is presented. This proposed implementation can achieve a speed-up of 117x compared to a single-threaded hybrid implementation that uses the CPU and GPU together by taking advantage of executing the rendering pipeline entirely on recent GPU architectures.

1. Introduction

Volume visualization is an essential tool for exploring and analysing the anatomy of complex structures and phenomena. It has been extensively used in various scientific and engineering arenas such as medical imaging, geoscience, microscopy, mechanical engineering, and others [1–3]. Several volume visualization techniques have been developed and extensively investigated. The main two categories that have gained broad acceptance by scientific communities were *volume* and *surface rendering*. Each technique has its specific area of application that is associated with its advantages, but in contrast, it also has its disadvantages that give the opportunity for other techniques to survive [4–6].

Volume rendering has shown great significance on the visual interpretation of large amount of 3D scalar and vector data generated by multidimensional sensors, acquisition devices, and supercomputer simulations. It concentrates on visualizing the desired internal features of volumetric objects and their bounding surfaces at the same time. In literature, several volume rendering algorithms have been presented either to improve the rendering speed of large datasets

or to enhance the rendering quality of their reconstructed images. By and large, the rendering speed and quality are *traded-off* and no single complete algorithm that can deliver the optimum quality associated with maximum interactivity exists [7].

A radical *domain-based* categorization of volume rendering algorithms classifies them into *spatial-domain* and *other-domain-based* techniques such as frequency domain, compression domain or the wavelet domain. The rendering pipeline of spatial domain techniques runs entirely in this domain. Domain-based methods operate by switching part of their computations to a different domain either to reduce the complexity of the rendering algorithm or to improve the performance of some operations that take considerable amount of time in the spatial domain. For a volume of size N^3, complexity of spatial-domain algorithms is of order $\mathcal{O}(N^3)$, since all the voxels composing this volume must be visited at least once to render a correct image. Although some algorithms use additional optimization techniques to reduce the number of traversed samples, this optimization is in general data dependent and subject to the size of the datasets. This time-complexity limits the usage of spatial domain rendering algorithms for interactive environments in some applications. In such cases, *frequency-domain-based* techniques can be used alternatively.

Frequency-domain volume rendering (FDVR) uses a 3D spectral representation of the volume to compute an image that looks like X-ray radiograph in $\mathcal{O}(N^2 \log N)$ time relying on the *projection-slice theorem*. It works by transforming the spatial volume into frequency domain. Then it reconstructs 2D projection at any viewing angle by resampling an extracted projection-slice along a perpendicular plane to the viewing direction followed by backtransforming this resampled slice to the spatial domain [8, 9].

Obtaining the spectral representation of the volume is the most computationally intensive step in the algorithm due to its $\mathcal{O}(N^3 \log N)$ complexity. Nevertheless, this rendering algorithm is extremely efficient because this step is executed once in a preprocessing stage. The rendering loop of this pipeline takes much less computing time.

FDVR is a generic technique that can work with any frequency transform to switch between the spatial and frequency domains. Our rendering pipeline will be based on Fourier transform and so, the rendering method can be called Fourier volume rendering.

The rest of the paper is organized as follows. Section 2 summarizes the related work in the literature. In Section 3, the rendering algorithm is demystified and our implementation strategy is presented. Section 4 elaborates the results gained by mapping the entire rendering pipeline to run on the GPU and Section 5 concludes the paper.

2. Fourier Volume Rendering Literature

Although the technique was introduced around 20 years ago, the literature behind FDVR in general and FVR in particular is quite scarce. In this section, we will try to summarize the most notable contributions that have been presented since that time in a nutshell.

In 1992, Dunne et al. introduced the fundamental idea behind frequency domain volume rendering and its advantages [8]. Malzbender systematically extended the projection-slice theorem to 3D to be a basis for volume rendering [9]. Based on FFT, he presented an implementation of the basic FVR pipeline and briefly discussed some considerations of resampling the frequency domain and their significant effects on the reconstruction quality of the generated projection image. He proposed to use a Hamming-windowed *sinc* reconstruction filter to reduce the aliasing accompanied with resampling the frequency spectrum. For the same mission, Grosso and Ertl proposed alternatively biorthognal wavelet reconstruction filters [10]. As a drawback, the basic FVR integral does not provide a direct way of modelling emission and scattering in the participating medium. This limitation was a fundamental disadvantage associated with frequency domain rendering that is reflected as lack of occlusion in the resulting reconstructions [11]. Levoy has partially restored the lost visual cues in the basic pipeline by applying several shading models that are linear combinations of Fourier projections [12]. His extension included depth cueing, directional shading, and Lambertian reflection with

spherical illumination. The result of Levoy's work did not exhibit real occlusion, yet it provided acceptable depth and shape cues that can simulate the existence of the missing occlusion. One significant disadvantage that limited the usage of his implementation was the demand of several copies of the volume, which consequently imposes high memory requirements for initial preprocessing. In cooperation with Totsuka, the same results have been obtained after considering alternative frequency domain methods by processing the frequency response of the volume data, which dramatically reduced the memory required before [13].

Until that time, FVR did not gain that broad acceptance by the scientific visualization and medical communities due to the lack of illumination models in the Fourier domain. In 2002, Entezari et al. enhanced the projections quality by incorporating various illumination models into the FVR pipeline [14]. The first model was based on Gamma-corrected hemispherical shading that was proposed by Scoggins et al. [15] and the second one adopted spherical harmonic functions for approximating cubic illumination shading. FVR suffered from reduced reconstruction quality that limited its usefulness in particular medical applications. In [16], a solution for enhancing FVR using contour extraction was proposed. It provided a flexible method for extracting material boundaries on surfaces in the Fourier space. Additionally, it included enhancement of several features for revealing important spatial relationships between interior and exterior structures making it an attractive tool for improved X-ray-like investigations for a given dataset. Cheng and Ching [17] also presented various methods for designing FVR transfer function based on Bezier curves and B-splines. Jansen et al. [18] partially accelerated the rendering pipeline on the GPU by mapping the Split-Stream-FFT on the GPU. As a major tool in digital radiography, Ntasis et al. [19] provided a web-based Fourier volume renderer for real-time preview of digital reconstructed radiographs (DRRs). Their implementation examined carefully the resampling issues of the frequency domain to generate remote high quality DRRs. Extending the technique beyond operating on volume data with regular grids, FVR has been adapted by Corrigan et al. [20, 21] to directly deal with meshless data. A high-level MATLAB-based FVR framework was presented in [22]. This framework abstracts the complex implementation details of the rendering pipeline to allow imaging researchers to develop image enhancement techniques without having prior knowledge of the OpenGL pipeline. Viola et al. have implemented a FVR heterogeneous rendering pipeline that uses the GPU to execute the rendering stage relying on fragment shaders [23]. However, this approach is limited if the current capabilities of unified computing GPU architectures are considered.

Practical implementation of FVR is complicated by two main factors which arise when the projection-slice theorem is applied to discrete sampled data [8]. First of all, conventional FFT algorithms yield frequency-domain output data which is not ideally structured for resampling. To mitigate this effect, it is necessary to add high performance multidimensional fft-shift stages to the rendering pipeline to rearrange the data. Moreover, sampling the frequency domain is equivalent to the replication of the signal in the spatial domain that ultimately accounts for the appearance of ghosting artifacts in the reconstructed images. This issue is resolved by zero-padding the volume in the spatial domain and using high-order interpolation filters in the frequency domain. Our CUDA-based implementation addresses all of these issues.

3. Algorithm and Implementation

The plain FVR algorithm is briefly illustrated to simplify the explanation of the contextual classification of the rendering pipeline. Based on this classification, an efficient strategy has been considered to map this pipeline to run entirely on the GPU.

3.1. Algorithm. The spatial volume must be shifted by a 3D *fft-shift* operation to set its center at the origin of the 3D space. The frequency spectrum of this volume is then obtained by a forward 3D FFT operation. This resulting spectrum is not centered at the origin of the frequency space. Consequently, another 3D fft-shift operation is required to center its zero-frequency component to prepare it for correct slice extraction. Afterwards, a 2D projection-slice passing through the origin of the spectral volume, with a normal that is parallel to the viewing direction, is carefully extracted. This slice represents the 2D FFT of the desired projection and thus, the reconstructed image can be directly obtained by a 2D inverse FFT operation. To reduce the aliasing and ghosting artifacts in the reconstructed image, this projection-slice is processed in a further step to have it resampled. The resampling stage is only mandatory if the desired projection was not orthogonal. After resampling the extracted slice, it is backtransformed to the spatial domain by an inverse 2D FFT operation. The resulting image from this inverse transformation is shifted by another 2D fft-shift operation to move the center of the image from the edge to origin of the grid used to display the image. Changing the viewing angle implies rotating the 3D spectrum to extract a new projection-slice that corresponds to this angle. The algorithm sequence is graphically depicted in Figure 1.

3.2. Pipeline Classification. According to the sequence of operations in this algorithm, the pipeline could be divided into two consecutive stages: a *preprocessing* stage and a *rendering loop*. The preprocessing stage is executed only once to prepare the 3D spectrum of the input spatial volume. The rendering loop is running continuously to generate different projections according to the input viewing angle. The main function of the preprocessing stage is limited to loading a volume of interest, obtaining its frequency spectrum and preparing it for slicing. After the preparation of the spectral volume, the rendering loop is executed to generate different projection images by extracting a projection-slice according to the input viewing angle, then resampling it, and finally backtransforming it to the spatial domain to generate the reconstructed image.

From another perspective, the pipeline could be split according to functionality into two complementary cores or contexts: a *computational* context and a *rendering* context. Cooperatively, both contexts complement each other

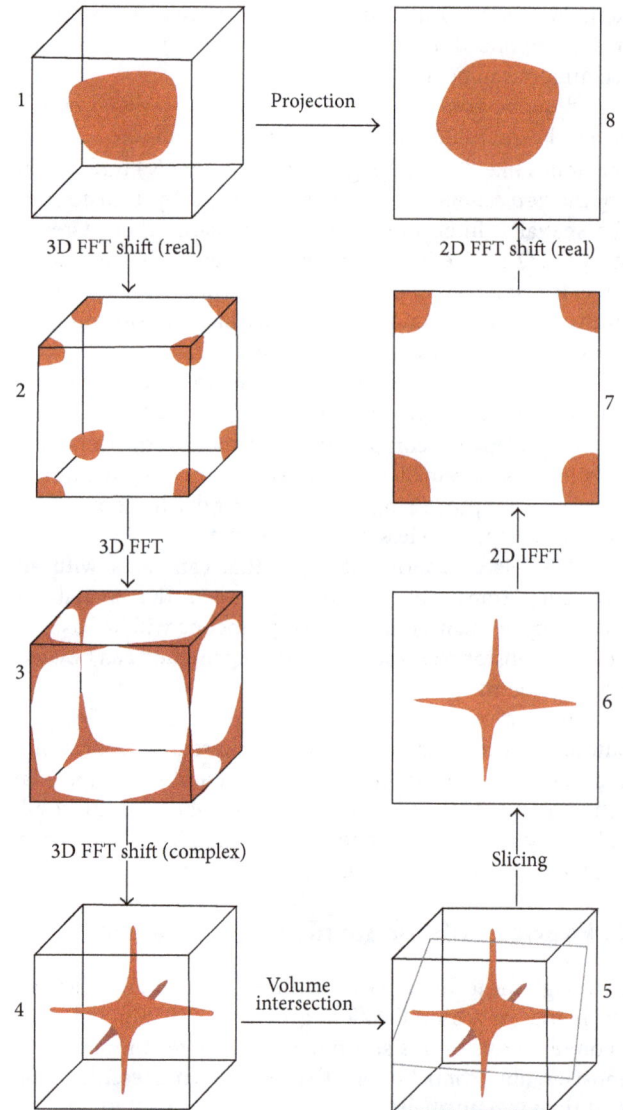

FIGURE 1: Graphical illustration of the FVR algorithm.

functional-wise, but from the sequence point of view, they are overlapping and one must switch from one context to the other to flow through the pipeline.

3.3. Implementation Strategy. Building the entire FVR pipeline on the GPU directly may be cumbersome and inefficient. In general, an adequate way of constructing GPU-based pipelines is to have a naïve and valid reference implementation of this pipeline on the CPU in advance. Having this CPU-based pipeline tested and validated, every stage of it can be afterwards implemented independently on the GPU and then validated to ensure similar results from the CPU-based implementation until getting the pipeline working integrally on the GPU. This implementation strategy is a rule of thumb to increases flexibility and efficiency for designing and building GPU pipelines. Our proposed FVR pipeline was built based on this strategy.

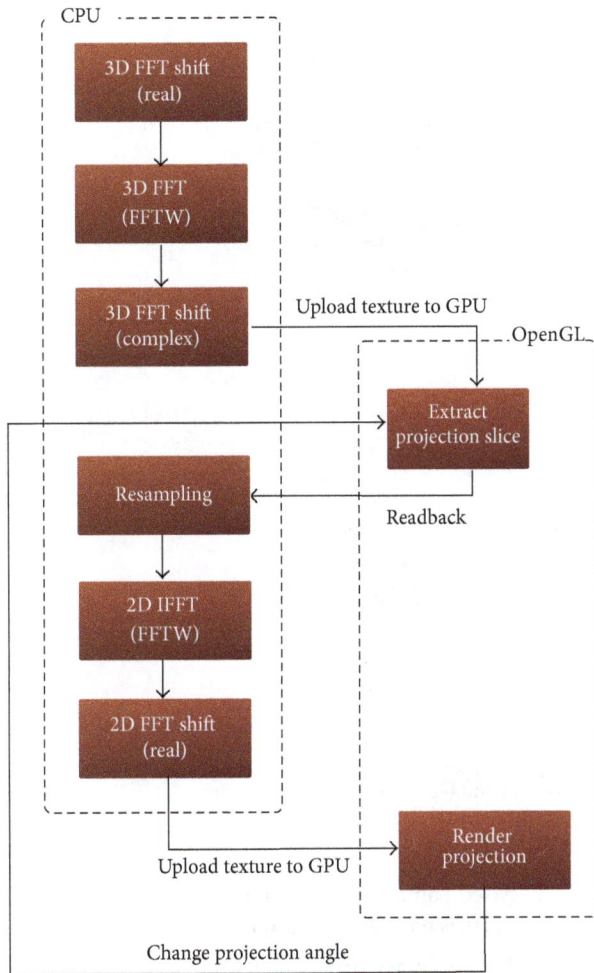

FIGURE 2: Heterogeneous implementation of the FVR pipeline. The computational context is executed on the CPU and the rendering contexts are executed in OpenGL contexts on the GPU.

According to the aforementioned contextual functional classification of the FVR pipeline, the CPU is employed for executing the computational context while the GPU can be used to implement the rendering contexts relying on any graphics application programming interface (API) like OpenGL or Direct 3D. This heterogeneous implementation is easier to handle than a full CPU-based pipeline because the 3D spectral volume can be efficiently represented by 3D OpenGL textures. This efficiency comes from their hardware-acceleration support and built-in interpolation schemes compared to using a 3D array on the CPU and doing the interpolation step manually.

3.4. Hybrid Pipeline. The reference hybrid implementation of the FVR pipeline has been adopted from a previous single threaded one discussed in [24]. This implementation is graphically illustrated in Figure 2. It starts its computational context on the CPU by loading a 3D datasets. This volume is then spatially shifted and its frequency spectrum is obtained by a forward 3D FFT operation. After activating the first

OpenGL off-screen rendering context, this spectral volume is mapped to a 3D texture that is allocated on and uploaded to the GPU memory. This texture is intersected with a proxy quadrant passing through the origin of the frequency domain. The resulting projection-slice is then directed to a frame buffer object (FBO) and packed in a 2-component 2D texture attached to this FBO. The contexts are then switched to move back to the computational context on the CPU, where the extracted projection-slice is downloaded from the 2D texture. The communication between the computational and off-screen rendering contexts is shown in Figure 3.

Afterwards, the computational context is resumed by resampling the projection-slice to remove the ghosting artifacts. The resampled slice is then back-transformed by an inverse 2D FFT operation to the spatial domain to produce a shifted image of the projection. This image is rearranged by a 2D fft-shift operation. The final reconstructed image is then packed into a 2D OpenGL texture and uploaded via the command *glTex2D* to reside on the GPU memory. Finally, the on-screen rendering context is activated and the texture that contains the final projection image is sent to the frame buffer to be displayed. This context is illustrated in Figure 4.

3.5. Hybrid Implementation Bottlenecks. As usual, each naïve approach has its accompanied bottlenecks that have to be investigated for either their complete removal or at least minimizing their performance overheads. The hybrid implementation of this technique obviously lacked the soul of interactivity due to several bottlenecks. In this section, the hybrid pipeline is analyzed to suppress its main bottlenecks and also to optimize its flow in order to get ready to have it entirely mapped to the GPU with both of its computational and rendering contexts.

A main concern that significantly affects the performance in the computational context is the FFT operations. These operations were expressed relying on the FFTW library [25–29]. The 3D FFT operation takes a considerable amount of time if the size of the input volume was 64^3 or more. Although it is executed once during the pre-processing stage, performing this operation on several volumes to reveal any depth cues will introduce a real bottleneck and this will consequently elongate the pre-processing stage. Additionally, the inverse 2D FFT operation is executed on a per-frame basis. In turn, reducing the time consumed by this operation will be reflected as an order of magnitude enhancement in the frame rate.

The performance of the rendering loop is affected by the resampling stage, which represents the most critical bottleneck in this pipeline. This operation involves four nested *for* loops. Two of them are used to iterate on each dimension of the slice and the other two are used for the filter kernel. For a projection-slice of size 512^2, the resampling operation takes a considerable amount of time that eventually blocks a real-time rendering loop. Additionally, executing the computational context on the CPU and the rendering ones on the GPU requires communicating each other to transfer the data back and forth between them. This transfer limits the overall performance of the pipeline to the bandwidth of

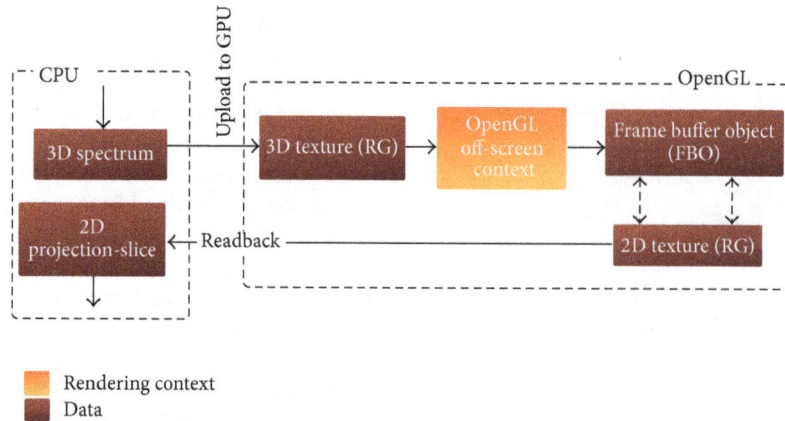

FIGURE 3: Communication between the computational context and OpenGL off-screen rendering context.

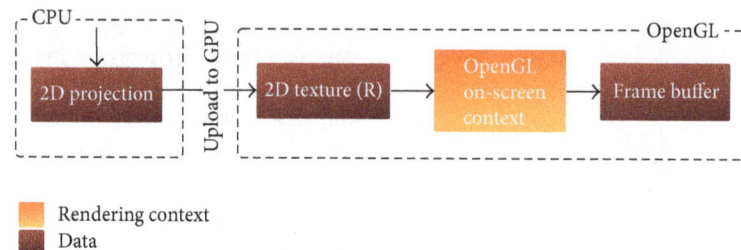

FIGURE 4: Communication between the computational context and OpenGL on-screen context.

the communication channel between the CPU and the GPU, which is much less than that on the GPU internally.

3.6. Algorithm Mapping to the GPU.

Mapping the FVR pipeline to be entirely running on the GPU is a significant step that will leverage the overall performance of the reconstruction process. This mapping procedure is feasible, yet, challenging. Although programming the GPU for executing nongraphics algorithms has been simplified by the introduction of generic GPU APIs like CUDA and OpenCL, but it is far from trivial to effectively exploit this titanic computing power provided by the GPU [30].

The hybrid implementation had a similar flow of typical OpenGL applications. This point makes the communication between OpenGL contexts and the CPU comparatively simple. In the GPU-based approach, the implementation of OpenGL contexts remains the same as that of the previous one, while the computational core of the pipeline will be implemented in a CUDA context. However, both contexts run on the GPU, but the interoperability between them takes a different mechanism and some workarounds for successful and efficient communication. The issues behind OpenGL interoperability with CUDA are discussed with some sort of details in [31, 32].

3.7. CUDA Kernels.

The first stage for mapping the computational core of the pipeline into a CUDA context is writing analogous device kernels to the respective C functions of the CPU-based computational context. In our mapping, the following kernels have been written.

(1) FFT_SHIFT_3D_REAL, which wraps around the 3D spatial volume.

(2) FFT_SHIFT_3D_COMPLEX, which wraps around the 3D complex spectrum.

(3) FFT_SHIFT_2D_REAL, which wraps around the resulting image from the inverse 2D FFT operation.

(4) RESAMPLE_SLICE, which executes the high-order resampling operation.

(5) REPACK_ARRAY, which replaces the complex array resulting from the 3D CUFFT operation by another 1D alternative to match the format of the OpenGL 3D spectrum texture.

The fft-shift kernels have been adopted from the proposed implementations in [33, 34]. The following FFT kernels were designed to encapsulate the FFT plans that were originally implemented within the CUFFT library [35].

(1) CUDA_FFT_3D, which executes the forward 3D FFT operation.

(2) CUDA_FFT_2D, which executes the inverse 2D FFT operation.

3.8. GPU-Based Pipeline.

In this GPU-accelerated pipeline, shown in Figure 5, the CPU is only used for loading the input volume and controlling the flow of the pipeline. This control

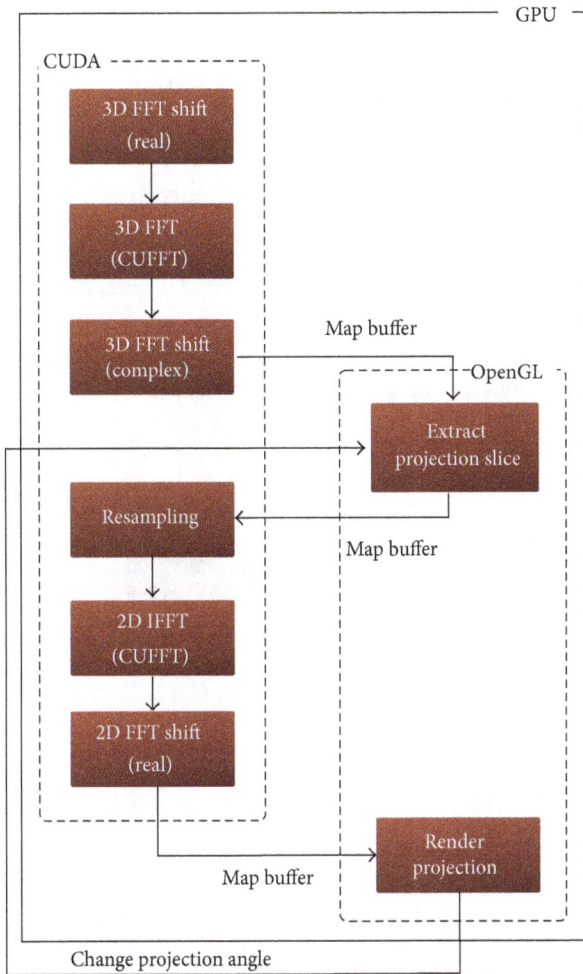

FIGURE 5: GPU-based implementation of the FVR pipeline. The rendering contexts of the hybrid implementation are reused and the computational one is reimplemented in a CUDA context.

includes switching between the different contexts, copying data from the CPU to the GPU, and dispatching OpenGL commands. Nevertheless, the entire flow of the pipeline is started and terminated on the GPU. The OpenGL rendering contexts employed in the hybrid pipeline will be reused in this implementation to interoperate with the CUDA computational context. However, there will be slight modifications concerned with the communication mechanisms between the different contexts.

Once the volume dataset of interest is loaded to the CPU side, it is directly shoved to reside on the GPU global memory by a *cudaMemcpy* operation. On the GPU side, a CUDA context is created and activated. Then the FFT_SHIFT_3D_REAL kernel is executed for centering the 3D spatial volume. CUDA_FFT_3D function is then invoked to obtain the 3D frequency spectrum of the input spatial volume. Afterwards, the FFT_SHIFT_3D_COMPLEX kernel is invoked to set the center of the spectral volume at the origin of the *k*-space. This array will be mapped to the OpenGL off-screen rendering context for performing the projection-slice extraction operation.

This complex array is converted to an alternative one that is compatible with an OpenGL 3D texture with two components using the REPACK_ARRAY kernel. Although the origin-aligned spectral volume array is located on the GPU memory, it cannot be accessed directly by OpenGL because it is located in the CUDA address space. This array can be read back to the CPU and then uploaded again to the GPU to reside on the texture memory of the CUDA context. This memory transfer operation is extremely useless and can be solved by using an OpenGL pixel buffer object (PBO) that is registered in the CUDA memory space. This workaround makes it possible to directly copy the spectral array to a buffer that is shared between the different contexts of the pipeline. This mechanism is illustrated in Figure 6.

After mapping the spectral texture to OpenGL memory space, we have to switch contexts to load the OpenGL off-screen rendering context. The 3D spectral texture is bound and intersected with a polygon, with the same sizes of the reconstructed image, and the result of this intersection is directed to the FBO and stored in the attached 2D texture. By projecting the desired slice in this FBO, the OpenGL off-screen rendering context is terminated and the rendering pipeline switches back to the CUDA context. A reference to the attached texture to the FBO is mapped to the CUDA context using CUDA array in order to be accessible for subsequent kernel calls. This CUDA array that carries the projection-slice is then mapped to a CUDA texture object. The RESAMPLE_SLICE kernel is then invoked, so the resampling operation is performed on this texture object and the results are stored directly into another 1D array with compatible format with the next CUFFT operation. Afterwards, the CUDA_FFT_2D function is executed on the resampled slice to generate the projection image. This resulting image is shifted, and thus, an fft-shift operation is considered by invoking the FFT_SHIFT_2D_REAL kernel. This correct image is ready to be displayed, but it has to be mapped in advance to an OpenGL 2D texture. This requires mapping the resulting array from the previous fft-shift operation to an OpenGL texture using a PBO.

After this mapping operation, the on-scree OpenGL rendering context is activated and the final image is pushed to the frame buffer for display. This context is illustrated in Figure 7. Changing the viewing angle repeats this flow by switching back to the OpenGL off-screen context to extract another projection-slice going through all the subsequent stages over and over until the termination of the running process.

3.9. GPU-Based Implementation Considerations. Although the OpenGL off-screen context is implemented the same way as it was done in the hybrid pipeline, the extracted projection-slice in the frame buffer object can not be read back by the CPU any more. Alternatively, it is mapped directly to the CUDA memory space by creating another PBO and registering this buffer object with the CUDA memory space. This allows direct attachment of the extracted slice data from the OpenGL off-screen context to be accessible and callable from the different CUDA kernels.

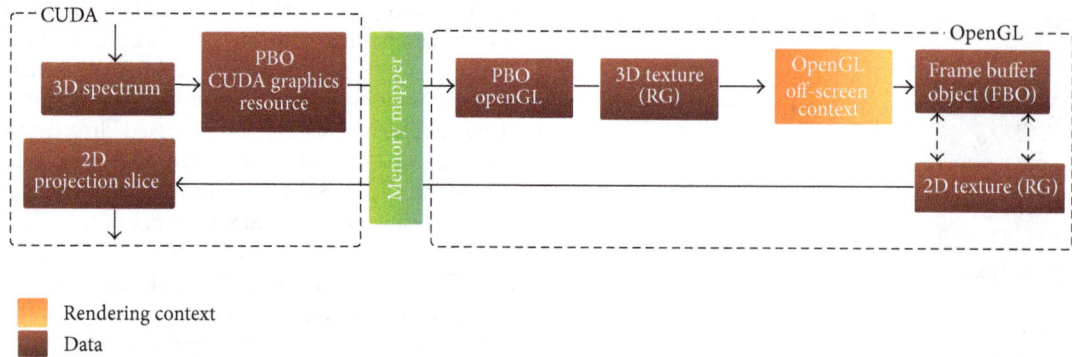

FIGURE 6: Communication between CUDA and OpenGL off-screen rendering contexts. The spectral volume is mapped between the two contexts via PBOs and the projection-slice is mapped to a 2D texture via CUDA array.

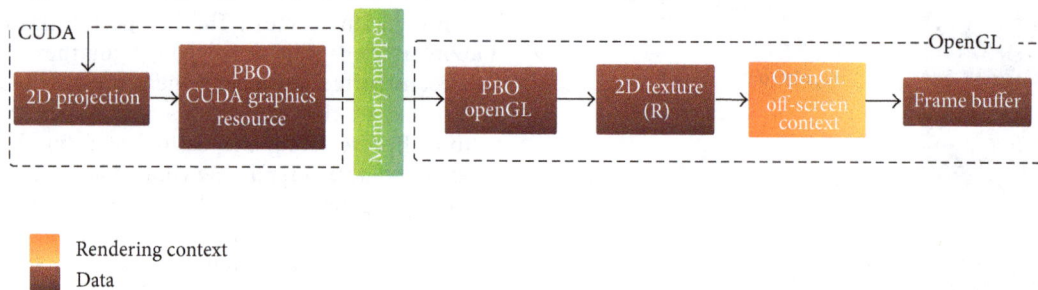

FIGURE 7: Communication between CUDA and OpenGL on-screen rendering context. The final projection is mapped between the two contexts via the PBO.

Due to the optimization of the texture caches for 2D spatial locality, reading device memory via texture fetches is more performing than reading from the global memory [36]. In that essence and to exploit the low-latency memory access associated with the texture memory, the extracted projection-slice is directly packed in a CUDA array. This array can be easily mapped to a CUDA texture which is writable from the OpenGL context via the CUDA array. It is only readable from the CUDA side. This texture leads to a significant speed-up in the resampling stage compared to the naïve *for* loop implementation in the hybrid pipeline.

The context switching operations were accelerated due to the direct connection between the different CUDA and OpenGL contexts relying on the shared buffer objects. These buffer objects are registered within all the contexts to allow direct mapping of the resulting textures from the computational context to the rendering ones. This permits efficient data sharing between the different contexts without any memory copies between the CPU and the CPU at all.

4. Results and Discussion

4.1. Reconstruction Results. Figure 8 shows the resulting radiographs of four medical datasets with different sizes and three intensity scaling factors. All the datasets are organized in regular 3D Cartesian grids [37, 38].

To show the artifacts associated with resampling the extracted projection slice, three different interpolation schemes have been applied: point-sampling, trilinear

interpolation, and windowed-*sinc* interpolation. Figure 9 reflects how the selection of the interpolation scheme can significantly affect the rendering quality of the projection image. The projection reconstructed in Figure 9(a) does not exhibit any ghosts because it is orthogonal and all the replicas are not present in the view. In Figure 9(b), the ghosting artifacts are very apparent due to the usage of the point sampling filter, which clamps the missing sample to the nearest available value. In Figure 9(c), the intensities of the replicas are reduced when trilinear interpolation scheme is applied. In fact, the nearest-neighbour and tri-linear interpolation schemes have almost the same performance for resampling projection-slices with sizes less than or equal to 512^2, but for larger volumes, the performance cost of trilinear interpolation is a bit high. However, this overhead is not significantly degrading the performance of the entire pipeline.

Figure 10 shows the result of zero-padding the spatial volume to suppress the overlapping between the central projection image and the surrounding replicas in the spatial domain. It has to be noticed that the zero-padding operation comes with no overhead on the performance although it dramatically increases the memory requirements by a factor of 8 for 100% zero-padding.

To minimize the artifacts associated with the nature of the technique, the rendering pipeline should afford a high order interpolation filter combined with a preprocessing zero-padding operation. A practical filter that can perform this operation is a Hamming windowed-*sinc* interpolation filter

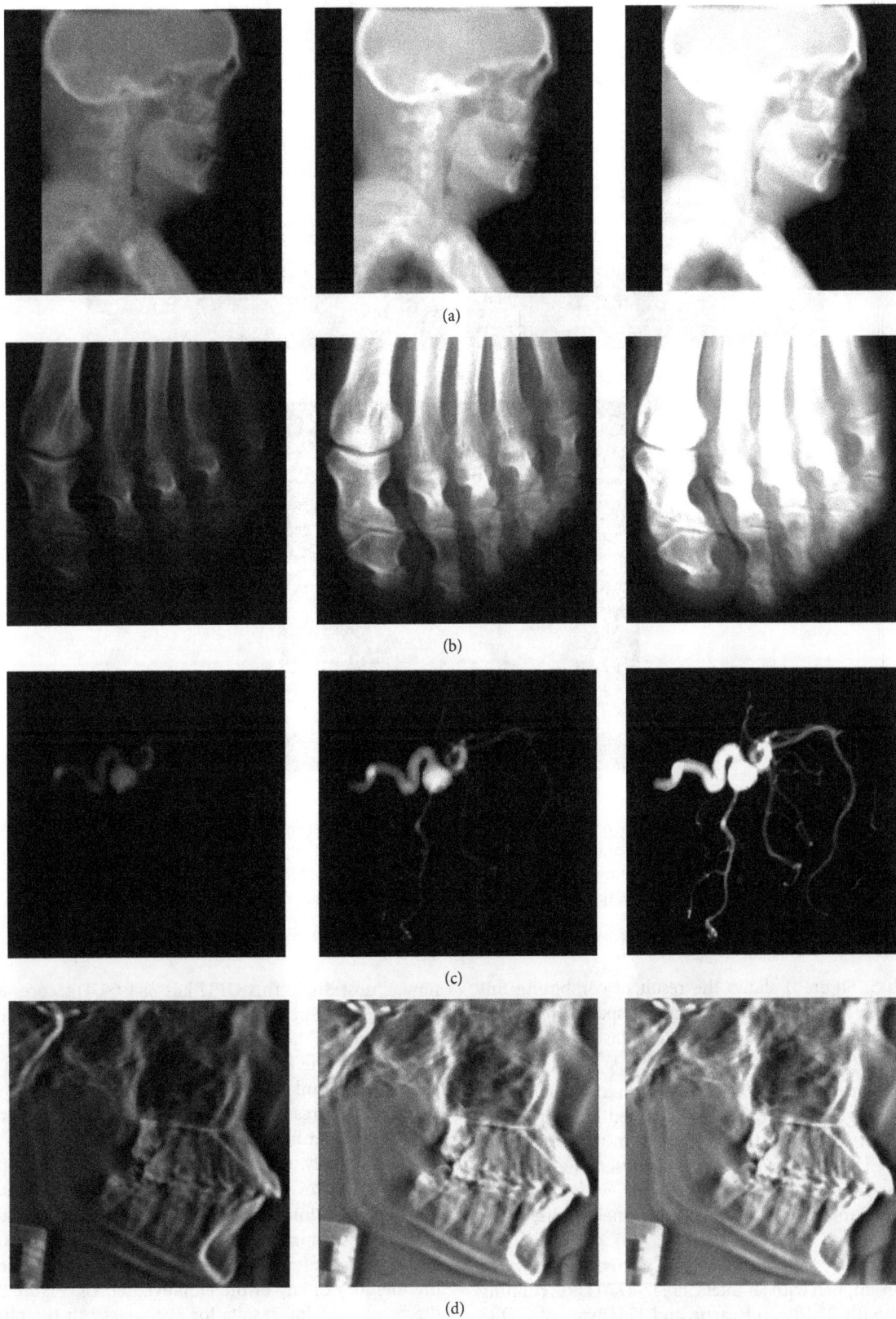

FIGURE 8: Reconstruction results of rendering several datasets with different projection-slice resolutions and multiple intensity scaling factors. In (a), a sagittal projection of the *visible male* dataset. In (b), an axial projection of a *foot* dataset. In (c), a front view of an *aneurysm* dataset. In (d), a sagittal projection of a *skull* dataset.

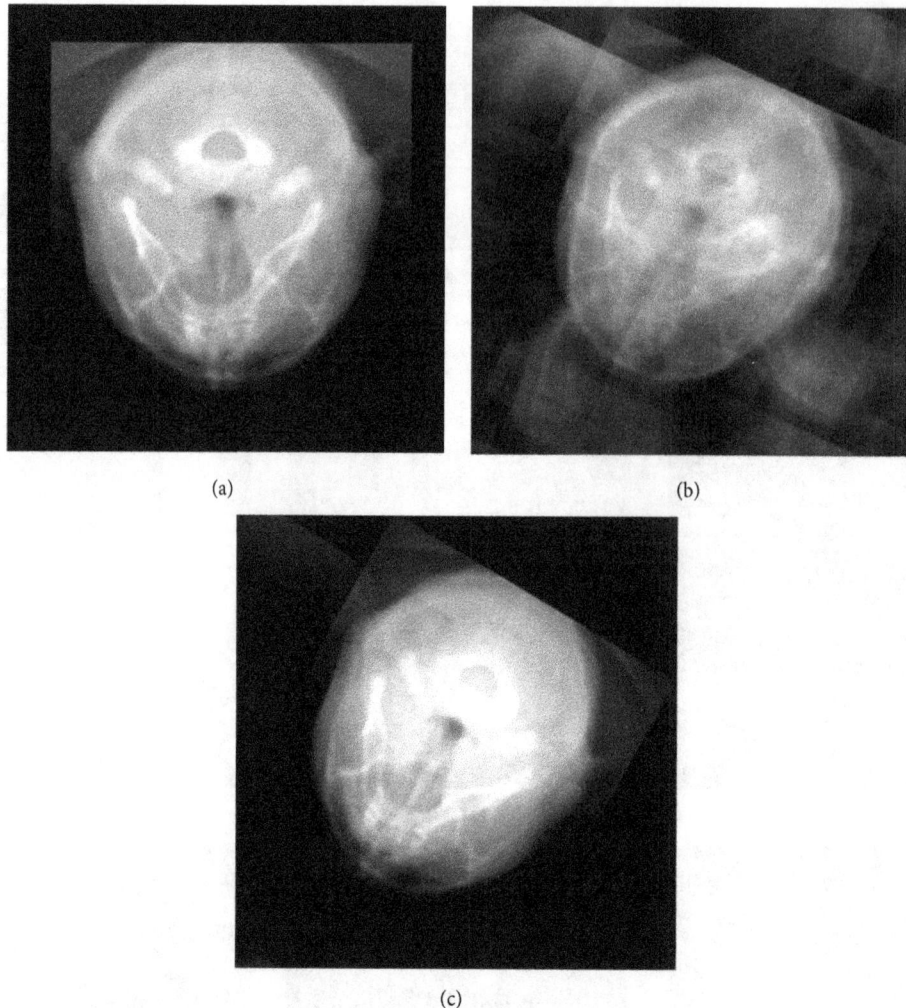

(a)

(b)

(c)

FIGURE 9: Results of rendering an axial projection of the *visible male* dataset with basic interpolation filters supported by OpenGL 3D textures. In (a), the projection of the dataset is orthogonal and the replicas are not shown. In (b) and (c), the volume is rotated and the ghosting artifacts are very apparent in (b) if a nearest-neighbour interpolation scheme is used and highly reduced if a trilinear interpolation filter is applied as shown in (c). Applying trilinear filtration on the spectral slice significantly affects the rendering performance if the slice size is greater than 512^2.

with width 5. Figure 11 shows the result of combining this reconstruction filter with zero-padding the spatial volume on an oblique projection of the *visible male* datasets.

4.2. Performance Analysis. On the performance side and in order to highlight the improvements gained by porting the computational context of the pipeline from the CPU to an alternative CUDA context, we have analysed the profiling results for every stage individually and then we demonstrate and accounted for the overall speed-ups gained for the entire pipeline.

The rendering pipeline has been benchmarked on a workstation shipped with an Intel Core i7-4770 CPU running at 3.4 GHz with 8 MByte of cache and 12 GBytes of DDR3 memory. The application was compiled on Ubuntu 14.04 using GCC 4.7.3 and NVIDIA CUDA compiler nvcc 6.0.1. Two GPUs have been selected to profile the accelerated pipeline. The first one was an NVIDIA GeForce GT 640, which is considered a midrange commodity GPU that costs

now almost $100. This GPU has 384 CUDA cores and four GBytes of 128-Bit DDR3 memory. It has been referred to in the text by GPU 1. The other GPU was an NVIDIA QUADRO K5000. This one is much more powerful than the first GPU and can be ranked as a state-of-the-art one since it has 1536 CUDA cores and four GBytes of GDDR5 memory. It will be referred later in the text and the benchmarks by GPU 2.

Additionally, and on the software side, the application was tested with CUDA 6.0. The benchmarks were generated for different volumes of sizes 128^3, 256^3, and 512^3. Although higher speed-ups can be achieved if the volume size goes beyond this limit, unfortunately, larger volumes cannot fit in the memory of any of the employed GPUs. Figure 12 shows the benchmarking results for every stage in the pipeline to elaborate the difference between the CPU performance in comparison to the two GPUs.

Table 1 summarizes the average execution times for the different stages of the pipeline and aggregates the entire pipeline performance for a volume dataset of size 512^3. We

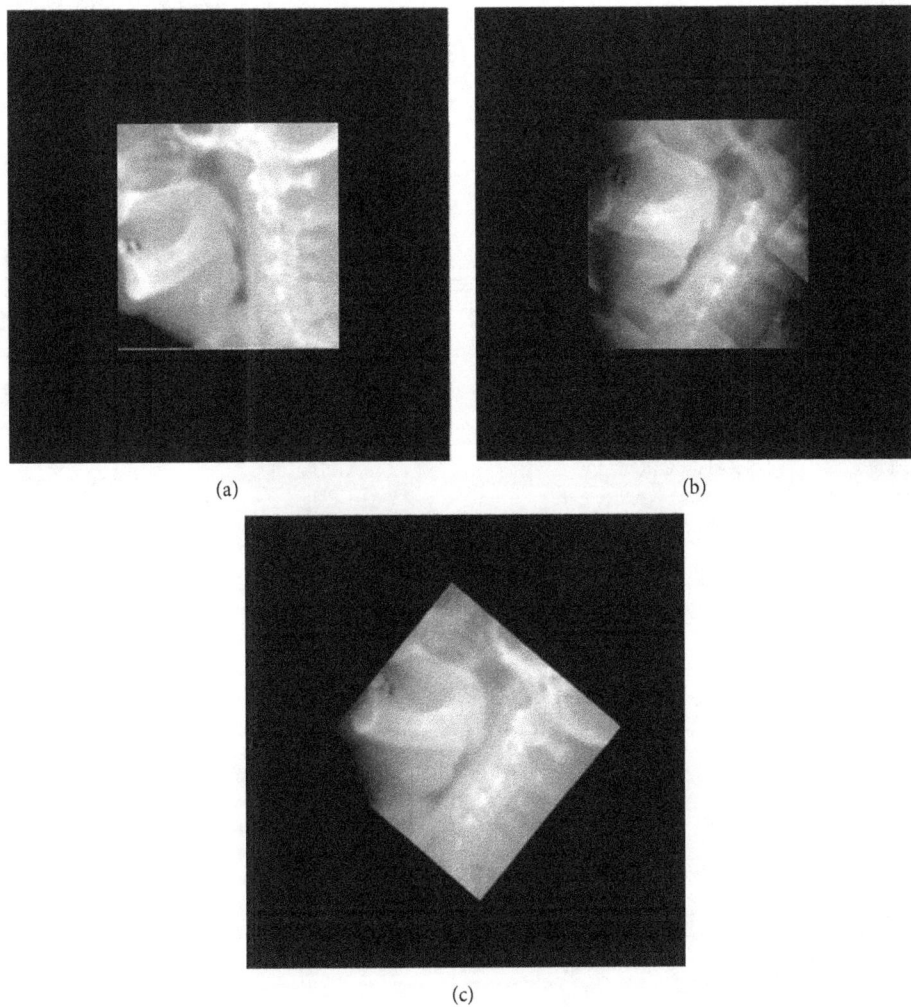

FIGURE 10: Zero-padding the spatial volume to remove the overlapping between the central image and the replicas. In (a), the central part of the *visible male* dataset is packed in a volume array of the same size. Rotating the volume in (b) results in overlapping. Zero-padding the subvolume removes all the overlapping after rotating the whole volume as shown in (c).

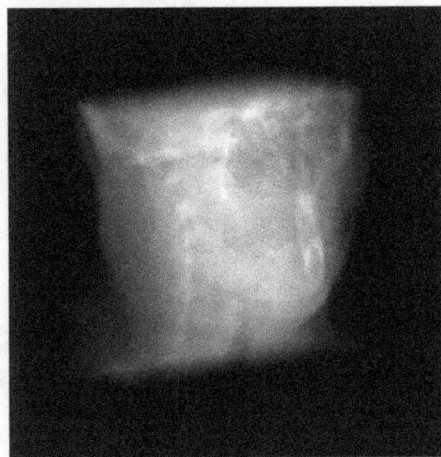

FIGURE 11: Rendering an oblique projection of the central part of the *visible male* dataset. The volume is zero-padded and the extracted slice undergoes a high-order resampling by applying a Hamming windowed-*sinc* reconstruction filter with order 5 to maximally reduce the ghosting artifacts.

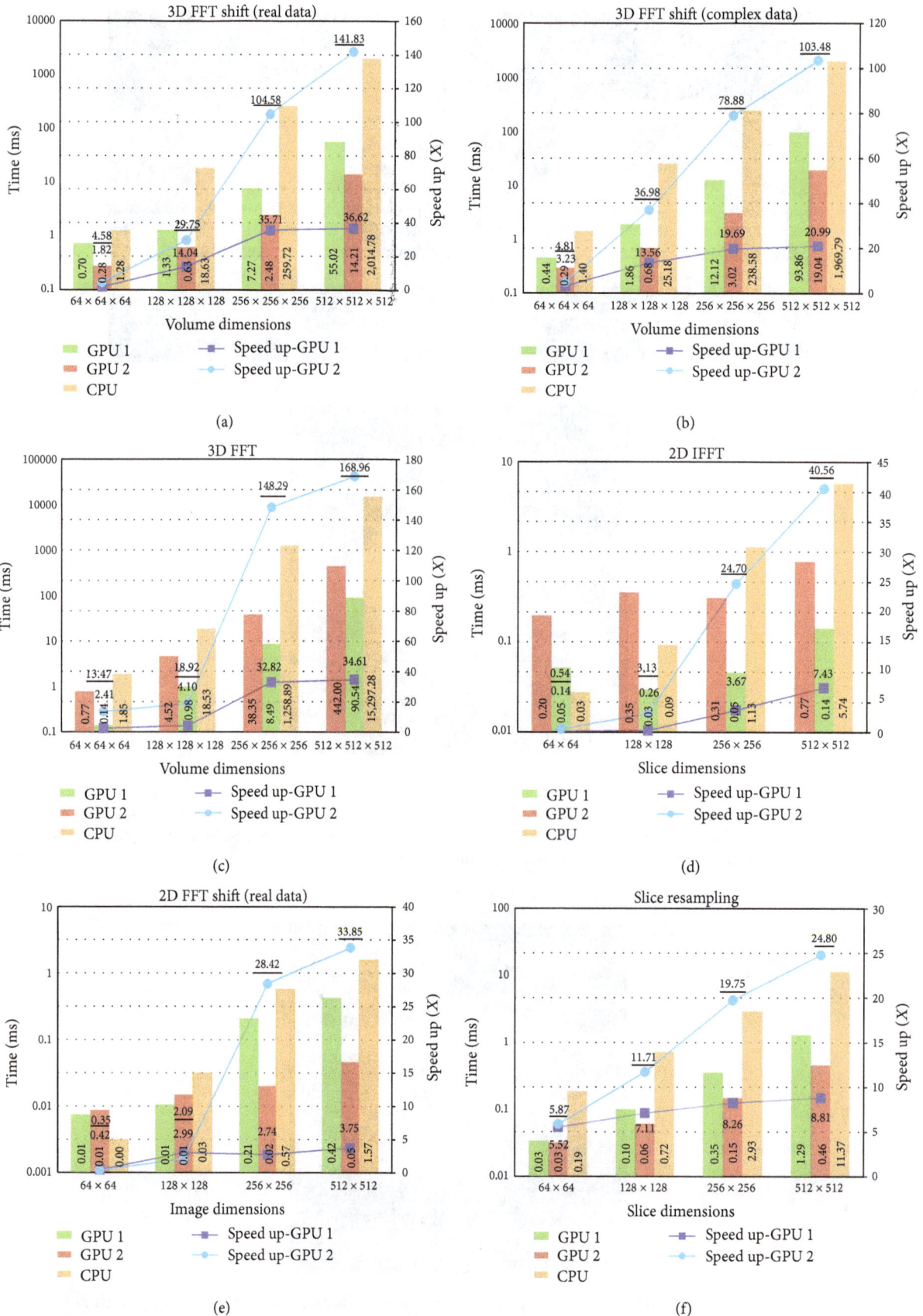

FIGURE 12: Benchmarking results of the different stages of the rendering pipeline executed on two different GPUs. GPU 1 is an NVIDIA GeForce GT 640, and GPU 2 is an NVIDIA QUADRO K5000.

TABLE 1: Performance benchmarks comparison between the different stages of the computational context on the CPU versus GPU for processing a volume of 512^3. All the results are in *milli-seconds*.

Operation	CPU	GPU 1	GPU 2
Volume uploading to GPU	—	100	40
3D real FFT shift	2014.778	55.01	14.2
3D FFT	15297.28	442.004	90.53
3D complex FFT shift	1969.79	93.86	19.03
Resampling	11.3	1.290	0.458
2D FFT	5.736	0.771	0.1414
2D real FFT shift	1.565	0.4175	0.04623
Preprocessing stage	**19281.847**	**690.886**	**163.78**
Rendering loop	**18.672**	**2.4796**	**0.6462**
Entire pipeline	**19300.5194**	**693.365**	**164.4**

also reference the hybrid implementation to relatively show that our implementation has gained a speed-up of 117x for the entire pipeline and 29x for the rendering loop. The GPU-accelerated pipeline requires uploading the spatial volume to the device global memory. This step takes on average less than 100 and 40 milli-seconds for a volume of size 512^3 on GPU 1 and GPU 2, respectively. Thanks to the interoperability mechanisms between CUDA and OpenGL, there are no further data transfer operations between the different stages of the rendering pipeline.

These profiles can be reduced if compared to a multithreaded implementation. However, building a multithreaded OpenGL application is quite complex, and thus a pure GPU implementation is much more appropriate to consider rather than constructing a multithreaded application for benchmarks comparison.

5. Conclusion and Future Work

This paper presented a high performance implementation of the Fourier volume rendering algorithm on CUDA-capable GPUs. The literature of FVR was briefly covered and followed by a detailed explanation of the plain rendering algorithm by introducing the notions of computational and rendering contexts. Our implementation strategy considered in advance building a reference hybrid rendering solution where the computational context is executed on the CPU and the rendering one on the GPU using OpenGL. This reference pipeline was then imported in a step-wise fashion to run entirely on the GPU by mapping the computational context to run within a CUDA context and redesigning the rendering contexts to communicate between CUDA and OpenGL to optimize the performance of the rendering loop. Using a 512^3 dataset, the pure GPU implementation outperformed the hybrid one by a factor of 117x for the entire pipeline and nearly 29x of speed up for the rendering loop. The GPU-accelerated pipeline will be extended in the future to include depth cues and different shading models that can improve the visual appearance of the resulting digital radiographs. A client-server distributed model of the pipeline will be also considered to allow rendering large-scale datasets on multiple computing nodes.

Acronyms

1D: One-dimensional
2D: Two-dimensional
3D: Three-dimensional
API: Application programming interface
CPU: Central processing unit
CUDA: Compute unified device architecture
DRR: Digital reconstructed radiograph
FDVR: Frequency domain volume rendering
FFT: Fast Fourier transform
FBO: Frame buffer object
FVR: Fourier volume rendering
GPU: Graphics processing unit
PBO: Pixel buffer object.

Conflict of Interests

The authors have declared no potential conflict of interests with respect to the authorship and/or publication of this paper.

Acknowledgment

The authors would like to gratefully thank the anonymous reviewers for their kind feedback and constructive comments that have helped them in improving the quality of the paper.

References

[1] T. T. Elvins, "A survey of algorithms for volume visualization," *ACM SIGGRAPH Computer Graphics*, vol. 26, pp. 194–201, 1992.

[2] M. Ikits, J. Kniss, A. Lefohn, and C. Hansen, "Volume rendering techniques," in *GPU Gems*, chapter 39, Addison-Wesley, 2007.

[3] B. Preim and D. Bartz, *Visualization in Medicine: Theory, Algorithms, and Applications*, The Morgan Kaufmann Series in Computer Graphics, Morgan Kaufmann, Boston, Mass, USA, 1st edition, 2007.

[4] G. Dougherty, *Digital Image Processing for Medical Applications*, chapter 12, Cambridge University Press, Cambridge, UK, 2009.

[5] K. H. Kim, M. J. Kwon, S. M. Kwon, J. B. Ra, and H. W. Park, "Fast surface and volume rendering based on shear-warp

factorization for a surgical simulator," *Computer Aided Surgery*, vol. 7, no. 5, pp. 268–278, 2002.

[6] J. K. Udupa, "Surface versus volume rendering: a comparative assessment," in *Proceedings of the 1st Conference on Visualization in Biomedical Computing*, pp. 83–91, May 1990.

[7] C. D. Hansen and C. R. Johnson, *The Visualization Handbook*, chapter 7, Elsevier, New York, NY, USA, 2005.

[8] S. Dunne, S. Napel, and B. Rutt, "Interactive display of volumetric data by fast fourier projection," *Computerized Medical Imaging and Graphics*, vol. 16, no. 4, pp. 237–251, 1992.

[9] T. Malzbender, "Fourier volume rendering," *ACM Transactions on Graphics*, vol. 9, no. 7, pp. 233–250, 2000.

[10] R. Grosso and T. Ertl, "Biorthogonal wavelet filters for frequency domain volume rendering," in *Visualization in Scientific Computing '95: Proceedings of the Eurographics Workshop in Chia, Italy, May 3–5, 1995*, Eurographics, pp. 81–95, Springer, Vienna, Austria, 1995.

[11] T. Theußl, "An implementation of frequency domain volume rendering using the Hartley transform," in *The Course of Special Topics in Computer Graphics*, 1999.

[12] M. Levoy, "Volume rendering using the Fourier projection-slice theorem," in *Proceedings of the Conference on Graphics Interface*, Technical Report from Stanford University CSL-TR-92-521, pp. 61–69, May 1992.

[13] T. Totsuka and M. Levoy, "Frequency domain volume rendering," in *Proceedings of the 20th Annual Conference on Computer Graphics and Interactive Techniques (SIGGRAPH '93)*, Technical Report from Stanford University CSL-TR-93-570, pp. 271–278, 1993.

[14] A. Entezari, R. Scoggins, T. Moller, and R. Machiraju, "Shading for Fourier volume rendering," in *Proceedings of the IEEE/ACM SIGGRAPH Symposium on Volume Visualization and Graphics*, pp. 131–138, Boston, Mass, USA, October 2002.

[15] R. K. Scoggins, R. Machiraju, and R. J. Moorhead, "Approximate shading for the re-illumination of synthetic images," in *Proceedings of the IEEE Visualization*, pp. 379–386, October 2001.

[16] Z. Nagy, M. Novotni, and R. Klein, "Enhancing Fourier volume rendering using contour extraction," in *Proceedings of the 7th International Conference on Medical Image Computingand Computer Assisted Intervention (MICCAI '04)*, pp. 470–477, September 2004.

[17] C.-C. Cheng and Y.-T. Ching, "Real-time adjustment of transfer function for Fourier volume rendering," *Journal of Electronic Imaging*, vol. 20, no. 4, Article ID 043004, 2011.

[18] T. Jansen, B. von Rymon-Lipinski, N. Hanssen, and E. Keeve, "Fourier volume rendering on the GPU using a split-stream-FFT," in *Proceedings of the 9th International Fall Workshop on Vision, Modeling, and Visualization (VMV '04)*, pp. 395–403, 2004.

[19] E. Ntasis, T. A. Maniatis, and K. S. Nikita, "Fourier volume rendering for real time preview of digital reconstructed radiographs: a web-based implementation," *Computerized Medical Imaging and Graphics*, vol. 26, no. 1, pp. 1–8, 2002.

[20] A. Corrigan and J. Wallin, "Visualization of meshless simulations using Fourier volume rendering," in *Proceedings of the ECCOMAS Thematic Conference on Meshless Methods*, pp. 65–70, July 2007.

[21] A. Corrigan, J. Wallin, and M. Vesenjak, "Visualization of meshless simulations using Fourier volume rendering," in *Progress on Meshless Methods*, vol. 11 of *Computational Methods in Applied Sciences*, pp. 291–305, Springer, Cham, Switzerland, 2009.

[22] M. Abdellah, A. Eldieb, and A. Sharawi, "Matlab-based Fourier volume rendering framework," in *Proceedings of the 7th Cairo International Biolmedical Engineering Conference (CIBEC '14)*, December 2014.

[23] I. Viola, A. Kanitsar, and M. E. Gröller, "GPU-based frequency domain volume rendering," in *Proceedings of the 20th Spring Conference on Computer Graphics (SCCG '04)*, pp. 55–64, April 2004.

[24] M. Abdellah, A. Eldeib, and A. Sharawi, "Offline large scale fourier volume rendering on low-end hardware," in *Proceedings of the Cairo International Biomedical Engineering Conference (CIBEC '14)*, pp. 59–62, Giza, Egypt, December 2014.

[25] M. Frigo and S. G. Johnson, "FFTW," V. 3.3, June 2014, http://www.fftw.org/.

[26] M. Frigo and S. G. Johnson, "The fastest Fourier transform in the west," Technical Report MIT-LCS-TR-728, Massachusetts Institute of Technology, Cambridge, Mass, USA, 1997.

[27] M. Frigo and S. G. Johnson, "FFTW: an adaptive software architecture for the FFT," in *Proceedings of the IEEE International Conference on Acoustics, Speech and Signal Processing*, vol. 3, pp. 1381–1384, IEEE, May 1998.

[28] S. G. Johnson and M. Frigo, "Implementing FFTs in practice," in *Fast Fourier Transforms*, C. S. Burrus, Ed., chapter 11, Connexions, Rice University, Houston, Tex, USA, 2008.

[29] M. Frigo and S. G. Johnson, "The design and implementation of FFTW3," *Proceedings of the IEEE*, vol. 93, no. 2, pp. 216–231, 2005.

[30] D. B. Kirk and W. W. Hwu, *Programming Massively Parallel Processors: A Hands-on Approach*, Morgan Kaufmann, San Francisco, Calif, USA, 1st edition, 2010.

[31] J. Stam, What every CUDA programmer should know about OpenGL, Online, Recorded Session ID 1055, 2009, http://developer.download.nvidia.com/compute/cuda/docs/GTC09Materials.htm.

[32] R. Farber, *CUDA Application Design and Development*, chapter 9, Elsevier, New York, NY, USA, 1st edition, 2011.

[33] M. Abdellah, S. Saleh, A. Eldeib, and A. Shaarawi, "High performance multi-dimensional (2D/3D) FFT-Shift implementation on Graphics Processing Units (GPUs)," in *Proceedings of the 6th Cairo International Biomedical Engineering Conference (CIBEC '12)*, pp. 171–174, Giza, Egypt, December 2012.

[34] M. Abdellah, "cufftShift: high performance CUDA-accelerated FFT-shift library," in *Proceedings of the High Performance Computing Symposium (HPC '14)*, pp. 5:1–5:8, Society for Computer Simulation International, San Diego, Calif, USA, 2014.

[35] NVIDIA, "CUFFT library," CUDA toolkit 6.0.

[36] NVIDIA, *CUDA C Best Practice Guide (Design Guide)*, 2012.

[37] The Volume Library, "Online library for Volume visualization datasets," http://lgdv.cs.fau.de/External/vollib/.

[38] "Online library for medical MR and CT datasets," January 2013, http://www.volvis.org/.

4

Automatic Classification of Normal and Cancer Lung CT Images Using Multiscale AM-FM Features

Eman Magdy, Nourhan Zayed, and Mahmoud Fakhr

Computer and Systems Department, Electronic Research Institute, Giza 12611, Egypt

Correspondence should be addressed to Eman Magdy; eman.magdy@eri.sci.eg

Academic Editor: Tiange Zhuang

Computer-aided diagnostic (CAD) systems provide fast and reliable diagnosis for medical images. In this paper, CAD system is proposed to analyze and automatically segment the lungs and classify each lung into normal or cancer. Using 70 different patients' lung CT dataset, Wiener filtering on the original CT images is applied firstly as a preprocessing step. Secondly, we combine histogram analysis with thresholding and morphological operations to segment the lung regions and extract each lung separately. Amplitude-Modulation Frequency-Modulation (AM-FM) method thirdly, has been used to extract features for ROIs. Then, the significant AM-FM features have been selected using Partial Least Squares Regression (PLSR) for classification step. Finally, *K*-nearest neighbour (*K*NN), support vector machine (SVM), naïve Bayes, and linear classifiers have been used with the selected AM-FM features. The performance of each classifier in terms of accuracy, sensitivity, and specificity is evaluated. The results indicate that our proposed CAD system succeeded to differentiate between normal and cancer lungs and achieved 95% accuracy in case of the linear classifier.

1. Introduction

Computed Tomography (CT) has outperformed conventional radiography in the screening of lungs because it generates very detailed high-resolution images and can show early-stage lesions that are too small to be detected by conventional X-ray. CT has been widely used to detect numerous lung diseases, including pneumoconiosis, pneumonia, pulmonary edema, and lung cancer [1]. Early detection of diseases is very crucial for treatment planning. However, it is considered one of the most challenging tasks performed by radiologists due to the huge amount of data generated by CT scan. Therefore, computer-aided diagnostic (CAD) systems are needed to assist radiologists in the analysis and evaluation of CT scans.

A CAD system analyzes medical images in several steps: first a preprocessing step for noise reduction and enhancing the image quality and then segmentation step to differentiate region of interest (ROI) from other structures in the image. After segmentation, different features such as geometrical, textural, and statistical features are extracted. Finally,

a classification/evaluation step is done to evaluate and diagnose the ROI based on extracted features.

Many efforts have been made to provide computer-aided diagnosis for lung images. Lung segmentation is a necessary step; it has progressed from manual tracing to semiautomated to fully automated segmentation. Here, some automated lung segmentation studies are presented [2–9]. Other studies present content-based image retrieval (CBIR) systems for lung images [10–15]. Earlier work in classification of lung cancer includes the work of Patil and Kuchanur [16] and Kuruvilla and Gunavathi [17] that used artificial neural networks to classify lung cancer images based on the features extracted from lung segmented images. Nevertheless, Patil and Kuchanur used geometrical features for classification and achieved only 83% accuracy of classification. And Kuruvilla and Gunavathi used statistical parameters as features for classification and achieved accuracy of 93.3%. Another work by Depeursinge et al. [18] classified different lung tissue patterns using discrete wavelet frames combined with gray-level histogram features. However, the main limitation of this work was the lack of resolution in scales with the decomposition,

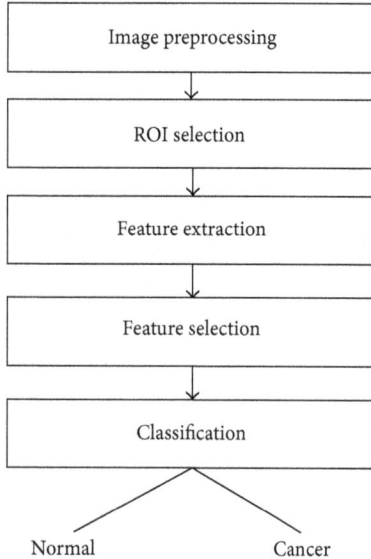

FIGURE 1: Block diagram of the proposed fully automated CAD system.

along with required feature weighting while merging features from different origins.

In this paper, we propose a CAD system for analysis, automatic segmentation, and classification of lung images into normal or cancer from CT dataset. The system is based on the multiscale Amplitude-Modulation Frequency-Modulation (AM-FM) approach. The lungs are firstly segmented from CT images and next left and right lungs are separated individually to be analyzed over a filterbank. Then, the AM-FM features are extracted and reduced for the classification step. Different classifiers are used to classify the images and the performance of each classifier has been evaluated.

2. Materials and Methods

Figure 1 shows the main block diagram of our proposed fully automated CAD system. As seen in this figure, the system is composed of five main steps: image preprocessing, select region of interest (ROI), feature extraction using AM-FM approach, feature selection to find the significant features, and finally a classification. The details of each step are discussed in the following sections.

2.1. Dataset. Data used in this research were obtained from The Cancer Imaging Archive (TCIA) sponsored by the SPIE, NCI/NIH, AAPM, and the University of Chicago [19]. A dataset of 83 CT images from 70 different patients was included. All images have a size of 512×512 pixels and are stored in Digital Imaging and Communication in Medicine (DICOM) format. An example of dataset is shown in Figure 2(a). In this figure, the right lung is abnormal as it has a cancer (the rounded gray shape), while the left lung is a normal one. For each lung CT image, we separate the left lung from the right lung automatically (as discussed later in

ROI Selection), and each separated lung is labelled as normal or cancer based on the dataset information.

2.2. Image Preprocessing. The objective of preprocessing step is to remove unwanted noise and enhance image quality. We have used a Wiener filter to remove noise while preserving the edges and fine details of lungs. The filter size of 3×3 is selected to avoid oversmoothing of the image. The result of Wiener filtering is shown in Figure 2(b).

Wiener filtering [20] is based on estimating the local mean and variance from a local neighborhood of each pixel. Then, it creates pixel-wise linear filtering using these estimates:

$$F(m,n) = \mu + \frac{\sigma^2 - \nu^2}{\sigma^2}(I(m,n) - \mu),\qquad(1)$$

where I and F denote the original and filtered images, respectively, μ and σ denote the mean and variance of a local neighborhood, respectively, and ν is the noise variance.

2.3. ROI Selection. Lung segmentation is a necessary step for any lung CAD system. We perform automatic segmentation of the lungs using successive steps. Then, the resulting segmented image is used to extract each lung separately (ROIs), producing two images: one for the left lung and the other for the right lung.

In the CT image, air appears in a mean intensity of approximately −3024 Hounsfield units (HU), and the lung tissue is in the range of −910 HU to −500 HU, while other structures are above −500 HU. The goal of segmentation step is to separate the lungs from both background and nonlung regions. To accomplish this, we propose a hybrid technique resulting from a combination of histogram analysis, thresholding, and morphological operations for automatic lung segmentation.

To simplify the segmentation process, the thorax region is firstly segmented from the background. A gray-level distribution (histogram) of the Wiener-filtered image is used to identify different regions in the image. The histogram has one peak corresponding to lung region and another two peaks for fat and muscle of thorax region and lung mediastinum. In addition, there is a spike at −3024 HU corresponding to background pixels. Figure 3 shows all peaks except for the background spike.

The threshold value is then computed from this histogram according to the following equation:

$$T = \frac{I_{\text{FM}} - I_L}{2} + I_L,\qquad(2)$$

where I_L denotes the peak intensity value of lung region and I_{FM} denotes the average intensity value of fat/muscle peaks.

Then, a binary image (Figure 4(a)) for segmented thorax region is created where the pixels with gray level greater than the selected threshold are set to "one" and other pixels are "zero."

After the thorax region is segmented, we perform a filling operation to fill the holes inside the binary image, so that the pixel values of lungs change from zero to one and produce

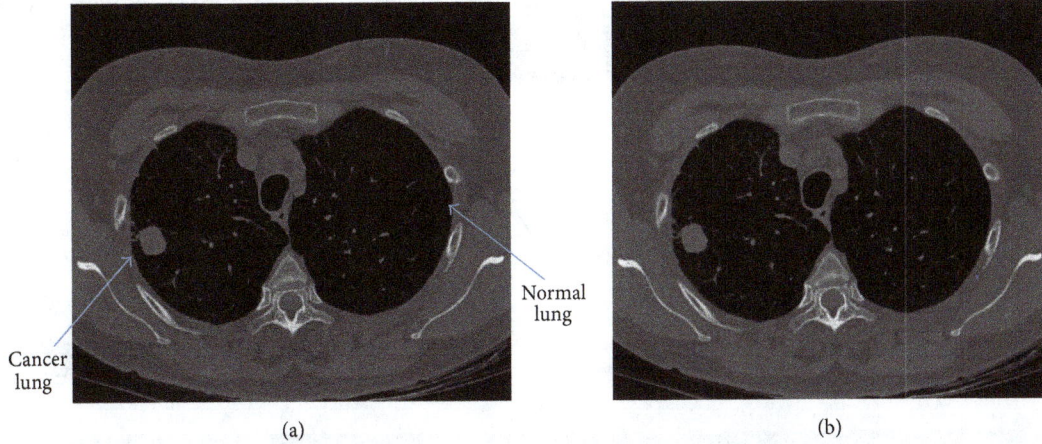

FIGURE 2: Image preprocessing: (a) original image and (b) filtered image.

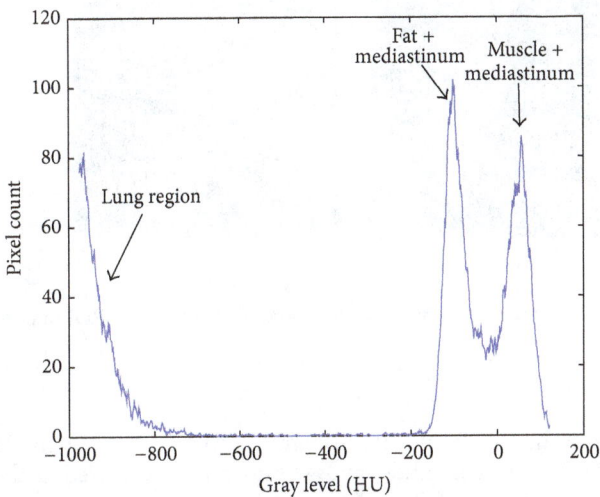

FIGURE 3: Histogram of the Wiener-filtered image.

a filled image (Figure 4(b)). Finally, the thorax binary image is subtracted from the filled image to obtain the segmented lungs as shown in Figure 4(c).

Once the image of lung segmentation is obtained, we used it to locate the left and right lungs in the filtered image, as seen in Figure 4(d). Then, this image is divided into two images for both lungs separately, each one covering the region of the lung as shown in Figures 4(e) and 4(f). From the 83 CT images, we obtained 166 different lung images after each image division, where 83 of them are normal lung images and the other 83 images are cancer lung images.

2.4. Feature Extraction. In this step, we apply the Amplitude-Modulation Frequency-Modulation (AM-FM) modeling techniques to extract features from lung images that will be used further in classification. A lot of research work has been made on AM-FM models [21–23].

2.4.1. AM-FM Methods. AM-FM is a technique that models nonstationary signals. Unlike Fourier transforms that provide

the frequency content of signal, AM-FM methods provide pixel-based information in terms of instantaneous amplitude (IA), instantaneous frequency (IF), and instantaneous phase (IP). And it does not have the main limitation found on wavelet when used to segment the lungs which was the lack of resolution in scales with the decomposition.

In 2D AM-FM model, a nonstationary image is represented by a sum of AM-FM components as [22]

$$I\left(k_1, k_2\right) = \sum_{n=1}^{M} a_n\left(k_1, k_2\right) \cos \varphi_n\left(k_1, k_2\right), \qquad (3)$$

where $n = 1, 2, \ldots, M$ denotes the different AM-FM harmonics, $a_n(k_1, k_2)$ denotes the instantaneous amplitude functions (IA), and $\varphi_n(k_1, k_2)$ denotes the instantaneous phase functions (IP).

For each AM-FM component, the instantaneous frequency (IF) is defined as the gradient of phase $\nabla \varphi_n(k_1, k_2) = (\partial \varphi_n(k_1, k_2) / \partial k_1, \partial \varphi_n(k_1, k_2) / \partial k_2)$. Here, the AM-FM demodulation problem is to estimate the IA, IF, and IP for the given input image.

In this work, AM-FM demodulation is achieved in several steps. First, we extend the input image to an analytic image by adding an imaginary part equal to the 2D Hilbert transform of the image [21]. Given a real-valued image $I(k_1, k_2)$, the analytic image $I_{AS}(k_1, k_2)$ is calculated as follows:

$$I_{AS}\left(k_1, k_2\right) = I\left(k_1, k_2\right) + jH_{2D}\left[I\left(k_1, k_2\right)\right], \qquad (4)$$

where H_{2D} denotes a two-dimensional extension of one-dimensional Hilbert transform.

Then, the analytic image is processed through a collection of band-pass filters (filterbank) (to be discussed in the next subsection) in order to isolate the AM-FM components.

And, from each filter response, we can estimate the IA and IP straightforwardly using these following equations:

$$\hat{a}\left(k_1, k_2\right) = \left|I_{AS}\left(k_1, k_2\right)\right|,$$

$$\hat{\varphi}\left(k_1, k_2\right) = \tan^{-1}\frac{\mathrm{imag}\left(I_{AS}\left(k_1, k_2\right)\right)}{\mathrm{real}\left(I_{AS}\left(k_1, k_2\right)\right)}. \qquad (5)$$

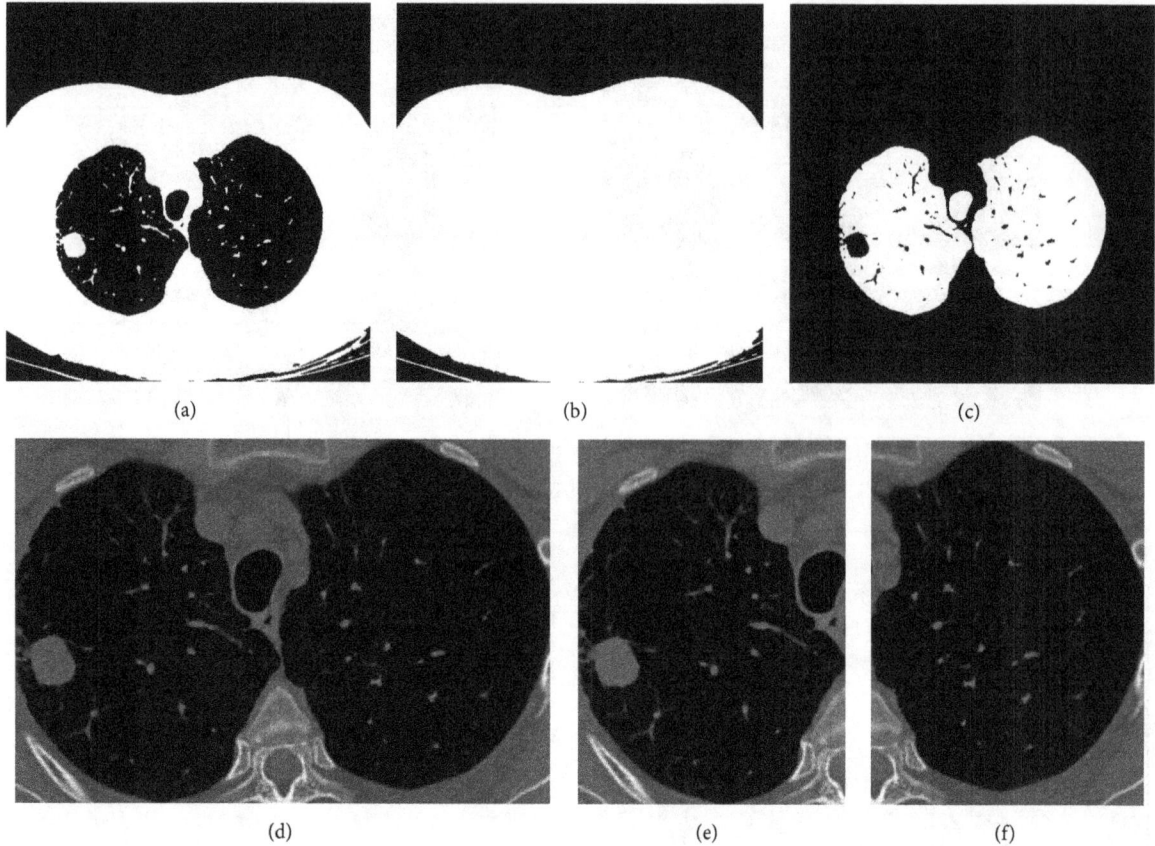

FIGURE 4: Segmentation and ROI selection. (a) Thorax binary image. (b) Filled image. (c) Lung segmentation. (d) Rectangular ROI of both lungs. (e) Right lung (cancer). (f) Left lung (normal).

To estimate the IF, we used a variable spacing local linear phase (VS-LLP) method as described in [23].

2.4.2. Filterbank Design. The purpose of multiscale filterbank is to isolate the AM-FM image components in model (3) prior to performing demodulation. Here, we use a four-scale filterbank developed by Murray [22] (see Figure 5).

In Figure 5, the frequency range of filterbank is depicted. Filter 1 is a low-pass filter (LPF), filters 2–7 are high frequency filters (H), filters 8–13 are medium frequency filters (M), filters 14–19 are low frequency filters (L), and filters 20–25 are very low frequency filters (VL). It can be noticed that the bandwidth is decreased by a factor of 1/2 for each added scale.

In this paper, we used different combinations of scales to extract the dominant AM-FM features. Here are the combinations used: (1) VL, L, M, and H; (2) LPF; (3) VL; (4) L; (5) M; (6) LPF, VL, L, M, and H; (7) LPF, VL; (8) VL, L; (9) L, M; (10) M, H; and (11) H. And, for each combination of scales, we estimate the IA, IP, and |IF| using (5) and the equations in [23].

2.4.3. Histogram Processing. For each combination of scales, we produce a histogram for AM-FM estimates: IA, IP, and |IF|. And all the computed histograms are normalized so that the area of each histogram is equal to one. Then, for each combination of scales, we create a 96-bin feature vector

from the IA, IP, and |IF| histograms, with 32 bins for IA, 32 bins for IF magnitude, and 32 bins for IP (centered at the maximum value). Therefore, each image produces 11 feature vectors corresponding to the 11 combinations of scales. We need to obtain a combined feature vector for each case by selecting the optimal and signification features from all over scales. Thus, we use Partial Least Squares Regression (PLSR) to achieve that.

2.4.4. Feature Selection. Feature selection is an important step that provides the significant features, which are used to differentiate between different classes accurately. We used Partial Least Squares Regression (PLSR) [24], which is a linear regression method that finds the relation between the predicted variables and observations. The regression problem is defined as

$$y = X\beta + \varepsilon, \tag{6}$$

where X is an $n \times p$ matrix of the extracted AM-FM features (n is the number of images and p is the number of features) and y is an $n \times 1$ vector of response or labels. We used label 0 for normal case and label 1 for abnormal case. β is $p \times 1$ vector of the regression parameters and ε is $n \times 1$ vector of the residuals.

We apply PLSR to determine the optimal number of features to be used. We select the PLSR factors number that

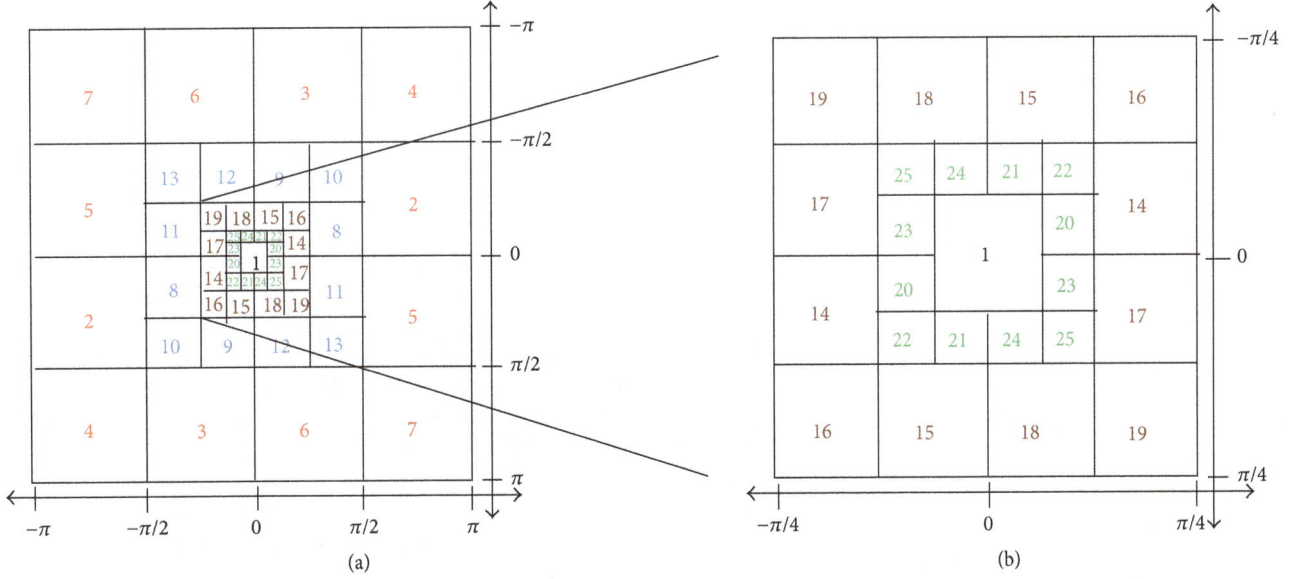

FIGURE 5: Four-scale filterbank [22]. (a) Complete frequency range of the filterbank. (b) Zoom on the low frequency filters (to be easily readable).

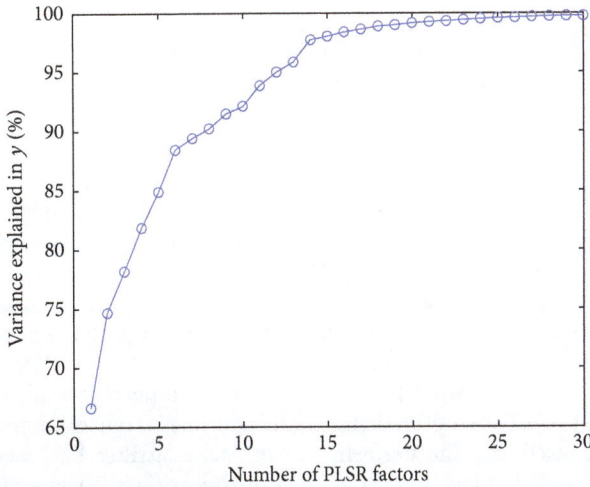

FIGURE 6: Plotting the number of PLSR factors with the cumulative variance percentage in the response variable y.

produces percentage of variance in response variable more than 90%. In Figure 6, we plot the percentage of variance in the response versus the number of PLSR factors. The plot shows that nearly 90% of the variance in y is given by the first eleven factors.

Once the optimal number of features is obtained, we form a feature vector to represent the selected features.

2.5. Classification. The final step of the proposed system is to correctly discriminate between normal and cancer lung images. The input to classification stage is the feature matrix from the previous step and the labeled vector (where 0 = normal and 1 = cancer).

Here, we have used four different classifiers: K-nearest neighbor (KNN) [25], support vector machine (SVM) [26], naïve Bayes [25], and linear classifier [25]. The basic idea of all of these classifiers depends on supervised learning; that is, each classifier takes a set of labeled images as a training set to build a model that is used further to assign new images (testing set) into classes. Out of 166 lung images, 100 images are selected as a training dataset and 66 other images are selected as a testing dataset.

3. Results and Discussion

The four classifiers are trained and their performance is evaluated with leave-M-out cross validation. We change the value of M to generate different sizes of testing and training sets, and, for each M value, the classification performance is evaluated by computing these different measures:

$$\text{Sensitivity (\%)} = \frac{\text{TP}}{\text{TP} + \text{FN}} \times 100,$$

$$\text{Specificity (\%)} = \frac{\text{TN}}{\text{FP} + \text{TN}} \times 100, \tag{7}$$

$$\text{Accuracy (\%)} = \frac{\text{TP} + \text{TN}}{\text{TP} + \text{FN} + \text{TN} + \text{FP}} \times 100,$$

where TP, TN, FN, and FP denote true positive, true negative, false negative, and false positive, respectively [27].

Figure 7 shows the computed accuracy, sensitivity, and specificity, respectively, for the four classifiers with the change in size of testing set. It can be noticed that the classifiers performances in terms of accuracy, sensitivity, and specificity are much better in case of small size of the testing set (when the classifiers got trained with large size of the training set). However, the performances of all classifiers decrease

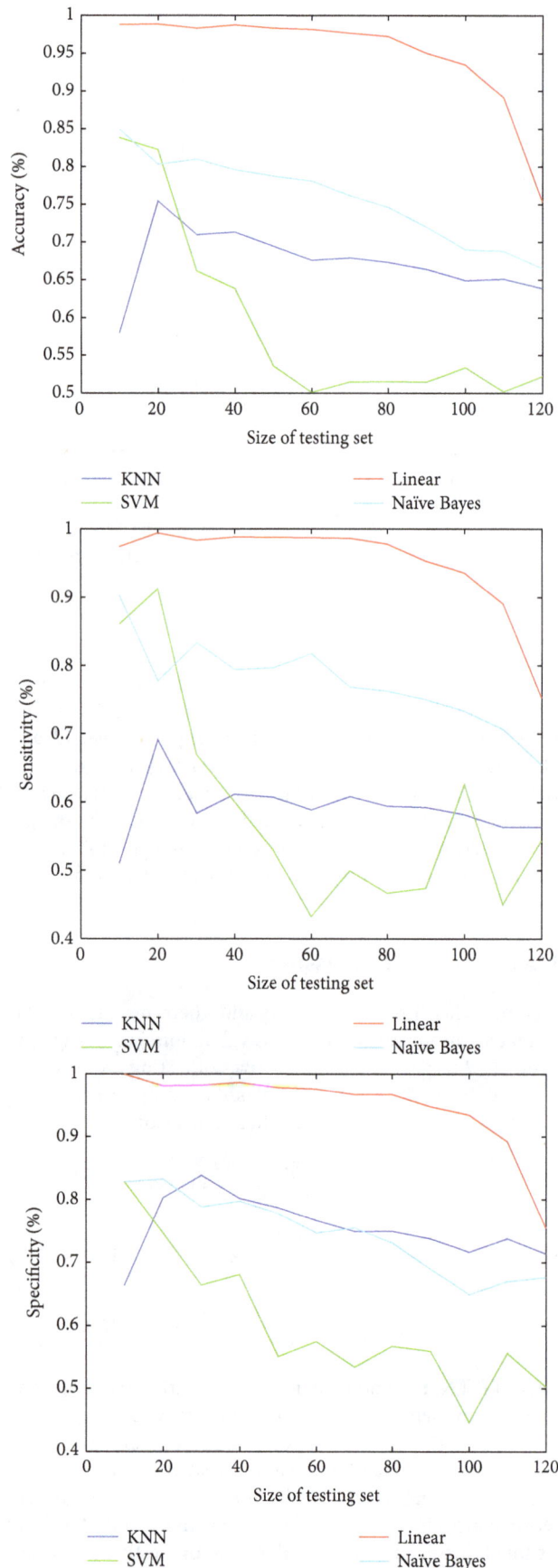

FIGURE 7: Comparison between accuracy, sensitivity, and specificity for the four classifiers with changing size of testing set.

TABLE 1: Classification performance measures for the four classifiers.

Classifier	Accuracy	Sensitivity	Specificity
KNN	64%	55%	72%
SVM	90%	85%	97%
Naïve Bayes	82%	82%	82%
Linear	95%	94%	97%

with increasing testing set size. From this figure, it is easily observed that the performance of SVM classifier is the least stable with increasing testing set size, while the other three classifiers are more stable. Moreover, it can be concluded that the linear classifier is the best one to discriminate between normal and cancer lungs.

Table 1 summarizes the performance measures for the four classifiers when the size of training set relative to the testing set is 60% to 40% of the total dataset size, respectively (i.e., training set = 100 images and test set = 66 images). As shown in Table 1, the linear classifier gives the best classification with 95% accuracy, 94% sensitivity, and 97% specificity. On the other hand, the KNN classifier is the worst classifier achieving only 64% accuracy, 55% sensitivity, and 72% specificity.

It is worth noting that the proposed CAD system is developed using MATLAB R2010a on Intel Core i5, 2.5 GHz, CPU, 6 GB RAM, Windows 7 64-bit PC.

4. Conclusions

In this paper, we develop a lung CAD system that analyzes and automatically segments the lungs and classifies each lung to normal or cancer. The system consists of five main steps: preprocessing, ROI selection, feature extraction, feature selection, and classification. AM-FM approach has been used to extract new features in terms of IA, IP, and IF. And PLSR is then used to reduce the large number of features and select the optimal and significant ones. Four classifiers are used and the performance of each classifier has been evaluated. It has been found that the linear classifier was the best one to discriminate between normal and cancer lungs with 95% accuracy.

Conflict of Interests

The authors declare that there is no conflict of interests regarding the publication of this paper.

Acknowledgments

The authors acknowledge the SPIE, the NCI, the AAPM, and The University of Chicago for making public access to the lung cancer dataset.

References

[1] N. Hollings and P. Shaw, "Diagnostic imaging of lung cancer," European Respiratory Journal, vol. 19, no. 4, pp. 722–742, 2002.

[2] W. Li, S. D. Nie, and J. J. Cheng, "A fast automatic method of lung segmentation in CT images using mathematical morphology," in *World Congress on Medical Physics and Biomedical Engineering 2006*, vol. 14 of *IFMBE Proceedings*, pp. 2419–2422, Springer, Berlin, Germany, 2007.

[3] S. Hu, E. A. Hoffman, and J. M. Reinhardt, "Automatic lung segmentation for accurate quantitation of volumetric X-ray CT images," *IEEE Transactions on Medical Imaging*, vol. 20, no. 6, pp. 490–498, 2001.

[4] J. K. Leader, B. Zheng, R. M. Rogers et al., "Automated lung segmentation in X-ray computed tomography: development and evaluation of a heuristic threshold-based scheme," *Academic Radiology*, vol. 10, no. 11, pp. 1224–1236, 2003.

[5] M. N. Prasad, M. S. Brown, S. Ahmad et al., "Automatic segmentation of lung parenchyma in the presence of diseases based on curvature of ribs," *Academic Radiology*, vol. 15, no. 9, pp. 1173–1180, 2008.

[6] J. Wang, F. Li, and Q. Li, "Automated segmentation of lungs with severe interstitial lung disease in CT," *Medical Physics*, vol. 36, no. 10, pp. 4592–4599, 2009.

[7] S. Armato and H. MacMahon, "Automated lung segmentation and computer-aided diagnosis for thoracic CT scans," *International Congress Series*, vol. 1256, pp. 977–982, 2003.

[8] S. G. Armato III and W. F. Sensakovic, "Automated lung segmentation for thoracic CT: impact on computer-aided diagnosis," *Academic Radiology*, vol. 11, no. 9, pp. 1011–1021, 2004.

[9] Y. Guo, Y. Feng, J. Sun et al., "Automatic lung tumor segmentation on PET/CT images using fuzzy markov random field model," *Computational and Mathematical Methods in Medicine*, vol. 2014, Article ID 401201, 6 pages, 2014.

[10] M. Lam, T. Disney, M. Pham, D. Raicu, J. Furst, and R. Susomboon, "Content-based image retrieval for pulmonary computed tomography nodule images," in *Medical Imaging 2007: PACS and Imaging Informatics*, vol. 6516 of *Proceedings of SPIE*, International Society for Optics and Photonics, March 2007.

[11] A. K. Dhara, C. K. Chama, S. Mukhopadhyay, and N. Khandelwal, "Content-based image retrieval system for differential diagnosis of lung cancer," *Indian Journal of Medical Informatics*, vol. 6, no. 1, article 1, 2012.

[12] J. B. Nirmala and S. Gowri, "A content based CT lung image retrieval by DCT matrix and feature vector technique," *International Journal of Computer Science Issues*, vol. 9, no. 2, 2012.

[13] H. Müller, N. Michoux, D. Bandon, and A. Geissbuhler, "A review of content-based image retrieval systems in medical applications—clinical benefits and future directions," *International Journal of Medical Informatics*, vol. 73, no. 1, pp. 1–23, 2004.

[14] C.-T. Liu, P.-L. Tai, A. Y.-J. Chen, C.-H. Peng, T. Lee, and J.-S. Wang, "A content-based CT lung image retrieval system for assisting differential diagnosis images collection," in *Proceedings of the IEEE International Conference on Multimedia and Expo (ICME 2001)*, pp. 174–177, August 2001.

[15] Y. Song, W. Cai, S. Eberl, M. J. Fulham, and D. Feng, "A content-based image retrieval framework for multi-modality lung images," in *Proceedings of the 23rd IEEE International Symposium on Computer-Based Medical Systems (CBMS '10)*, pp. 285–290, October 2010.

[16] S. A. Patil and M. B. Kuchanur, "Lung cancer classification using image processing," *International Journal of Engineering and Innovative Technology*, vol. 2, no. 3, 2012.

[17] J. Kuruvilla and K. Gunavathi, "Lung cancer classification using neural networks for CT images," *Computer Methods and Programs in Biomedicine*, vol. 113, no. 1, pp. 202–209, 2014.

[18] A. Depeursinge, D. Sage, A. Hidki et al., "Lung tissue classification using wavelet frames," in *Proceedings of the 29th Annual International Conference of IEEE Engineering in Medicine and Biology Society (EMBC '07)*, pp. 6259–6262, IEEE, Lyon, France, August 2007.

[19] *SPIE-AAPM-NCI Lung Nodule Classification Challenge Dataset*, The Cancer Imaging Archive, 2015.

[20] H. Shao, L. Cao, and Y. Liu, "A detection approach for solitary pulmonary nodules based on CT images," in *Proceedings of the 2nd International Conference on Computer Science and Network Technology (ICCSNT '12)*, pp. 1253–1257, Changchun, China, December 2012.

[21] J. Havlicek, *AM-FM image models [Ph.D. thesis]*, University of Texas at Austin, Austin, Tex, USA, 1996.

[22] V. Murray, *AM-FM methods for image and video processing [Ph.D. thesis]*, University of New Mexico, Albuquerque, NM, USA, 2008.

[23] V. Murray, P. Rodriguez, and M. S. Pattichis, "Multiscale AM-FM demodulation and image reconstruction methods with improved accuracy," *IEEE Transactions on Image Processing*, vol. 19, no. 5, pp. 1138–1152, 2010.

[24] R. Rosipal and N. Krämer, "Overview and recent advances in partial least squares," in *Subspace, Latent Structure and Feature Selection*, vol. 3940, pp. 34–51, Springer, 2006.

[25] T. Mitchell, *Machine Learning*, 1997.

[26] C. Campbell and Y. Ying, *Learning with Support Vector Machines*, 2011.

[27] N. A. Papadopoulos, E. M. Plissiti, and I. D. Fotiadis, "Medical-image processing and analysis for CAD systems," in *Medical Image Analysis Methods*, L. Costaridou, Ed., pp. 51–86, Taylor & Francis, CRC Press, Boca Raton, Fla, USA, 2005.

5

Imaging Performance of Quantitative Transmission Ultrasound

Mark W. Lenox,[1] **James Wiskin,**[1] **Matthew A. Lewis,**[2] **Stephen Darrouzet,**[1]
David Borup,[1] **and Scott Hsieh**[1]

[1]*QT Ultrasound, LLC, Novato, CA 94949, USA*
[2]*Department of Radiology, University of Texas Southwestern Medical Center, Dallas, TX 75390, USA*

Correspondence should be addressed to Mark W. Lenox; mark.lenox@qtultrasound.com

Academic Editor: Jyh-Cheng Chen

Quantitative Transmission Ultrasound (QTUS) is a tomographic transmission ultrasound modality that is capable of generating 3D speed-of-sound maps of objects in the field of view. It performs this measurement by propagating a plane wave through the medium from a transmitter on one side of a water tank to a high resolution receiver on the opposite side. This information is then used via inverse scattering to compute a speed map. In addition, the presence of reflection transducers allows the creation of a high resolution, spatially compounded reflection map that is natively coregistered to the speed map. A prototype QTUS system was evaluated for measurement and geometric accuracy as well as for the ability to correctly determine speed of sound.

1. Introduction

Quantitative Transmission Ultrasound (QTUS) is an imaging modality based on tomographic techniques extended to ultrasound. In such a system, images are generated using both reflection and transmission techniques. While transmission ultrasound has been investigated as an adjunct to mammography for quite some time [1, 2], recent developments in hardware and imaging algorithms have enabled marked improvements in spatial resolution and clinical utility. Physically, a transmitter and receiver pair is colocated with multiple transducers with various focal lengths in a U-shaped arrangement as shown in Figure 1.

This type of device has been shown to work well in breast imaging applications [3–6]. Early work to characterize systems of this nature has been performed [7], but much remains to be done to move toward reproducible methods that can be applied to all systems of this type. No NEMA standards have been developed for 3D tomographic ultrasound methods. There are a number of characteristics of QTUS systems that make them neither entirely tomographic in the normal sense, nor standard B-mode, and this represents a challenge to properly evaluate their performance. For example, typical ultrasound characteristics, like speckle, are eliminated by the B-mode compounding, so alternatives must be developed

to give potential users a better grasp of what contrast to noise type characteristics might mean in a clinical setting. Furthermore, shadowing is also severely depressed and this makes the measurement of system resolution in plane a true 2D problem instead of a 1D problem, even against a hard fast target. This paper proposes methods to evaluate such systems in ways that would be familiar to those working in other modalities and presents preliminary findings for such a system.

In transmission mode, the transmitter emits a plane wave that is received by the receiver. In this case, the receiver is a 1536 element PZT array with custom data acquisition electronics package that supports real-time RF data acquisition at rates of 33.3 Ms/s at 14 bits per sample. Multiple acquisitions at frequencies ranging from 300 kHz to 1.5 MHz are acquired for 180 angles as the U-channel is rotated around the subject. Once acquired, the projection information is reconstructed using nonlinear inverse scattering in 3D [3–6]. The result of this reconstruction is a quantitative volume map of speed of sound (measured at 1.5 MHz), with units of meters per second (m/s), and attenuation with units of dB/m/MHz.

In reflection mode, each of the three reflection transducers (4 MHz center frequency) with different focal lengths are alternately fired between transmission measurements in a B-mode acquisition. The resulting images (60 per transducer)

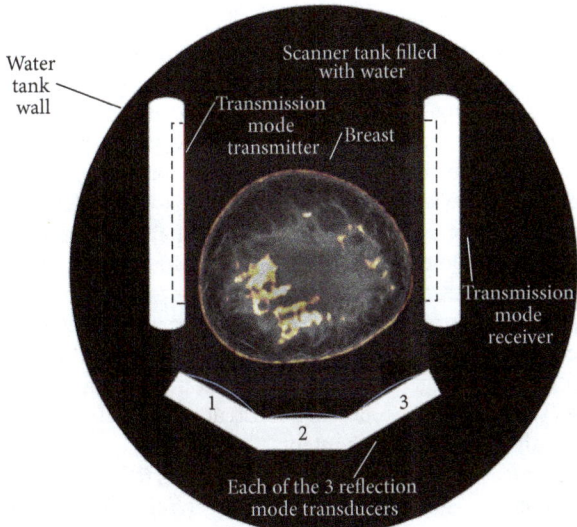

FIGURE 1: System geometry.

are compounded together and corrected for refraction using the speed map computed in the transmission phase. This compounding produces a nonquantitative image that is proportional to impedance mismatch, referred to simply as reflection units (RUs). Since impedance mismatch for ultrasound waves indicates a change in tissue type, these images have high resolution and are very instructive of anatomical reference. Due to the nature of this type of compounding, speckle is dramatically reduced, but the resulting image can be read very much like a traditional B-mode image.

The end result of each scan is a 3D volume of three different types, speed, attenuation, and reflection. These image stacks are precisely coregistered since they were acquired at the same time and can be put together to form a 3D view of the object in the field of view (FOV). The 3D nature of the device allows the evaluation of both 2D qualities, like dimension and relative placement, as well as 3D physical qualities, such as the volume of a structure and the quantitative evaluation of the speed of sound within the entirety of that volume. To date, internal research studies have concentrated on the use of speed-of-sound information and this paper will concentrate on the accuracies of those measurements; however, future studies are planned to include analysis of attenuation information.

2. Materials and Methods

In this experiment, the current generation QT Ultrasound system (QT Ultrasound LLC, Novato, CA) was evaluated in both transmission and reflection modes for geometric accuracy and uniformity over the field of view and for quantitative accuracy of the speed-of-sound maps. Several phantoms were constructed to test speed-of-sound quantitative accuracy, geometric accuracy, contrast resolution, contrast to noise ratio, and uniformity. In addition, laboratory experiments were performed to independently evaluate the expected

speed values of the various materials used to construct the phantoms.

2.1. Speed of Sound. A phantom was constructed and evaluated using the QTUS system as well as analytic methods. This particular phantom contains inclusions 15 mm in diameter with different speeds to simulate cyst and solid lesion pathologies. It is designed to mimic soft tissue regions such as breast as there are no high speed structures to simulate bone.

All materials are custom formulated polyurethanes designed for a specific speed with the high speed material provided by Yezitronix (Yezitronix Group Inc., Canada) and the low speed and background materials were supplied by Conversion Technology (Conversion Technology Inc., Boulder, USA). Samples of each material in the speed phantom were provided separately in the form of a $2''$ diameter cylinder with a $1''$ thickness. These samples could be independently evaluated by measuring the change in signal phase when the sample is placed between two 5 MHz pistons, relative to the water path signal phase with the sample removed.

2.2. Spatial Measurements. Tests are included to measure both the spatial resolution of the device and the spatial accuracy when measuring distances between varieties of object sizes across the field of view.

Spatial resolution is patterned after the NEMA standards for other tomographic modalities [8], with measurements in the center as well as at varying radii from the center in the transaxial direction as well as a slice thickness definition. Unlike modalities such as PET, where it is physically possible to build point sources that are substantially smaller than the intrinsic resolution and measure the system response directly as an impulse response, QTUS has very high theoretical resolution and thus determining the intrinsic resolution from the impulse response of the system is problematic. Previous work has relied on a single step edge method [7] to perform this evaluation; however, it is possible to bias that measurement in the direction of the step and it also requires exceptionally small voxels to properly compute the derivative of the gradient function. In order to get around these limitations we propose to evaluate the square step response and remove the step width using the sum of squares approach. This approach involves measuring the gradient in two opposing directions to eliminate bias. In this method, the measured response, R_{meas}, is the convolution of the intrinsic resolution R_{int} and the actual object size S_{obj}. Since these represent Gaussian functions, then their relationship can be expressed as the sum of squares:

$$R_{int}{}^2 + S_{obj}{}^2 = R_{meas}{}^2. \tag{1}$$

Since the spread of the object is precisely determined by the actual known size, determination of R_{int} becomes straightforward. With this method, the intrinsic resolution can be evaluated without dependence on the ability to construct a particular sized target to evaluate the system response function. It is potentially possible to bias this measurement by choosing an object of a specific size, so it is important to specify completely the size of the object used when specifying the resolution.

For this evaluation in transmission mode, a spatial measurement phantom is used. This phantom consists of styrene monofilament stretched between two styrene plates arrayed in a nautilus spiral starting at the center. The diameter of the monofilament can be easily changed depending on the type of imaging performed. We choose 608 microns for speed measurements to achieve the necessary contrast. As the ability to perform full resolution measurements improves, it is likely that this measurement standard will change, and the monofilament will get smaller. Full width at half maximum (FWHM) width measurements are made in both the X and Y dimensions as shown in Figure 4, measured by linearly interpolating known data points on each side [8], and then deconvolved from the object size using (1). By choosing a nautilus spiral, it is possible to get a relatively clear view of all filaments with a minimum of interference. Since transmission measurements are made in a line through the object, a thin cylindrical target performs well and does not require precise vertical positioning to get consistent results.

It is important to consider that resolution enhancing methods like point-spread-function modeling can sharpen the resulting clinical images; however, the use of PSF modeling in the reconstruction will interfere with these measurement methods. The desired result of this measurement is the intrinsic resolution of the system which could then be used for PSF modeling and further improvements in clinical utility. Thus, for the purposes of this paper, all PSF modeling is disabled within the reconstruction.

Measurement of reflection spatial resolution requires the use of spherical targets because the geometry of a line crossing the beam causes reflections that can vary considerably with the initial angle of incidence of the beam to the monofilament line and this makes an unbiased measurement very difficult. One family of phantoms developed in collaboration with colleagues at UT Southwestern Medical Center is comprised of a gelatin outer layer with an inner core comprised of the synthetic clay Laponite XLG (BYK Additives, Gonzales, TX). Using tweezers, soda lime glass beads with nominal diameter of 500 micrometers (Cospheric LLC, Santa Barbara, CA) were manually placed in a plane in the middle of the Laponite at coordinates $(0, 0)$, $(0.8660, 0.500)$, $(1.4141, -1,4142)$, and $(-1.500, -2.5981)$ cm. The gelatin skin is formed in a 90 mm inner diameter disposable 8 oz cup (http://www.us.huhtamaki.com/) using a glass beaker coated with nonstick spray oil to form the inner chamber. The gelatin powder (Type B from bovine skin, Sigma Aldrich) is mixed in a 1 : 5 ratio with deionized and degassed water in a larger beaker and heated under mild stirring to at least 35 Celsius. After 30 minutes, the beaker is further degassed, and remaining bubbles and detritus on the surface are removed with suction. As the gelatin cools to below 32 Celsius, the gelatin stock is titrated with formalin (Sigma Aldrich) at 1.4 mL per 40 mL of water. This amount of formalin is known to cross-link gelatin such that the melting temperature is increased above the 31 Celsius temperature of the ultrasound tomography water bath [9].

The inner chamber is filled with Laponite XLG, a magnesium silicate gel with baseline speed of sound below 1500 m/s [10]. The Laponite powder is rapidly mixed with water under vigorous stirring. After some time, the mixture becomes clear, at which point the stock material is treated similarly for bubble removal. The inner chamber of the phantom is filled with Laponite to the level where inclusions are to be added. After the soda lime glass beads are placed, the partially assembled phantom is cooled in a refrigerator for 10 minutes so that the beads adhere to the Laponite. Then they are covered with additional Laponite material. The phantom is completed with a second formulation of gelatin to pour a top for the phantom. Some changes in the Laponite compartment size are observed in the days following construction, presumably due to equalization of water content.

To measure slice thickness, a dual inverted comb phantom is used. A series of 2 mm diameter styrene rods are positioned linearly with a 0.5/10 mm gradient such that the imaging plane covers both combs as in Figure 5. The slice thickness is defined by the thickest point where it is possible to resolve the ends of one of both combs.

To compute slice thickness, an image plane is selected that cuts across both of the comb gradients perpendicular to the rods. The upper level and lower level included in the slice are noted by observing which rods are present in the image. As the rods subside from the plane at a rate of 0.5 mm per 10.0 mm a linear relationship is established to interpolate submillimeter changes in the plane boundaries. The difference in the plane boundaries is the slice thickness.

2.3. Uniformity. Uniformity for speed measurements is patterned after the other NEMA uniformity performance measurement protocols [8]. A uniform phantom (8 cm diameter, 4 cm axial extent) made of polyurethane is scanned, and a volume region of interest (ROI) is made 2 mm inside of the outer edge for all planes that are completely inclusive. The polyurethane has a low uniform speed of 1430 m/s, and, since there are no changes in material, there should be very low reflectivity throughout the object. It is important that there be no gasses present as air bubbles can significantly alter the measurement. It is recommended that the phantom be soaked in the water tank for at least an hour prior to this test to assure uniform temperature distribution and absorption of any exterior bubbles.

We define that the uniformity U of the region is expressed as a percentage of the standard deviation σ_{roi} divided by the mean value μ_{roi} of the region of interest:

$$U = \frac{\sigma_{\text{roi}}}{\mu_{\text{roi}}} * 100. \tag{2}$$

Uniformity for reflection images is not well defined. Since reflection is a measure of impedance mismatch, a truly anechoic cylinder volume will have a mean value of zero. This makes (2) unstable in this case. Further work in measurement of reflection uniformity is needed but is beyond the scope of this paper.

2.4. Contrast to Noise Ratio and Contrast Resolution. Contrast to noise ratio (CNR) expresses the potential to detect

TABLE 1: Speed-of-sound accuracy against the speed phantom measured with twin pistons.

Area	Mean (M/S)	SD (M/S)	Uniformity (%)	Actual (M/S)	Error (M/S)	Error (% actual)	Error (SD)
High	1571.9	18.1	1.15%	1566	5.9	0.37%	0.33
Low	1418.8	5.69	0.40%	1406	12.8	0.91%	2.25
Water	1508.6	7.09	0.46%	1510	1.4	0.09%	0.20
Background	1447.9	6.24	0.43%	1445	2.9	0.02%	0.46

an object against a background that contains a noise component. In this case, we define CNR as the difference between a region containing the object and the background, divided by the standard deviation of the background:

$$\text{CNR} = \frac{S_{\text{obj}} - S_{\text{bkd}}}{\delta_{\text{bkd}}}. \qquad (3)$$

A contrast phantom, made up of styrene rods placed in a circle, shown in Figure 6, is used to evaluate CNR against multiple targets at the same time. The contrast resolution (CR) of a device is defined to be the point in which the CNR no longer allows identification of an object smaller than that dimension.

3. Discussion

3.1. Results

3.1.1. Speed-of-Sound Accuracy. Speed-of-sound measurements were performed on the speed phantom shown in Figure 2. Actual speeds were measured with the piston setup shown in Figure 3. Error was computed as difference from the actual values measured with the pistons and expressed as the percentage of the actual value as well as in standard deviations from the region-of-interest (ROI) measurement. The percentage of actual error provides the overall magnitude of the possible error. The error expressed in standard deviations provides a measure of accuracy relative to the expected accuracy within the ROI. Values less than 1.0 indicate that the error is less than the measured noise in the ROI. As reported in Table 1, in the range of typical tissue values (water speed and faster), the system was able to accurately determine speed of sound within 1% of the actual value in all cases.

3.1.2. Transmission Resolution Measurements. Transmission measurements were performed on the nautilus phantom using 608-micron styrene monofilament submerged in water. As constructed, the nautilus phantom is shown in Figure 7.

Good contrast was achieved against the water background as shown in Figure 8, allowing accurate measurements at all radius values. Measured FWHM values were corrected with (1) and the resulting intrinsic resolution values are given in Table 2.

FWHM values were relatively flat across the FOV, varying from 1.870 mm to 2.490 mm with an average of 2.335 mm in both X and Y. Measurements performed with the dual inverted comb phantom yielded an actual slice thickness of 2 mm in transmission (speed-of-sound) mode.

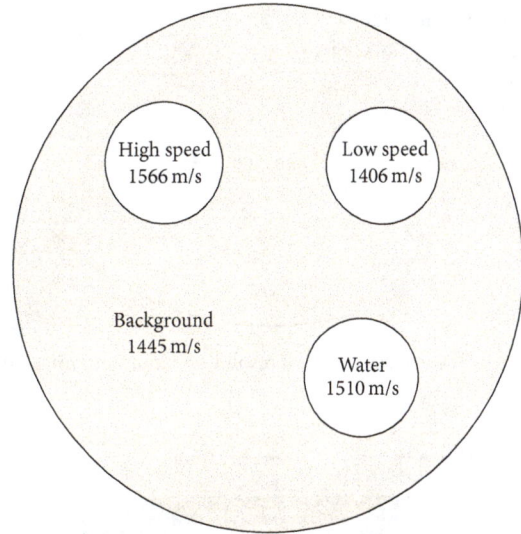

FIGURE 2: Speed phantom specifications.

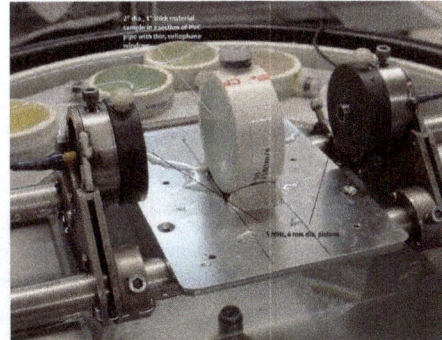

FIGURE 3: Experimental setup. Two, colinear, 5 MHz, 6 mm diameter piston transducers are mounted 100 mm apart. The 2″ diameter, 1″ thick material sample is placed between them normal to the beam axis.

3.1.3. Reflection Resolution Measurements. The reflection resolution phantom with embedded 500-micron beads was scanned. The results are shown in Table 3.

Resolution results were relatively flat across the field of view with the exception of the exact center where they were slightly degraded as would be expected due to additional scattering at depth and residual refraction effects. Average resolution across the entire FOV was 543 microns in the X direction and 557 microns in the Y direction. However, average resolution of all areas except the exact center is significantly better

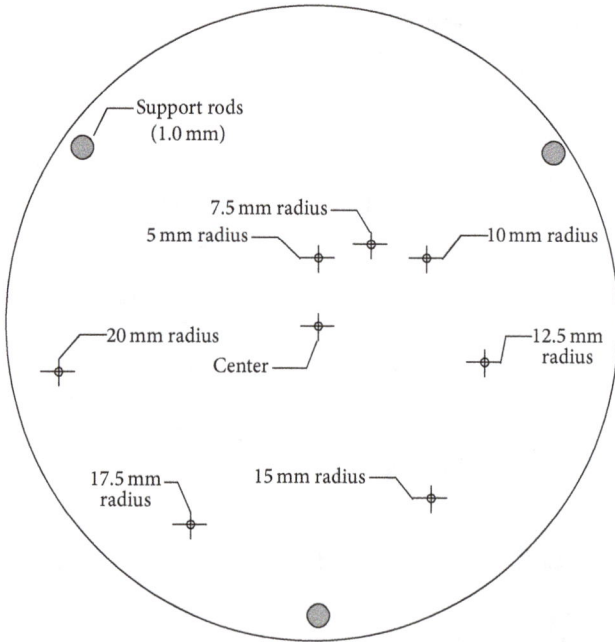

FIGURE 4: Transmission spatial resolution phantom dimensions.

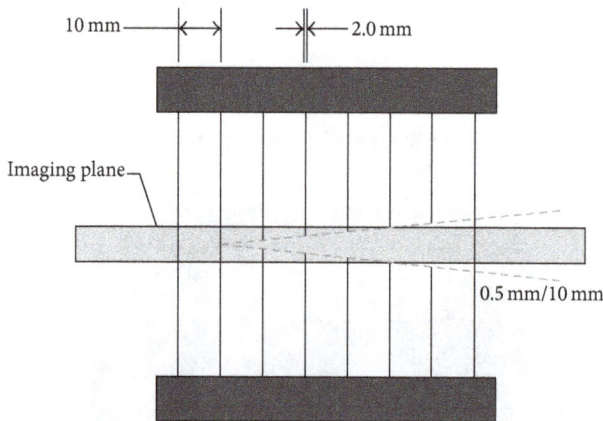

FIGURE 5: Slice thickness phantom. Dual inverted comb gradients locate the upper and lower edge of the imaging plane to determine actual slice thickness.

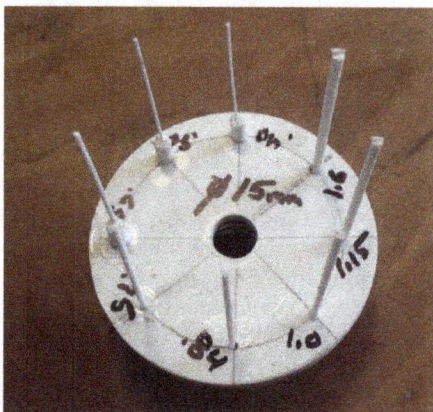

FIGURE 6: Contrast phantom.

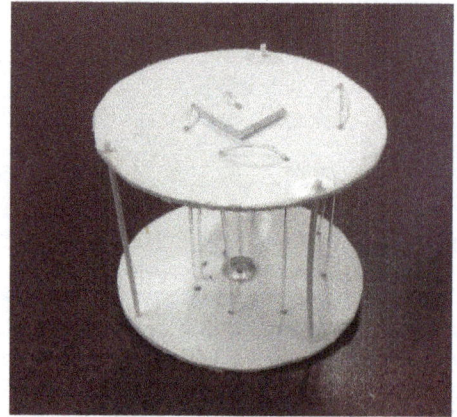

FIGURE 7: Nautilus phantom.

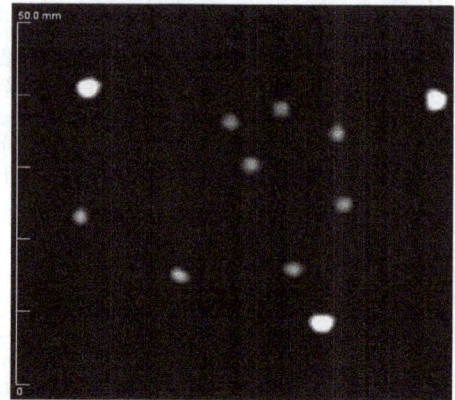

FIGURE 8: Speed-of-sound image of nautilus phantom showing 608-micron monofilament structures window leveled to show maximum contrast against a water background (grayscale in m/s).

TABLE 2: Transmission resolution measurements.

Position	X FWHM (mm)	Y FWHM (mm)
Center	2.11	2.06
5 mm	2.45	2.36
7.5 mm	2.18	2.40
10 mm	2.13	2.49
12.5 mm	2.31	2.03
15 mm	2.41	1.94
17.5 mm	2.20	2.10
20 mm	1.87	2.32

TABLE 3: Reflection resolution measurements.

Position	X FWHM (mm)	Y FWHM (mm)
Center	0.771	0.751
10 mm	0.346	0.543
20 mm	0.536	0.373
30 mm	0.478	0.531

at 453 microns in the X direction and 482 microns in the Y direction. As this represents the field of view most commonly used in normal observations, this is the level of performance

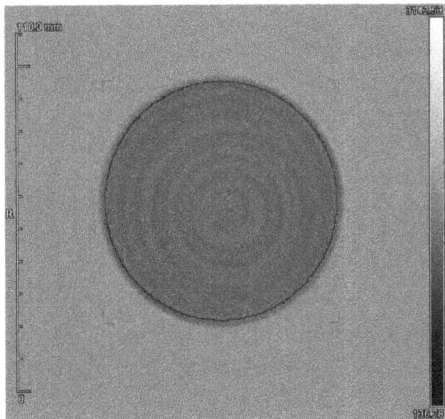

FIGURE 9: Speed-of-sound image of a uniform phantom (grayscale in m/s, max 3142 m/s, min 136 m/s).

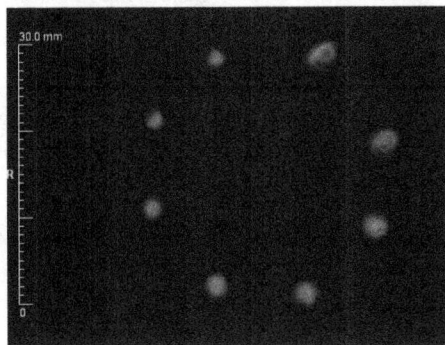

FIGURE 10: Contrast resolution reflection results.

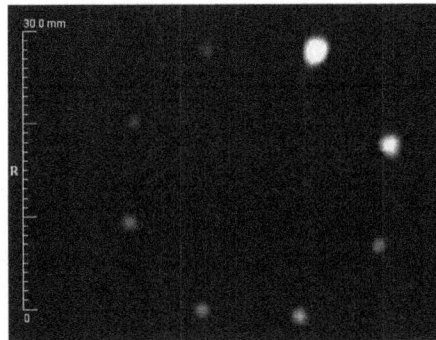

FIGURE 11: Contrast resolution speed results window leveled to highlight maximum available contrast.

TABLE 4: Speed and reflection CNR.

Object	Speed CNR	Reflection CNR	Speed m/s
1.6 mm	28.4	2.7	1949
1.15 mm	21.5	3.6	1786
1.0 mm	15.5	5.9	1657
0.84 mm	15.7	3.8	1626
0.75 mm	14.4	4.5	1611
0.65 mm	13.5	4.2	1610
0.50 mm	10.8	4.3	1582
0.40 mm	10.2	4.0	1574

that should be expected in general operation. Measurements performed with the dual inverted comb phantom yielded a slice thickness of 6 mm in reflection mode.

3.1.4. Uniformity. An 80 mm uniform phantom made of T2039-6634 polyurethane (Conversion Technology Inc., Boulder, CO, USA) was scanned in both reflection and transmission modes as shown in Figure 9.

Overall, the mean speed of a region 2 mm inside of the outside edge of the phantom was measured to be 1401.9 m/s with a standard deviation of 44.1. According to (2), this yields a uniformity of 3.1%.

3.1.5. Contrast to Noise Ratio and Contrast Resolution. The contrast resolution phantom was scanned in both reflection and transmission modes. Reflection mode, shown in Figure 10, yields excellent results from 1.6 mm down to 400 microns. Performance is essentially flat down to 400 microns for these high speed targets against a water background. This result suggests a contrast resolution better than 400 microns in reflection mode. Reflection mode measures impedance mismatch, so since the material in each rod is the same, the mismatch against water should also be the same and all intensities should match. The larger rods, 1.6 mm and 1.15 mm, show slight nonuniformities due to the 10-degree angle of

incidence that the reflection transducers have against the vertical rods.

Contrast resolution in transmission mode is shown in Figure 11. All rods are visible from 1.6 mm down to 0.4 mm with expected degradation in signal strength/contrast as the object size decreases. The actual speed of the styrene plastic samples measured with the previously described piston method on a large sample indicates 2000 m/s. The largest sample size of 1.6 mm diameter indicates a speed of 1949 m/s, slowly degrading to 1574 m/s for the 400-micron pin due to partial volume effects. These results are summarized in Table 4.

Contrast resolution performance overall indicates that detectability of dense structures should be very good, even in the submillimeter range.

3.1.6. Contrast to Noise Ratio. The design of the CNR phantom with 8 separate targets integrated allows a single scan to yield 8 individual measurements under exactly the same conditions (i.e., temperature). Contrast to noise ratio was measured by drawing regions surrounding the rods with an isocontour. All regions used the same arbitrary lower limit, with no effective upper limit so that the mean value can be compared directly. The background region was chosen to be inside the objects as shown in Figure 12.

After applying (3), CNR values were computed from 1.4 mm to 0.4 mm for both speed of sound and reflection information with results given in Table 4.

The actual speed of styrene was measured using the dual-piston method previously described as 2002 m/s. In speed

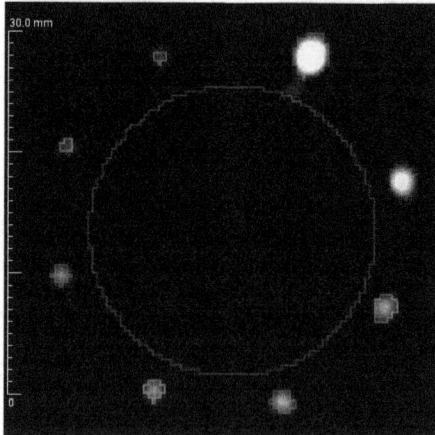

FIGURE 12: Contrast to noise ratio ROI measurement locations (grayscale in m/s).

mode, the CNR steadily deteriorates as the size of the object becomes smaller, but it remains better than 10 : 1 even on objects as small as 400 microns. As would be expected, the algorithm underestimates the actual values as the size gets smaller and partial volume effects come into play.

Reflection performs very well across the entire range, staying essentially flat down to 400 microns. This result is expected and in fact is one of the more powerful applications of ultrasound. Under most conditions, objects will cause a discernable reflection between adjacent neighboring scatterers as long as their size is greater than half the wavelength of the wave. In this case, at 4 MHz, the wavelength is approximately 0.382 mm, so, theoretically, objects should provide signal at 0.191 mm. This theoretical minimum is smaller than the 0.40 mm objects used in this test.

4. Conclusions

It has been shown in the literature that ultrasound can be used to evaluate the pathology of lesions in a variety of cancers [11]. The ability to perform this evaluation is largely due to both the fact that the speed of sound is directly related to the bulk and shear modulus of the material and the fact that the structural changes to the tissue that arise from various pathologies affect the bulk modulus. This relationship suggests that direct speed-of-sound measurements have positive potential to discriminate various pathologies, including those that exhibit some type of calcification similar to elastography.

QTUS provides a stable measure of both geometry and speed of sound on objects as small as 0.4 mm in diameter, and possibly smaller. Contrast resolution and CNR experiments, in particular, show considerable promise in reflection as well as transmission modes of operation when high speed contrast targets are present. These conditions are very similar to conditions present when imaging calcifications based on Calcium Oxalate and Calcium Hydroxyapatite, the typical pathologies present in calcified breast lesions, and Ductile Carcinoma In Situ (DCIS) [12]. In addition, spatial resolution and accuracy are good enough to encourage accurate location and biopsy of extremely small lesions.

As a first step, future work should include more phantom studies with smaller structures to fully define the limits of the technology. In addition to that, work should include clinical trials to perform a proper receiver operating characteristic (ROC) analysis of a QT Ultrasound system in evaluating calcifications.

Conflict of Interests

The authors declare that there is no conflict of interests regarding the publication of this paper.

References

[1] G. H. Glover, "Computerized time-of-flight ultrasonic tomography for breast examination," *Ultrasound in Medicine & Biology*, vol. 3, no. 2, pp. 117–127, 1977.

[2] J. F. Greenleaf and R. C. Bahn, "Clinical imaging with transmissive ultrasonic computerized tomography," *IEEE Transactions on Biomedical Engineering*, vol. 28, no. 2, pp. 177–185, 1981.

[3] J. Wiskin, D. Borup, M. Andre et al., "Three-dimensional non-linear inverse scattering: quantitative transmission algorithms, refraction corrected reflection, scanner design and clinical results," *Proceedings of Meetings on Acoustics*, vol. 19, no. 1, Article ID 075001, 2013.

[4] M. Andre, J. Wiskin, and D. Borup, "Clinical results with ultrasound computed tomography of the breast," in *Quantitative Ultrasound in Soft Tissue*, J. Mamou and M. L. Oelze, Eds., chapter 15, pp. 395–432, Springer, 2013.

[5] M. André, J. Wiskin, D. Borup, S. Johnson, H. Ojeda-Fournier, and L. Olson, "Quantitative volumetric breast imaging with 3D inverse scatter computed tomography," in *Proceedings of the Annual International Conference of the IEEE Engineering in Medicine and Biology Society (EMBC '12)*, pp. 1110–1113, IEEE, San Diego, Calif, USA, August-September 2012.

[6] J. Wiskin, D. Borup, S. Johnson, and M. Berggren, "Non-linear inverse scattering: high resolution quantitative breast tissue tomography," *The Journal of the Acoustical Society of America*, vol. 131, no. 5, article 3802, 2012, also in (*Virtual Journal of Biological Physics Research*, vol. 23, no. 10, 2012).

[7] R. R. Leach Jr., S. G. Azevedo, J. G. Berryman et al., "Comparison of ultrasound tomography methods in circular geometry," in *Medical Imaging 2002: Ultrasonic Imaging and Signal Processing, 362*, vol. 4687 of *Proceedings of SPIE*, San Diego, Calif, USA, April 2002.

[8] National Electrical Manufacturers Association, *NEMA Standards Publication NU 2-2007*, National Electrical Manufacturers Association, Rosslyn, Va, USA, 2007.

[9] J. P. Fernandes, B. F. Pastorello, D. B. de Araujo, and O. Baffa, "Formaldehyde increases MAGIC gel dosimeter melting point and sensitivity," *Physics in Medicine and Biology*, vol. 53, no. 4, pp. N53–N58, 2008.

[10] J. Sheppard and F. A. Duck, "Ultrasonic tissue-equivalent materials using inorganic gel mixtures," *The British Journal of Radiology*, vol. 55, no. 657, pp. 667–669, 1982.

[11] A. T. Stavros, D. Thickman, C. L. Rapp, M. A. Dennis, S. H. Parker, and G. A. Sisney, "Solid breast nodules: use of sonography to distinguish between benign and malignant lesions," *Radiology*, vol. 196, no. 1, pp. 123–134, 1995.

[12] M. Scimeca, E. Giannini, C. Antonacci, C. A. Pistolese, L. G. Spagnoli, and E. Bonanno, "Microcalcifications in breast cancer: an active phenomenon mediated by epithelial cells with mesenchymal characteristics," *BMC Cancer*, vol. 14, article 286, 2014.

Incidence of Brain Abnormalities Detected on Preoperative Brain MR Imaging and Their Effect on the Outcome of Cochlear Implantation in Children with Sensorineural Hearing Loss

Xiao-Quan Xu, Fei-Yun Wu, Hao Hu, Guo-Yi Su, and Jie Shen

Department of Radiology, The First Affiliated Hospital of Nanjing Medical University, No. 300, Guangzhou Road, Nanjing 210029, China

Correspondence should be addressed to Fei-Yun Wu; wfy_njmu@163.com

Academic Editor: Guowei Wei

The incidence of sensorineural hearing loss (SNHL) increased gradually in the past decades. High-resolution computed tomography (HRCT) and magnetic resonance (MR) imaging, as an important part of preimplantation evaluation for children with SNHL, could provide the detailed information about the inner ear, the vestibulocochlear nerve, and the brain, so as to select suitable candidate for cochlear implantation (CI). Brain abnormalities were not rare in the brain MR imaging of SNHL children; however, its influence on the effect of CI has not been clarified. After retrospectively analyzing the CT and MR imaging of 157 children with SNHL that accepted preoperative evaluation from June 2011 to February 2013 in our hospital and following them during a period of 14.09 ± 5.08 months, we found that the white matter change, which might be associated with the history of medical condition, was the most common brain abnormality. Usually CI was still beneficial to the children with brain abnormalities, and the short-term hearing improvement could be achieved. Further study with more patients and longer follow-up time was needed to confirm our results.

1. Introduction

The incidence of sensorineural hearing loss (SNHL) was about 1/1000 in the newborns and about 9/1000 in the school age children, and it was still increasing gradually in the past decades [1]. Although previous studies indicated that the injury or infection during the parturition might be associated with the occurrence of SNHL, no definite pathogenesis was identified [2]. Nowadays, cochlear implantation (CI) has been accepted as the first-line treatment option for pediatric profound SNHL [3].

Imaging examination played an important role in the preimplantation evaluation of pediatric SNHL [4, 5]. High-resolution computed tomography (HRCT) and magnetic resonance (MR) imaging could provide the detailed information about the inner ear, the vestibulocochlear nerve, and the brain, which could help to select suitable candidate for CI and to predict whether CI would be beneficial or not.

Till now, several studies had clarified the incidence of the inner ear malformation or vestibulocochlear nerve deficiency

and their influence on CI [6]. However, few studies focused on the effect of brain abnormalities detected on preoperative brain MR imaging on CI, although several studies had introduced its incidence.

Therefore, based on a large cohort of 157 patients who accepted preimplantation evaluation for SNHL in our hospital, we try to study the incidence of brain abnormalities and to clarify the influence of brain abnormalities on the hearing improvement after CI, further to clarify whether the brain abnormalities should be viewed as the contraindication of CI.

2. Material and Methods

2.1. Patients Group. This study was approved by our institutional review board. From June 2011 to February 2013, 157 children with SNHL accepted HRCT and MR scan as a part of preoperative evaluation. The 157 patients consisted of 89 boys and 68 girls with a mean age of 4.3 years (range: 1–15 years). Audiological evaluation indicated that there were 137 children with bilateral SNHL and 20 children with unilateral SNHL. Among all the 157 children with SNHL, 26 brain abnormalities were found on the brain MR imaging of 23 patients, and the incidence was 14.6% (23/157).

2.2. Data Acquisition. All patients underwent both HRCT and MR scans of the temporal bone. The HRCT scans were performed using a 16-slice spiral CT scanner (SOMATOM Emotion, Siemens, Germany). Parameters for the CT scanning are kV: 120, mAs: 28, and slice thickness: 1 mm. Volumetric acquisitions were reconstructed with 0.75 mm slice thickness throughout the temporal bone contiguously. The transverse imaging plane was parallel to the supraorbital-meatal line. This allowed creating multiplanar reconstructions in any plane. Bone window settings were designed as window level of +700 Hounsfield unit (HU) and window width of +4000 HU.

MR imaging was obtained on a 3.0 Tesla MR scanner (Siemens, Germany) with the matched eight-channel phased array coils. The MR protocol included axial T2-weighted imaging and axial T1-weighted imaging, as well as axial three-dimension sampling perfection with application optimized contrasts using different flip angle evolutions (3D-SPACE) imaging of temporal bones. Parameters for the T1 sequence are TR/TE, 250/2.5 ms; slice thickness, 5 mm. Parameters for the T2 sequence are TR/TE, 5000/100 ms; slice thickness, 5 mm. Parameters for the 3D-SPACE sequence are TR/TE, 1000/131 ms; flip angle, 120; averages, 2; field of view, 200 mm; matrix size, 384 * 384; slice thickness, 0.5 mm; slice gap, 0 mm. The total scanning time was approximately 10 min for each patient. The 3D-SPACE sequences were reconstructed in the axial plane as well as in an oblique sagittal plane, approximately perpendicular to the long axis of each internal auditory canal (IAC) for viewing.

2.3. Image Assessment and Follow-Up. CT and MR imaging were assessed on a clinical picture archiving and communication system (PACS) workstation by two radiologists (Wu FY, Xu XQ). Brain abnormality was defined as any abnormal signal or structural abnormality demonstrated on the brain MR imaging. If the volume of the white matter lesion was less than 10% of that of the whole white matter, the lesion was categorized as a "focal lesion." Otherwise, the lesion was classified as a "diffuse lesion."

Patients were followed up mainly through the manner of phone calls. Except that one patient with bilateral SNHL was lost during the follow-up, we successfully followed up the other 22 patients with SNHL within a period of 14.09 ± 5.08 months (range: 7–27 months). Follow-up focused on evaluation of hearing improvement before and after CI. Children's parents were asked to finish the infant toddler-meaningful auditory integration scale (IT-MAIS) to evaluate the patients' ability to make meaningful use of sound before and after CI [7, 8].

IT-MAIS consisted of a series of 10 questions. Questions 1 and 2 related the bonding of the child to the device, including the willingness of the child to wear it and his ability to recognize and identify device malfunction. Questions 3 to 6 related

the alerting to sound of the child when not in a "listening set." Questions 7 to 10 related to the ability of the child to derive meaning from the auditory phenomena (Table 1). Response to each question was scored on a scale from 0 to 4, based on the frequency of reported behavior (0 = never, 1 = rarely, 2 = occasionally, 3 = frequently, and 4 = always). Therefore, a copy of IT-MAIS would score from 0 to 40. A score of 0 indicates the inability of the child to make use of sounds in his or her everyday environment, and a score of 40 indicates that the child can consistently understand and make use of sounds.

2.4. Statistical Analysis. The numerical data were averaged and reported as means ± standard deviation (SD). Improvement of IT-MALS score in "diffuse lesion" group and "focal lesion" group before and after CI was compared with Wilcoxon analysis. $P < 0.05$ was considered statistically significant. Statistical analysis was carried out with the SPSS 17.0 (Chicago, IL, USA).

3. Results

3.1. Incidence and Description of Brain Abnormalities. Among all the 157 patients with SNHL, 26 brain abnormalities were found on the MR imaging of 23 patients, and the incidence was 14.6% (23/157). The most common abnormality was pure white matter changes ($n = 13$), followed by pure structural abnormalities ($n = 3$), combination of white matter changes and structural abnormalities ($n = 3$), intraparenchymal cystic lesions ($n = 3$), and others (abnormal enlargement of subarachnoid space) ($n = 1$).

Among the 23 patients with brain abnormalities, concurrent abnormalities were found in 6 children, including bilateral mastoiditis ($n = 3$), malformed semicircular canal ($n = 1$), cochlear hypoplasia, absence of cochlear nerve ($n = 1$), and enlarged vestibular aqueduct ($n = 1$). The detailed demographic, clinical, and follow-up results of all the 23 patients were listed in Table 1.

3.2. Medical History during the Gestation and Perinatal Period. Among the 16 patients with white matter changes, 15 patients were successfully followed up. Among the 15 patients, 13 patients or their mothers had a history of medical condition that could be associated with the brain abnormalities, including viral influenza ($n = 6$), premature delivery ($n = 4$), cytomegalovirus ($n = 3$), rubella virus ($n = 2$), measles virus ($n = 1$), kernicterus ($n = 1$), and hypoxic ischemic encephalopathy ($n = 1$). The other SNHL patients had no history of medical condition that could be associated with the brain abnormalities.

3.3. Follow-Up of SNHL Children with Brain Abnormalities after CI. Twenty-three patients with brain abnormalities included 20 patients with bilateral SNHL and 3 patients with unilateral SNHL. After excluding the 3 unilateral cases that did not accept CI, one bilateral SNHL patient who gave up CI due to the complicated inner ear malformation, and one

TABLE 1: Follow-up of 23 SNHL patients with brain abnormalities after cochlear implantation.

Abnormal brain MRI findings	Concurrent abnormalities	Y/S	U/B	CI	IT-MAIS Before	IT-MAIS After	FU (Mon)	Focal/diffuse
White matter changes								
Bilateral frontal and temporal subcortical area Bilateral periventricular area Ventriculomegaly	—	1/M	B	Yes	0	10	15	Diffuse
Multiple WMC lesions	—	1/M	U	No	—	—	12	—
Right posterior horn of lateral ventricle	—	4/M	B	Yes	3	31	14	Focal
Bilateral posterior horn of lateral ventricle	Malformed semicircular canal	2/F	B	Yes	1	34	16	Focal
Bilateral periventricular area Bilateral centrum semiovale	—	1/M	U	No	—	—	9	—
Bilateral frontal and parietal subcortical area	—	1/M	B	Yes	1	29	27	Focal
Bilateral posterior horn of lateral ventricle	Bilateral mastoiditis	1/M	B	Yes	2	27	18	Focal
Multiple WMC lesions	—	1/F	B	Yes	1	23	12	Diffuse
Multiple WMC lesions Arachnoid cyst (left temporal area)	—	15/F	B	Yes	2	16	20	Diffuse
Multiple WMC lesions	Bilateral mastoiditis	1/M	B	Yes	2	24	8	Diffuse
Bilateral periventricular area	—	1/M	B	Yes	2	25	7	Focal
Bilateral frontal subcortical area Bilateral posterior horn of lateral ventricle Arachnoid cyst (left temporal area)	Bilateral mastoiditis	5/M	B	Yes	1	24	11	Diffuse
Bilateral periventricular area	—	3/M	U	No	—	—	18	—
Right posterior horn of lateral ventricle	—	4/F	B	Yes	2	27	18	Focal
Bilateral posterior horn of lateral ventricle Bilateral centrum semiovale	Cochlear hypoplasia Absence of cochlear nerve	3/F	B	No	—	—	11	—
Bilateral periventricular area	—	1/M	B	L*	—	—	—	—
Structural abnormalities								
Cisterna magna enlargement	—	2/M	B	Yes	1	28	15	—
Arachnoid cyst (left temporal area)	—	1/M	B	Yes	1	24	12	—
Arachnoid cyst (left temporal area)	—	3/F	B	Yes	2	29	9	—
Intraparenchymal cystic lesions								
Intraparenchymal cystic lesions (left lateral ventricular trigone)	—	1/M	B	Yes	2	22	7	—
Intraparenchymal cystic lesions (right occipital area)	—	3/F	B	Yes	3	25	22	—
Intraparenchymal cystic lesions (right centrum semiovale)	—	3/M	B	Yes	2	26	13	—
Others								
Abnormal enlargement of subarachnoid space (bilateral frontal and temporal area)	Enlarged vestibular aqueduct	1/F	B	Yes	0	17	16	—

Y, year old; S, sex; U, unilateral SNHL; B, bilateral SNHL; CI, cochlear implantation; FU, follow-up.
L* means the patient was lost during the follow-up.

bilateral SNHL patient who was lost during the follow-up, a total of 18 patients with bilateral SNHL accepted CI.

Among the 18 patients, the IT-MAIS score improved from 1.55 ± 0.86 to 24.50 ± 5.68 after CI. Among the 18 patients, 11 patients with the white matter changes received CI, and the IT-MAIS score improved from 1.54 ± 0.82 to 24.55 ± 6.71. A representative case is shown in Figure 1.

Eleven patients with white matter changes included 5 patients with "diffuse lesion" and 6 patients with "focal lesion." In the "diffuse lesions" group, except one patient who was 15 years old, the other 4 patients were 1, 1, 1, and 5 years old, respectively, with a mean age of 2.00 ± 2.00 years. In the "focal lesions" group, the mean age of the 6 patients was 2.17 ± 1.47 years. Meanwhile, in the "focal lesions" group, 2 patients

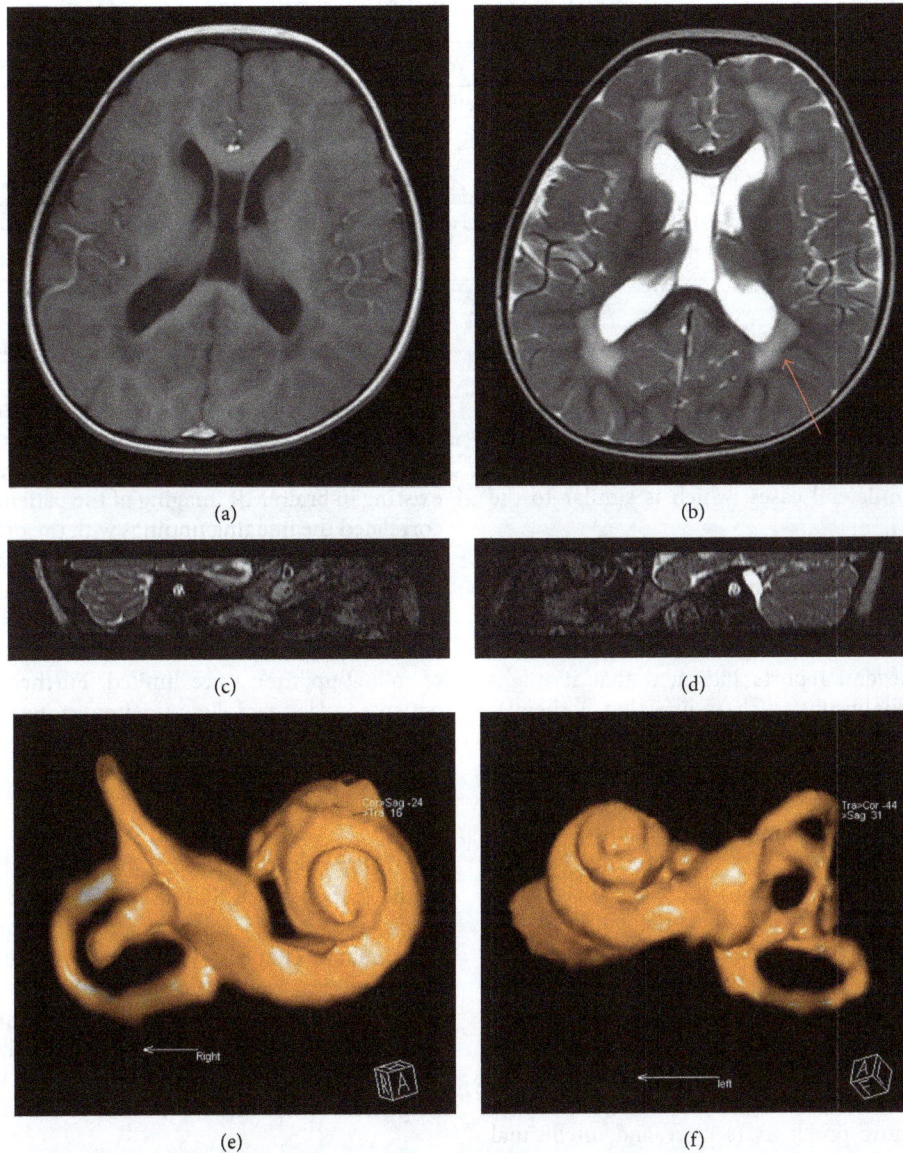

FIGURE 1: MR imaging of a representative patient with SNHL. (a, b) Axial T1 and T2 weighted imaging showed abnormal signal in the white matter in the bilateral periventricular area and enlargement of septum pellucidum. (c, d) Sagittal 3D-SPACE imaging showed the normal facial nerve, cochlear nerve, and vestibular nerves in the internal auditory canal. (e, f) Volume rendering imaging showed the normal structure of the inner ear. IT-MAIS score of this patient improved from 0 to 10 after CI.

had the concomitant abnormalities, including semicircular canal malformation in one patient and bilateral mastoiditis in another patient. In the "diffuse lesions" group, also 2 patients had the concomitant abnormalities, combined with bilateral mastoiditis in both of them. There were no other neurologic deficits or developmental delays associated with the brain abnormalities shown on the brain MR imaging in both of the two groups. In addition, there was no significant difference about the IT-MAIS score between two groups before CI (1.20 ± 1.41 versus 1.83 ± 0.71; $P > 0.05$). However, better hearing improvement was found in the "focal lesion" group than the "diffuse lesion" group after CI (27.00 ± 3.10 versus 18.20 ± 5.85; $P < 0.05$). Detailed IT-MAIS score change for children with SNHL before and after CI was showed in Table 2.

4. Discussion

The incidence of brain abnormalities in our study was 14.6%, relatively lower than previous studies, which demonstrated that the incidence of brain abnormalities varied from 20% to 56% [1, 9, 10]. The relative lower incidence might be explained that our hospital is the sole unit responsible for preoperative evaluation in our geographic region. The relative bigger base number of children with SNHL might reduce

TABLE 2: IT-MAIS score of children with SNHL before and after cochlear implantation.

Group	All SNHL children ($n = 18$)		WMC group ($n = 11$)		WMC group ($n = 11$)	
IT-MAIS score	Before	After	Before	After	Diffuse ($n = 5$)	Focal ($n = 6$)
	1.55 ± 0.86	24.50 ± 5.68	1.54 ± 0.82	24.55 ± 6.71	18.20 ± 5.85^{a}	27.00 ± 3.10^{b}
P	$P < 0.05$		$P < 0.05$		$P < 0.05$	

WMC indicates white mater change. The number in the parenthesis means the number of the patients in each group. [a,b]The score means the improvement of IT-MAIS score in the two groups.

the incidence of brain abnormalities detected to a certain extent. Meanwhile, another study indicated that the brain abnormalities appeared more in the brain MR imaging of patients with bilateral rather than unilateral SNHL [11]. In our study, 23 SNHL patients with brain abnormalities included 20 bilateral and 3 unilateral cases, which is similar to the previous study.

The white matter changes were the most common brain abnormality. In our study, the incidence of white matter changes was 69.6%, which was similar to previous studies [1, 12]. The pathogenesis of white matter changes remains unclear, although several reports indicated that it might be related to previous insults, such as infection, ischemia, hypoxia, or prematurity [13]. In our study, 13 children or their mothers had an exact history of medical condition that could be associated with the white matter changes, including viral influenza in 6 patients, premature delivery in 4 patients, cytomegalovirus in 3 patients, rubella virus in 2 patients, measles virus in one patient, kernicterus in one patient, and hypoxic ischemic encephalopathy in one patient. No exact history of medical condition was found in the other 10 patients. Therefore, we speculated that the white matter changes might be partly associated with the history of medical condition during the gestation and perinatal period.

The white matter changes were viewed as an important marker of abnormal neurodevelopment and might help to predict potential future problems (seizure and intellectual impairment) in certain patients [14]. However, the impact of white matter changes on the hearing improvement after CI was still unclear. In our study, a total of 11 patients with the white matter changes accepted CI, and IT-MAIS score improved from 1.54 ± 0.82 to 24.55 ± 6.71 after CI. Therefore, we insisted that the SNHL patients with white matter changes could also acquire hearing improvement after CI. White matter changes should not be viewed as the absolute contraindication of CI. Meanwhile, we found that the patients in the "focal lesion" group could acquire probable better improvement than the patients in the "diffuse lesion" group (27.00 ± 3.10 versus 18.20 ± 5.85). In addition, as to the patients in whom SNHL was combined with other abnormalities, including arachnoid cyst or intraparenchymal cystic lesions, they also acquired the hearing improvement after CI. Therefore, these kinds of abnormalities should also not be viewed as the absolute contraindication of CI. However, due to the rarity of the SNHL patients with brain abnormalities and relatively short follow-up time, it might be difficult to make a definite conclusion regarding the impact of brain abnormalities on CI. Further study with

more patients and longer follow-up time was needed to confirm our results.

Our study had several limitations. First, our study was a retrospectively clinical observational and descriptive study. We could just describe the different brain abnormalities existing in brain MR imaging of the patients with SNHL and correlated the imaging findings with the medical histories, so as to analyze the potential cause of the brain abnormalities. However, no exact pathological evidence could be achieved for supporting our research result. Secondly, the number of the SNHL patients with brain abnormalities and the period of follow-up time were limited. Further study with more patients and longer follow-up time was needed to confirm our results.

5. Conclusion

Brain abnormalities were common on the brain MR imaging of the patients with SNHL; therefore, the whole brain MR scan was necessary in the preimplantation evaluation. The white matter changes, which were the most common brain abnormalities, might be associated with the history of medical condition during the gestation and perinatal period. Brain abnormalities might not influence the short-term hearing improvement after CI. Further study with more patients and longer follow-up time was needed to confirm our results.

Conflict of Interests

None of the authors has identified a potential conflict of interests.

Authors' Contribution

Xiao-Quan Xu assessed images and wrote the paper, Fei-Yun Wu designed the paper and assessed images, Hao Hu followed up all the patients in the study, Guo-Yi Su helped with MR scan for all the patients, and Jie Shen helped with CT scan for all the patients.

References

[1] N. E. Jonas, J. Ahmed, J. Grainger et al., "MRI brain abnormalities in cochlear implant candidates: how common and how important are they?" *International Journal of Pediatric Otorhinolaryngology*, vol. 76, no. 7, pp. 927–929, 2012.

[2] V. M. Joshi, S. K. Navlekar, G. R. Kishore, K. J. Reddy, and E. C. V. Kumar, "CT and MR imaging of the inner ear and

brain in children with congenital sensorineural hearing loss," *Radiographics*, vol. 32, no. 3, pp. 683–698, 2012.

[3] J. B. Fallon, D. R. F. Irvine, and R. K. Shepherd, "Cochlear implants and brain plasticity," *Hearing Research*, vol. 238, no. 1-2, pp. 110–117, 2008.

[4] F. Yan, J. Li, J. Xian, Z. Wang, and L. Mo, "The cochlear nerve canal and internal auditory canal in children with normal cochlea but cochlear nerve deficiency," *Acta Radiologica*, vol. 54, no. 3, pp. 292–298, 2013.

[5] M. Miyasaka, S. Nosaka, N. Morimoto, H. Taiji, and H. Masaki, "CT and MR imaging for pediatric cochlear implantation: emphasis on the relationship between the cochlear nerve canal and the cochlear nerve," *Pediatric Radiology*, vol. 40, no. 9, pp. 1509–1516, 2010.

[6] J. W. Kutz Jr., K. H. Lee, B. Isaacson, T. N. Booth, M. H. Sweeney, and P. S. Roland, "Cochlear implantation in children with cochlear nerve absence or deficiency," *Otology & Neurotology*, vol. 32, no. 6, pp. 956–961, 2011.

[7] G. Ricci, F. Trabalzini, M. Faralli, L. D'Ascanio, C. Cristi, and E. Molini, "Cochlear implantation in children with "CHARGE syndrome": surgical options and outcomes," *European Archives of Oto-Rhino-Laryngology*, vol. 271, no. 3, pp. 489–493, 2014.

[8] A. M. Robbins, J. J. Renshaw, and S. W. Berry, "Evaluating meaningful auditory integration in profoundly hearing-impaired children," *American Journal of Otology*, vol. 12, no. Supplement, pp. 144–150, 1991.

[9] A. Lapointe, C. Viamonte, M. C. Morriss, and S. Manolidis, "Central nervous system findings by magnetic resonance in children with profound sensorineural hearing loss," *International Journal of Pediatric Otorhinolaryngology*, vol. 70, no. 5, pp. 863–868, 2006.

[10] J. Walton, W. P. Gibson, H. Sanli, and K. Prelog, "Predicting cochlear implant outcomes in children with auditory neuropathy," *Otology & Neurotology*, vol. 29, no. 3, pp. 302–309, 2008.

[11] H. F. B. Teagle, P. A. Roush, J. S. Woodard et al., "Cochlear implantation in children with auditory neuropathy spectrum disorder," *Ear and Hearing*, vol. 31, no. 3, pp. 325–335, 2010.

[12] R. D. Proctor, M. L. Gawne-Cain, J. Eyles, T. E. Mitchell, and V. B. Batty, "MRI during cochlear implant assessment: should we image the whole brain?" *Cochlear Implants International*, vol. 14, no. 1, pp. 2–6, 2013.

[13] V. M. Joshi, S. K. Navlekar, G. R. Kishore, K. J. Reddy, and E. C. V. Kumar, "CT and MR imaging of the inner ear and brain in children with congenital sensorineural hearing loss," *Radiographics*, vol. 32, no. 3, pp. 683–698, 2012.

[14] J. M. Perlman, "White matter injury in the preterm infant: an important determination of abnormal neurodevelopment outcome," *Early Human Development*, vol. 53, no. 2, pp. 99–120, 1998.

7

Learned Shrinkage Approach for Low-Dose Reconstruction in Computed Tomography

Joseph Shtok, Michael Elad, and Michael Zibulevsky

Computer Science Department, Technion - Israel Institute of Technology, Haifa 32000, Israel

Correspondence should be addressed to Joseph Shtok; shtok@cs.technion.ac.il

Academic Editor: Jun Zhao

We propose a direct nonlinear reconstruction algorithm for Computed Tomography (CT), designed to handle low-dose measurements. It involves the filtered back-projection and adaptive nonlinear filtering in both the projection and the image domains. The filter is an extension of the learned shrinkage method by Hel-Or and Shaked to the case of indirect observations. The shrinkage functions are learned using a training set of reference CT images. The optimization is performed with respect to an error functional in the image domain that combines the mean square error with a gradient-based penalty, promoting image sharpness. Our numerical simulations indicate that the proposed algorithm can manage well with noisy measurements, allowing a dose reduction by a factor of 4, while reducing noise and streak artifacts in the FBP reconstruction, comparable to the performance of a statistically based iterative algorithm.

1. Introduction

1.1. Problem Statement. Computed tomography (CT) imaging produces a 3D map of the scanned object, where the different materials are distinguished by their X-ray attenuation properties. In medicine, such a map has a great diagnostic value, making the CT scan one of the most frequent noninvasive exploration procedures practiced in almost every hospital. The attenuation of biological tissues is measured by comparing the intensity of the X-rays entering and leaving the body. The main problem precluding pervasive use of the CT scan for diagnostics and monitoring is the damage caused to the tissues by the X-ray radiation. CT manufacturers make great efforts to reduce the X-ray dose required for images of diagnostic quality. In this work we propose an algorithm that enables a high-quality reconstruction from low-dose (and thus noisy) measurements.

In ideal conditions, the information obtained in the scan suffices to build an exact attenuation map, called the CT image. In practice, the measurements are degraded by a number of physical phenomena. The main factors are off-focal radiation, afterglow and crosstalk in the detectors, beam hardening, and Compton scattering (see [1] for a detailed overview). These introduce a structured error into the measurements, mostly the type that is modeled by a convolution with some kernel. Another source of deterioration, dominant in the low-dose scenario, is the stochastic noise. One type of such noise stems from the low photon counts, which occur when the X-rays pass through high-attenuation areas. This phenomenon is similar to the shot noise, encountered in photo cameras in poor lighting conditions. Statistically, the photon counts are modeled as instances of Poisson random variables. Another type of the stochastic noise originates from dark currents in the detectors, interference noise from interconnecting cables, and other hardware sources. This electronic noise is modeled in the measurements as an additive Gaussian random variable.

In this work we aim to reduce the influence of the stochastic noise on the image quality, with the assumption that the structured error components, mentioned above, are treated by the existing methods. Explicitly, we use the well-accepted compound Poisson-Gaussian statistical model and propose a new noniterative method for image reconstruction, based on the concept of sparse representations [2] and involving machine learning concepts.

1.2. Present Reconstruction Algorithms. The basic linear reconstruction method, filtered back projection (FBP) [3], makes a very limited account of the noise structure in the data: it employs a low-pass 1D convolution filter in the Radon domain, whose parameters are preset for specific anatomical regions and standard scan protocols. Errors in the photon counts manifest in the output CT image in the form of streak artifacts, which corrupt its content and jeopardize its diagnostic value. Accordingly, each measured line integral is effectively smeared back over that line by the back projection; an incorrect measurement results in a line of wrong intensity in the image. Typically, the streaks radiate from bone regions or metal implants, which corrupt its content and jeopardize its diagnostic value. Images of better quality—with reduced artifacts and increased spatial resolution—are obtained with a statistically-based approach, where the maximum a posteriori (MAP) is optimized with respect to the sought image. This problem is converted to a minimization of the penalized likelihood (PL) objective function [1], (1). The likelihood expression models the physical process of CT scan, which allows interpreting the measurements more correctly. The likelihood component expresses the expected statistical behavior of the data. The penalty component models the expected properties of the CT images (i.e., contains a *prior* information about the image to be reconstructed). The PL objective can be designed to restore the measurements from noisy observations [1, 4, 5] or to reconstruct directly the CT image [6]. In most cases, the optimization problem is difficult to solve, so it is sometimes replaced by a second-order approximation, the penalized weighted least squares (PWLS) [6, 7]. A drawback of a reconstruction based on explicit statistical modeling is the computationally heavy iterative solution.

To improve the performance of the fast FBP reconstruction, adaptive signal processing techniques, implicitly modeling the noise statistics, have been proposed. These are applied to the measurements data in a noniterative fashion and have computational complexity comparable to that of the FBP. Hsieh employs a trimmed mean filter, adaptive to the noise variance [8]. For each detector reading x, the algorithm adaptively chooses a number of its neighbors participating in the filtering operation. The value of x is replaced with the average of these neighbors after a portion of their highest and lowest values is discarded. To some extent, the aforementioned statistical model of the scan is used: the noisy samples get a stronger filtering than the more reliable ones. The experimental results in this work are very impressive. A similar concept, with a different kind of filter, is adopted by the work of Kachelrieß et al. who apply adaptive convolution-based filtering in the sinogram domain [9]. The filter width is data dependent and also it is applied only where the data intensity is below a threshold, so the algorithm processes only the regions where the noise is substantial. In [10], two signal processing steps are introduced to improve the performance of FBP. The measurements' data is processed by the penalized weighted least squares filter in a Karhunen-Loeve domain (more familiar under the name of principal component analysis, PCA). An additional step of image postprocessing is performed by edge-preserving smoothing with locally adaptive parameters.

Beyond the use of general-purpose tools, there are algorithms applying machine learning methods for adaptive processing of the tomographic data. Close in its spirit to our work is the algorithm described in [11]. Here, the measured projections are locally filtered according to a preliminary classification of its regions. The classes and the corresponding filters are derived automatically, via an offline example-based training process. Thus, the standard smoothing by the low-pass convolution filter is replaced with locally adaptive filtering, optimized for the minimal mean square error in the training images.

1.3. Our Work. Our method employs an adaptive local processing of the measurements and a matched postprocessing stage in the CT image domain. Those steps are intended to enable the FBP to deal with the noisy measurements. The technique employed in both stages is a learned shrinkage in the transform domain, following the ideas outlined in the work by Hel-Or and Shaked in [12].

The learned shrinkage filter was originally designed for noise reduction and is employed in our work to reduce an error measure in the CT image domain, while acting on the raw measurements (at the first stage) and on the reconstructed image (at the second). In a nutshell, the learned shrinkage operator is a nonlinear adaptive filter, applied locally to the signal data. It requires an example-based training of the filter's defining parameters, which minimizes a desired reconstruction error with respect to reference CT images.

Due to the fact that the noise in the measurements is data dependent, we introduce a scalar transformation which normalizes the noise variance according to its statistical model. The aforementioned filter is applied after this transformation. The error measure in the image domain, used in the training objective, is a function of the reconstructed CT image and its ground truth—a high quality reference image. The measure consists of two components, the standard mean square error and a gradient-based expression capturing the amount of blur at fine edges of the image. Filters, optimized with respect to this error measure, are shown to produce CT images with low spatial noise and artifacts, while producing sharp edges.

On one hand, our approach accounts for the statistical model of the noise, as used by the iterative algorithms; on the other, the computationally heavy learning procedure is performed once offline, at the calibration stage, while the processing of the new data is done very fast, on par with the FBP algorithm. This gives a hope to bridge the gap between the slow high-quality statistical algorithms and the fast linear reconstruction. We also mention that in the learning process our algorithm has the potential to adjust to additional unknown degradation factors and hardware specifications.

One possible application of the proposed method is to exploit the adaptive nature of its filtering stages to taylor the filter parameters to an individual patient, in a specific scan setup. Such step can be made in the scenario where repeated

CT scans are performed, for reasons of monitoring. Thus after the first full-dose scan, the X-ray exposure in the following procedures can be reduced by using filters trained on the image data very similar to that which is expected in the next scan. With the correct training protocol, there is no danger of overfitting the filters to the "healthy" images and thus to jeopardise detection of anomalies (an experiment, suggesting this fact, is reported later in this paper). In this way, a patient can avoid a substantial amount of X-ray exposure.

In our numerical experiments we compare the proposed algorithm against three existing ones. First is the optimally tuned FBP, which serves as a baseline; another is the nonlinear ATM filter for CT reconstruction, proposed by Hsieh in [8], and the third is the iterative, statistically-based PWLS reconstruction [6]. Our method is shown to outperform both the FBP and the ATM in the sense of image quality and robustness to changes of the anatomical region, and it is comparable to the statistically-based reconstruction. The comparison includes a visual display, a number of quantitative measures and evaluation of the local impulse response for each algorithm.

The paper is organized as follows. The mathematical description of the CT scan is given in Section 2. The learned shrinkage method is presented in Section 3. The new error measure is described in Section 4, laying the ground for our method for CT reconstruction, described in Section 5. A numerical study is given in Section 6. Section 7 concludes the paper.

2. Mathematical Model of the CT Scan

Our algorithm is designed in the setup of two-dimensional, parallel-beam scan geometry. An example of a scanned object is an axial slice (axial plane is the one parallel to the floor when the patient is standing) of the patient's body. The main part of a CT scanner is a rotating gantry, which has the X-ray source mounted against an array of detectors. During the scan, the gantry sweeps the angular range of $[0, \pi]$, equally divided into a large number of projections or "views". For each angle θ, the one-dimensional array of detectors produces photon counts from rays that arrive in a fan-shaped beam from the source. Via a rebinning step, the rays are rearranged so that there is a comb of parallel rays for each projection. The acquired data is arranged into a 2D matrix, whose columns correspond to different angles, and the rows are assigned to different bins in each projection.

To describe the nature of measured data we use the compound Poisson-Gaussian statistical model that is assumed in [1, 13] and is also empirically verified in [8]. Each measured photon count y_ℓ is viewed as an instance of the random variable Y_ℓ given by

$$Y_\ell \sim \text{Poiss}\left(\lambda_\ell\right) + \text{Gauss}\left(d, \sigma_n\right), \quad \text{where}$$
$$\lambda_\ell = \lambda_0 \cdot \exp\left(-[\mathbf{R}f]_\ell\right), \tag{1}$$

where $\mathbf{R}f$ is the Radon transform of the scanned image f and the constant λ_0 is the photon count at the X-ray source. The Radon transform is defined on the collection of all straight lines ℓ through the object. For each ℓ, its value is the linear integral:

$$[\mathbf{R}f]_\ell = \int_\ell f\left(\ell\right) d\ell. \tag{2}$$

The log-transformed photon counts $g_\ell = -\log(y_\ell/\lambda_0)$ are the approximate line integrals; the corresponding data matrix g is called a *sinogram* since every point in the image space traces a sine curve in this domain.

The filtered back-projection algorithm is based on the Radon inversion formula. First, the measurements are transformed to the Radon domain by the logarithm function: $g = -\log(y/\lambda_0)$. Then, a linear operator implementing the inverse of Radon transform is applied as follows:

$$\tilde{f} = \mathbf{R}^* \mathbf{F}_{\text{RL}}\left(g\right), \tag{3}$$

where $\mathbf{R}^*$ is the adjoint of the Radon transform, also known as the back-projection operator:

$$\left(\mathbf{R}^* g\right) x = \int_\theta g\left(\theta, x \cdot \theta\right) d\theta. \tag{4}$$

The filter $\mathbf{F}_{\text{RL}}$ uses the Ram-Lak kernel κ [14], defined in the Fourier domain by

$$\hat{\kappa}\left(\omega\right) = |\omega|. \tag{5}$$

In practice, an additional, low-pass filtering is performed in the Radon domain to reduce the high-frequency noise amplified by the Ram-Lak kernel. It is usually implemented by applying a Butterworth or a Shepp-Logan window in the frequency domain. The optimal parameters of the low-pass filter differ from one anatomical region to another. Their preset values are kept fixed in the clinical CT scanners, and the radiologist selects an appropriate one for each clinical study. As a study in [15] shows, the image properties depend nonnegligibly on this parameter.

3. Learned Shrinkage in a Transform Domain

We describe the learned shrinkage algorithm proposed by Hel-Or and Shaked in [12] for signal denoising. A popular Bayesian approach for recovery of a signal x from measurements $y = x + \xi$, contaminated with i.i.d. Gaussian noise, consists in solving the penalized least squares optimization problem,

$$\hat{\alpha} = \arg\min_\alpha \|y - \mathbf{D}\alpha\|_2^2 + \lambda\rho\left(\alpha\right), \tag{6}$$

and computing the signal estimate by $\hat{x} = \mathbf{D}\hat{\alpha}$ [16]. Effectively, the sought signal is encoded in terms of the dictionary $\mathbf{D}$ (a linear transform, e.g., wavelets), whose properties encourage noise reduction. The left summand in this expression is a data fidelity term, and the right one expresses expected properties of the signal's coefficients. The classical assumption of a rapid decay of their magnitudes corresponds to the following penalty expression [17, Section 1.3]:

$$\rho\left(\alpha\right) = \|\alpha\|_p^p, \quad \text{with } 0 \le p \le 1. \tag{7}$$

For a unitary transform $\mathbf{D}$, the problem (6) is separable and admits a simple closed-form solution, which is described by a scalar *shrinkage* function $\mathcal{S}$ applied elementwise to the vector of coefficients $\mathbf{D}^{-1}y$. The formula for the shrinkage function is derived analytically from the expression for $\rho(\alpha)$ [18]. Thus, the signal estimate $\hat{x}$ has the formula:

$$\hat{x} = \mathbf{D}\mathcal{S}\mathbf{D}^{-1}y. \qquad (8)$$

This technique was pioneered by Donoho and Johnston [19], who developed it for the wavelet transform, and it is now widely applied in the broader context of nonunitary operators and even redundant dictionaries which are tight frames (see [12, 16] for an overview). In those cases, any shrinkage operation can provide only an approximate solution to (6).

For image denoising, the data dimensions are too large to process the entire image if $\mathbf{D}$ is not a computationally efficient structured transformation and also, while images vary wildly, small image patches fall into a well-structured statistical pattern. Therefore, the shrinkage idea is applied to an image denoising by extracting overlapping square patches and processing each of them separately. The overlaps help avoiding block artifacts and stabilize the filtering action. Each pixel is altered differently in each patch it belongs to; strong differences are tamed by averaging over all those patches.

Technically, a patch p of size $d \times d$, corresponding to location k in the signal matrix y, is extracted by the linear operator $\mathbf{E}_k$ and is reinstalled (after a processing) into a signal-sized empty matrix by its transpose $\mathbf{E}_k^\top$. Thus, the patchwise denoising action for a 2D signal is described by

$$\hat{x} = \mathbf{G}_\mathbf{D}\left(y\right) = \mathbf{M}_\mathbf{E}^{-1}\sum_k \mathbf{E}_k^\top \mathbf{D}\mathcal{S}\mathbf{D}^{-1}\mathbf{E}_k y. \qquad (9)$$

Here $\mathbf{M}_\mathbf{E} = \sum_k \mathbf{E}_k^\top \mathbf{E}_k$ is compensating for the overlapping by dividing each pixel by the number of patches containing it.

When the dictionary $\mathbf{D}$ is a nonunitary full-rank matrix, the vector of coefficients is computed using the pseudoinverse $\mathbf{D}^+$ of the dictionary. As mentioned before, in this case no exact solution for the shape of the shrinkage function is available. A practical solution for denoising in this setting is proposed in [12]: the shape of the shrinkage function in (9) is learned in an example-based process (rather than being defined descriptively), by optimizing an objective function. Also, for better results, it is preferable to use an array of shrinkage functions, corresponding to the structure of the transform $\mathbf{D}$, rather than a single one. For instance, when an N-levels wavelet transform is used, separate functions are dedicated to each level. The vector α in this case is partitioned into N subsets, each processed with an individual shrinkage function.

In [12], the shrinkage functions are modeled as linear combinations of splines of order 1. In other words, these are piecewise linear functions whose joints are configurable. The N shrinkage functions $\mathcal{S}_1, \ldots, \mathcal{S}_N$ are defined by two sets of vectors, $\mathbf{q} = [\mathbf{q}_1, \ldots, \mathbf{q}_N]$ and $\mathbf{p} = [\mathbf{p}_1, \ldots, \mathbf{p}_N]$. The vector $\mathbf{q}_i$ is an evenly spaced sequence of numbers, covering the dynamic range of the ith subset in α; each $\mathcal{S}_i$ is the

antisymmetric piecewise linear function determined by the following equations:

$$\mathcal{S}_i\left(\mathbf{q}_i\left(j\right)\right) = \mathbf{p}_i\left(j\right), \quad \mathcal{S}_i\left(-\mathbf{q}_i\left(j\right)\right) = -\mathbf{p}_i\left(j\right), \quad \forall j$$
$$\mathcal{S}_i\left(0\right) = 0. \qquad (10)$$

The antisymmetry assumption comes from the belief that only the absolute values of the coefficients should affect the amount of shrinkage applied. It was verified experimentally both in the work of Hel-Or and Shaked and in ours.

The shrinkage operator now has a parameter set $\mathbf{p}$, assuming a fixed set of domains $\mathbf{q}$. We define an estimator $\mathbf{G}_{\mathbf{p},\mathbf{D}}$ for the signal x, based on (9) with this addition:

$$\hat{x} = \mathbf{G}_{\mathbf{p},\mathbf{D}}\left(y\right) = \mathbf{M}_\mathbf{E}^{-1}\sum_k \mathbf{E}_k^\top \mathbf{D}\mathcal{S}_\mathbf{p}\mathbf{D}^+\mathbf{E}_k y. \qquad (11)$$

Let us denote by $\alpha_k = (\mathbf{D}^+\mathbf{E}_k y)$ the representation of the kth patch in the noisy signal.

The objective function for tuning the parameter set $\mathbf{p}$ is the mean square error (MSE) of the signal estimate $\tilde{x} = \mathbf{G}_{\mathbf{p},\mathbf{D}}(y)$, with respect to the true signal x available at the training stage:

$$\mathbf{p}^* = \arg\min_\mathbf{p} \left\| \mathbf{G}_{\mathbf{p},\mathbf{D}}(y) - x \right\|_2^2$$
$$= \arg\min_\mathbf{p} \left\| \mathbf{M}_\mathbf{E}^{-1}\sum_k \mathbf{E}_k^\top \mathbf{D}\mathcal{S}_\mathbf{p}(\alpha_k) - x \right\|_2^2, \qquad (12)$$
$$\alpha_k = \mathbf{D}^+\mathbf{E}_k y.$$

Hel-Or and Shaked define the *slice transform* (SLT) which is applied to α_k in order to reformulate the shrinkage operation as a linear function in $\mathbf{p}$. Explicitly, a large sparse matrix $U_{\mathbf{q},\alpha_k}$ encoding this data is designed ([12, Section IV]) to perform the shrinkage via a matrix-vector product:

$$U_{\mathbf{q},\alpha_k} \cdot \mathbf{q} = \alpha_k, \quad U_{\mathbf{q},\alpha_k} \cdot \mathbf{p} = \mathcal{S}_\mathbf{p}\left(\alpha_k\right). \qquad (13)$$

Using this approach, the optimization of the objective function (12) turns into a simple least squares problem,

$$\mathbf{p}^* = \arg\min_\mathbf{p} \left\| \mathbf{M}_\mathbf{E}^{-1}\sum_k \mathbf{E}_k^\top \mathbf{D}U_{\mathbf{q},\alpha_k} \cdot \mathbf{p} - x \right\|_2^2. \qquad (14)$$

It is easily solved for $\mathbf{p}$ using the pseudo-inverse operator.

An application of this method to image denoising, demonstrated in [12], shows very promising results. Moreover, the use of custom-built functions makes the shrinkage operation more robust and suitable for signal processing problems other than noise reduction. For instance, an algorithm for single image super resolution, proposed in [20] and based on the same principles, exhibits a state-of-the-art performance.

4. Error Measure in the Image Domain

4.1. Constructing the Error Measure. Before considering an example-based training for CT reconstruction, one must establish a viable error measure in the image domain, minimization of which would lead to radiological images of a good quality. We consider a quantitative error measure for the deteriorated CT image $\tilde{f}$ (reconstructed with some algorithm), which uses the ground truth image f. The basic choice for such measure is the mean square error (MSE):

$$\text{MSE}\left(\tilde{f}\right) = \left\|f - \tilde{f}\right\|_2^2. \tag{15}$$

Pursuing a low MSE value is an accepted goal in the general field of image processing; however, we observe in our experiments that algorithms optimized for minimal MSE produce images with reduced spatial resolution. The reason is that the true image often contains large nearly constant regions, which calls for extensive smoothing. Fine details, washed off by this smoothing, do not increase the MSE notably, so its net value over the entire image is low. We therefore introduce an additional component to the error measure, which encourages the preservation of fine edges in the image.

Consider an edge between two homogeneous regions in the image, where the change in intensity is small comparing to the global dynamic range. If the filter applied blurs this edge, the MSE value is increased by a small amount; however, the gradient norm at the edge is much smaller than in the original image. Thus, it makes sense to penalize not only for difference in intensity values between the reference image f_0 and the reconstruction $\tilde{f}$ but for the difference in gradient norms:

$$\mathbf{Q}_1\left(f_0, \tilde{f}\right) = \sum_x \left| \left\|\nabla f_0(x)\right\|_2^2 - \left\|\nabla \tilde{f}(x)\right\|_2^2 \right|. \tag{16}$$

However, the stated error measure is still reduced by over-smoothing the image: wherever the value of $\left\|\nabla \tilde{f}(x)\right\|_2^2$ is larger than $\left\|\nabla f_0(x)\right\|_2^2$ (which happens a lot in the noisy image $\tilde{f}$), smoothing the image $\tilde{f}$ will reduce the error. Therefore, we restrict our error measure only to the regions where the original gradient norm is larger than the reconstructed one; those regions are most problematic in the sense of lost details. Thus, the following formula for a penalty component is proposed:

$$\mathbf{Q}\left(f_0, \tilde{f}\right) = \sum_x W(x) \max\left(0, \left\|\nabla f_0(x)\right\|_2^2 - \left\|\nabla \tilde{f}(x)\right\|_2^2\right). \tag{17}$$

The weight matrix W, introduced here, is designed to remove all the locations where the reference gradient norm is above 2% of its maximal value. This (empirically chosen) threshold is applied in order to focus on the low-contrast edges and not to waste the learning capacity of the filter on the strong flesh-bone transitions. For a practical optimization we replace the function (max$(0, x)$ has a noncontinuous derivative in

0) max$(0, x)$ with a smoothed version $\psi(x, \delta)$, based on the Huber penalty function [21]:

$$\psi_\delta(x) = \begin{cases} 0, & x < 0 \\ \dfrac{x^2}{2}, & 0 \le x < \delta \\ \delta|x| - \dfrac{\delta^2}{2}. & x \ge \delta. \end{cases} \tag{18}$$

Another modification to the formula is introduced. Often the radiologist is primarily interested in observing the clinical images in a specific dynamic range; for instance, if soft tissues are of interest, the relevant range seldom exceeds the window of $[-300, 300]$ Hounsfield units (HU). On other hand, if bones are observed, the range should cover the bone intensity; in this case, a range of $[0, 1500]$ HU may be relevant. We provide the ability to use this information in order to concentrate the learning capacity of the filter in the required dynamic range. Thus we introduce a binary mask $\mathbf{H}$ in the image domain, which (in the training stage) is set to exhibit only those image regions which fall into the relevant dynamic range. Bottom line, we set the main penalty component to the form of weighted L_2 norm, $\left\|f - \tilde{f}\right\|_{2,\mathbf{H}}^2 = (f - \tilde{f})^T \mathbf{H}(f - \tilde{f})$. The obtained error measure is named MSEg (mean square error, augmented with the g gradient), and its final expression is

$$\text{MSEg}\left(f_0, \tilde{f}\right) = \left\|f_0 - \tilde{f}\right\|_{2,\mathbf{H}}^2 + \mu \mathbf{Q}\left(f_0, \tilde{f}\right),$$

$$\text{where } \mathbf{Q}\left(f_0, \tilde{f}\right) = \sum_x W(x)\,\psi_\delta\left(\left\|\nabla f_0(x)\right\|_2^2 - \left\|\nabla \tilde{f}(x)\right\|_2^2\right). \tag{19}$$

The reference image f_0 will be omitted from the notation from now on. Using this function for training of data filters produces CT images, which combine low MSE value with high spatial resolution measure. In the following principle experiment, it is compared to the basic MSE penalty in order to demonstrate the effect of the proposed gradient-based term.

4.2. Empirical Evaluation of the Proposed Measure. The following experiment shows the effect of the gradient-based term in (19) on the visual impression from the "optimized" image. The FBP algorithm is employed to perform CT reconstruction from noisy observations. The cutoff frequency ϕ_0 of the low-pass filter in the Radon domain is gradually increased to alter the variance-resolution tradeoff in the reconstructed image. In Figure 1 we display a graph of MSE values of the obtained image as a function of ϕ_0 and a graph of $\mathbf{Q}(f_0, \tilde{f})$ values. Both are unimodal graphs with a single minimum. For $\mathbf{Q}(f_0, \tilde{f})$, the minimum is obtained at a higher frequency than for the MSE measure. In Figure 2 we display reconstructions corresponding to these two optimal frequencies. A visual inspection led us to the conclusion that the minimal-MSE version (upper row, on the right) is a blurred image, where spatial resolution is sacrificed for noise reduction. The version minimizing the $\mathbf{Q}(f_0, \tilde{f})$ penalty (lower row, on the left) is visually more appealing since it has a higher spatial resolution at the expense of stronger noise that is managed well by the human eye. For comparison, we also display the reference image (upper left) and two extreme cases corresponding to low/high cutoff frequency (middle column).

The two conclusions drawn from this experiment are (1) if we add the gradient-based penalty $\mathbf{Q}(f_0, \tilde{f})$ to the error measure and train the reconstruction chain to minimize its value, the obtained images are more informative to the human eye, with higher spatial resolution, and the cost is a higher noise level and (2) the values of $\mathbf{Q}(f_0, \tilde{f})$ are lower by two orders of magnitude than the MSE; therefore, in a balanced total error term (19), the value of the weight μ should be around 100 in order for $\mathbf{Q}(f_0, \tilde{f})$ to have an effect.

5. The Algorithm for CT Reconstruction

The algorithm consists of the sequence of steps, producing a CT image from the measured photon counts. They are stated here and detailed in the sequel.

(i) *Data adjustment for signal processing*: the photon counts are altered so as to enable an approximate modeling with only the Poisson random variable; then, they undergo the Anscombe transform [22] to normalize the noise variance.

(ii) *Learned Shrinkage in the measurements domain*: the 2D matrix of the adjusted measurements data is processed patchwise using the learned shrinkage algorithm (we modify the original method of Hel-Or and Shaked, adjusting it to indirect measurements).

(iii) *Standard FBP*: the FBP transform with no low-pass filter reconstructs the CT image from the restored measurements data.

(iv) *Learned Shrinkage in the image domain*: a different instance of the learned shrinkage algorithm is applied on the obtained image, producing the final outcome.

We now extend the discussion on each of these steps.

5.1. Adjusted Measurements. The first step is to remove the Gaussian component from the measurements model stated in (1). Following [1], we compute the adjusted variables $\hat{y}$:

$$\hat{y}_\ell = \left[y_\ell - d + \sigma_n^2\right]_+, \qquad (20)$$

where the $[x]_+ = \max\{x, 0\}$. It is easily seen that the expectation and the variance of this distribution are equal to those of the single Poisson variable with the parameter $\hat{\lambda}_\ell = \lambda_\ell + \sigma_n^2$, and so for the purposes of noise normalization, we will assume that this is the distribution modeling for the adjusted measurements $\hat{y}_\ell$. Also, we assume a zero-mean electronic noise ($d = 0$), and therefore the positivity correction is not relevant.

The variance of the Poisson random variable equals its expectation $\hat{\lambda}_\ell = \lambda_\ell + \sigma_n^2$ and can be approximated by the measured value $\hat{y}_\ell$. We assume that the noise reduction by the learned shrinkage works best when the noise is homogeneous (constant variance in all points). The reason is that the representations of all the patches in the data matrix are processed by the same scalar function, and if the noise energy in each patch was different, it would require a spatially varying shrinkage. In order to achieve unit variance in all the measurements, we use the Anscombe transform [22], intended to normalize the Poisson variable:

$$\phi(x) = 2\sqrt{x + \frac{3}{8}}. \qquad (21)$$

To summarize, the overall data adjustment is performed elementwise by the following scalar function $\omega(x)$:

$$z_\ell = \omega(y_\ell) = \phi\left(y_\ell + \sigma_n^2\right) = 2\sqrt{y_\ell + \sigma_n^2 + \frac{3}{8}}. \qquad (22)$$

5.2. The Objective Function for Training. Let $z = \omega(y)$ denote the matrix of adjusted measurements. We state the expression for the image $\tilde{f}$ reconstructed with our algorithm, before the postprocessing stage. The noise reduction in z is done by the nonlinear filter $\mathbf{G_p} = \mathbf{G_{p,D}}$, defined in (11). Here the dictionary $\mathbf{D}$ is a fixed linear transformation (we use the unitary discrete cosine transform), and therefore it is omitted from the notation. After the filtering, the data is transformed to the Radon domain by applying the $\omega^{-1}(x)$, followed by the $-\log$ function. Then the FBP operator $\mathbf{T}$ is applied to produce the CT image $\tilde{f}$. To summarize, the image is computed as follows:

$$\tilde{f}_\mathbf{p}(z) = -\mathbf{T}\left(\log\left(\frac{1}{\lambda_0}\omega^{-1}\mathbf{G_p}(z)\right)\right). \qquad (23)$$

The objective function for the training of the parameter set $\mathbf{p}$ is the proposed error measure from (19), regularized with an additional factor:

$$\begin{aligned}
\mathbf{\Gamma_p}(z) &\equiv \mathrm{MSEg}\left(f, \tilde{f}_\mathbf{p}(z)\right) + \gamma\|\mathbf{p} - \mathbf{q}\|_2 \\
&= \left\|f - \tilde{f}_\mathbf{p}(z)\right\|_{2,\mathbf{H}}^2 + \mu\mathbf{Q}\left(f_0, \tilde{f}_\mathbf{p}(z)\right) \\
&\quad + \gamma\|\mathbf{p} - \mathbf{q}\|_2.
\end{aligned} \qquad (24)$$

Here $\gamma\|\mathbf{p} - \mathbf{q}\|_2$ is a regularization term penalizing the deviation of each shrinkage function from the identity. Its purpose is to make the shape of the shrinkage functions more robust to outlier examples.

In order to minimize the function $\mathbf{\Gamma_p}(z)$ with respect to the argument $\mathbf{p}$, we use the memory-efficient ℓ-BFGS convex optimization method [23], which requires computing the value and the gradient of the function being minimized. The implementation of the algorithm is by the courtesy of Mark Schmidt (see http://www.di.ens.fr/mschmidt/Software/minFunc.html). Since our objective function is not

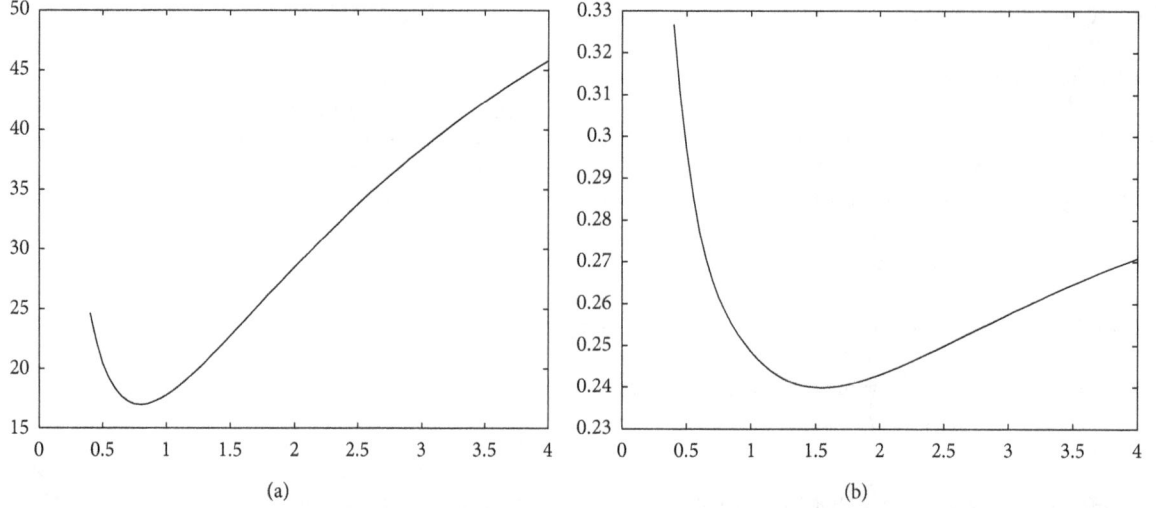

FIGURE 1: Graphs of the MSE values $\|f_0 - \tilde{f}\|_2^2$ (a) and the gradient penalty values $\mathbf{Q}(f_0, \tilde{f})$ (b) as a function of the cutoff frequency.

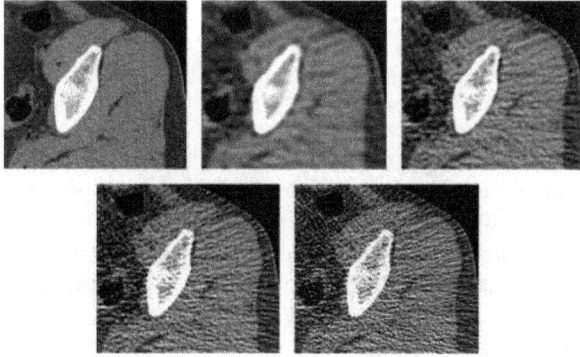

FIGURE 2: Left to right, upper to lower: reference image, FBP reconstructions obtained with low-pass filter with $\phi_0 = 0.4$ (very low), $\phi_0 = 0.8$ (optimal for MSE), $\phi_0 = 1.55$ (optimal for gradient-based measure $\mathbf{Q}(f_0, \tilde{f})$), and $\phi_0 = 4$ (very high).

convex, there is a theoretical question regarding the convergence of this numerical scheme. In practice, we have observed that the method converges in ~100 iterations, and the obtained parameter set enables producing CT images of a good quality (in comparison to other reconstruction methods).

The gradient of the function $\mathbf{G}_p(z)$ (defined in (11)) with respect to $\mathbf{p}$ can be expressed with the help of the slice transform proposed in [12]. Recall that $\alpha_k = \mathbf{D}^+ \mathbf{E}_k z$ is a representation of the kth patch in z. The shrinkage operation $\mathcal{S}_{\mathbf{p}} \alpha_k$ is replaced by an equivalent matrix-vector multiplication $U_{\mathbf{q}, \alpha_k} \mathbf{p}$. Then $\mathbf{G}_p(z)$ has the form

$$\mathbf{G}_{\mathbf{p}}(y) = \mathbf{M}_{\mathbf{E}}^{-1} \sum_k \mathbf{E}_k^\top \mathbf{D} U_{\mathbf{q}, \alpha_k} \mathbf{p}, \qquad (25)$$

which is linear in $\mathbf{p}$. Now, if we consider the estimator $\tilde{f}_{\mathbf{p}}(z)$ as a function of $\tilde{z} = \mathbf{G}_p(z)$, we see that this is a composition

of elementwise scalar function $-\log(1/\lambda_0)\omega^{-1}$ and the linear operator $\mathbf{T}$. Thus, the gradient here is also easily computed. Finally, the gradient of the functional MSEg with respect to $\tilde{f}$ consists of L_2 norms and derivative operators, so its expression is derived using standard methods. We conclude that the gradient $\nabla_{\mathbf{p}} \mathbf{\Gamma}_{\mathbf{p}}(z)$ has a closed-form analytical expression and can be readily computed.

The expressions presented above involve only one image f, just for a better readability; in practice, we may sum the errors over a training set of many images f.

Another important remark is this: when this training objective is used, the parameters of the shrinkage operator $\mathcal{S}_{\mathbf{p}}$ are tuned to not to reduce the photon count noise in the measured data y (via the processing of the adjusted data z) but to prepare the data in the best way for the specific reconstruction operator $\mathbf{T}$. Here lies the key difference between this algorithm and existing methods for measurements denoising, which target high signal quality in the raw data but do not consider the final CT image.

5.3. *Image Postprocessing*. At this point, after the preprocessing filter is tuned, we have a working reconstruction chain that produces CT images. The stated objective is pursued by its components somewhat indirectly, by changing the raw measurements. A further reduction of the reconstruction error can be achieved by administering another filter, acting on the obtained CT images themselves. We use again the method of learned shrinkage. The training data comprises of the set of CT images $\tilde{f}_{\mathbf{p}}(z)$, reconstructed from the original noisy measurements, as described before. The corresponding reference images serve again as the ground truth. Overlapping patches are extracted from an image, processed by the shrinkage functions in the transform domain and are reinstalled back. The noise statistics in the obtained CT images are difficult to estimate because of the preprocessing stage. Therefore, we do not attempt to normalize the noise in the image patches.

We formulate the training objective for the parameter set $\mathbf{p}^I$ of the image domain shrinkage similarl to the case of measurements domain:

$$
\begin{aligned}
\Gamma_{\mathbf{p}^I}^I \left(\tilde{f} \right) &= \mathrm{MSEg} \left(f, \mathbf{G}_{\mathbf{p}^I} \left(\tilde{f} \right) \right) + \gamma_I \left\| \mathbf{p}^I - \mathbf{q}^I \right\|_2 \\
&= \left\| f - \mathbf{G}_{\mathbf{p}^I} \left(\tilde{f} \right) \right\|_{2,\mathbf{H}}^2 + \mu \mathbf{Q} \left(f_0, \mathbf{G}_{\mathbf{p}^I} \left(\tilde{f} \right) \right) \quad (26) \\
&\quad + \gamma_I \left\| \mathbf{p}^I - \mathbf{q}^I \right\|_2 .
\end{aligned}
$$

Here the upper script I denotes the image domain. The input image $\tilde{f}$ is computed via the formula in (23) using the vector $\mathbf{p}$ of shrinkage parameters, learned earlier. This way the postprocessing is tuned for the very same kind of images it will be getting in the operational mode. As previously stated, the training stage consists of minimizing the value of $\Gamma_{\mathbf{p}^I}^I(\tilde{f})$ with respect to $\mathbf{p}^I$. This task is simpler than the optimization in the measurements' domain since no data adjustment or reconstruction is required. Using an expression for the gradient $\nabla_{\mathbf{p}^I} \Gamma^I$, we invoke again the ℓ-BFGS method to solve the optimization problem. The convergence here is faster than in the measurements domain, and it takes about 30 iterations to the convergence.

We remark that the postprocessing method could be evaluated in its own right, when the corrupted input images may come from the standard FBP or from any other reconstruction method. This evaluation is left for a future study.

5.4. The Training Set. The example-based training approach requires a collection of high quality reference images, each accompanied with a degraded set of measurements. It is preferable to compose the training set from clinical images obtained from a CT scan of a human body, rather than from images of synthetic phantoms. In any case, the example object has to be scanned twice: one time with a very high X-ray dose to compute a high-quality reference image (using standard FBP, for instance), and another time with the low dose desired for the practical scan performed on patients. This configuration is feasible with human cadavers: there is no restriction on the X-ray dosage, and there is no problem of registration between the two consecutive scans for a still object (in our experience, with a clinical scanner of General Electric). Another approach for producing the training pairs is to start with given high-quality CT slices and simulate the low-dose measurements by reproducing the machine's X-ray operation as faithfully as possible. This is the approach we took in our work.

We suggest that the training set should be composed of CT images representing a specific anatomical region. This is in light of the observation that the characteristics of CT images vary substantially between different such regions. This leads to building a collection of learned parameter sets, specialized for head, lungs, abdomen, arms, and so forth. During the reconstruction, the operator of the CT scanner should choose the relevant version of the parameter set, just like it is done today with the different smoothing filters for the standard FBP. Nevertheless, in our numerical experiments we also show that a filter specialized on one anatomic region also makes a good performance on other ones. A deeper study of dependence of the learned filter on the training set should be carried out by professional radiologists.

A training set we build for a specific anatomic region consists of a sequence of axial slices from that region, uniformly distributed in z-axis. The size of the training set is also a parameter to be investigated; we found that 9–12 images suffice for a stable optimization and a consecutive robust reconstruction of the thighs or the abdomen regions. However, in regions rich with small details where there are important but subtle differences between nearby slices (the brain, for instance) a larger collection of images is possibly required.

5.5. Computational Complexity. The number of operations required for the $n \times n$ image reconstruction with our algorithm is $\mathcal{O}(n^3)$, which is the same complexity as required by the regular FBP alone.

The measurements' matrix consists of $2n \times \sqrt{2}n = 2.82n^2$ elements. The learned shrinkage applied to the measurements consists in applying the analysis operator $\mathbf{D}^+$ at each patch of size $d \times d$, then applying the scalar shrinkage function on each of the d^2 coefficients and recomputing the patch by a multiplication with $\mathbf{D}$. The dictionary $\mathbf{D}$ we use is the unitary 2D discrete cosine transform (DCT), which requires $\mathcal{O}(2d^2 \log(d))$ operations. We use patches of size $d = 11$; thus, computing a representation of each patch requires about $2d^2 \log(d) = 580$ operations and the same amount of work to convert the representation back to the signal. Further, applying a shrinkage function takes $\mathcal{O}(c \cdot d^2)$ operations, where the constant c is about 20, governed by the length of the vector $\mathbf{q}$ in (10). The number of patches, extracted from an $n \times n$ image, depends on the chosen amount of overlapping; up to n^2 patches can be processed. To summarize, the application of the learned shrinkage filter has the computational complexity of $\mathcal{O}(4c \cdot n^2 d^2 (\log(d) + 1))$. The standard size of clinical CT images is $n = 512$, so the number $d^2(\log(d) + 1)$ is of the same order of magnitude as n (for $d = 11$, this number equals 822). Therefore, it takes about $80n^3$ operations, which is comparable to the $\mathcal{O}(n^3)$ complexity of the FBP transform.

We notice that the processing of individual patches can be naturally parallelized on multiple core or GPU, reducing the computation time by a nonnegligible factor (depending on the available hardware).

6. Empirical Study

6.1. Experimental Setup. The algorithm was implemented using the Matlab environment and tested on sets of clinical CT images (axial slices). These were extracted from a CT scan of a male, from regions of the head, abdomen, and thighs. The images are courtesy of the Visible Human Project (See http://www.nlm.nih.gov/research/visible/visible_human .html). The images are of dimensions 512 × 512, acquired with 1 mm intervals along the z-axis. The intensity levels

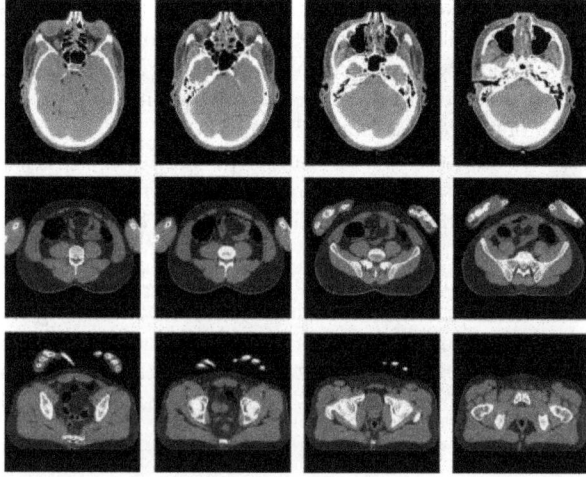

FIGURE 3: Examples of clinical images used in the experiments. Upper row: axial head slices displayed in the range (HU window) of $[-170, 250]$), middle row: abdomen images, lower row: thigh images. The two lower rows are displayed in the HU window $[-220, 350]$. Head images are slightly enlarged relative to other regions for better visibility.

correspond to Hounsfield units (HU), given with the accuracy of 12 bits per pixel. Representatives of these sets we have assembled are displayed in Figure 3. We wish to point out that the reference images used for the training stage are not perfect since they were obtained using a standard X-ray dosage. If very-high-quality images were available for the training, we would expect our algorithm to perform better.

In absence of raw measurements' data from a CT scanner we simulate the scan process by computing projections of given CT images (considered to be the ground truth) as follows. First, the intensity values in the image are converted from the Hounsfield units to the units of reciprocal length, corresponding to the linear attenuation coefficient μ. The relation between the two scales is (http://www.medcyclopaedia.com/library/topics/volume_i/ h/hounsfield_unit.aspx/)

$$\text{HU}(x) = \frac{\mu(x) - \mu(\text{water})}{\mu(\text{water}) - \mu(\text{air})} \cdot 1000, \qquad (27)$$

where $\mu(\text{water}) = 0.19 \, \text{cm}^{-1}$, $\mu(\text{air}) = 0 \, \text{cm}^{-1}$. The original 512×512 images are cropped to dimensions 461×461 by removing the empty background (to save computation time). Then, noiseless sinogram $\overline{g} = \mathbf{R}f$ is simulated by applying to the reference image a pixel-driven implementation of the discrete 2D Radon transform. The algorithm for forward- and back projection uses linear interpolation in the locations of bins/pixels. Explicitly, each bin in a projection is a weighted sum of a few (temporary) finer bins, which are computed by integrating image intensities over a narrow (quarter of a pixel) ray in the image domain. The weights are linear in the distance between the center of the coarse bin and the centers of the fine bins.

For $n \times n$ images, we have used n views (projections), evenly distributed over the angle range $[0, \pi]$. Each projection

consists of $\sqrt{2}n$ bins. Ideal photon counts are computed from the sinogram entries via the relation $\lambda_\ell = \lambda_0 e^{-\overline{g}_\ell}$. The measured photon counts y_ℓ are produced by generating random Poisson variables with expectations λ_ℓ and zero-mean Gaussian variables with a chosen standard deviation σ_n. The X-ray dose is controlled by the maximal photon count λ_0 and the value of σ_n.

The design parameters of the proposed algorithm are set as follows. The filter, based on the learned shrinkage, is implemented using the 2D unitary discrete cosine transform (DCT) (see Figure 5). It is implemented using d^2 elements composing a linear basis, which are matrices of dimensions $d \times d$. The representation of a $d \times d$ signal is computed as the set of inner products between the signal and each basis element. This approach allows computing the representation of the entire collection of image patches in a batch, by convolving the image with each basis element. In our work we set $d = 11$.

Each of the 121 corresponding shrinkage functions of the operator $\mathcal{S}_\mathbf{p}$ consists of 2×20 linear pieces (the factor of 2 is for the negative and the positive parts; recall that the shrinkage functions are antisymmetric by design, so there is just 20 degrees of freedom); this number was established empirically and is similar to the one used in [12]. Graphs of shrinkage functions, obtained in one of the training sessions, are displayed in Figure 4. The regularization parameters in (24), (26) were set to $\gamma = 10^{-4}$, $\gamma_I = 250$. Use of the regularization has helped to constrain the shapes of the pre- and postprocessing shrinkage functions, avoiding jumps resulting from outlier samples. We discuss the process of their tuning in the sequel.

We mention that numerical experiments were also carried out with the nondecimated 3-level Haar Wavelet frame, but they are not presented here due to slightly inferior results (comparing to those obtained with the DCT). However, our impression is that a particular choice of the transform is not of a crucial importance. Another remark we shall make concerns the redundancy of the dictionary. We have compared the performance of the algorithm using the unitary DCT against its version with an overcomplete DCT. In our experiments, no improvement was induced by this change.

6.2. Implementation of the Existing Algorithms. We implement three existing reconstruction algorithms. First is the standard FBP, with the classical noise reduction done by a sinogram smoothing. Second is an iterative, statistically-based algorithm, approximating the penalized likelihood solution; specifically, it is the penalized weighted least squares (PWLS), proposed in [6]. The third method is the adaptive truncated median (ATM) filter [8]. It is close in its spirit to our work—a fast nonlinear preprocessing method, designed to improve the performance of FBP in a low-dose scan scenario.

6.2.1. Implementation of the FBP Algorithm. The FBP was realized according to the following formula:

$$\mathbf{T} = \mathbf{R}^* \circ \mathbf{F}_{\text{low}} \circ \mathbf{F}_{\text{RL}}. \qquad (28)$$

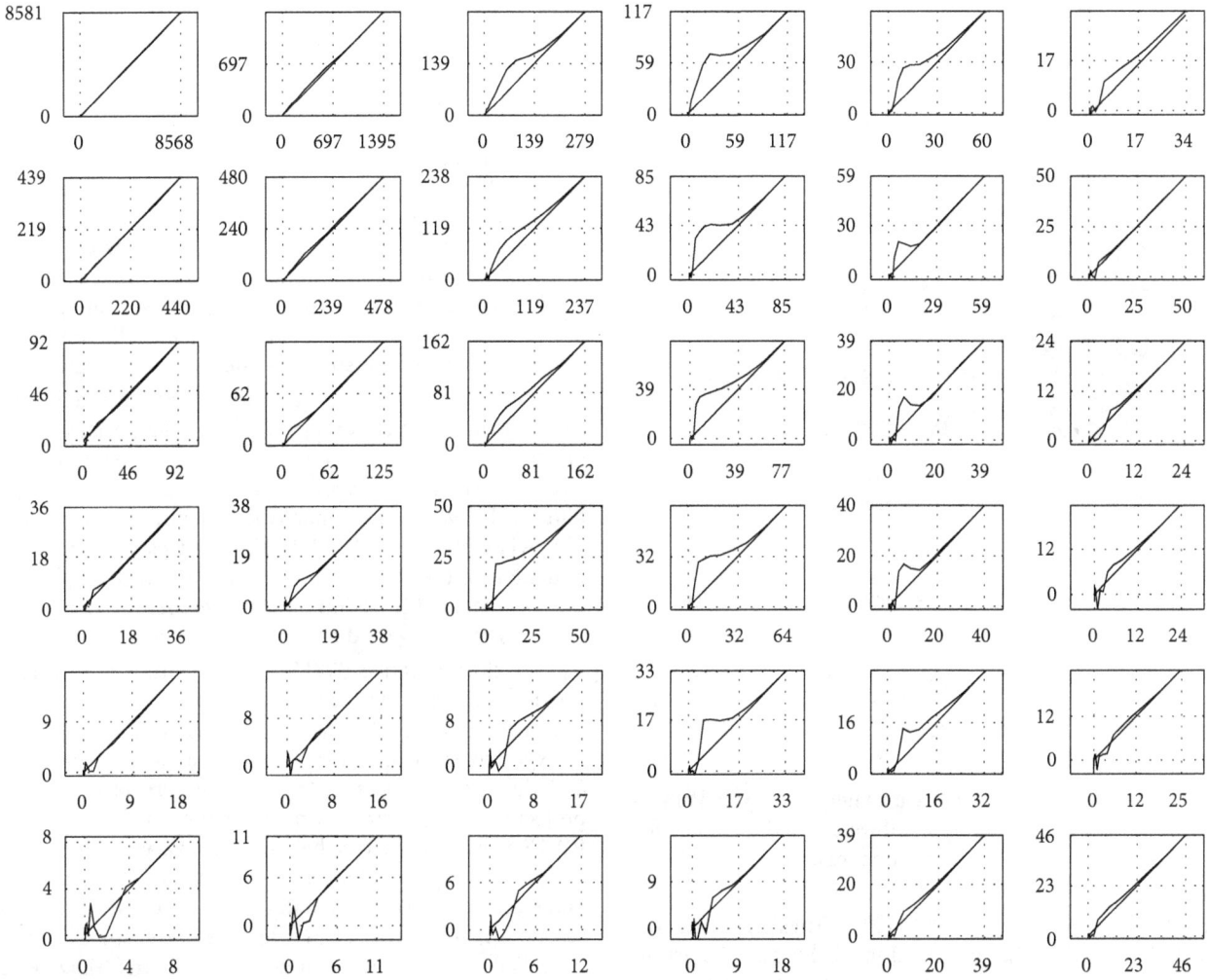

FIGURE 4: Shrinkage functions obtained via the learning process on a training set consisting of male thighs images. Only the odd rows and columns from the original 11×11 array of functions are displayed due to space considerations. Due to the antisymmetry, only the positive half of the x-axis is drawn.

$\mathbf{F}_{RL}$ is a convolution filter with the discrete Ram-Lak kernel κ of m taps, computed via the following formula ([24, equation (5.5)]):

$$\kappa(p) = \operatorname{sinc}(p) - \frac{1}{2}\left(\operatorname{sinc}\left(\frac{p}{2}\right)\right)^2, \quad p = -\frac{m}{2} : \frac{m}{2}, \tag{29}$$

$$\operatorname{sinc}(x) = \frac{\sin(x)}{x}.$$

The low-pass filter $\mathbf{F}_{low}$ is implemented by composing the Ram-Lak filter with the Butterworth window [25] in the Fourier domain. An expression for this window is

$$|H(\omega)| = \left(1 + \left(\frac{\omega}{\phi_0}\right)^{2p}\right)^{-1/2}. \tag{30}$$

The two defining parameters are the cutoff frequency ϕ_0, which controls the frequency response of the filter and the order p, which affects the steepness of its roll-off. In the experiments, these two parameters are tuned manually for

the best visual impression on the training set (this issue is discussed in the sequel).

6.2.2. Implementation of the PWLS Algorithm. We used the objective function stated in Equation (14) of [6], which represents an approximation to the log-likelihood function of the CT image $\tilde{f}$, with an addition of a penalty component $R_\delta(\tilde{f})$. In our notation it is stated as follows:

$$L(y \mid \tilde{f}) = \frac{1}{2}\sum_\ell W_\ell\left([\mathbf{R}\tilde{f}]_\ell - g_\ell\right)^2 + \gamma R_\delta(\tilde{f}), \quad \text{where}$$

$$W_\ell = \frac{y_\ell^2}{y_\ell + \sigma_n^2}, \quad g_\ell = -\log\frac{y_\ell}{\lambda_0}. \tag{31}$$

The expression for the regularization is

$$R(\tilde{f}) = \sum_p \sum_{k \in \mathcal{N}(p)} \psi\left(\tilde{f}_p - \tilde{f}_k\right). \tag{32}$$

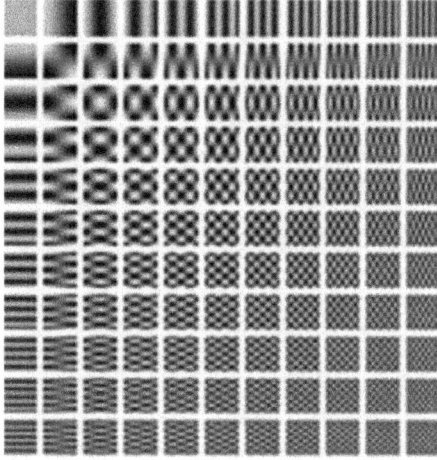

FIGURE 5: Two-dimensional discrete cosines basis. Each square in the 11×11 array is a 2D function representing a basis element.

Here $\psi(x)$ is the convex edge-preserving Huber penalty

$$\psi(x, \delta) = \begin{cases} \dfrac{x^2}{2}, & x < \delta \\ \delta |x| - \dfrac{\delta^2}{2}, & x \geq \delta \end{cases} \tag{33}$$

and $\mathcal{N}(p)$ is the set of the four nearest neighbors of p. Parameters γ, δ of the penalty component were tuned manually for best the visual impression on training images.

6.2.3. Implementation of the ATM Filter. The ATM filter was briefly described in the introduction. Technically, its action on a location p in a signal S is defined by two parameters: the number M of data values in the neighborhood of p, involved in the filtering and the fraction α of outliers assumed in this data. The filtered value at p is computed as the average of this neighborhood, taken after removing the $M\alpha$ highest and the $M\alpha$ lowest values. This filter is made adaptive by using data-dependent parameters M and α, computed for each location of the measurements matrix. The formulas for ATM parameters, given in [8], involve the signal value (photon count) $x = S(p)$:

$$M = \frac{2\beta\lambda}{2\lambda + \max(0, x - \delta)}, \qquad \alpha = \frac{\alpha_m x}{\lambda}. \tag{34}$$

In [8] it is not specified what is the shape of the neighborhood of the pixel p, involved in its filtering. In our implementation, we assume it is a discrete disc. Also, no method for computing the inner parameters β, λ, δ, α_m is proposed; a set of prescribed values is given instead. In our implementation, these parameters are tuned to minimize the net MSE on the training set, by sweeping two-dimensional grids, built for different pairs of parameters. This is done in iterations, each time a different pair out of the four parameters is changed.

6.3. Visual Evaluation and Comparison of the Algorithms. The existing and proposed methods are compared on the

reconstruction of a test image of thighs' section. The noise on the projection data was generated by setting $\lambda_0 = 1.5 \cdot 10^5$, $\sigma_n = 5$. The visual comparison of is given in Figure 7, where the corresponding reconstructed images are presented. We display an enlarged region of the image, for better observability. The displayed dynamic range is set to $[-220, 350]$ Hounsfield units (HU), chosen for best visualization of the particular axial slice. In general, there is no predefined HU-window radiologists use to look at the CT images; the window is tuned manually in an interactive fashion, and it depends on the anatomical region, diagnostic purposes, and personal preferences. The reference image is depicted in Figure 6 in few different windows to display the effect of such tuning.

The FBP image (Figure 7, lower right) suffers from streak artifacts, which corrupt its content—especially, the fine details. The strength of the artifacts can be reduced at the cost of blurring the image; here the strength of the low-pass filter in FBP was tuned manually for visually plausible images. The ATM algorithm (middle right) displays a significant reduction in the strength of the streaks, which implies that most outliers in the Radon domain were removed. However, some residual noise and detailed corruption are still present.

The slow, iterative PWLS algorithm (upper row, right) provides a better version of the image, with improved sharpness and complete lack of streaks. The latter property is expected since the image is built as a MAP optimizer and there is no smear of the raw-data errors by the back projection. Still, there is a noise texture in the image. The PWLS performance can be tuned by varying the penalty weight, Huber parameter, and the number of iterations. These parameters were set manually to produce a high spatial resolution, at the cost of manageable noise; specifically, we used 90 iterations, and the value $\gamma = 8 \cdot 10^{-5}$ in (31). Different, MSE-optimized reconstructions by the compared methods are given in Figure 16.

Finally, we refer to the two images produced by our method. The stage-I image (lower left) was obtained by applying the FBP to the preprocessed data. The postprocessing of this image results in the stage-II version (middle left). The FBP streaks are significantly reduced in stage-I image, similarl to the ATM method; however, some of the streaks are sharply visible around the bone area. The reason for their appearance is that the filter is not removing all of the problematic streak effects; since our method is based on FBP, some of its artifacts remain. Moreover, they are better visible on resulting the image due to reduced background noise and lack of the rest of the streaks. We should note that the general noise level is visibly lower than that appearing in the rest of the images. The noise is further reduced in stage-II image, without introducing additional blur.

The error images are displayed in Figure 8. With our method (stage II), the error image has less of the uniform noise than any of the three compared methods, and the edges appearing in the error image (they point to the loss of spatial resolution) are as weak as those observed in the PWLS reconstruction.

In Table 1, some quantitative measures of reconstruction quality are provided. The signal-to-noise Ratio (SNR) is

TABLE 1: Quantitative measures for the compared algorithms.

Method	FBP	ATM	PWLS	Shrinkage
Thighs				
MSEg =				
MSE + grad	16.12 + 11.64	11.81 + 12.54	7.98 + 5.31	6.99 + 11.17
MSEg total	27.76	14.35	13.29	18.16
SNR (dB)	26.56	28.70	29.56	30.73
SSIM	0.8643	0.9124	0.9219	0.9398
Abdomen				
MSEg =				
MSE + grad	14.96 + 6.88	11.78 + 6.73	7.12 + 7.49	6.80 + 7.18
MSEg total	21.83	18.52	14.61	13.99
SNR (dB)	26.42	27.34	29.53	30.41
SSIM	0.8832	0.8985	0.9326	0.9483
Head				
MSEg =				
MSE + grad	6.99 + 11.40	6.99 + 11.39	3.31 + 7.99	2.77 + 6.38
MSEg total	18.40	18.38	11.30	9.15
SNR (dB)	30.84	30.84	31.94	33.74
SSIM	0.9764	0.9764	0.9783	0.9864

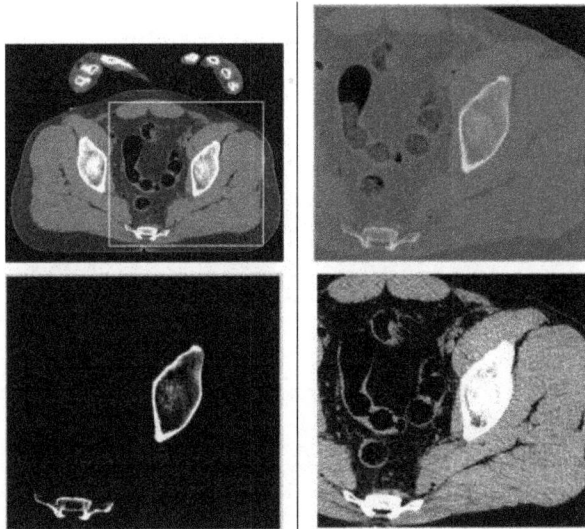

FIGURE 6: Left to right, upper to lower: test image with a marked zoom-in window, a zoom-in region depicted in dynamic ranges $[-1000, 1500]$, $[100, 700]$, $[-100, 150]$ HU, respectively. Yet another version of this image appears in Figure 7 (upper left), in $[-220, 350]$ HU.

defined for the ideal signal f and a deteriorated version $\hat{f}$ by $\text{SNR}(f, \hat{f}) = -20 \log_{10}(\|f - \hat{f}\|_2/\|f\|_2)$. In practice, we consider the signal $\hat{f}$ up to a multiplicative constant and compute

$$\text{SNR}\left(f, \hat{f}\right) = \min_{\alpha} -20 \log_{10}\left(\frac{\|f - \alpha\hat{f}\|_2}{\|f\|_2}\right). \quad (35)$$

The structured similarity (SSIM) measure was introduced in [26] as an alternative to MSE which is more relevant to human perception of the images. The explicit formula involves first and second moments of the local image statistics and the correlation between the two compared images. In our numerical experiments, we have used the Matlab code provided by the authors of [26], which is available at http://www.cns.nyu.edu/~lcv/ssim/.

Finally, the MSEg measure is introduced in this paper, (19).

The SNR and MSEg values are measured in the range of $[-220, 350]$ (HU). The MSEg value is detailed as a sum of the MSE component and the gradient-based component in order to show the balance between the two factors in the different cases. All three of the computed measure consistently point to the gradual quality improvement as one passes from FBP to ATM and to PWLS and finally to the proposed method.

To appreciate the effect of the postprocessing (stage II of our method), we display the absolute-valued difference between the two stages in Figure 9. Almost no structure can be observed in this error image, and this implies that very little of the image content is lost during the postprocessing.

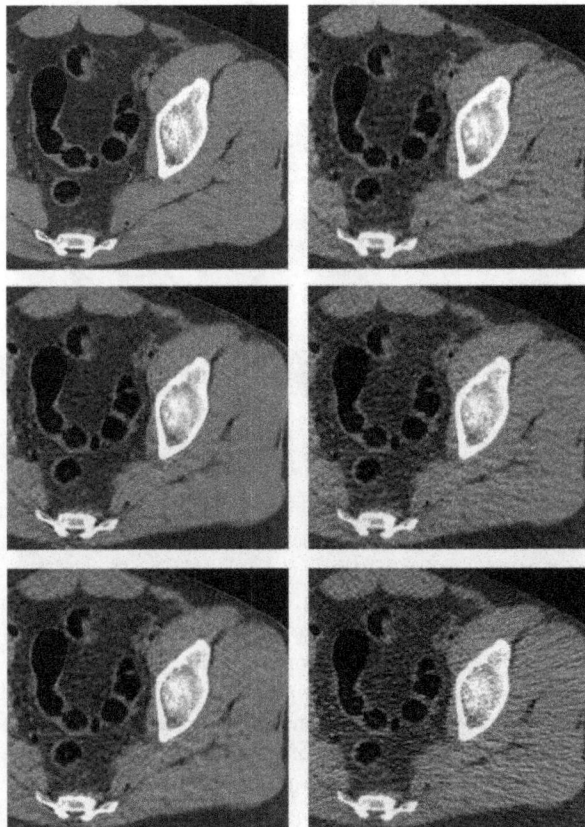

FIGURE 7: Reconstruction of a test image (thighs' section). Images are listed left to right and displayed in HU range of $[-220, 350]$. Upper row: reference image, PWLS. Middle row: our method (stage II), ATM. Lower row: our method (stage I), FBP.

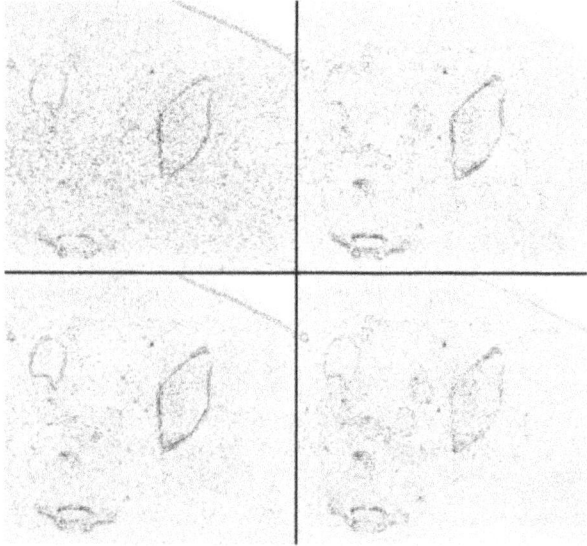

FIGURE 8: Absolute-valued differences between the reconstructions and the reference image. Darker shade corresponds to a larger error. Left to right, upper to lower: FBP, PWLS, ATM, and our method (stage II).

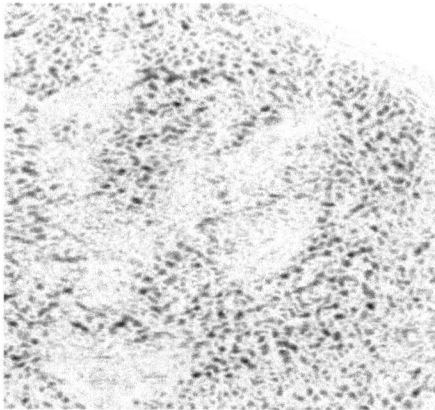

FIGURE 9: Absolute-valued difference between stage-I and stage-II of our method.

6.4. Behavior in Different Anatomical Regions.

An important issue of the example-based training approach is the dependence of the reconstruction quality on the training set and the anatomical region. Recall that the reference images for training were taken from the thighs' region; we now use the trained shrinkage functions to restore axial head and abdomen sections. The compared reconstruction methods are also applied (without changing their parameters) to the new regions. The results are displayed in Figures 10–13. The test image from the head region, along with some other examples of head sections, is given in Figure 10. In the FBP reconstruction (Figure 11, lower right), the quality of the fine details is reduced due to the streak noise; both PWLS (upper right) and our method (middle and lower left) exhibit better restoration of these details (see, for instance, the thin vein-like lines on the left and right sides of the image, as well as

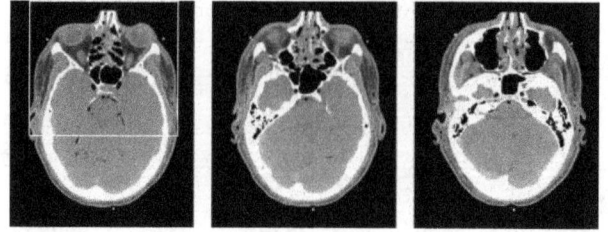

FIGURE 10: Few example images of head sections. The marked region in the test image (on the left) is zoomed on in Figure 11.

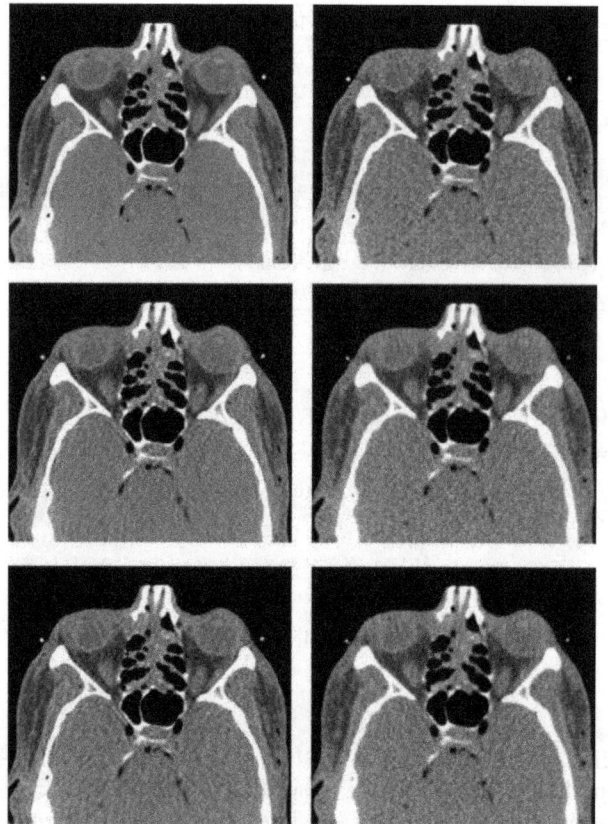

FIGURE 11: Head reconstruction. Images are listed left to right and displayed in HU range of [−170, 250]. First row: reference image, PWLS. Second row: our method (stage II), ATM. Third row: our method (stage I), FBP.

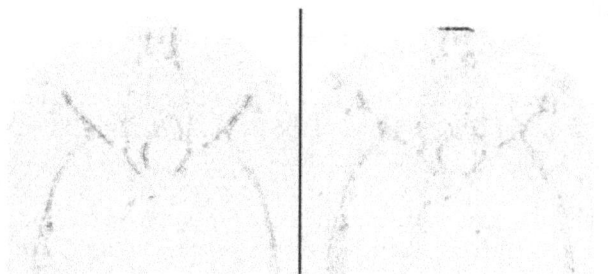

FIGURE 12: Head reconstruction errors with respect to the reference image (darker shade corresponds to a larger error). Left: PWLS, right: our method (stage II).

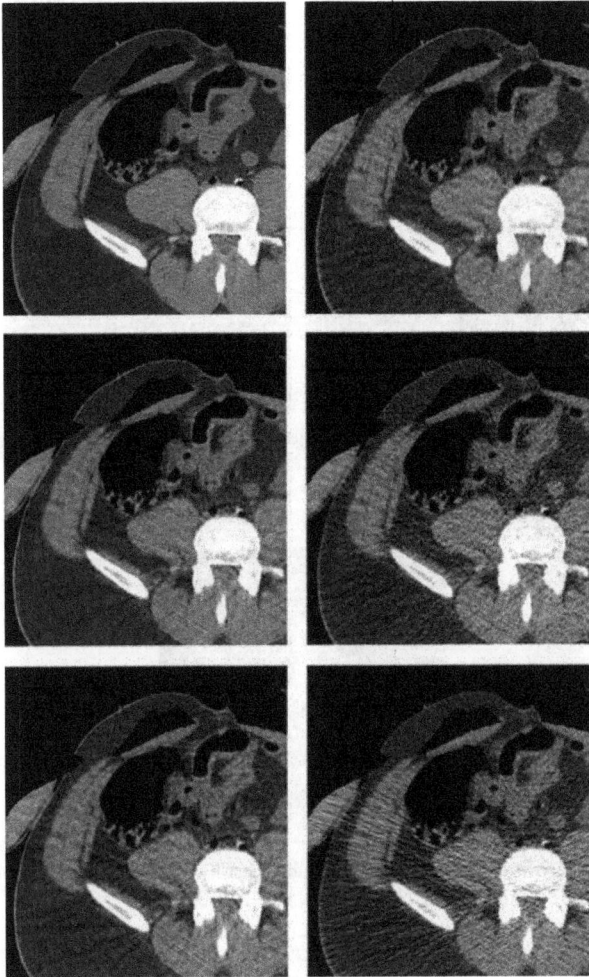

FIGURE 14: Abdomen reconstruction errors with respect to the reference image (darker shade corresponds to a larger error). Left: PWLS, right: our method (stage II).

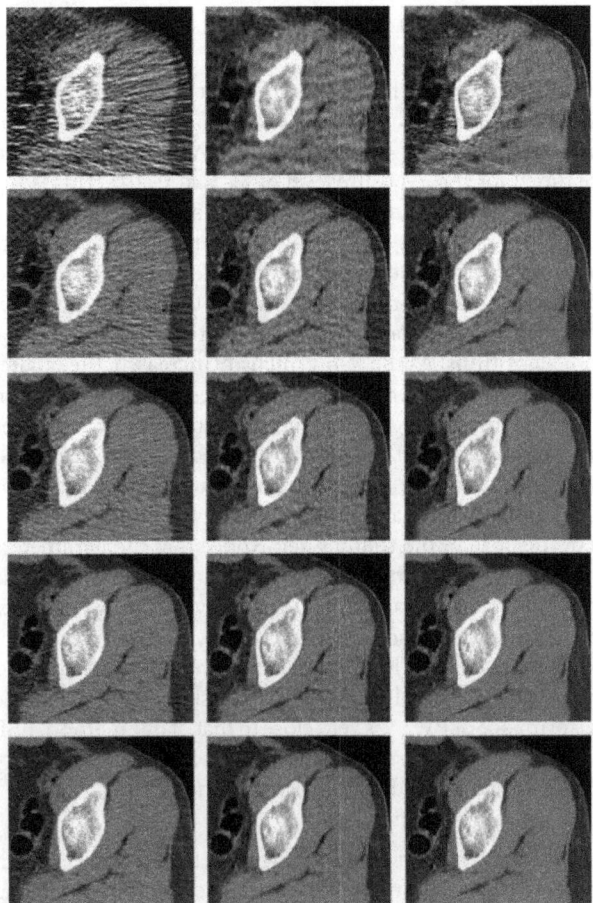

FIGURE 13: Abdomen reconstruction. Images are listed left to right and displayed in HU range of $[-220, 350]$. First row: reference image, PWLS. Second row: our method (stage II), ATM. Third row: our method (stage I), FBP.

the small bright spots in the upper central region). With our method the noise texture still exhibits streaks (since this is an FBP-based method), but the noise energy is lower than that in the PWLS, which is reflected in higher SNR value. The parameters of the ATM method should apparently be different for the head scan data since the resulting image is almost the same as the FBP without preprocessing. We conclude that ATM is sensitive to the choice of an anatomical region and has to be tuned using relevant training sets. Quantitative measures, presented in Table 1, also show the similarity between FBP and ATM images and point to improved quality of images produced by the shrinkage method. An exception is the MSEg measurement in the thighs' image, where the PWLS achieves a lower value of the gradient-based penalty.

In the abdomen image reconstruction (Figure 13) the ATM performs better than the FBP but both ATM and PWLS do not succeed to reduce the noise like the shrinkage method does. Figures 12 and 14 depict the reconstruction error for the PWLS and our algorithm (other methods are omitted here out of space economy) and support the observations above.

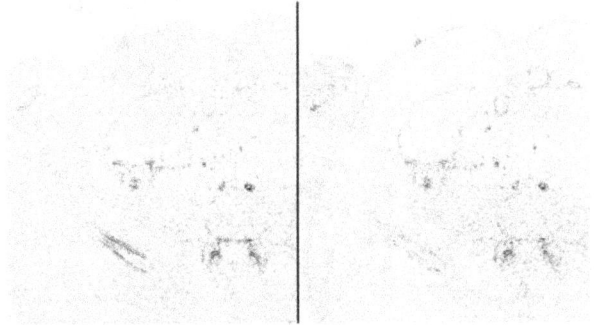

FIGURE 15: Columns, left to right: reconstruction by FBP, PWLS, and stage-II of our method. Rows, upper to lower: increasing signal energy corresponding to exposure levels of $\lambda_0 = [3 \cdot 10^4, 9.5 \cdot 10^4, 3 \cdot 10^5, 9.5 \cdot 10^5, 3 \cdot 10^6]$.

6.5. *Behavior at Different Noise Levels.* The impact of noise level on reconstruction quality is demonstrated via an array of images in Figure 15 with FBP, PWLS, and our method. Table 2 contains the standard quality measures—MSE and SSIM values for each noise level. The X-ray dose is increased exponentially from $\lambda_0 = 3 \cdot 10^4$ to $\lambda_0 = 3 \cdot 10^6$ (first to last

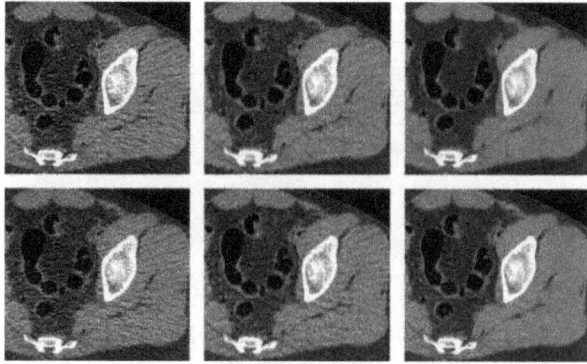

FIGURE 16: Upper row, left to right: reconstructions optimized for SNR values—FBP (28.5 dB), PWLS (30.6 dB), our method (31.41 dB). Lower row: reconstruction with higher spatial resolution—FBP (26.5 dB), PWLS (29.6 dB), our method (30.73 dB).

rows in the figure), which results in linear improvement of the visual perception. The parameters of FBP were adjusted for each noise level; the parameters of the PWLS and our method are tuned for the exposure level of $\lambda_0 = 1.5 \cdot 10^5$. This is the noise level used to simulate the training set in our algorithm.

In the strongest noise (row 1), our approach exhibits more streaks than the PWLS version since it is an FBP-based method (because our methods was not trained for this level of noise). In other cases the visual impression is similar for both algorithms. As the X-ray intensity increased, the quality of images produced by our method rises promptly to attain a nearly perfect image at the highest exposure. This testifies for the robustness of the training procedure with respect to noise level since the reconstruction results are adequate for X-ray doses which are either significantly higher or lower than the dose in the training set. Notice that the parameters of the PWLS algorithm are not optimal for the lowest noise level, where an oversmoothing is observed. The SNR values of PWLS images lead the charts at very low and very high exposure levels, while in rows 2, 3 of the table our method shows superior results. The SSIM measure implies that the performance of PWLS is very close to that of our method. FBP is comparable to these two algorithms at high X-ray intensity and is way below in the low-dose scenario.

6.6. Aiming for Lowest MSE. Now we return to the question of whether MSE is an error measure relevant to radiological images. The images, presented earlier in Figure 7, were obtained by tuning the algorithms for high spatial resolution, at the price of noise level and the SNR value. Here we display three algorithms—FBP, PWLS, and our method—with parameters optimized for maximal SNR (we were not able to control the ATM filter behavior that way). With FBP, it is achieved by tuning the cut-off frequency of its sinogram filter; for PWLS, we have increased the weight of the Huber penalty component. Our method is manipulated by tuning the weight μ of the gradient-based component in (24), (26). In the upper row of Figure 16, reconstruction of the test image by those three methods with SNR-optimized parameters is displayed. The lower row contains the image versions from

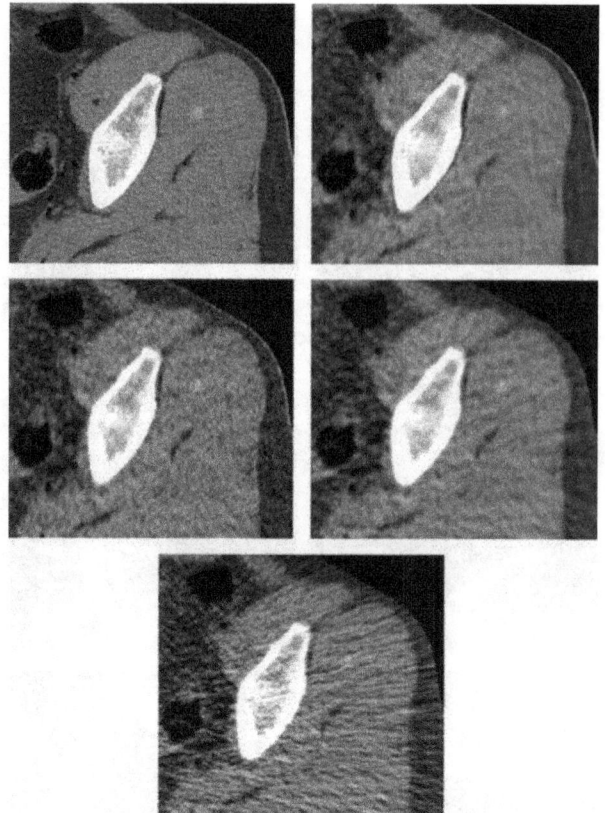

FIGURE 17: Detectability test for a small inserted lesion. Upper to lower rows, right to left: reference image, our method, PWLS, ATM, and FBP images. The HU window is [−220, 350].

Figure 7; they were produced with parameters optimized for visual perception. Specifically, the spatial resolution was improved at expense of a tolerable additional noise. This display is given to show the tradeoff between the noise reduction and spatial resolution and visualize our stimulus in pursuing the latter virtue rather than the former.

6.7. Detecting Lesions in Noisy Images. A lesion detectability experiment is designed as follows: we add a small disk-shaped blob in the homogeneous region of test image. The average intensity of the lesion is 105 HU on the background tissue of average 54 HU. The experiment is conducted in conditions of strong noise, concealing the lesion spot in the FBP reconstruction. Explicitly, it corresponds to $\lambda_0 = 7 \cdot 10^4$ photons. In Figure 17 the reconstruction of a region, containing the lesion, is displayed. We compare our algorithm with the PWLS, ATM, and the FBP. The parameters of the learned shrinkage were trained offline on the training data with the same noise energy; the PWLS and ATM were used with the same parameters as earlier for the following reasons. For PWLS, a manual tuning of the smoothing weight did not result in any improvement of visibility. For ATM, there is no intuitive way to change the four parameters for a higher noise level. The FBP was used with same cut-off frequency but higher order of the Butterworth window, which made the lesion more observable.

TABLE 2: Quantitative measures corresponding to the image array in Figure 15. The SNR is measured in HU window of $[-220, 350]$.

Noise level λ_0	FBP		PWLS		Shrinkage	
	SNR	SSIM	SNR	SSIM	SNR	SSIM
$3 \cdot 10^4$	21.87	0.75	27.82	0.90	25.39	0.86
$9.5 \cdot 10^4$	26.53	0.86	28.97	0.91	29.88	0.92
$3 \cdot 10^5$	28.86	0.91	30.59	0.93	31.65	0.94
$9.5 \cdot 10^5$	30.67	0.93	32.62	0.95	32.43	0.95
$3 \cdot 10^6$	32.29	0.95	33.93	0.96	32.85	0.96

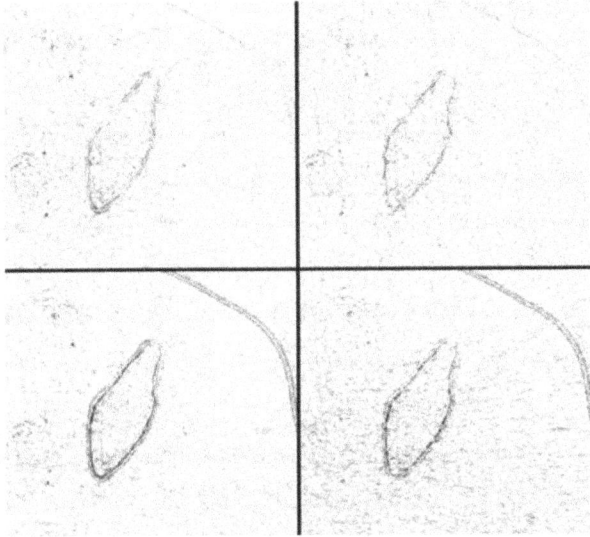

FIGURE 18: Error maps for the lesion detectability test, built with respect to the reference image. Upper to lower rows, left to right: our method, PWLS, ATM, and FBP images. Darker shade corresponds to higher error. The lesion is not observed in any version, which means it is recovered correctly by all the methods; however, in FBP image the lesion is obscured by streaks.

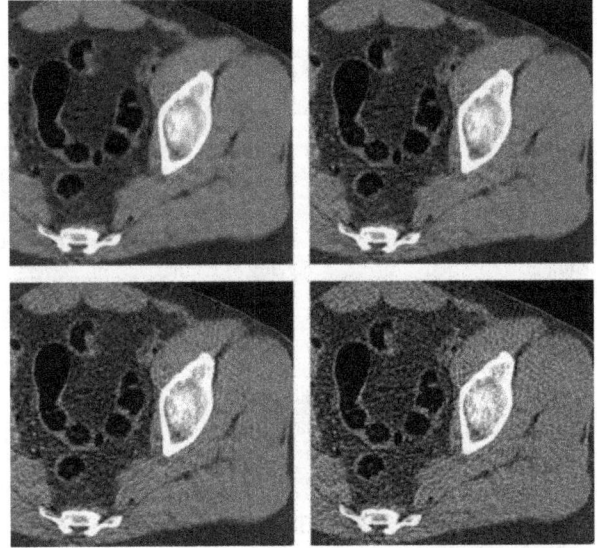

FIGURE 19: Reconstruction with learned shrinkage trained with the different values of the weight μ. Upper to lower rows, left to right: images corresponding to $\mu = [14.3, 105.6, 205.5, 400]$.

One can observe that the synthetic lesion (no similar structure was present in the training data) is recovered correctly and, in contrast with the FBP image, it can be clearly observed. PWLS produces an image which is more sharp and noisy than our result, and the ATM image is of a lower quality. The error images in Figure 18 (difference between the reconstruction and the reference) imply that the noise in the image produced by our method is lower than that in the PWLS reconstruction (this experiment is also the chance to compare the algorithms at a stronger noise). The lesion is not observed in any error image which means it is not lost in reconstruction; the problem with FBP is not that it fails to recover the lesion but the high streak-shaped noise obscuring it.

6.8. Design Parameters of the Proposed Method. We now study the impact of various parameters appearing in the reconstruction chain. First we consider the objective function in (24). The weight μ controls the influence of the gradient-based component; when set to zero, the training leads to best MSE reduction. The influence of this component on the

visual appearance of the image is observed in Figure 19. The presented sequence of images corresponds to values (these values are a subset of an exponential sequence of the μ range, swept in a numerical experiment. We chose these four values because they provide visibly different reconstructions.) $\mu = [14.3, 105.6, 205.5, 400]$. As μ grows, the blur, introduced by the reconstruction, is reduced; however, new artifacts arise. They result from strong influence of the gradient-based component. After a finer tuning we chose to use $\mu = 100$, which produces the most visually appealing image. Its sharpness is near best, and artifacts are on the level of background noise. For real-life application, a more elaborate study by a radiologist may be needed to tune this parameter for clinical needs.

Another aspect of the training process is the regularization weights γ in (24) and γ_I in (26), which restrict the deviation of the shrinkage functions from identity. In general, using such regularization is a good practice to increase the robustness of the method by preventing the overfitting. Also, this helps reducing the impact of outlier examples on the shape of shrinkage functions. In our experiments, the influence of those regularization terms was not significant: when the weights γ, γ_I are decreased, the effect of learned shrinkage becomes stronger but no negative phenomena

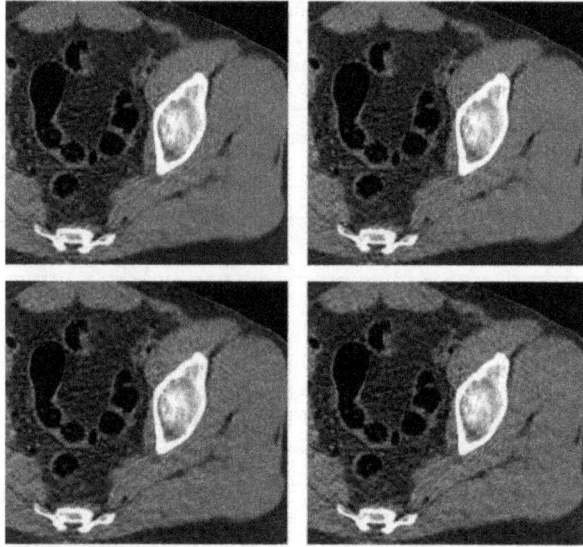

FIGURE 20: Left to right: reconstruction with learned shrinkage trained using varying regularization weight, $\gamma_I = [0.001, 0.0032, 0.0316, 0.1]$.

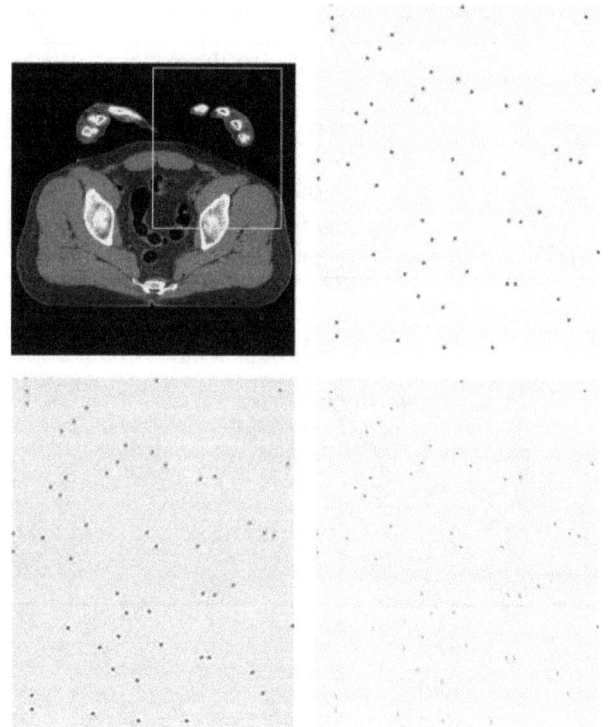

FIGURE 21: Upper left: reference image with added spikes. The LIR maps are shown in the marked region. Upper right: LIRs obtained with FBP reconstruction. Lower row, left to right: LIR maps obtained with our algorithm and the PWLS.

appear. This is observed in Figure 20, where a number of versions of a test image, associated with different values of γ_I, are shown.

6.9. Local Impulse Response. The evaluation of spatial resolution in the CT images is carried out by computing the local impulse responses (LIR) of the projection-reconstruction operator in the image domain. The reference image is projected twice, one time in its original form and another with a random set of 212 single-pixel implants, scattered randomly in the image. The intensity of the implants is set to the maximal value present in the image. In Figure 21 we display an example region in a test image with added spikes and the corresponding maps of LIRs obtained by subtracting the two reconstructions—with and without spikes—by the compared methods. All the parameters of the compared methods are set as in the very first experiment. For each method, the full-width half-maximum (FWHM) measure is computed in all the locations and averaged. It is defined as follows: first, a 2-D image patch containing the response spot is resized into a ×16 larger image in order to reduce the discretization effect. Then, the number of pixels, which intensity is higher than half of the maximal value in the patch, is counted and divided by the refinement factor of 16.

The computation was done for FBP, PLWS, and our algorithm. An average FWHM value produced by stage I of our method is 2.11 pixels; the resolution is slightly improved to 2.06 pixels by the stage II. Notice that this postprocessing step simultaneously reduces the noise and increases the image sharpness; this virtue is attributed to the design of our error measure. The FBP exhibits the same average FWHM value—2.04 pixels. In Figure 21 both FBP and our method are seen to produce disk-shaped LIRs without distortions everywhere in the image. The situation is different with the data-adaptive PWLS, which achieves lower FWHM values—1.61 pixels on

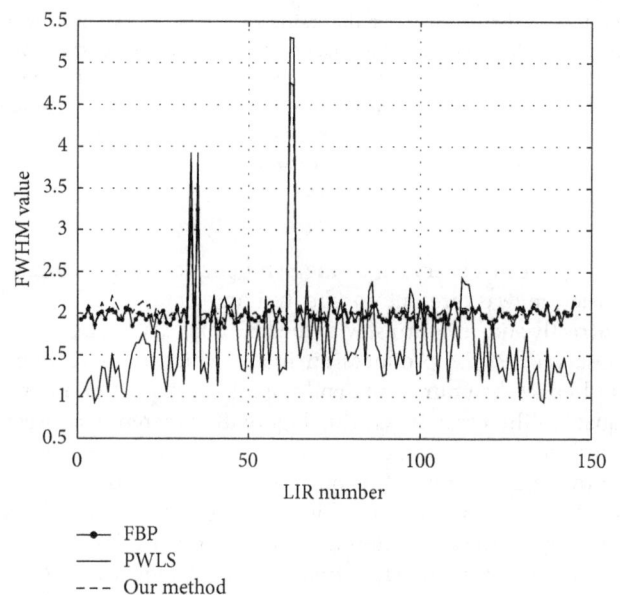

FIGURE 22: FWHM values in 212 random image locations.

average—but displays an anisotropic smearing of the spikes. The graphs of FWHM values for all the LIRs are given in the Figure 22.

6.10. Effective X-Ray Dose Reduction. The reduction of noise and artifacts enables, effectively, reduction of the X-ray dose

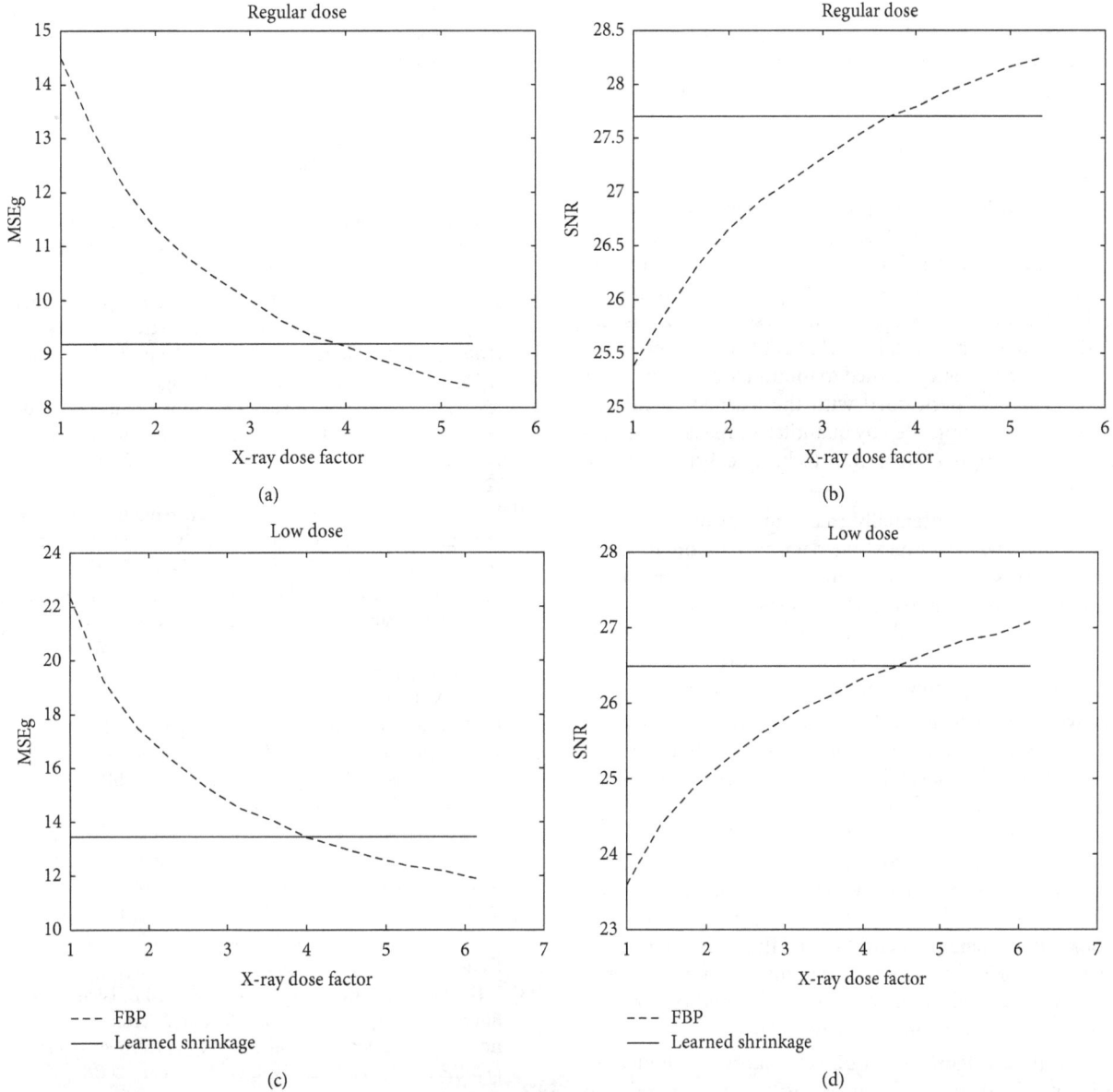

FIGURE 23: Effective dose reduction by the proposed method, with respect to the optimally tuned FBP algorithm. (a), (b) Regular X-ray dose. (c), (d) low X-ray dose. (a), (c) MSEg measure. (b), (d): SNR measure.

while keeping the level of image quality. We estimate the reduction factor by comparing the SNR and MSEg values of the reconstructed image, acquired with different X-ray doses (controlled by the source intensity λ_0). The comparison is conducted between the standard FBP and the proposed reconstruction method.

For each dose level, we tune the FBP parameters to choose a reconstruction with minimal MSEg value. In a second experiment, for each noise level, the FBP is tuned to maximize the SNR value. In Figure 23 we present the resulting comparison of these two measures for a low dose and a regular dose scan. The x-axis is scaled to show the dose reduction factor, while the MSEg or SNR values change along the y-axis. In the SNR graph we plot the values achieved by SNR-optimized FBP, and, in MSEg graph, the performance

of MSEg-optimized FBP is displayed. Those are compared to the single SNR/MSEg value, achieved by our algorithm in the noise level it was trained for; the x-axis of the graphs was scaled to display the ratio between the X-ray dose levels for FBP and our method. All the four graphs point to the effective dose savings of factor ~4 when switching from the optimally tuned FBP to our method.

7. Discussion and Conclusions

We have introduced a practical CT reconstruction algorithm which performs a non linear processing of the measurements and the reconstructed image. Both actions are aimed at high-quality reconstruction from data corrupted with shot noise and electronic noise. The defining parameters of the learned shrinkage are trained in an offline session on a set of available reference images. When applied to deteriorated measurements of new images, the algorithm produces a reconstruction which improves upon the standard FBP output and the nonlinear ATM filter and is comparable to the iterative PWLS reconstruction.

The learned shrinkage in the transform domain is a nonlinear two-dimensional filter applied in the domain of the noisy measurements. It is shown to be capable of substantially reducing the streak artifacts caused by the measurements' noise. Further postprocessing action is essentially a classical image denoising task, which is carried out without a comprehensive noise model and is aimed to minimize a specific error measure. It is also performed with the learned shrinkage. Our observations, supported by quantitative measures, point to the quality improvement this technique brings to the reconstructed images.

We remark that a potentially greater quality improvement would be achieved by exploiting data correlation in three dimensions (instead of processing 2D slices), similarl to three-dimensional adaptive filtering presented in [9]. Our algorithm naturally generalizes to the 3D setup—the extension would involve 3D discrete cosine transform and a quality measure computed in some volumes of the training data.

As with any algorithm, based on supervised learning, there is a concern of whether the medical anomalies and special objects will be faithfully recovered. In our simulations, the visual comparison of the images reconstructed with our method to the reference images confirms that the content is faithfully recovered. Also, we point to the fact that the processing is performed locally (11×11 squares) and in a transform domain; the action of the shrinkage operation is of statistical rather than geometric nature; thus it is improbable and it will be biased by specific anatomical structures. Still, only the practical realization of the algorithm and verification by clinical radiologists can resolve this concern.

The proposed algorithm requires no hardware changes in a working CT scanner and can be easily incorporated into the reconstruction software of one; thus, in practice it can be implemented in existing clinical machinery with small effort.

Acknowledgment

The research leading to these results has received funding from the European Research Council under European Union's Seventh Framework Programme, ERC Grant agreement no. 320649.

References

[1] P. J. La Rivière, J. Bian, and P. A. Vargas, "Penalized-likelihood sinogram restoration for computed tomography," *IEEE Transactions on Medical Imaging*, vol. 25, no. 8, pp. 1022–1036, 2006.

[2] M. Elad, *Sparse and Redundant Representations: From Theory to Applications in Signal and Image Processing*, Springer, Berlin, Germany, 2010.

[3] F. Natterer and F. Wübbeling, "Mathematical methods in image reconstruction," *SIAM Monographs on Mathematical Modeling and Computation*, pp. 1–207, 2001.

[4] P. J. La Rivière, J. Bian, and P. A. Vargas, "Comparison of quadratic- and median-based roughness penalties for penalized-likelihood sinogram restoration in computed tomography," *International Journal of Biomedical Imaging*, vol. 2006, Article ID 41380, 7 pages, 2006.

[5] T. Li, X. Li, J. Wang et al., "Nonlinear sinogram smoothing for low-dose X-ray CT," *IEEE Transactions on Nuclear Science*, vol. 51, no. 5, pp. 2505–2513, 2004.

[6] I. A. Elbakri and J. A. Fessler, "Statistical image reconstruction for polyenergetic X-ray computed tomography," *IEEE Transactions on Medical Imaging*, vol. 21, no. 2, pp. 89–99, 2002.

[7] J. Wang, T. Li, H. Lu, and Z. Liang, "Penalized weighted least-squares approach to sinogram noise reduction and image reconstruction for low-dose X-ray computed tomography," *IEEE Transactions on Medical Imaging*, vol. 25, no. 10, pp. 1272–1283, 2006.

[8] J. Hsieh, "Adaptive streak artifact reduction in computed tomography resulting from excessive x-ray photon noise," *Medical Physics*, vol. 25, no. 11, pp. 2139–2147, 1998.

[9] M. Kachelrieß, O. Watzke, and W. A. Kalender, "Generalized multi-dimensional adaptive filtering for conventional and spiral single-slice, multi-slice, and cone-beam CT," *Medical Physics*, vol. 28, no. 4, pp. 475–490, 2001.

[10] H. Lu, X. Li, I. Hsiao, and Z. Liang, "Analytical noise treatment for low-dose CT projection data by penalized weighted least-square smoothing in the K-L domain," in *Medical Imaging 2002: Physics of Medical Imaging*, Proceedings of SPIE, pp. 146–152, San Diego, Calif, USA, February 2002.

[11] B. I. Andía, K. D. Sauer, and C. A. Bouman, "Nonlinear back-projection for tomographic reconstruction," *IEEE Transactions on Nuclear Science*, vol. 49, no. 1 I, pp. 61–68, 2002.

[12] Y. Hel-Or and D. Shaked, "A discriminative approach for wavelet denoising," *IEEE Transactions on Image Processing*, vol. 17, no. 4, pp. 443–457, 2008.

[13] J. Thibault, C. A. Bouman, K. D. Sauer, and J. Hsieh, "A recursive filter for noise reduction in statistical iterative tomographic imaging," in *Computational Imaging IV*, vol. 6065 of *Proceedings of SPIE/IS&T*, San Jose, Calif, USA, January 2006.

[14] G. N. Ramachandran and A. V. Lakshminarayanan, "Three-dimensional reconstruction from radiographs and electron micrographs: application of convolutions instead of Fourier transforms," *Proceedings of the National Academy of Sciences of the United States of America*, vol. 68, no. 9, pp. 2236–2240, 1971.

[15] J. H. Kim, K. I. Kim, and C. E. Kwark, "Filter design for optimization of lesion detection in SPECT," in *Proceedings of the 1996 IEEE Nuclear Science Symposium*, vol. 3, pp. 1683–1687, November 1996.

[16] M. Elad, "Why simple shrinkage is still relevant for redundant representations?" *IEEE Transactions on Information Theory*, vol. 52, no. 12, pp. 5559–5569, 2006.

[17] A. M. Bruckstein, D. L. Donoho, and M. Elad, "From sparse solutions of systems of equations to sparse modeling of signals and images," *SIAM Review*, vol. 51, no. 1, pp. 34–81, 2009.

[18] M. Elad, B. Matalon, J. Shtok, and M. Zibulevsky, "A wide-angle view at iterated shrinkage algorithms," in *Wavelets XII*, Proceedings of SPIE, pp. 26–29, San Diego, Calif, USA, August 2007.

[19] D. L. Donoho and J. M. Johnstone, "Ideal spatial adaptation by wavelet shrinkage," *Biometrika*, vol. 81, no. 3, pp. 425–455, 1994.

[20] Y. Hel-Or, A. Adler, and M. Elad, "A shrinkage learning approach for single image super-resolution with overcomplete representations," in *Computer Vision—ECCV 2010*, vol. 6312, pp. 622–635, Springer, Berlin, Germany, 2010.

[21] P. J. Huber, "Robust estimation of a location parameter," *Annals of Statistics*, vol. 53, pp. 73–101, 1964.

[22] F. J. Anscombe, "The transformation of poisson, binomial and negativebinomial data," *Biometrika*, vol. 35, no. 3-4, pp. 246–254, 1948.

[23] D. C. Liu and J. Nocedal, "On the limited memory BFGS method for large scale optimization," *Mathematical Programming B*, vol. 45, no. 3, pp. 503–528, 1989.

[24] F. Wubbeling and F. Natterer, *Mathematical Methods in Image Reconstruction*, SIAM, Philadelphia, Pa, USA, 2001.

[25] T. H. Yoon and E. K. Joo, "Butterworth window for power spectral density estimation," *ETRI Journal*, vol. 31, no. 3, pp. 292–297, 2009.

[26] Z. Wang, A. C. Bovik, H. R. Sheikh, and E. P. Simoncelli, "Image quality assessment: from error visibility to structural similarity," *IEEE Transactions on Image Processing*, vol. 13, no. 4, pp. 600–612, 2004.

8

Statistical Analysis of Haralick Texture Features to Discriminate Lung Abnormalities

Nourhan Zayed and Heba A. Elnemr

Computer & Systems Department, Electronics Research Institute, Cairo 12611, Egypt

Correspondence should be addressed to Nourhan Zayed; nourhan@eri.sci.eg

Academic Editor: Tiange Zhuang

The Haralick texture features are a well-known mathematical method to detect the lung abnormalities and give the opportunity to the physician to localize the abnormality tissue type, either lung tumor or pulmonary edema. In this paper, statistical evaluation of the different features will represent the reported performance of the proposed method. Thirty-seven patients CT datasets with either lung tumor or pulmonary edema were included in this study. The CT images are first preprocessed for noise reduction and image enhancement, followed by segmentation techniques to segment the lungs, and finally Haralick texture features to detect the type of the abnormality within the lungs. In spite of the presence of low contrast and high noise in images, the proposed algorithms introduce promising results in detecting the abnormality of lungs in most of the patients in comparison with the normal and suggest that some of the features are significantly recommended than others.

1. Introduction

The lung is an organ that performs a multitude of vital functions every second of our lives. This fact leads to considering lung abnormalities, life-sustained diseases that have high priority in detection, diagnosis, and treatment if possible. Our focus in this paper will be on two popular abnormalities within the lung, which are pulmonary edema and lung tumor. Pulmonary edema (water in the lungs) is caused by fluid building up in the air sacs of the lungs [1, 2]. On the other hand, lung cancer/tumor is a disease where uncontrolled cell growth in tissues of the lung occurred [3].

Computer-aided diagnosis (CAD) schemes for thoracic computed tomography (CT) are widely used to characterize, quantify, and detect numerous lung abnormalities, such as pulmonary edema and lung cancer [4, 5]. An accurate lung segmentation method is always a critical first step in these CAD schemes and can significantly improve the performance level of these schemes. Although manual or semiautomatic lung segmentation methods for CT images were used in some early CAD schemes [6–10], they are impractical for current CAD schemes because multidetector CT (MDCT)

scanners can generate hundreds of CT slices for a patient. An automated method for lung segmentation is needed for MDCT. In addition, the eye identification/detection of the abnormality type (pulmonary edema or tumors) in computed tomography (CT) images is very difficult even for the experienced clinicians because of its variable shape along with low contrast and high noise associated with it. As the final stage of treating the lung cancer is surgical removal of the diseased lung, hence it is necessary to identify the cancer location, which can be useful before they plan for the surgery.

The aim of our work is to develop an automated novel texture analysis based method for the segmentation of the lungs and the detection of the abnormalities, whether pulmonary edema or lung tumor. Haralick's features based on the gray level cooccurrence matrix (GLCM) are applied to capture textural patterns in lung images. The objective of this work is the selection of the most discriminating and finding out the significant texture features that can differentiate between these two types of abnormalities, in comparison to normal.

Haralick features are statistical features that are computed over the entire image. These measurements are utilized to describe the overall texture of the image using measures

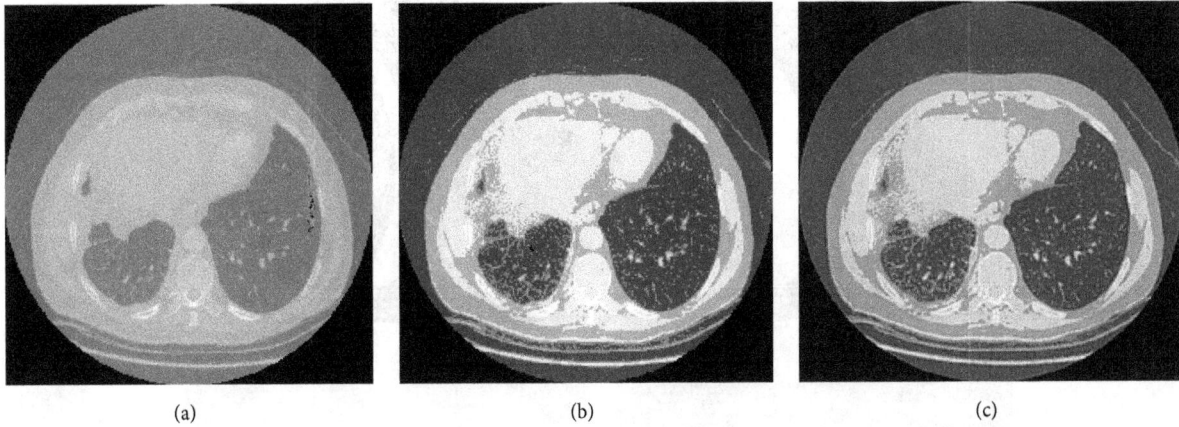

FIGURE 1: (a) The lung CT image; (b) the histogram equalized image; (c) the Weiner filtered output image.

such as entropy and sum of variance. Chaddad et al. propose an approach, based on Haralick's features, to detect and classify colon cancer cells. This work aimed to select the most discriminating parameters for cancer cells [11]. A study to investigate the feasibility of using Haralick features to discriminate between "cancer" and "normal" subimages within a patient is illustrated in [12].

In this paper, CT images are first preprocessed for noise reduction and image enhancement, followed by segmentation techniques, as the tools to segment the lungs, and finally Haralick texture features [13–15] are calculated. Statistical analysis is done to detect the most significant Haralick features that will characterize the type of the abnormality within the lungs. Despite the low contrast and high noise existence in the images, the proposed algorithms introduce promising results in detecting the abnormality of lungs in most of the patients in comparison with the normal.

2. Materials and Methods

This paper presents a new automatic lung cancer detection system based on Haralick texture features extracted from the slice of DICOM Lung CT images. The proposed system is accomplished in four stages: image preprocessing, lung image segmentation, feature extraction, and classification. Statistical analysis is used to obtain the best features for classification to differentiate between lung cancer patients, ordered edema patients, and control subjects. The following sections will describe in detail these stages. All image analyses were achieved without any knowledge of patient clinical characteristics or status.

2.1. Dataset. Patients with either a lung cancer tumor or pulmonary edema were encompassed in the study. This study included two datasets, the first dataset referred to the Radiology Department at New Elkasr ElAiny teaching hospital, University of Cairo. The other dataset was obtained from The Cancer Imaging Archive (TCIA) sponsored by the SPIE, NCI/NIH, AAPM, and the University of Chicago [16]. The two datasets of 532 CT images from 37 different patients

were included. The images are 512 × 512 stored in DICOM format. For each lung CT image, we separate the left lung from the right lung automatically, and each separated lung is labeled as normal or edema/cancer based on the dataset information.

2.2. Preprocessing. The main goal of preprocessing is to improve the quality of an image as well as make it in a form suited for further processing by human or machine [17]. This is accomplished by enhancing the visual appearance of an image besides removing the irrelevant noise and unwanted parts in the background. The proposed enhancement process, which is based on combining filters and noise reduction techniques for pre- and postprocessing as well, is carried out applying histogram equalization (HE) [18–20] followed by Wiener filtering [21, 22].

Figure 1 presents the enhancement in the lung image contrast attained by applying the histogram equalization. However, the obtained gray scale image contains noises such as white noise and salt and pepper noise. Thus, Wiener filter is utilized to remove these noises from the enhanced lung image. Figure 1(c) shows the effect of applying Weiner filter on the contrast enhanced lung image.

2.3. Lung Segmentation. Lung segmentation step aims to basically extract the voxels corresponding to the lung cavity in the axial CT scan slices from the surrounding lung anatomy. The segmentation technique proposed in [23] is utilized. This technique is based on the fact that there is a large density difference between air-filled lung tissues and surrounding tissues. Furthermore, both lungs are almost looking like mirror images of themselves in a human body. The segmentation of lung regions is achieved through the following steps. In the first step, the preprocessed CT image is converted into a binary image; a threshold of 128 was selected. Values greater than the threshold are mapped to white, while others less than that are marked as black. Consequently, the two lungs are marked and the area around them is cropped out. Second, an erosion morphological operation is employed in order to eliminate any white pixels within the two lungs. Afterward,

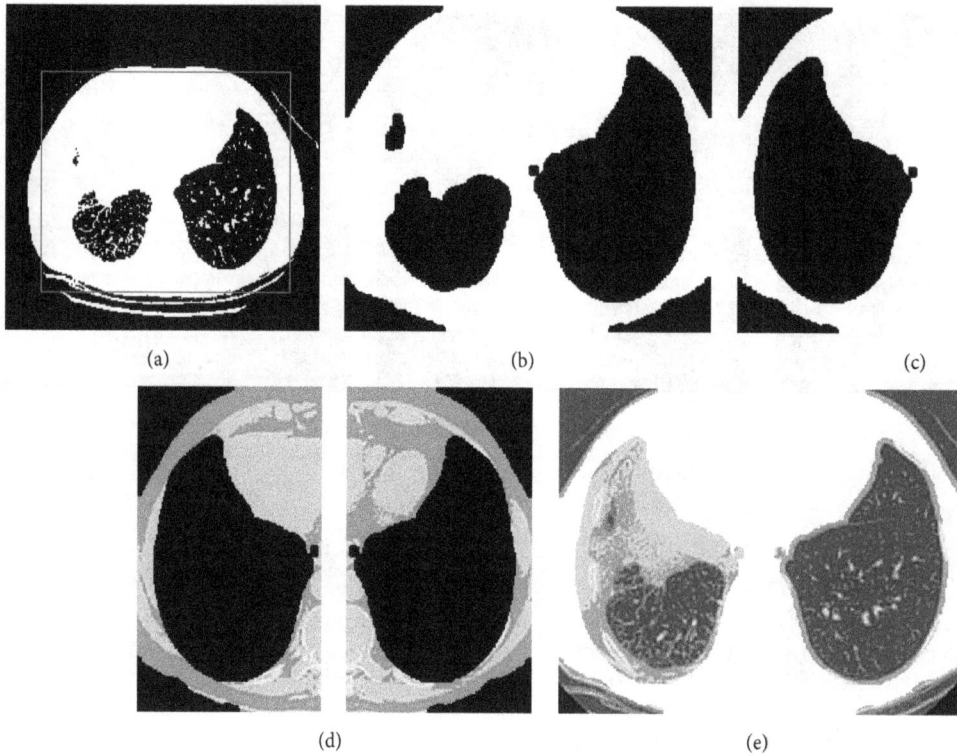

FIGURE 2: (a) The threshold image; (b) the eroded image; (c) the lung mask mirror; (d) the mask projection of the corresponding lungs images; (e) the extracted lungs.

the eroded and the original images are both divided into two equal regions. Black pixels for each region in the eroded image are counted; the region with the largest black area will be deemed as a lung mask. The attained lung mask is reflected in the opposite direction. As a result, right and left lung masks are obtained. These masks are multiplied with the corresponding original image regions; this will project the lung masks on the original two lungs images. Finally, update each black pixel in the obtained images by its original value; other pixels are set to 255. Figure 2 illustrates the lung extraction process.

2.4. Feature Extraction. Feature extraction is the process of obtaining higher-level information of an image such as color, shape, and texture. Texture is a key component of human visual perception. Statistical texture methods analyze the spatial distribution of gray values, by computing local features at each point in the image and inferring a set of statistics from the distributions of the local features. Haralick et al. introduced Gray Level Cooccurrence Matrix (GLCM) and texture features back in 1973 [13]. This technique has been widely used in image analysis applications, especially in the biomedical field. It consists of two steps for feature extraction. The GLCM is computed in the first step, while the texture features based on the GLCM are calculated in the second step.

GLCM shows how often each gray level occurs at a pixel located at a fixed geometric position relative to each other pixel, as a function of the gray level [13]. The horizontal direction 00 with a range of 1 (nearest neighbor) was used

in this work. The 9 texture descriptions used are presented in (4) to (13), where N_g is the number of gray levels, p_d is the normalized symmetric GLCM of dimension $N_g \times N_g$, and $p_d(i, j)$ is the (i, j)th element of the normalized GLCM [13].

Contrast (Moment 2 or standard deviation) is a measure of intensity or gray level variations between the reference pixel and its neighbor. Large contrast reflects large intensity differences in GLCM:

$$\text{Contrast} = \sum_i \sum_j (i - j)^2 p_d(i, j). \tag{1}$$

Homogeneity measures how close the distribution of elements in the GLCM is to the diagonal of GLCM. As homogeneity increases, the contrast, typically, decreases:

$$\text{Homogeneity} = \sum_i \sum_j \frac{1}{1 + (i - j)^2} p_d(i, j). \tag{2}$$

Entropy is the randomness or the degree of disorder present in the image. The value of entropy is the largest when all elements of the cooccurrence matrix are the same and small when elements are unequal:

$$\text{Entropy} = -\sum_i \sum_j p_d(i, j) \ln p_d(i, j). \tag{3}$$

Energy is derived from the Angular Second Moment (ASM). The ASM measures the local uniformity of the gray levels.

When pixels are very similar, the ASM value will be large. Consider

$$\text{Energy} = \sqrt{\text{ASM}}$$

$$\text{ASM} = \sum_i \sum_j p_d^2(i, j). \tag{4}$$

Correlation feature shows the linear dependency of gray level values in the cooccurrence matrix:

$$\text{Correlation} = \sum_i \sum_j p_d(i, j) \frac{(i - \mu_x)(j - \mu_y)}{\sigma_x \sigma_y}, \tag{5}$$

where μ_x; μ_y and σ_x; σ_y are the means and standard deviations and are expressed as

$$\mu_x = \sum_i \sum_j i p_d(i, j)$$

$$\mu_y = \sum_i \sum_j j p_d(i, j)$$

$$\sigma_x = \sqrt{\sum_i \sum_j (i - \mu_x)^2 p_d(i, j)} \tag{6}$$

$$\sigma_y = \sqrt{\sum_i \sum_j (j - \mu_y)^2 p_d(i, j)}.$$

The moments are the statistical expectation of certain power functions of a random variable and are characterized as follows.

Moment 1 (m_1) is the mean which is the average of pixel values in an image and it is represented as

$$m_1 = \sum_i \sum_j (i - j) p_d(i, j). \tag{7}$$

Moment 2 (m_2) is the standard deviation that can be denoted as

$$m_2 = \sum_i \sum_j (i - j)^2 p_d(i, j). \tag{8}$$

Moment 3 (m_3) measures the degree of asymmetry in the distribution and it is defined as

$$m_3 = \sum_i \sum_j (i - j)^3 p_d(i, j). \tag{9}$$

And finally Moment 4 (m_4) measures the relative peak or flatness of a distribution and is also known as kurtosis:

$$m_4 = \sum_i \sum_j (i - j)^4 p_d(i, j). \tag{10}$$

Furthermore, difference statistics that are a subset of the cooccurrence matrix are also used. These features are based on the distribution of probability $P_{x-y}(k)$ which is defined as follows:

$$P_{x-y}(k) = \sum \sum C_d(i, j), \quad k = 0, 1, \dots, N_g - 1, \tag{11}$$

where $C_d(i, j)$ is the (i, j)th element of the GLCM. The most basic difference statistic texture descriptions are the ASM, mean, and entropy:

$$\text{ASM} = \sum_k \left(P_{x-y}(k) \right)^2. \tag{12}$$

When the $P_{x-y}(k)$ values are very similar or close, ASM is small. ASM is large when certain values are high and others are low:

$$\text{Mean} = \sum_k k P_{x-y}(k). \tag{13}$$

When $P_{x-y}(k)$ values are concentrated near the origin, mean is small and mean is large when they are far from the origin:

$$\text{Entropy} = -\sum_k P_{x-y}(k) \log P_{x-y}(k). \tag{14}$$

Entropy is smallest when $P_{x-y}(k)$ values are unequal and largest when $P_{x-y}(k)$ values are equal.

The calculation of the Haralick texture features using the previous equations for the CT images volume sequences for every segmented lung (right and left) separately was performed. For each participant the gray level cooccurrence texture features: contrast, homogeneity, entropy, energy, correlation, and m_1, m_2, m_3, and m_4 accompanied by the difference statistical features: ASM, contrast, mean, and entropy were obtained for each segmented lung (right and left).

2.5. Statistical Analysis. For the purpose of random lung assignment in healthy volunteers, the left lung represented the diseased lung in the same percentage of cases as the patient population. For the acute data, two single factor analyses of variance (ANOVA) tests were conducted for each Haralick texture feature measurement between affected (either left or right) and fellow lung (either left or right) for both categories cancer and edema patients. A single factor analysis of variance (ANOVA) was conducted as well between patients and controls. Other between-subject single factor analyses were conducted to find out the significant Haralick features that could differentiate cancer from edema.

3. Experimental Results

Two datasets of 532 CT images were included. For each lung CT preprocessed image, we separate the left lung from the right lung automatically as discussed before in Section 2.3, and each separated lung is labeled as normal or edema/cancer based on the dataset information. The Haralick texture features measurements for each lung separately are calculated (the gray level cooccurrence texture features: contrast, homogeneity, entropy, energy, correlation, and moments along with the difference statistical features: ASM, mean, and entropy). The mean and the standard deviation of the Haralick texture features measurements calculated as well as the ANOVA results are given for tumor patients affected lung versus fellow lung in Table 1 and for pulmonary edema patients in Table 2. The ANOVA summary of statistics for either pulmonary

TABLE 1: ANOVA (1 within-subject factor) results for cancer patients Haralick texture features (comparison between AL and FL). AL: affected lung; FL: fellow lung.

Feature name	AL (average ± SEM)	FL (average ± SEM)	AL versus FL
Homogeneity	0.511 ± 0.01	0.517 ± 0.01	$\mathbf{F(1, 426) = 22.0\ p < 0.000004}$
Energy	0.372 ± 0.01	0.374 ± 0.01	$\mathbf{F(1, 426) = 15.1\ p < 0.0001}$
Correlation	0.964 ± 0.001	0.965 ± 0.001	$\mathbf{F(1, 426) = 6.15\ p < 0.013}$
Contrast	231.98 ± 4.54	231.76 ± 4.54	$F(1, 426) = 0.012\ p < 0.911$
Entropy	8.0 ± 0.19	7.94 ± 0.19	$\mathbf{F(1, 426) = 11.8\ p < 0.0007}$
m_1	0.003 ± 0.02	0.007 ± 0.02	$F(1, 426) = 0.029\ p < 0.88$
m_2	231.13 ± 4.54	231.75 ± 4.01	$F(1, 426) = 0.012\ p < 0.911$
m_3	-164 ± 190.79	-683.99 ± 155.33	$F(1, 426) = 2.65\ p < 0.09$
m_4	1784467 ± 83311	1654941 ± 56455	$F(1, 426) = 6.25\ p < 0.19$
Diff_ASM	0.226963389 ± 0.006	0.229353096 ± 0.005	$F(1, 426) = 3.18\ p < 0.06$
Diff_Mean	6.195 ± 0.08	6.28 ± 0.09	$F(1, 426) = 2.16\ p < 0.12$
Diff_Entropy	3.159 ± 0.03	3.55 ± 0.03	$F(1, 426) = 2.32\ p < 0.10$

TABLE 2: ANOVA (1 within-subject factor) results for edema patients Haralick texture features (comparison between AL and FL). AL: affected lung; FL: fellow lung.

Feature name	AL (average ± SEM)	FL (average ± SEM)	AL versus FL
Homogeneity	0.64 ± 0.013	0.60 ± 0.020	$F(1, 105) = 2.16\ p < 0.15$
Energy	0.428 ± 0.01	$0.429.01 \pm 0.01$	$F(1, 105) = 0.029\ p < 0.87$
Correlation	0.006 ± 0.001	0.008 ± 0.001	$F(1, 105) = 2.32\ p < 0.141$
Contrast	177.07 ± 5.89	188.58 ± 4.26	$\mathbf{F(1, 105) = 15.1\ p < 0.0002}$
Entropy	2.10 ± 0.04	2.19 ± 0.067	$\mathbf{F(1, 105) = 1.28\ p < 0.269}$
m_1	0.52 ± 0.03	-0.47 ± 0.02	$\mathbf{F(1, 105) = 41.8\ p < 0.000001}$
m_2	199.975 ± 9.658	218.583 ± 10.085	$F(1, 105) = 2.20\ p < 0.152$
m_3	5219 ± 1436	-7539 ± 885	$\mathbf{F(1, 105) = 41.8\ p < 0.000001}$
m_4	2854294 ± 208886	2382237 ± 263250	$F(1, 105) = 2.12\ p < 0.158$
Diff_ASM	0.377 ± 0.01	0.288 ± 0.08	$\mathbf{F(1, 105) = 4.56\ p < 0.043}$
Diff_Mean	4.07 ± 0.4379	4.89 ± 0.48478	$\mathbf{F(1, 105) = 7.87\ p < 0.01}$
Diff_Entropy	2.96 ± 0.05	3.29 ± 0.05	$\mathbf{F(1, 105) = 4.73\ p < 0.039}$

edema or tumor patients versus normal is given in Table 3. The significant Haralick texture features that can differentiate between pulmonary edema and tumor are found in Table 4.

From Table 1, we can conclude that Haralick texture features measurements (homogeneity, energy, correlation, and entropy) of the affected cancer lung were significantly different than that of the fellow lung. The homogeneity, energy, and correlation were significantly less than those of the normal fellow lung. While entropy of the cancerous lung is approaching being significantly more than that of the fellow lung, Moment 3 and the difference statistical feature ASM (diff_ASM) texture feature measurement of the cancerous lung is approaching being significantly less than that of the normal lung.

Table 2 showed that Haralick texture features measurements (homogeneity, entropy, and moments calculated from the cooccurrence matrix as well as mean and ASM computed from the difference statistics) of the pulmonary edema affected lung were also significantly different than those of the control subject lung; moreover contrast and entropy computed from the difference statistics were significantly more than those of the fellow lung.

Considering Tables 1 and 2, we can conclude from Table 3 that the homogeneity, energy, entropy, m_3, m_4, diff_ASM, diff_mean, and diff_entropy are good biomarkers to significantly differentiate between diseased and normal lungs without any disease specification. On the other hand, the results illustrated in Tables 1, 2, and 4 show that entropy and the entropy calculated from the difference statistics would be a good candidate to significantly differentiate between pulmonary edema and cancer.

4. Conclusion and Discussion

The texture features analyses are well known approaches to quantify and express the heterogeneity that may not be appreciated by clinical naked eyes, and it was presented before as good imaging biomarkers to differentiate between diseases. In this paper an evaluation of the Haralick texture features is done in order to identify the most significant features that can be used in order to detect and differentiate abnormalities within the lungs for cancer and edema versus normal. Our results indicate that entropy determined by gray level cooccurrence matrix and ASM is significantly different in

TABLE 3: ANOVA (1 within-subject factor) results summary of statistics p value for patients (either edema or cancer) Haralick texture features versus normal controls.

Feature name	Diseased versus normal controls (p value)	Feature name	Diseased versus normal controls (p value)
Homogeneity	$p < 0.00002$	m_2	$p < 0.229$
Energy	$p < 0.0006$	m_3	$p < 0.0002$
Correlation	$p < 0.485$	m_4	$p < 0.002$
Contrast	$p < 0.229$	Diff_ASM	$p < 0.000001$
Entropy	$p < 0.0004$	Diff_Mean	$p < 0.000005$
m_1	$p < 0.0007$	Diff_Entropy	$p < 0.0004$

TABLE 4: ANOVA (1 between-subject factor) results summary of statistics p value for patients Haralick texture features cancer versus edema patients.

Feature name	Cancer versus edema patients (p value)	Feature name	Cancer versus edema patients (p value)
Homogeneity	$p < 0.0002$	m_2	$p < 0.69$
Energy	$p < 0.065$	m_3	$p < 0.01$
Correlation	$p < 0.179$	m_4	$p < 0.89$
Contrast	$p < 0.699$	ASM	$p < 0.73$
Entropy	$p < 0.017$	Mean	$p < 0.032$
m_1	$p < 0.0004$	Entropy	$p < 0.007$

edema patients versus normal while it is not in cancer patients versus normal. Since the entropy is the degree of randomness or the degree of disorder in the image, and the angular second moment represents the uniformity in the image, this may be interpreted as the cancer disease causing a localized heterogeneity in the diseased specified area in the lung while the edema causes heterogeneous disorder in the whole lung image. High entropy values calculated implies that the elevated level of disorder and disorganization occurred due to the edema diseased lung versus the cancer diseased lung. The energy feature that is derived from the angular second moment measures and representing the local uniformity of the gray levels is a good biomarker to differentiate between cancer and edema diseases. From Table 2, contrast is a good biomarker for the pulmonary edema disease and this agrees with the texture feature meaning which means high contrast values for heavy texture changes. Gray level cooccurrence matrix textural properties such as homogeneity, correlation, mean, and moments are good significant biomarkers for diseased lung versus normal ones in general without any specification for the disease type. Our results agree with other articles indicating that textural analysis has the potential to develop into a valuable clinical tool that improves the diagnosis, tumor staging, and therapy assessment.

While our results are promising, there is still further work that can be done in the detecting of the abnormality within the lungs to detect the type of that abnormality whether it will be a lung cancer or edema. A preliminary investigation has been done using statistical analysis to identify the most useful texture features that can be fed to any classification technique later. This statistical analysis is done using ANOVA. After selecting these features we can feed them for better localization and classification as further work.

Conflict of Interests

The authors declare that there is no conflict of interests regarding the publication of this paper.

Acknowledgments

The authors acknowledge the SPIE, the NCI, the AAPM, and The University of Chicago for providing public access to the lung cancer dataset.

References

[1] L. B. Ware and M. A. Matthay, "Acute pulmonary edema," *The New England Journal of Medicine*, vol. 353, no. 26, pp. 2788–2796, 2005.

[2] J. Šedý, J. Zicha, J. Kuneš, P. Jendelová, and E. Syková, "Mechanisms of neurogenic pulmonary edema development," *Physiological Research*, vol. 57, no. 4, pp. 499–506, 2008.

[3] R. S. Herbst, J. V. Heymach, and S. M. Lippman, "Lung cancer," *The New England Journal of Medicine*, vol. 359, no. 13, pp. 1367–1380, 2008.

[4] N. Hollings and P. Shaw, "Diagnostic imaging of lung cancer," *European Respiratory Journal*, vol. 19, no. 4, pp. 722–742, 2002.

[5] T. Manikandan and N. Bharathi, "Lobar fissure extraction in isotropic CT lung images—an application to cancer identification," *International Journal of Computer Applications*, vol. 33, no. 6, pp. 17–21, 2011.

[6] J. Wang, F. Li, and Q. Li, "Automated segmentation of lungs with severe interstitial lung disease in CT," *Medical Physics*, vol. 36, no. 10, pp. 4592–4599, 2009.

[7] U. Bağci, M. Bray, J. Caban, J. Yao, and D. J. Mollura, "Computer-assisted detection of infectious lung diseases: a review," *Computerized Medical Imaging and Graphics*, vol. 36, no. 1, pp. 72–84, 2012.

[8] D. Sharma and G. Jindal, "Computer aided diagnosis system for detection of lung cancer in CT scan images," *International Journal of Computer and Electrical Engineering*, vol. 3, no. 5, pp. 714–718, 2011.

[9] J. Wang, F. Li, K. Doi, and Q. Li, "Computerized detection of diffuse lung disease in MDCT: the usefulness of statistical texture features," *Physics in Medicine and Biology*, vol. 54, no. 22, pp. 6881–6899, 2009.

[10] J. Wang, F. Li, K. Doi, and Q. Li, "A novel scheme for detection of diffuse lung disease in MDCT by use of statistical texture features," in *Medical Imaging 2009: Computer-Aided Diagnosis, 726039*, vol. 7260 of *Proceedings of SPIE*, Lake Buena Vista, Fla, USA, February 2009.

[11] A. Chaddad, C. Tanougast, A. Dandache, and A. Bouridane, "Extraction of haralick features from segmented texture multispectral bio-images for detection of colon cancer cells," in *Proceedings of the 1st International Conference on Informatics and Computational Intelligence (ICI '11)*, pp. 55–59, Bandung, Indonesia, December 2011.

[12] B. D. Fleet, J. Yan, D. B. Knoester, M. Yao, J. R. Deller Jr., and E. D. Goodman, "Breast cancer detection using haralick features of images reconstructed from ultra wideband microwave scans," in *Clinical Image-Based Procedures. Translational Research in Medical Imaging*, vol. 8680 of *Lecture Notes in Computer Science*, pp. 9–16, Springer International, Cham, Switzerland, 2014.

[13] R. M. Haralick, K. Shanmugam, and I. Dinstein, "Textural features for image classification," *IEEE Transactions on Systems, Man and Cybernetics*, vol. 3, no. 6, pp. 610–621, 1973.

[14] R. M. Haralick, "Statistical and structural approaches to texture," *Proceedings of the IEEE*, vol. 67, no. 5, pp. 786–804, 1979.

[15] J. M. H. du Buf, M. Kardan, and M. Spann, "Texture feature performance for image segmentation," *Pattern Recognition*, vol. 23, no. 3-4, pp. 291–309, 1990.

[16] S. G. Armato III, *SPIE-AAPM-NCI Lung Nodule Classification Challenge Dataset*, The Cancer Imaging Archive, 2015.

[17] R. C. Gonzalez and R. E. Woods, *Digital Image Processing*, Addison-Wesley, 1992.

[18] C. Wang and Z. Ye, "Brightness preserving histogram equalization with maximum entropy: a variational perspective," *IEEE Transactions on Consumer Electronics*, vol. 51, no. 4, pp. 1326–1334, 2005.

[19] I. Jafar and H. Ying, "Image contrast enhancement by constrained variational histogram equalization," in *Proceedings of the IEEE International Conference on Electro/Information Technology (EIT '07)*, pp. 120–125, IEEE, Chicago, Ill, USA, May 2007.

[20] S.-D. Chen and A. R. Ramli, "Minimum mean brightness error bi-histogram equalization in contrast enhancement," *IEEE Transactions on Consumer Electronics*, vol. 49, no. 4, pp. 1310–1319, 2003.

[21] D. Sharma and G. Jindal, "Computer aided diagnosis system for detection of lung cancer in CT scan images," *International Journal of Computer and Electrical Engineering*, vol. 3, no. 5, 2011.

[22] S. V. Vaseghi, *Advanced Digital Signal Processing and Noise Reduction*, John Wiley & Sons, New York, NY, USA, 2nd edition, 2000.

[23] H. A. Elnemr, "Statistical analysis of law's mask texture features for cancer and water lung detection," *International Journal of Computer Science Issues*, vol. 10, no. 6, 2013.

9

Automated Feature Extraction in Brain Tumor by Magnetic Resonance Imaging Using Gaussian Mixture Models

Ahmad Chaddad

Department of Diagnostic Radiology, University of Texas MD Anderson Cancer Center, 1400 Pressler Street, Houston, TX 77030, USA

Correspondence should be addressed to Ahmad Chaddad; ahmad.chaddad@univ-lorraine.fr

Academic Editor: Habib Zaidi

This paper presents a novel method for Glioblastoma (GBM) feature extraction based on Gaussian mixture model (GMM) features using MRI. We addressed the task of the new features to identify GBM using T1 and T2 weighted images (T1-WI, T2-WI) and Fluid-Attenuated Inversion Recovery (FLAIR) MR images. A pathologic area was detected using multithresholding segmentation with morphological operations of MR images. Multiclassifier techniques were considered to evaluate the performance of the feature based scheme in terms of its capability to discriminate GBM and normal tissue. GMM features demonstrated the best performance by the comparative study using principal component analysis (PCA) and wavelet based features. For the T1-WI, the accuracy performance was 97.05% (AUC = 92.73%) with 0.00% missed detection and 2.95% false alarm. In the T2-WI, the same accuracy (97.05%, AUC = 91.70%) value was achieved with 2.95% missed detection and 0.00% false alarm. In FLAIR mode the accuracy decreased to 94.11% (AUC = 95.85%) with 0.00% missed detection and 5.89% false alarm. These experimental results are promising to enhance the characteristics of heterogeneity and hence early treatment of GBM.

1. Introduction

Providing quantitative and accurate information for medical diagnosis, Magnetic Resonance Imaging (MRI) plays an essential role in medical imaging [1]. MRI has several advantages over other medical imaging techniques regarding its multiple applications, namely, for cardiovascular, musculoskeletal, and, in particular, for imaging of the brain and neurological systems [2, 3]. However, a bottleneck of MR image processing arises from variations in intensity due to B1 and B0 field inhomogeneity [4, 5]. This is manifested by the nonuniform appearance even of a single tissue which may mislead image analysis algorithms, which enhance abnormality area detection by a segmentation model [2, 6].

In the last decade, MR imaging established itself as key imaging modality in diagnosis and follow-up of brain tumors including Glioblastoma (GBM) [7]. GBM is the most common primary malignant brain tumor in adults [8]. It is characterized by abnormal and uncontrolled cell proliferation, necrosis, and vascular proliferation [9]. Despite the ongoing research and clinical trials, GBM remains one of the most aggressive malignant tumors with less than 5% of patients surviving five years after diagnosis [10]. This is attributed to the highly infiltrative nature and the heterogeneity that Glioblastoma exhibits on molecular and genomic levels which lead to differences in individual treatment response and prognosis [11].

Accordingly, research has focused on exploring associations between certain imaging features and the underlying genomic profiles of GBM in a new branch in clinical radiology known as "imaging genomics" [12, 13]. Using a GMM, Simon et al. recently showed that delineation and quantification of apparent diffusion coefficient in gliomas can be performed reliably and fast and demonstrated how thereby user-dependent variability can automatically be removed [14]. Consequently, recent work has focused on developing robust methods for reading and imaging features extraction from such MR images.

Automatic reading algorithms can foster faster and more precise readings of MR images as well as segmenting the abnormal imaging areas to classify them as GBM or not.

(a)   (b)   (c)

(d)

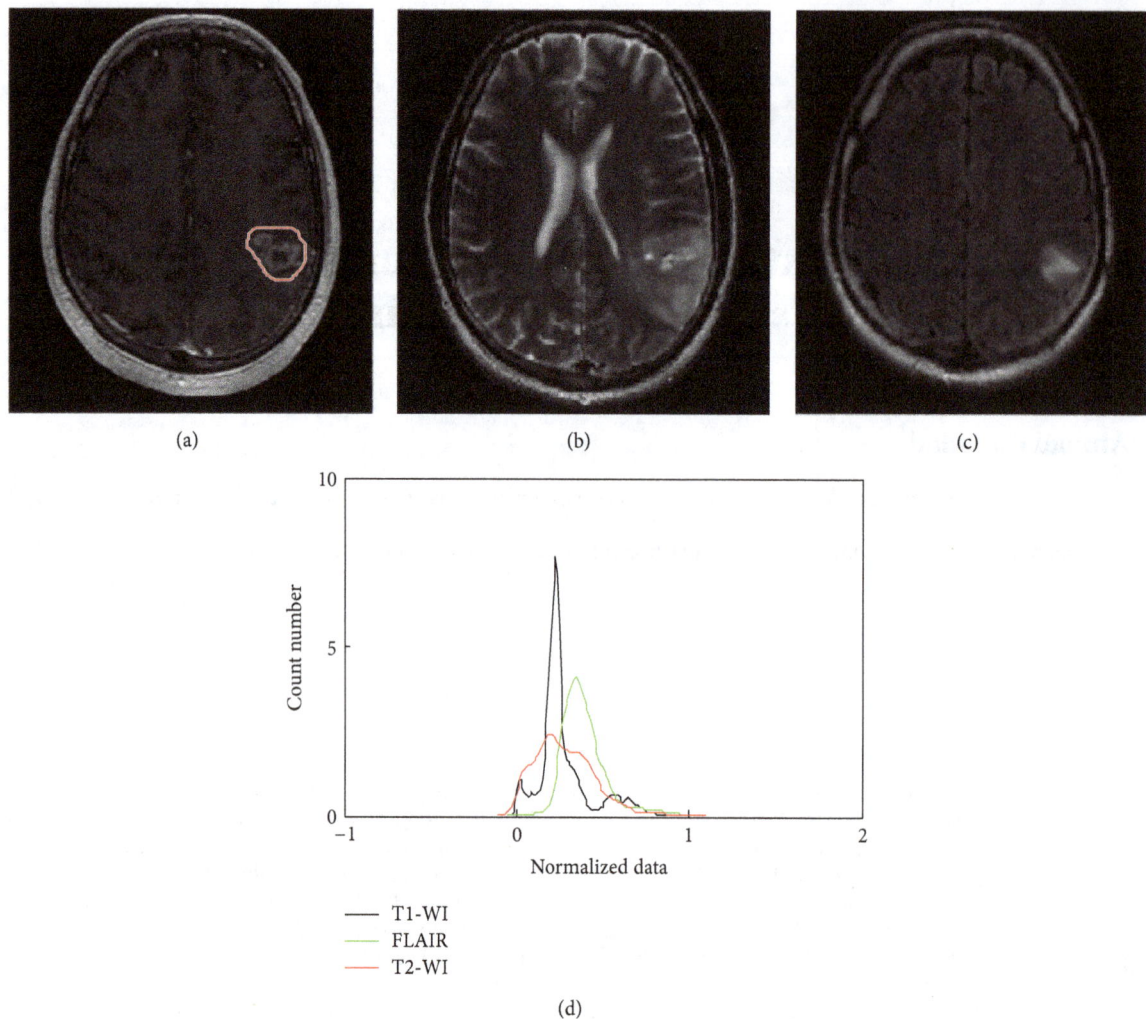

FIGURE 1: Analysis of GBM schema: (a) brain tumor image on axial T1-WI, (b) axial T2-WI, (c) axial FLAIR sequence, and (d) GBM data fitting in three MR sequences.

Robust reading of MR images includes several consecutive steps. The system must first segment the image by detecting and extracting the abnormal area from their surrounding medium using multithresholding segmentation and morphological image processing. This step requires careful selection of the appropriate segmentation methodology for processing of high resolution grayscale MR images. While several segmentation methods based on MR images have been proposed using filtering to remove noise, these techniques are not generally applicable to automated detection of GBM as the tumor can be unintentionally eliminated during the process of noise reduction. Segmentation methods based on thresholding or multithresholding are thus preferred.

That way, it is likely that GBM and the normal brain tissue "survive" the thresholding. This method divides an image into several regions using multithresholding [15–18]. The second step following the detection of area of imaging abnormality, representing GBM, involves extraction of some characteristic parameters and texture features that are specific for GBM [19–26]. Plurals based on the texture features were proposed where the visual analysis of texture is a difficult task,

particularly with GBM. The texture analysis based on gray level cooccurrence matrix (GLCM) determines neighborhoods around pixels (texture elements) where the GLCM is counted using the specific offset and phases [27]. Also, shape and texture feature were used to classify the brain tumor type and grade using SVM model; however the classifier accuracy was limited by 85% [28].

Moreover, the feature quality is essential to improve the classifier accuracy and accordingly the applications. For example, wavelet based classification has proven to be a powerful technique [29–31]. However, due to its comparatively low classification accuracy this approach was not promising to follow in our MRI data. We therefore aimed to investigate GBM tumor features that may have the potential to measure specific GBM characteristics. To achieve this, we focused on features derived from Gaussian mixture model (GMM) analysis on both weighted T1 and T2 and FLAIR sequences.

Figure 1 shows 2D axial image of brain within GBM region indicated by the red line in Figure 1(a). Clearly, GBM area has higher intensity on the grayscale level brain MR image, but some pixels of normal brain share the same

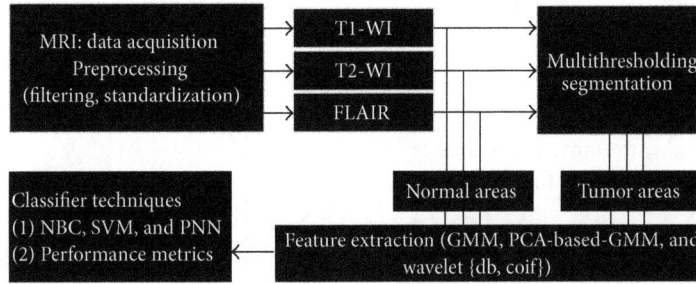

FIGURE 2: Schematic diagram of the proposed method for automatic feature extraction.

intensity values as the GBM pixels. These pixels closely resemble the GBM pixels in terms of their intensity, rendering GBM detection a difficult task. Also, histogram of GBM area is not similar in the three MRI sequences.

2. Materials and Methods

The schematic of the proposed method is shown in Figure 2: (1) preprocessing to normalize grayscales and filtering to remove the noise from images in the three MRI sequences, T1-WI, T2-WI, and FLAIR; (2) tumor (GBM) areas detection by multithresholding segmentation and normal areas determined from the normal brain material; (3) feature extraction from the GMM curve fitting of the grayscale histogram on T1-WI, T2-WI, and FLAIR images; (4) applying three classifier techniques to discriminate between the tumor areas and normal areas based on GMM features; and (5) validating the effect of GMM features by comparative study with PCA and wavelet features. The details of the schematic are given below.

2.1. Data Acquisition. A data set of 17 patients was collected by November 2013 from the publicly available Cancer Imaging Archive (http://www.cancerimagingarchive.net/) database for our preliminary study. We excluded patients with incomplete imaging data set. All of the images had 512×512 pixels acquisition matrices and were converted into grayscale before further processing. MRI raw data were filtered to remove noise and standardized by the linear normalization, followed by multithreshold-based segmentation. This technique was applied to determine the tumor position and was successfully applied for the GBM data collection process. Note that preprocessing of skull stripping is required; it is necessary to obtain only the brain material without the skull bone; however, multithresholding segmentation with morphological operation filter may be detecting GBM area in two-dimension axial image. In this context, automated operation can be a difficult task if the GBM area is smaller than skull thickness.

2.2. Multithresholding Segmentation. Single threshold segmentation for GBM region pixels may resemble normal brain pixels. Segmentation based on multithresholding resolved this problem. Accordingly, we carried out an initial estimation of GBM localization by using multithresholding (multilevel image thresholds) segmentation method proposed by Otsu [32]. This approach enabled the definition of thresholds

that maximize the interclass variances, thus also minimizing the intraclass variances. It can offer multilevel image thresholds in order to segment the desired object (brain tumor). In our case, we adjusted the multithresholding of an image for skull stripping and tumor detection. In order to robustly detect GBM, we had to resolve the problem arising from resembling pixels spots. This could be easily resolved by median filter depending on the window size.

2.3. GMM Feature Extracted. Many GMM had previously been considered in the literature for face identification [27], which was found to offer the best trade-off in terms of complexity, robustness, and discrimination. It has also been used for voice identification based on the feature and score normalization techniques [33, 34]. Also, GMM based features show promise accuracy classifier to distinguish between target and ghost/clutter regions [35].

GMM is a parametric probability density function represented as a weighted sum of K Gaussian component densities according to

$$p(x \setminus \lambda) = \sum_{i=1}^{K} w_i g(x \setminus \mu_i, \Sigma_i),$$ (1)

where x represented the N dimensional continuous valued data vector, w_i the mixture weight, and g the component Gaussian densities.

Each component density was controlled by the N-variate Gaussian function according to

$$g(x \setminus \mu_i, \Sigma_i)$$
$$= \frac{1}{(2\pi)^{N/2} |\Sigma_i|^{1/2}} \exp\left\{ -\frac{1}{2} (x - \mu_i)^T (\Sigma_i)^{-1} (x - \mu_i) \right\},$$ (2)

where μ_i was the average of a vector, T is the transpose, and Σ_i is the covariance matrix.

The complete Gaussian mixture model was parameterized by the mean vectors, covariance matrices, and mixture weights from all component densities. These parameters can be expressed according to

$$\lambda = \{w_i, \mu_i, \Sigma_i\}.$$ (3)

The variance (v_i) of components was represented by the diagonal of the covariance matrix Σ_i. We extracted then a feature vector R from three components of GMM according to

$$R = \{w_1 \cdots w_3, \mu_1 \cdots \mu_3, v_1 \cdots v_3\}, \quad (4)$$

where w, μ, and v are the weight, average, and variance of GMM components (indexes 1, 2, and 3 are the first, second, and third component of GMM).

Each segmented GBM area could be represented by the feature vector R_{GBM} that is of size 1 by 9 elements. A similar feature vector size (R_N) for normal area was computed.

For n GBM areas, we had Rt_{GBM} matrix that was of size n by 9 elements, meaning n samples. Similar matrix for the area of normal brain was Rt_N. When computing the matrixes Rt_{GBM} and Rt_N, the classification operation became ready.

2.4. Principal Component Analysis Applied on GMM Features.
In the following, we present a principal component analysis technique to reduce the data and to get the appropriate feature from each vector feature.

Each feature vector of GBM and of normal brain was extracted from several Gaussian distributions which were represented by the average, standard deviation, and weight. Concatenating the parameters of GMM, this technique could show the correlation between the features extracted. Further, it could have been a good factor classifier to distinguish between GBM and normal brain tissue. Two matrixes (Rt_{GBM}) and (Rt_N) of n GBM and normal samples were n by 9, where each feature row concerns 9 elements. GBM and normal area samples of $n = 17$ patients were arranged into data matrixes Rt_{GBM} and Rt_N according to

$$Rt_{GBM} = [R_{1G} \cdots R_{nG}]$$
$$Rt_N = [R_{1N} \cdots R_{nN}], \quad (5)$$

where $[R_{1G} \cdots R_{nG}]$ and $[R_{1N} \cdots R_{nN}]$ were the GMM features of GBM and normal area, respectively.

Training data were received by Rt_{GBM} and Rt_N. PCA was employed, where the covariance of Rt_{GBM} and Rt_N was computed. The covariance matrix could be found according to

$$C_{GBM} = \text{cov}(Rt_{GBM}),$$
$$C_N = \text{cov}(Rt_N), \quad (6)$$

where cov was the covariance. C_{GBM} and C_N are the same size 9 by 9.

According to the following equation, the eigenvalues and eigenvectors could be computed according to

$$CV = \Lambda V, \quad (7)$$

where V was the matrix of principal component and each column in V was an eigenvector. Λ was the diagonal matrix where the diagonal elements were the values of the eigenvalues.

We organized the eigenvectors by their corresponding eigenvalues and we retained three eigenvectors as the PCs of the data from C_{GBM} and C_N, respectively, where the higher variance represented the three largest eigenvalues. Figure 3

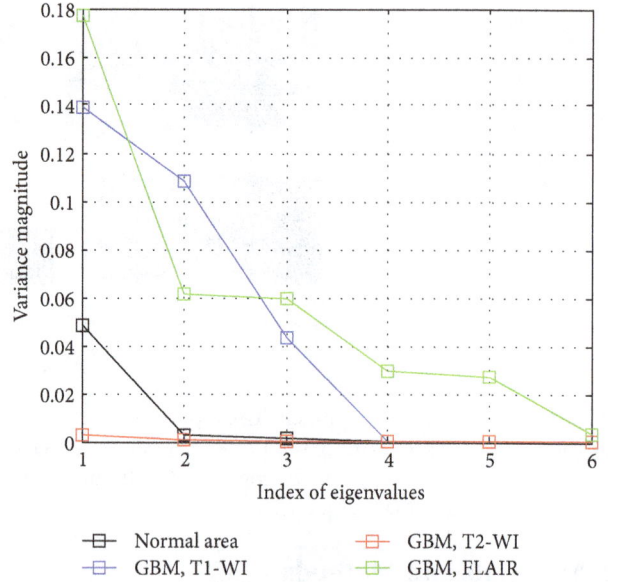

FIGURE 3: Principal components based on higher variance of GBM and normal areas: (black curve) variance magnitude of 17 normal areas from T1-WI, T2-WI, and FLAIR, (blue curve) variance magnitude of 17 GBMs chosen from T1-WI, (red curve) variance magnitude of 17 GBMs chosen from T2-WI, and (green curve) variance magnitude of 17 chosen GBMs chosen from FLAIR mode of MRI.

shows the variance of eigenvalues of three MRI modes. Clearly, the maximum variances common between T1-WI, T2-WI, and FLAIR were located in the first three indexes of eigenvalues. The matrix dimension of Rt_{GBM} and Rt_N was reduced by the projection of each row according to

$$P_i^{GBM} = \text{PC}_{GBM}^T (Rt_{GBM}),$$
$$P_i^N = \text{PC}_N^T (Rt_N), \quad (8)$$

where $\{\}^T$ was the transpose indicator, PC_{GBM}^T and PC_N^T were the transpose of principal components of GBM and normal area, respectively, and i was the index of row in GBM matrix Rt_{GBM} and normal area matrix Rt_N, respectively.

Using 3 PCs, a new matrix P^{GBM} of GBM that was of size 17 by 3 and matrix P^N of normal area had a similar size. We considered then three classifier models to evaluate GBM and normal areas discrimination based on GMM features and their three principal components, respectively.

2.5. Classifier Setting.
In general, the goal of a learning/classification algorithm is to build a set of training examples with class labels. In this context, we implemented three classifier techniques, namely, naïve Bayes (NB) [36], support vector machine (SVM) [37], and probabilistic neural network (PNN) [38]. The implementation of NB is performed using a kernel estimation method which approximated the complex distributions of the data. Then, SVM was implemented using the Gaussian radial basis function, and radial basis network based PNN was employed which is a fast classifier technique.

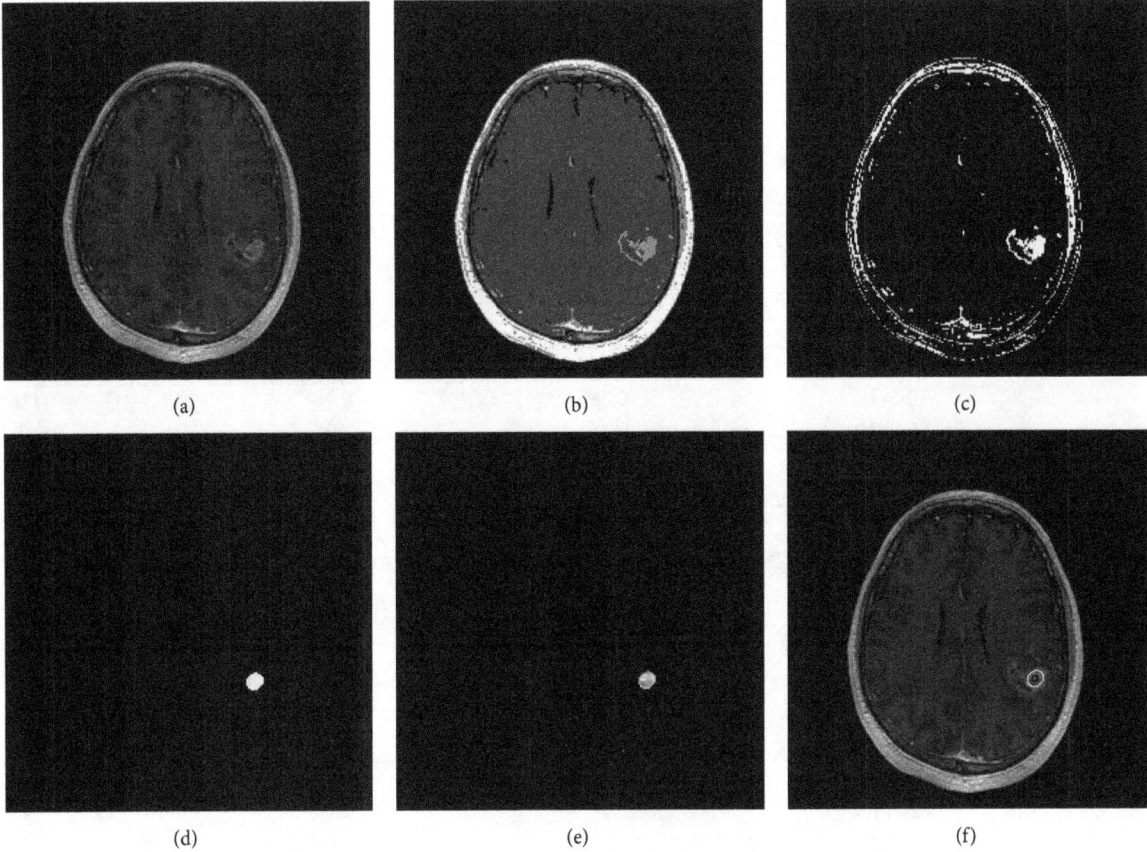

FIGURE 4: GBM detection by segmentation and morphology operations: (a) T1-MR image, (b) image segmented by four levels, (c) range of GBM gray level conserve, (d) filtering of (c), (e) raw GBM data detected, and (f) GBM located on the brain image.

The reason for using these specific classifier methods is to achieve the trade-off performance which is reported.

Due to the limited data available (17 patients), validation data sets were performed based on leave-one-out cross-validation [39]. Performance metrics are expressed by the following equations:

False Alarm

$$= \frac{\text{number of normal samples uncorrectly classified}}{\text{total number of sample cases}},$$

Missed Detection

$$= \frac{\text{number of GBM samples uncorrectly classified}}{\text{total number of sample cases}}, \quad (9)$$

Accuracy

$$= \frac{\text{number of GBM and normal samples correctly classified}}{\text{total number of sample cases}}.$$

Moreover, receiver operating characteristic (ROC) curves and the associated area under the curve (AUC) values were computed to assess the discrimination between GBM and normal areas [40]. The results of the performance metrics reflected the succeeding GMM features for discrimination between GBM and normal area. Note that the training data set of the normal brain tissue regions represent different normal regions within the MR image.

3. Experimental Results and Discussions

3.1. Segmentation of the GBM. GBM tumor tissue was detected using the multithresholding segmentation based on Otsu's technique and the morphology operation to obtain only the abnormal brain regions in robust term. Figure 4 shows GBM tumor segmented using several steps. The process of tumor detection from MR images may appear to be a difficult task as MR images contained some areas which have a similar range of gray color (Figure 4(b)). Morphology operators or filtering was necessary to remove noise like the boundary of skull and brain (Figures 4(c) and 4(d)). Then GBM was detected and located (Figures 4(e) and 4(f)).

3.2. GMM Feature Extraction and Classification. Three GMM curve fittings based on the histogram analysis showed three components of GBM (see Figure 5). Three Gaussian components were chosen based on the empirical metrics which showed three components of GBM. GMM features were shown to be feasible for discriminating between GBM and normal brain.

Table 1 shows a comparative study between the three modes of MR images based on the classifier accuracy, false alarm, and missed detection. These metrics represented the

TABLE 1: Performance metrics (%) based on the GMM features.

Classifier	Sequence	Accuracy	False alarm	Missed detection
NB	T1-WI	97.05	2.95	0
	T2-WI	97.05	0	2.95
	FLAIR	94.11	5.89	0
	*Entire GBM	86.27	2.94	10.78
SVM	T1-WI	70.58	0	29.41
	T2-WI	64.70	5.88	29.41
	FLAIR	67.64	2.94	29.41
	*Entire GBM	66.66	4.90	28.43
PNN	T1-WI	94.11	5.89	0
	T2-WI	70.58	11.76	17.64
	FLAIR	94.11	2.94	2.94
	*Entire GBM	86.27	2.94	10.78

*Entire GBM refers to T1-WI, T2-WI, and FLAIR features combined together.

TABLE 2: Performance metrics (%) based on the PCA features.

Classifier	Sequence	Accuracy	False alarm	Missed detection
NB	T1-WI	73.52	8.82	17.64
	T2-WI	79.41	2.94	17.64
	FLAIR	82.35	5.88	11.76
	Entire GBM	68.62	15.68	15.68
SVM	T1-WI	55.88	0	44.11
	T2-WI	61.76	8.82	29.41
	FLAIR	85.29	0	14.70
	Entire GBM	35.29	20.58	44.11
PNN	T1-WI	61.76	8.82	29.41
	T2-WI	52.94	14.70	32.35
	FLAIR	94.11	0	5.88
	Entire GBM	51.96	9.80	38.23

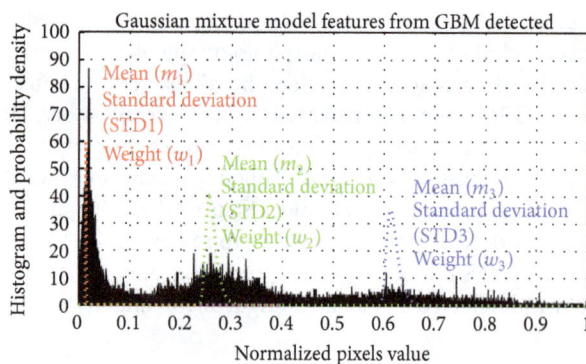

FIGURE 5: GMM curve fitting: example of GBM based GMM features.

highest performance using NB classifier with the classification accuracy range between 94.00 and 97.00%, false alarm range between 0.00 (which means that the normal area samples were correctly classified without error) and 5.89%, and missed detection range between 0.00 (which means that the GBM samples were correctly classified without error) and 2.95%. This latter value of missed detection represented the one GBM sample from 17 that was incorrectly classified (or classified as normal area).

GMM features were reduced with a PCA, which accounted for 97% of the cumulative variance from these features. Table 2 shows the performance metrics of the classifier accuracy based on the PCA. Clearly, the accuracy was decreased in the two MRI sequences T1-WI and T2-WI with the best performance achieved using BN classifier, where the accuracy ranged between 73.52 and 79.41%, false alarm ranged between 2.94 and 8.82%, and missed detection is 17.64%. In FLAIR sequence, PNN model showed highest value (94.11%, 0.00%, and 5.88%) of accuracy, false alarm, and missed detection, respectively.

Clearly, the accuracy decreased in T1-WI and T2-WI which reflected the lack of PCA features. In other words, GBM features provided from GMM were likely independent which was represented by the decrease accuracy value when we applied the PCA, while FLAIR sequence showed a similar value of 94.11% with GMM and PCA features which represent the correlation between the features. This is also represented by the highest correlation value of GMM features in the FLAIR sequence (Figure 6), while the heat map of correlation shows a less value in T1-WI and T2-WI sequences.

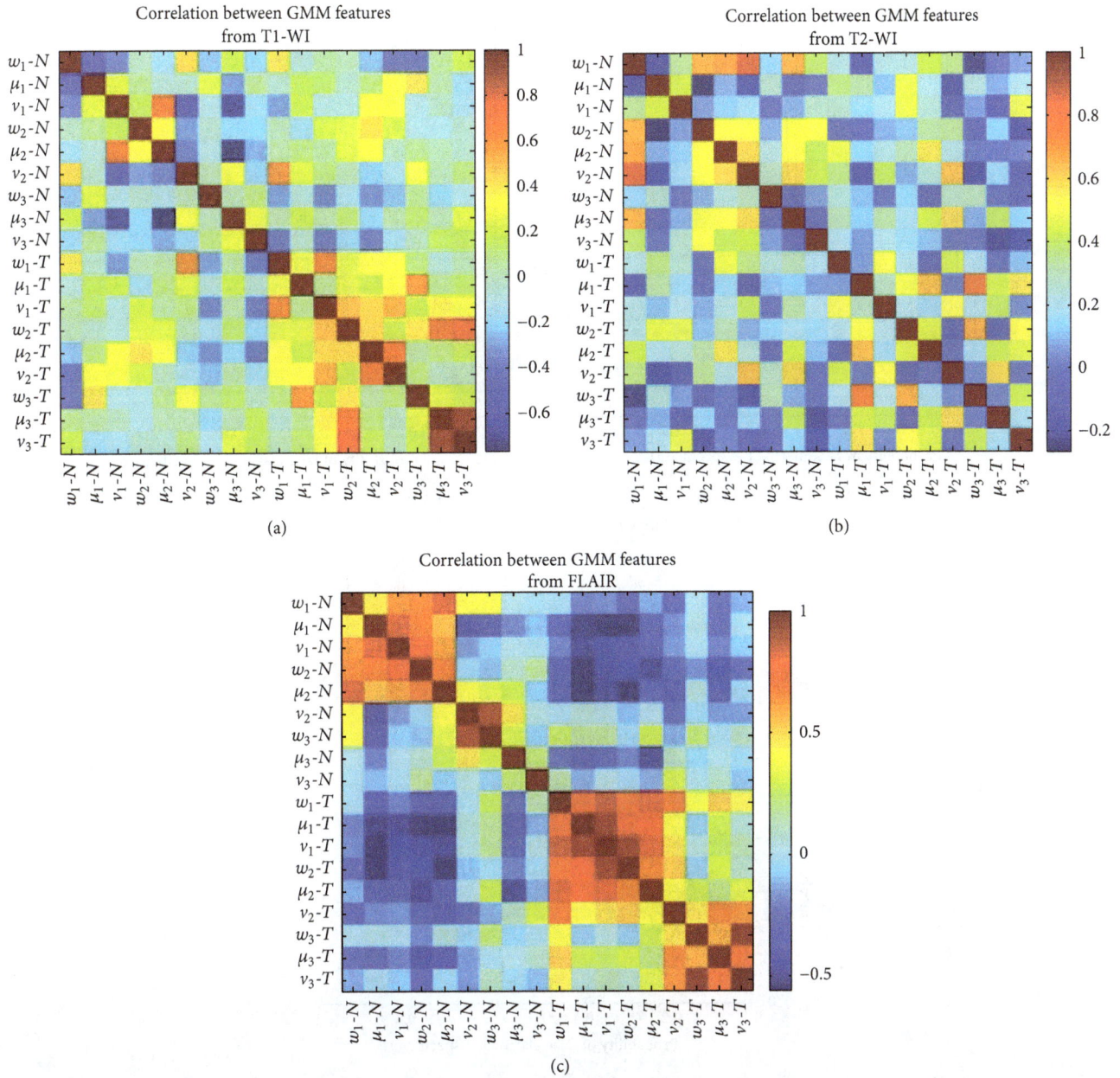

FIGURE 6: Heat map with correlation coefficients between GMM features: w, μ, and v are the weight, average, and variance, respectively; N and T are the index of normal and tumor (GBM) areas, respectively.

Another aspect of the classification was considered by using all data based on 51 images (entire GBM) including 17 images T1-WI, T2-WI, and FLAIR. Table 1 shows the classifier accuracy decrease to 86.27% with 2.94% false alarm and 10.78% missed detection using BN classifier. Clearly, the discrimination between GBM and normal brain tissue using single MR sequence was better than using all together. The classifier accuracy decreased to 68.62% (see Table 2) when we applied the PCA which proved again that the GMM features had no redundancy information in T1-WI and T2-WI and are better to be used for the discrimination of GBM from normal brain based on single MRI sequence. Note that BN classifier

showed a better performance than SVM and PNN classifier model.

Moreover, ROC curves and the associated AUC have been computed. Figure 7 shows the ROC curves to evaluate the quality of a classifier. Table 4 shows that AUC values of 95.85% based on GMM features are better than PCA (AUC = 86.16%) using FLAIR sequence. Clearly, the AUC obtained by using GMM features were better than those from PCA.

3.3. Comparatives and Discussions. A comparative study was employed using wavelet based feature [29–31]. Two wavelets,

(a)

(b)

(c)

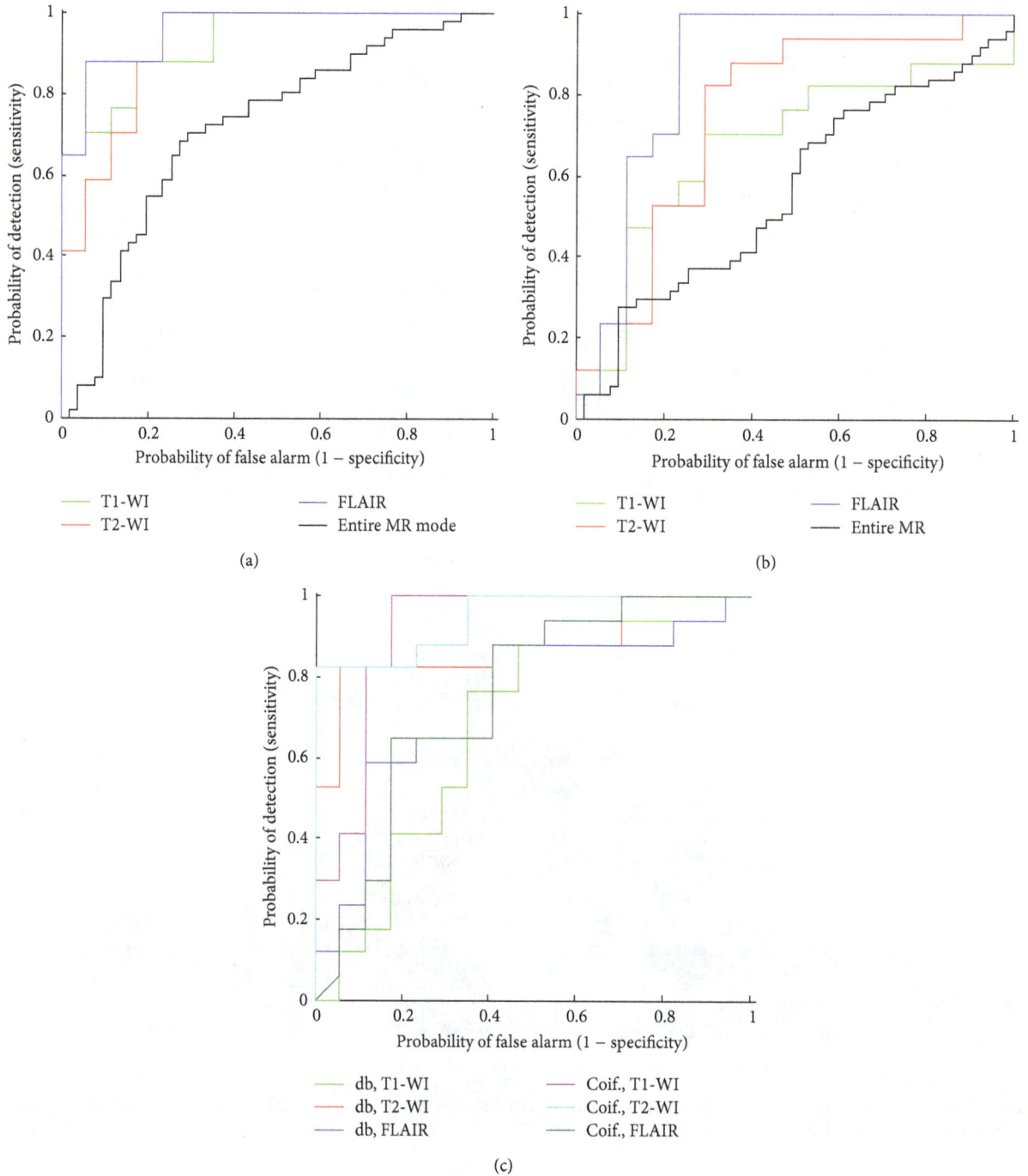

FIGURE 7: ROC curves of GBM and normal area discrimination based on T1-WI, T2-WI, FLAIR, and entire MR mode (T1-WI, T2-WI, and FLAIR, 51 images): (a) GMM features, (b) PCA features, and (c) Daubechies (*db1*) and Coiflets (*coif1*) wavelet features.

namely, *Daubechies (db1)* and *Coiflets (coif1)*, were considered [41, 42]. Three quantified functions were computed, namely, average, standard deviation, and entropy. Classifier accuracy based on the wavelet features showed the highest accuracy value of 88.23% (*coif1*) in T2-WI using SVM and PNN, 79.41% (*coif1*) in T1-WI, and 70.58% (*db1*) in FLAIR sequence using PNN and NB (see Table 3). ROC curves were associated with AUC based on wavelet feature (*coif1*) with range value 74.50–94.46% better than those based on wavelet feature

(*db1*) which showed values of 68.51–87.54% (Figure 7(c) and Table 4). We note that the main goal of the feature extraction using discrete wavelet transform technique is that the approximation coefficients usually contain the most important information (low frequency). Hence they constitute one part of the extracted features and another represented by the critical information from the high-frequency part (details). In comparison, GBM identification is more promising using the GMM features with highest accuracy classifier.

TABLE 3: Performance metrics (%) based on the wavelets.

Classifier	Metrics	T1-WI		T2-WI		FLAIR	
		db1	*coif1*	*db1*	*coif1*	*db1*	*coif1*
NB	Accuracy	67.64	79.41	82.35	85.29	70.58	64.70
	False alarm	17.64	8.82	8.82	8.88	8.82	14.70
	Missed detection	14.70	8.8235	8.82	8.82	20.58	20.58
SVM	Accuracy	50	76.47	85.29	88.23	58.82	55.88
	False alarm	20.58	14.70	2.94	0	8.82	8.82
	Missed detection	29.41	8.82	11.76	11.76	32.35	35.29
PNN	Accuracy	70.58	79.41	82.35	88.23	70.588	58.82
	False alarm	20.58	20.58	11.76	5.88	20.58	29.41
	Missed detection	8.82	0	5.88	5.88	8.82	11.76

*db1 and coif1 are the first order of Daubechies and Coiflet wavelet, respectively.

TABLE 4: Comparison of area under (%) ROC curve between three feature types.

Feature		T1-WI	T2-WI	FLAIR
Wavelets	*coif1*	91.35	94.46	74.5
	db1	68.51	87.54	73.7
GMM		92.73	91.70	95.85
PCA		67.82	75.43	86.16

This work is the first focusing on the robust GBM characteristics using the GMM features, while previous literature showed the efficiency of the texture and statistical features analysis to discover brain tumors heterogeneity [24–27, 38]. Through the texture analysis we find that this changes depending on the size and number of the pixels in the determined region. For example, cooccurrence matrix provides valuable information about the relative position of the neighboring pixels in an image. It has been proved that the texture descriptors improve performance of diagnosis where texture is an important source of image characteristics [24, 25]. However, GBM region can be easily distinguished from normal brain areas using the GMM features because we determined the number of Gaussian components (three components in this work [43]), and the number or swap of pixels did not affect the accuracy result. In other words, the number of features is independent of the pixels in the brain tumor image. All GBM tumor regions being diagnosed following MR imaging, the big advantage of this technique derives from the robust processing of MRI data to the final decision.

Obviously, neuroradiologists are becoming more and more important players to early diagnose GBM. Our vision is to integrate engineering based methods as described in daily practice to enhance radiologists' performance beyond their routine "vision." In particular in utterly devastating diseases, like GBM, improvement in any medical specialty involved is of utmost essence.

As a limitation, this study is based on a single cohort design and subject to its respective limitations. Second, the number of 17 patients limited our analysis of the GBM heterogeneity. However, there is currently no consensus on how to assess GBM heterogeneity. Third, the goal of this study was to analyze the number of images features to determine the efficiency of the GMM features as prognostic indicator. And last, the entire algorithm worked and collected data automatically.

4. Conclusions

This paper implements the GMM features extracted from GBM tumor using MR images to assist in radiologic GBM heterogeneity recognition. By a comparative study of other features types as PCA and wavelet, this technique resides in its ability to detect GBM automatically with high accuracy performance which was difficult previously. Turning to the future, it is the authors' intentions to extend this work to implement a full algorithm integrated on MRI equipment in order to identify the GBM robustly using GMM features.

Ethical Approval

The materials are in compliance with all applicable laws, regulations, and policies for the protection of medical data, and any necessary approvals, authorizations, and informed consent documents were obtained.

Consent

Informed consent was obtained from all patients for being included in the study.

Conflict of Interests

The author declares that there is no conflict of interests regarding the publication of this paper.

References

[1] C.-C. Chen, Y.-L. Wan, Y.-Y. Wai, and H.-L. Liu, "Quality assurance of clinical MRI scanners using ACR MRI phantom: preliminary results," *Journal of Digital Imaging*, vol. 17, no. 4, pp. 279–284, 2004.

[2] J. Sachdeva, V. Kumar, I. Gupta, N. Khandelwal, and C. K. Ahuja, "Segmentation, feature extraction, and multiclass brain tumor classification," *Journal of Digital Imaging*, vol. 26, no. 6, pp. 1141–1150, 2013.

[3] J. W. Patriarche and B. J. Erickson, "Part 1. Automated change detection and characterization in serial MR studies of brain-tumor patients," *Journal of Digital Imaging*, vol. 20, no. 3, pp. 203–222, 2007.

[4] B. Likar, M. A. Viergever, and F. Pernuš, "Retrospective correction of MR intensity inhomogeneity by information minimization," *IEEE Transactions on Medical Imaging*, vol. 20, no. 12, pp. 1398–1410, 2001.

[5] F. Yang, M. A. Thomas, F. Dehdashti, and P. W. Grigsby, "Temporal analysis of intratumoral metabolic heterogeneity characterized by textural features in cervical cancer," *European Journal of Nuclear Medicine and Molecular Imaging*, vol. 40, no. 5, pp. 716–727, 2013.

[6] J. J. Caban, J. Yao, and D. J. Mollura, "Enhancing image analytic tools by fusing quantitative physiological values with image features," *Journal of Digital Imaging*, vol. 25, no. 4, pp. 550–557, 2012.

[7] D. S. Nachimuthu and A. Baladhandapani, "Multidimensional texture characterization: on analysis for brain tumor tissues using MRS and MRI," *Journal of Digital Imaging*, vol. 27, no. 4, pp. 496–506, 2014.

[8] D. A. Hamstra, C. J. Galbán, C. R. Meyer et al., "Functional diffusion map as an early imaging biomarker for high-grade glioma: correlation with conventional radiologic response and overall survival," *Journal of Clinical Oncology*, vol. 26, no. 20, pp. 3387–3394, 2008.

[9] E. Helseth, G. Unsgaard, A. Dalen, and R. Vik, "Effects of type beta transforming growth factor in combination with retinoic acid or tumor necrosis factor on proliferation of a human glioblastoma cell line and clonogenic cells from freshly resected human brain tumors," *Cancer Immunology Immunotherapy*, vol. 26, no. 3, pp. 273–279, 1988.

[10] Q. T. Ostrom, H. Gittleman, P. Farah et al., "CBTRUS statistical report: primary brain and central nervous system tumors diagnosed in the United States in 2006–2010," *Neuro-Oncology*, vol. 15, supplement 2, pp. ii1–ii56, 2013.

[11] R. G. W. Verhaak, K. A. Hoadley, E. Purdom et al., "Integrated genomic analysis identifies clinically relevant subtypes of glioblastoma characterized by abnormalities in PDGFRA, IDH1, EGFR, and NF1," *Cancer Cell*, vol. 17, no. 1, pp. 98–110, 2010.

[12] P. O. Zinn and R. R. Colen, "Imaging genomic mapping in glioblastoma," *Neurosurgery*, vol. 60, no. 1, pp. 126–130, 2013.

[13] P. O. Zinn, B. Majadan, P. Sathyan et al., "Radiogenomic mapping of edema/cellular invasion MRI-phenotypes in glioblastoma multiforme," *PLoS ONE*, vol. 6, no. 10, Article ID e25451, 2011.

[14] D. Simon, K. H. Fritzsche, C. Thieke et al., "Diffusion-weighted imaging-based probabilistic segmentation of high- and low-proliferative areas in high-grade gliomas," *Cancer Imaging*, vol. 12, no. 1, pp. 89–99, 2012.

[15] S. Balla-Arabé and X. Gao, "Image multi-thresholding by combining the lattice Boltzmann model and a localized level set algorithm," *Neurocomputing*, vol. 93, pp. 106–114, 2012.

[16] A. Rojas Domínguez and A. K. Nandi, "Detection of masses in mammograms via statistically based enhancement, multilevel-thresholding segmentation, and region selection," *Computerized Medical Imaging and Graphics*, vol. 32, no. 4, pp. 304–315, 2008.

[17] L. Hertz and R. W. Schafer, "Multilevel thresholding using edge matching," *Computer Vision, Graphics, & Image Processing*, vol. 44, no. 3, pp. 279–295, 1988.

[18] N. Otsu, "A threshold selection method from Gray-Level histograms," *IEEE Transactions on Systems, Man, and Cybernetics*, vol. 9, no. 1, pp. 62–66, 1979.

[19] A. Chaddad, C. Tanougast, A. Golato, and A. Dandache, "Carcinoma cell identification via optical microscopy and shape feature analysis," *Journal of Biomedical Science and Engineering*, vol. 6, no. 11, pp. 1029–1033, 2013.

[20] G. Castellano, L. Bonilha, L. M. Li, and F. Cendes, "Texture analysis of medical images," *Clinical Radiology*, vol. 59, no. 12, pp. 1061–1069, 2004.

[21] D. Mahmoud-Ghoneim, M. K. Alkaabi, J. D. de Certaines, and F.-M. Goettsche, "The impact of image dynamic range on texture classification of brain white matter," *BMC Medical Imaging*, vol. 8, article 18, 2008.

[22] M. Sasikala and N. Kumaravel, "A wavelet-based optimal texture feature set for classification of brain tumours," *Journal of Medical Engineering and Technology*, vol. 32, no. 3, pp. 198–205, 2008.

[23] O. Yu, Y. Mauss, G. Zollner, I. J. Namer, and J. Chambron, "Distinct patterns of active and non-active plaques using texture analysis on brain NMR images in multiple sclerosis patients: preliminary results," *Magnetic Resonance Imaging*, vol. 17, no. 9, pp. 1261–1267, 1999.

[24] L. Dettori and L. Semler, "A comparison of wavelet, ridgelet, and curvelet-based texture classification algorithms in computed tomography," *Computers in Biology and Medicine*, vol. 37, no. 4, pp. 486–498, 2007.

[25] P. Georgiadis, D. Cavouras, I. Kalatzis et al., "Improving brain tumor characterization on MRI by probabilistic neural networks and non-linear transformation of textural features," *Computer Methods and Programs in Biomedicine*, vol. 89, no. 1, pp. 24–32, 2008.

[26] A. Chaddad, C. Tanougast, A. Dandache, A. Al Houseini, and A. Bouridane, "Improving of colon cancer cells detection based on Haralick's features on segmented histopathological images," in *Proceedings of the IEEE Conference on Computer Applications and Industrial Electronics (ICCAIE '11)*, pp. 87–90, IEEE, Penang, Malaysia, December 2011.

[27] F. Cardinaux, C. Sanderson, and S. Bengio, "User authentication via adapted statistical models of face images," *IEEE Transactions on Signal Processing*, vol. 54, no. 1, pp. 361–373, 2006.

[28] E. I. Zacharaki, S. Wang, S. Chawla et al., "Classification of brain tumor type and grade using MRI texture and shape in a machine learning scheme," *Magnetic Resonance in Medicine*, vol. 62, no. 6, pp. 1609–1618, 2009.

[29] J. K. Dash and L. Sahoo, "Wavelet based features of circular scan lines for mammographic mass classification," in *Proceedings of the 1st International Conference on Recent Advances in Information Technology (RAIT '12)*, pp. 58–61, March 2012.

[30] S. Dua, U. Rajendra Acharya, P. Chowriappa, and S. Vinitha Sree, "Wavelet-based energy features for glaucomatous image classification," *IEEE Transactions on Information Technology in Biomedicine*, vol. 16, no. 1, pp. 80–87, 2012.

[31] S. Li, C. Liao, and J. T. Kwok, "Wavelet-based feature extraction for microarray data classification," in *Proceedings of the International Joint Conference on Neural Networks (IJCNN '06)*, pp. 5028–5033, July 2006.

[32] N. Otsu, "A threshold selection method from gray-level histograms," *IEEE Transactions on Systems, Man and Cybernetics*, vol. 9, no. 1, pp. 62–66, 1979.

[33] T. Kinnunen and H. Li, "An overview of text-independent speaker recognition: from features to supervectors," *Speech Communication*, vol. 52, no. 1, pp. 12–40, 2010.

[34] C. Barras and J. Gauvain, "Feature and score normalization for speaker verification of cellular data," in *Proceedings of the IEEE International Conference on Acoustics, Speech, and Signal Processing (ICASSP '03)*, vol. 2, pp. II49–II52, IEEE, April 2003.

[35] V. Kilaru, M. Amin, F. Ahmad, P. Sévigny, and D. DiFilippo, "Gaussian mixture modeling approach for stationary human identification in through-the-wall radar imagery," *Journal of Electronic Imaging*, vol. 24, no. 1, Article ID 013028, 2015.

[36] C. C. Aggarwal, *Data Classification: Algorithms and Applications*, CRC Press, 2014.

[37] M. Hearst, S. Dumais, E. Osman, J. Platt, and B. Scholkopf, "Support vector machines," *IEEE Intelligent Systems and their Applications*, vol. 13, no. 4, pp. 18–28, 1998.

[38] D. F. Specht, "Probabilistic neural networks," *Neural Networks*, vol. 3, no. 1, pp. 109–118, 1990.

[39] M. Stone, "Cross-validatory choice and assessment of statistical predictions," *Journal of the Royal Statistical Society. Series B. Methodological*, vol. 36, pp. 111–147, 1974.

[40] S. H. Park, J. M. Goo, and C.-H. Jo, "Receiver operating characteristic (ROC) curve: practical review for radiologists," *Korean Journal of Radiology*, vol. 5, no. 1, pp. 11–18, 2004.

[41] S. G. Mallat, "Theory for multiresolution signal decomposition: the wavelet representation," *IEEE Transactions on Pattern Analysis and Machine Intelligence*, vol. 11, no. 7, pp. 674–693, 1989.

[42] I. Daubechies, *Ten Lectures on Wavelets*, vol. 61 of *CBMS-NSF Regional Conference Series in Applied Mathematics*, SIAM, Philadelphia, Pa, USA, 1992.

[43] A. Chaddad, P. O. Zinn, and R. R. Colen, "Brain tumor identification using Gaussian Mixture Model features and Decision Trees classifier," in *Proceedings of the 48th Annual Conference on Information Sciences and Systems (CISS '14)*, pp. 1–4, IEEE, Princeton, NJ, USA, March 2014.

10

Evaluation of Algebraic Iterative Image Reconstruction Methods for Tetrahedron Beam Computed Tomography Systems

Joshua Kim,[1,2] **Huaiqun Guan,**[3] **David Gersten,**[4] **and Tiezhi Zhang**[1,2,4]

[1] *TetraImaging, 4591 Bentley Drive, Troy, MI 48098, USA*

[2] *Department of Physics, Oakland University, 2200 N. Squirrel Road, Rochester, MI 48309, USA*

[3] *21st Century Oncology Inc., 4274 W. Main Street, Dothan, AL 36305, USA*

[4] *Department of Radiation Oncology, William Beaumont Hospital, 3601 W. Thirteen Mile Road, Royal Oak, MI 48073, USA*

Correspondence should be addressed to Tiezhi Zhang; tiezhi.zhang@beaumont.edu

Academic Editor: Habib Zaidi

Tetrahedron beam computed tomography (TBCT) performs volumetric imaging using a stack of fan beams generated by a multiple pixel X-ray source. While the TBCT system was designed to overcome the scatter and detector issues faced by cone beam computed tomography (CBCT), it still suffers the same large cone angle artifacts as CBCT due to the use of approximate reconstruction algorithms. It has been shown that iterative reconstruction algorithms are better able to model irregular system geometries and that algebraic iterative algorithms in particular have been able to reduce cone artifacts appearing at large cone angles. In this paper, the SART algorithm is modified for the use with the different TBCT geometries and is tested using both simulated projection data and data acquired using the TBCT benchtop system. The modified SART reconstruction algorithms were able to mitigate the effects of using data generated at large cone angles and were also able to reconstruct CT images without the introduction of artifacts due to either the longitudinal or transverse truncation in the data sets. Algebraic iterative reconstruction can be especially useful for dual-source dual-detector TBCT, wherein the cone angle is the largest in the center of the field of view.

1. Introduction

Image-guided radiation therapy (IGRT) is essential to ensure proper dose delivery to the target while sparing the surrounding tissue [1, 2]. Cone beam CT (CBCT) is a popular online imaging modality used for LINAC-based IGRT [3, 4]. Although CBCT is convenient to use, the performance of CBCT systems is less than ideal. The image quality for the CBCT is significantly degraded due to excessive scattered photons [5–8] as well as suboptimal performance of the flat panel detector [9]. These issues limit the use of CBCT for certain advanced radiation therapy techniques such as online adaptive radiotherapy [8, 10]. It is also well known that at large cone angles, there are artifacts caused by using approximate reconstruction methods that appear in CBCT reconstructions [11], but this issue has largely been ignored in IGRT because the scatter and detector issues are the dominant factors in the degradation of CBCT image quality.

Tetrahedron beam computed tomography (TBCT) is a novel volumetric CT modality that overcomes the scatter and detector problems of CBCT [12, 13]. A TBCT system is composed of a minimum of one linear source array with one linear detector array positioned opposite and orthogonal to it. In TBCT, scattered photons are largely rejected due to the fan-beam geometry of the system. A TBCT system also uses the same high performance detectors that are used for helical CT scanners. Therefore, TBCT should be equivalent to diagnostic helical CT with regard to scatter rejection and detector performance. However, similar to CBCT, the data sufficiency condition [14, 15] is not satisfied with a single axial TBCT scan. TBCT still suffers from the same large cone angle artifacts that are present in CBCT images reconstructed using the conventional Feldkamp-Davis-Kress (FDK)-type approximate filtered backprojection (FBP) algorithm [16]. More importantly, in a TBCT system that is composed of two source arrays and two detector arrays, the cone

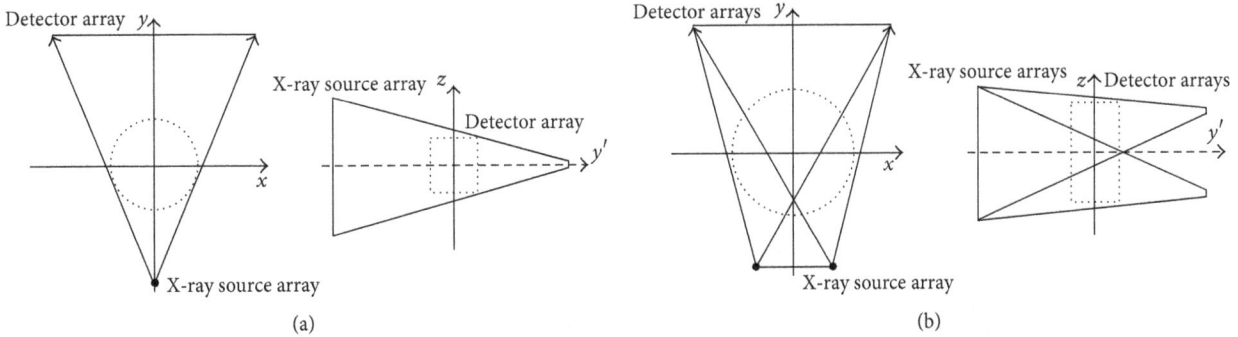

(a)

(b)

FIGURE 1: Single-source single-detector TBCT geometry (a). Dual-source dual-detector TBCT geometry (b).

reconstruction artifact is most significant in the center of the field of view (FOV). Therefore, reducing cone artifacts is more important for this arrangement.

Owing to the rapid improvement in computational power, it has become practical to use iterative reconstruction methods in the clinic. Iterative imaging reconstruction methods have been proven to be capable of reducing imaging dose [17, 18], increasing image resolution [19, 20], and reducing artifacts [21, 22]. Most CT vendors provide different iterative image reconstruction solutions for their diagnostic CT scanners. The algebraic reconstruction technique (ART) [23] and the simultaneous ART (SART) [24] algebraic iterative methods, in particular, have been shown to reconstruct cone beam data with minimal artifacts at large cone angles [21].

In order to further improve TBCT image quality and reduce reconstruction artifacts at larger cone angles, we implemented iterative algebraic reconstruction methods for different TBCT geometries in this study. We evaluated the performance of these algorithms using various numerical phantoms as well as digitally-projected patient images. The patient reconstruction results were then compared to the reconstructed images produced using a fan-beam reconstruction method that was considered to be the ground truth for this study.

2. Material and Methods

2.1. TBCT Geometries. The TBCT system geometry is flexible enough to incorporate multiple source and detector arrays if the need arises. Figure 1 shows a comparison of the geometries for the [single-source single-detector] TBCT system and for the dual-source dual-detector TBCT system. With the dual-source dual-detector geometry, the length of the detector and source arrays can be reduced while still being able to achieve the same FOV. However, for a TBCT system that uses two detector arrays, the approximate reconstruction artifacts would be most prominent in the central transverse plane of the image instead of at the top and bottom of the image. Therefore, reducing the cone artifact is especially important for the [dual-source dual-detector] TBCT system.

2.2. Algebraic Reconstruction Algorithms. Detector projection measurements during a CT scan are represented by the linear system equation

$$\mathbf{p} = \mathbf{A}\mathbf{x}, \qquad (1)$$

where $\mathbf{x} = (x_1, x_2, \ldots, x_N)$ represents the image to be reconstructed and $\mathbf{p} = (p_1, p_2, \ldots, p_M)$ represents the measured projection data. M and N are the total number of line integral measurements and total number of image voxels, respectively. The total number of measurements, M, is the product of the number of detectors and the number of projections per detector. The system matrix $\mathbf{A} \in \mathbb{R}^{M \times N}$ has matrix elements $a_{ij} \geq 0$ that map the image voxel i onto the projection measurement j. In iterative reconstruction, the image voxel values are treated as unknowns in the system of equations given by (1). For a 3D CT scan, the dimensions of the system matrix $\mathbf{A}$ are enormous. Both M and N could be in the order of hundreds of millions.

To calculate the elements of the system matrix, we implemented the distance-driven method introduced by De Man and Basu [25]. For this method, the boundaries of the detectors and voxels are mapped onto a common plane. The lengths of overlap of the detector and voxel boundaries along each of the axes of the plane are then calculated. These two values are then multiplied together to determine the value of the system matrix elements.

This system of equations cannot be solved directly due to the ill-posedness of the problem, the noise in the data, and the immense size of the system matrix, but it can be solved iteratively using an algebraic approach. Iterative methods begin with an initial guess of the image voxel values, which is then forward projected using the system matrix to produce an estimate of the projection data. The differences between the estimated and measured projection data are calculated and used to determine correction terms which are then back projected onto the image. This process is iteratively repeated until some convergence criteria have been satisfied or a preset number of iterations has completed. For this study, we have chosen to implement the well-known SART algorithm [24] which has been shown to converge to the weighted least squares solution from any initial guess [26]. It has also been demonstrated in previous studies that the convergence of algebraic methods could be improved by varying the order in which projections are processed [27], and so we implement the SART both with and without the use of the multilevel access ordering scheme (MAS) developed by Guan and Gordon [27].

2.2.1. Simultaneous Algebraic Reconstruction Technique. The forward projection of each measurement is calculated using $\widehat{p}_j = \sum_i a_{ij} x_i$ and then compared to the measured projection value p_j. The difference between these values is then weighted and backprojected over the image. For the SART algorithm, all projection measurements collected at a single projection image are used to simultaneously update each image voxel value. The update term is given by

$$x_i^{n+1} = x_i^n + \lambda \frac{\sum_{j=A}^{B} a_{ij} \left(\left(p_j - \widehat{p}_j \right) / \sum_{i=1}^{N} a_{ij} \right)}{\sum_{j=A}^{B} a_{ij}}, \qquad (2)$$

where n is the update step, i is the image voxel index, j is the projection data index, λ is the relaxation parameter, and A and B are the indices of the first and last projection data elements used for the nth update step. These values are defined by $A = (n-1)K$ and $B = nK$ where K is the number of projection data elements that make up a single projection image. One iteration is completed after all projection images have been used to update the image. The image **x** converges to a stable solution after a few iterations. The relaxation parameter value that was chosen for this study was 0.08, which was selected by trial and error and falls within the range suggested in the literature [28, 29].

2.2.2. Multilevel Projection Ordering Scheme. The MAS ordering system was developed for algebraic reconstruction algorithms in order to minimize the correlation between sequential projection images that are used to update the image [27]. This leads to an improvement in the convergence speed of the algebraic methods. This method has been evaluated and compared against alternate ordering systems and has been shown to provide the greatest benefit in improving the efficiency of the reconstruction algorithms [30]. For a system with V projection views ordered sequentially as $0, 1, \ldots, V - 1$, this system determines a number of levels according to $L = \log_2 V$. If V is not a power of two, then one is added to the number of levels. The levels are ordered so that any two sequential views are chosen for maximum orthogonality between them. The order of the indices in the first level is set as 0 ($0°$) followed by $V/2$ ($90°$). The second level again has two elements and the indices are set as $V/4$ ($45°$) followed by $3V/4$ ($135°$). The order of the indices in the third level is $V/8$, $5V/8$, $3V/8$, and then $7V/8$. The value of the index is rounded down to the nearest integer if the division results in a decimal. This process is repeated until all L levels are complete. This system was originally developed for a set of projections that covers the range 0 to $180°$. For the projection set that covers a full rotation, the scheme would be used to calculate the order for the projections that cover the first $180°$. The indices for the set of projections that cover the 180 to $360°$ range can be found by adding 180 to the set of indices covering the first $180°$. No change needs to be made to (2) when using the MAS ordering

scheme. To implement the MAS scheme, only the indices A and B need to be redefined so that $A = (v-1)K$ and $B = vK$ where v is the projection view index determined according to the MAS scheme.

2.2.3. Image Reconstruction for Dual-Source Dual-Detector TBCT. In the dual-source dual-detector configuration, four projection images are generated at each rotation angle. Each of the projection images collected at a given rotation angle is truncated both longitudinally and transversely as can be seen in the diagram shown in Figure 1(b). This leads to the center region of the FOV being covered by more than one source array detector array pair. Sequentially, backprojecting equally weighted correction terms calculated from each of the four projection images will cause artifacts. Instead, the correction terms from each of the four projection images are first weighted and then simultaneously backprojected onto the image. The weights applied to the correction terms for image voxel i are given by

$$w_{1,1,i} = \frac{e^{-k_{x'} x_i'} e^{-k_z z_i}}{\left(1 + e^{-k_{x'} x_i'}\right)\left(1 + e^{-k_z z_i}\right)}$$

$$w_{1,2,i} = \frac{e^{-k_{x'} x_i'}}{\left(1 + e^{-k_{x'} x_i'}\right)\left(1 + e^{-k_z z_i}\right)}$$

$$w_{2,1,i} = \frac{e^{-k_z z_i}}{\left(1 + e^{-k_{x'} x_i'}\right)\left(1 + e^{-k_z z_i}\right)} \qquad (3)$$

$$w_{2,2,i} = \frac{1}{\left(1 + e^{-k_{x'} x_i'}\right)\left(1 + e^{-k_z z_i}\right)},$$

where $w_{\alpha,\beta,i}$ is the weight applied to the update term from the projection set collected using source array α and detector array β. x_i' is the transverse position of voxel i in the rotated reference frame, z_i is the longitudinal position of voxel i, $k_{x'}$ is a constant used to vary the rate at which the transverse contribution fades out, and k_z is the constant used to vary the rate at which the longitudinal contribution fades out. Therefore, the new expression for the update term for the SART reconstruction method using the dual-source dual-detector configuration is

$$x_i^{n+1} = x_i^n + \lambda$$

$$\times \sum_{\alpha=1:2} \sum_{\beta=1:2} w_{\alpha,\beta,i} \frac{\sum_{j=A}^{B} a_{ij} \left(\left(p_j - \widehat{p}_j \right) / \sum_{i=1}^{N} a_{ij} \right)}{\sum_{j=A}^{B} a_{ij}}, \qquad (4)$$

where $w_{\alpha,\beta,i}$ is the weighting factor defined by (3), $a_{i,j}$ is an element of the system matrix $\mathbf{A}_{\alpha,\beta}$, p_j is an element of the measured projection data set $\mathbf{p}_{\alpha,\beta}$, and $\widehat{p}_j$ is an element of the estimated projection set calculated using the system matrix $\mathbf{A}_{\alpha,\beta}$.

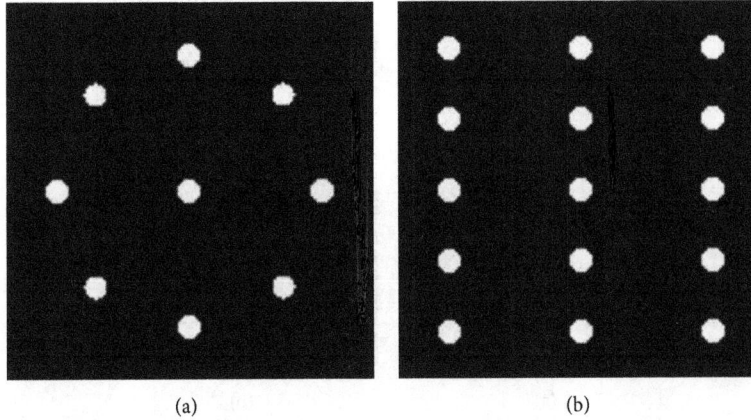

FIGURE 2: Transverse (a) and coronal (b) views of the spherical phantom.

2.3. Evaluation Method

2.3.1. System Parameters.
We employed the same geometry that was used in our TBCT benchtop system [13]. The reconstructed images had dimensions $256 \times 256 \times 128$ with an isotropic voxel size of 1 mm. A total of 360 projections were generated at one degree intervals. For a TBCT system that incorporates a multirow detector array, each TBCT projection is a 3D matrix whose dimensions correspond to the number of sources, the number of detector columns, and the number of detector rows. Therefore, the TBCT projection data dimensions for our system containing 75 field emission X-ray sources and five detector rows with 275 detector columns per row were $75 \times 275 \times 5$. The X-ray source spacing was 4 mm, and the isotropic detector pixel size was 2.54 mm. These projections were reconstructed using a modified FDK filtered backprojection algorithm and the SART algorithm both with and without the MAS ordering scheme.

2.3.2. Phantom.
The three-dimensional Shepp-Logan phantom [31] was used to test the performance of the reconstruction algorithms. The parameters were taken from this reference except that the density values of the ellipsoids were magnified to increase the contrast. Patient projection data were also generated by forward projecting the CT image of a real patient. The same matrix that was used for image reconstruction was also used to forward project the patient image for generation of the patient projection set. The resolution of the reconstructed image was 1 mm $\times$ 1 mm $\times$ 1.5 mm.

It has been shown that the use of the SART algorithm can mitigate the large cone angle artifacts that are produced when using approximate reconstruction methods such as the FDK algorithm [11]. In order to test the effectiveness of our modified algebraic reconstruction methods at reducing the cone angle artifacts, a numerical Defrise-like phantom was created [32]. The seven identical, longitudinally stacked ellipses of uniform density that compose this phantom provided a cone angle of 20 degrees. The phantom was positioned at the isocenter, which was set to be equidistant from both source and detector positions. The distance from the source to the detector was set at 64 cm.

The linear system of equations when using the disk phantom has a very low rank due to the longitudinal symmetry of the phantom. We believe that the cone artifacts appearing in the reconstructions are exaggerated due to the atypical geometry of the disk phantom. In reality, the symmetry and shape of the disks do not appear in regular patients' images. To test the cone artifact using a phantom with a different configuration, we created a phantom where each disk was replaced by a set of nine small spheres. For this configuration, there is one central sphere and eight spheres equally spaced in a circle pattern around it as shown in Figure 2. Five sets of these sphere configurations were stacked longitudinally at equal intervals and together provided the same 20 degree cone angle that was provided by the disk phantom. Similar to the disk phantom, the sphere phantom is also longitudinally symmetric, but while the disk phantom generated identical projection images at every projection angle, the sphere phantom generated data that was sinusoidally varying as a function of projection angle. Figure 3 compares the sinograms of the central slices for the two phantoms. The disk and sphere projection data were generated using the same method that was used to generate the Shepp-Logan projection data.

2.3.3. Image Evaluation Metrics.
The figures of merit (FOM) chosen for quantitative evaluation of the reconstructed images are the relative root mean square error (RRME) and the square Euclidean distance, which are defined by

$$\mathrm{RRME} = \sqrt{\frac{\sum_{i \in I} \left(x_i - x_i^{\mathrm{ref}} \right)^2}{\sum_{i \in I} \left(x_i^{\mathrm{ref}} \right)^2}},$$

$$\mathrm{sqEuc} = 1 - \frac{1}{N} \sum_{i \in I} \left(x_i - x_i^{\mathrm{ref}} \right)^2, \tag{5}$$

where x^{ref} is the reference image.

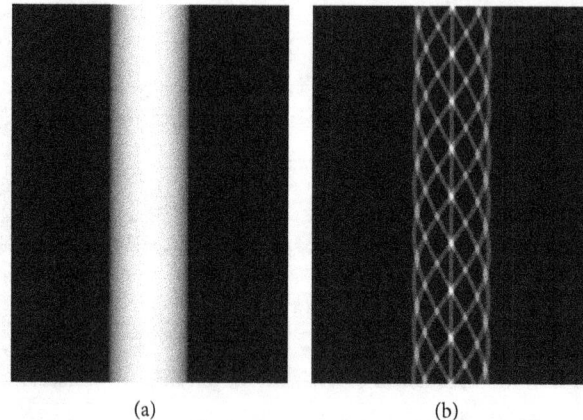

(a)   (b)

FIGURE 3: CBCT sinograms for the central slice of the (a) disk phantom and the (b) sphere phantom.

3. Results

3.1. Evaluation of the Algebraic Reconstruction Methods. We first tested the SART algorithms with data created using the [single-source single-detector] TBCT geometry. SART reconstructions of a transverse slice of the Shepp-Logan phantom after 1, 5, 10, and 15 iterations are displayed in Figure 4. The results are given for the SART method both with and without the MAS ordering scheme. The numerical phantom image and FDK reconstruction are also displayed for comparison. In Figure 5, the convergence rates of the algebraic methods are compared using the square Euclidean distance and RRME. The FOM values for the FDK reconstruction are displayed as reference lines on the graphs. Both metrics indicate that the algebraic methods achieved their best results between four and six iterations and that the FOM values for the algebraic methods were comparable to the FDK results in that region.

The SART method converged at approximately the same rate whether or not the MAS ordering scheme was used, but the SART method using the MAS scheme clearly gave better initial results. After five iterations, the SART method with the MAS ordering scheme was chosen as the method for providing the best balance between convergence speed and image quality. The reconstructions using the FDK and SART with MAS algorithms were then compared to the original phantom by evaluating a line integral taken through different views of the image. As shown in Figure 6, the line profile results from the sagittal and coronal views show good agreement between the reconstructed images and the numerical phantom.

In the images reconstructed using the SART algorithm, ringing artifacts can be seen at both the top and bottom of the phantom in both the coronal and sagittal views. This artifact is a result of using a cubic voxel discretization of the image space [24, 33–35]. Because of discretization of the continuous object, the modeled object edges are blurred and therefore the projection values calculated after forward projecting the image voxels will not match the measured values. Ringing artifacts will then result in areas with very high image gradients because the corrections to these voxels

will be incorrectly weighted, and the resulting overshoot and undershoot in the voxels at the edges will then propagate to the neighboring voxels that are under a non-negativity constraint during further iterations. This effect is usually controlled by selecting a number of iterations that qualitatively provide the best tradeoff between edge sharpness and ringing artifact. The simplest way to mitigate this effect is to use a finer grid size [34], but this would lead to an increase in the computational expense of the algorithm. Other possible methods used to reduce these artifacts include the use of a spherically symmetric basis for the voxels instead of the cubic basis that is conventionally used [33, 36] and the use of a smoothing method during reconstruction [35].

A pig's head was scanned using our TBCT benchtop system. The projections were reconstructed using the FDK and SART algorithms. With no image to use as a ground truth image, the reconstructions were evaluated qualitatively. Based on the results of the Shepp-Logan phantom, we used five iterations of the SART algorithm and used the MAS projection ordering scheme. A transverse image of the pig's head reconstructions is displayed in Figure 7 for comparison. There is close visual agreement between the images reconstructed using the different methods with slightly better contrast seen in the SART images.

3.2. Evaluation of the Cone Artifact. Projection images of the Defrise-like phantom were generated for both CBCT and TBCT geometries. Coronal images of the original phantom as well as reconstructions produced using the regular FDK method for CBCT, the modified FDK method for the TBCT, and the SART with MAS method for TBCT are shown in Figures 8(a)–8(d). Line profiles taken through the center and edges of the coronal image are displayed in Figures 8(e) and 8(f), respectively. When using the FDK method, cone artifacts appeared in the reconstructions at the larger cone angles when using either of the TBCT and CBCT geometries. By contrast, the reconstructions produced using the SART algorithm did not suffer from large cone angle artifacts. There was, however, slight elongation of the disks along the longitudinal axis and a corresponding drop in CT values at

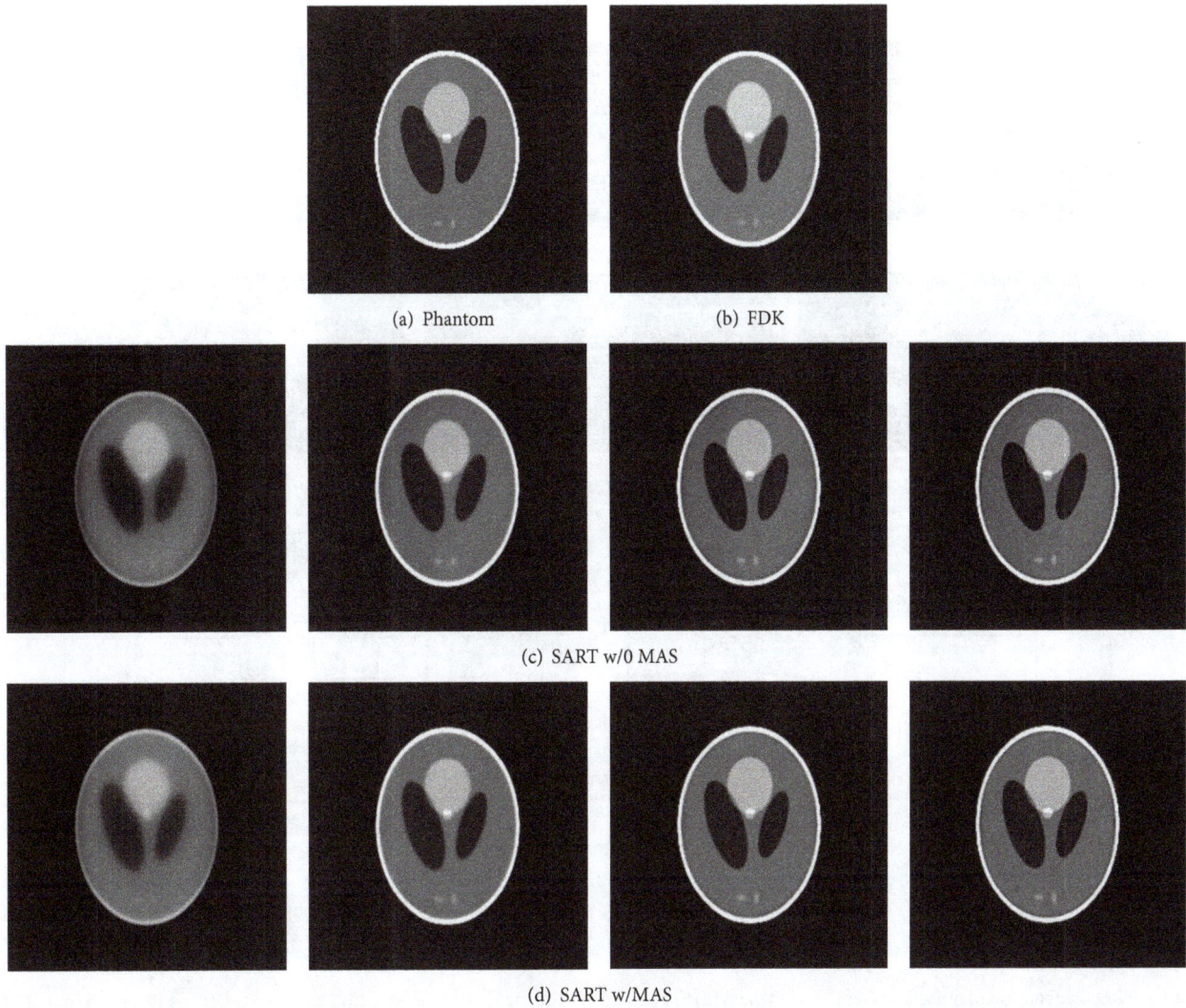

(a) Phantom   (b) FDK

(c) SART w/0 MAS

(d) SART w/MAS

FIGURE 4: Reconstructions of the (a) Shepp-Logan phantom using the (b) FDK, (c) SART without the MAS ordering scheme, and (d) SART with the MAS ordering scheme. The four columns in (c) and (d) show reconstructed images after 1, 5, 10, and 15 iterations for the SART methods. The display window is set to [0.99 1.05].

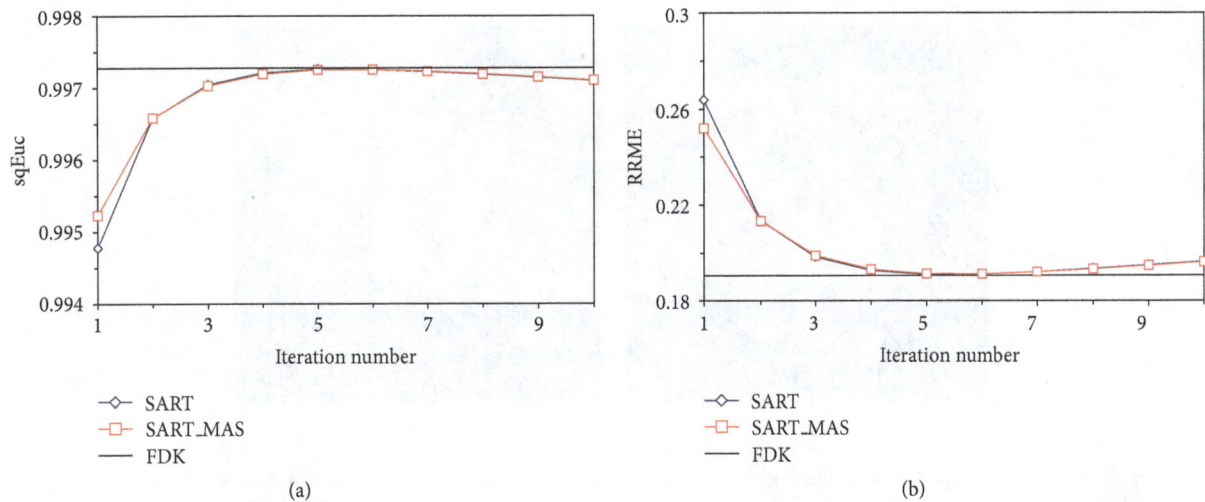

(a)   (b)

FIGURE 5: Comparison of convergence rates of three algebra reconstructions with (a) square Euclidean distance and (b) RRME.

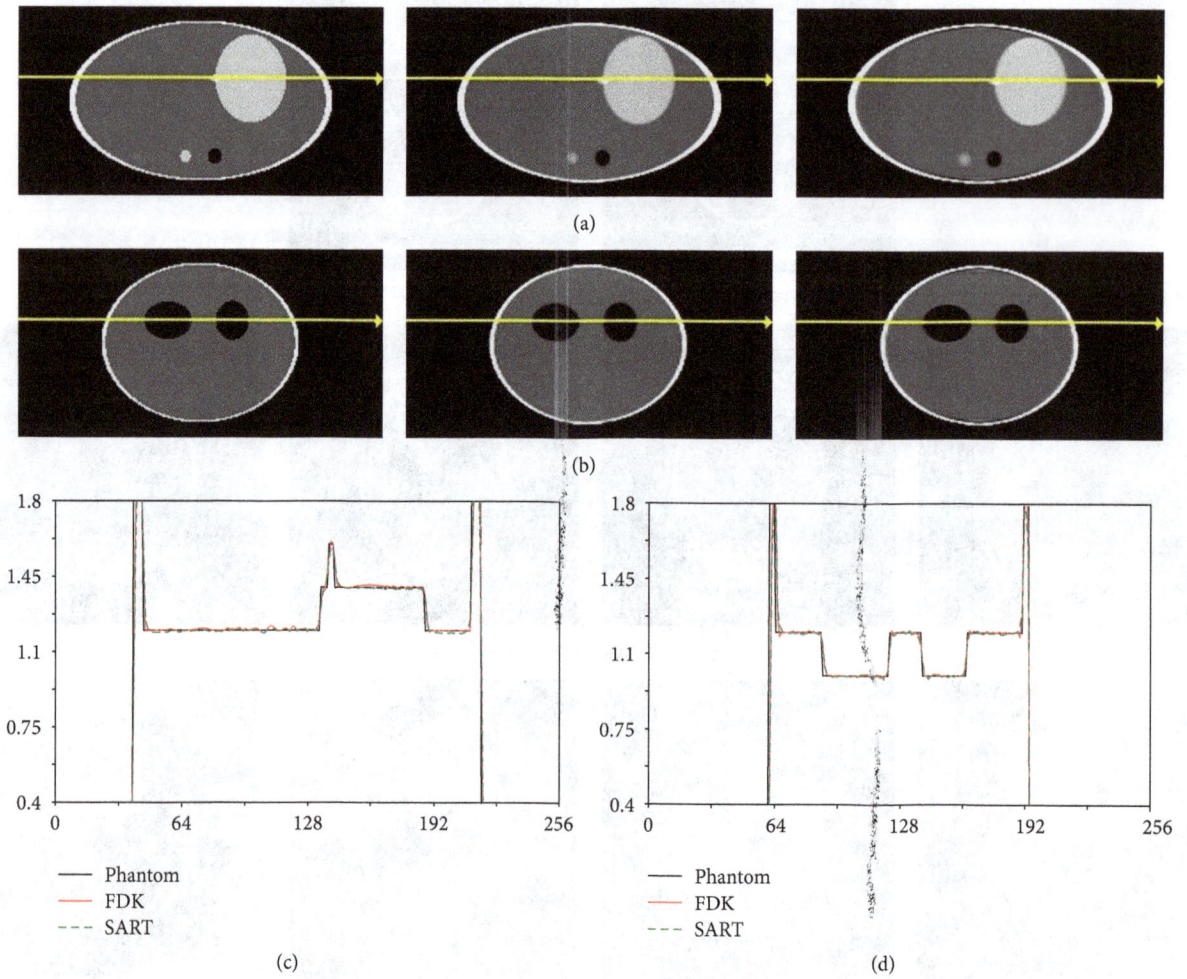

FIGURE 6: Reconstruction of noiseless Shepp-Logan data. (a) Sagittal and (b) coronal views of reconstructed images. (c) Sagittal and (d) coronal profiles of reconstructed images. In (a) and (b), from left to right are phantom, FDK reconstruction, and SART reconstruction images. For both the coronal and sagittal SART reconstructions, overshoot artifacts can be observed at the top and bottom edges of the phantom.

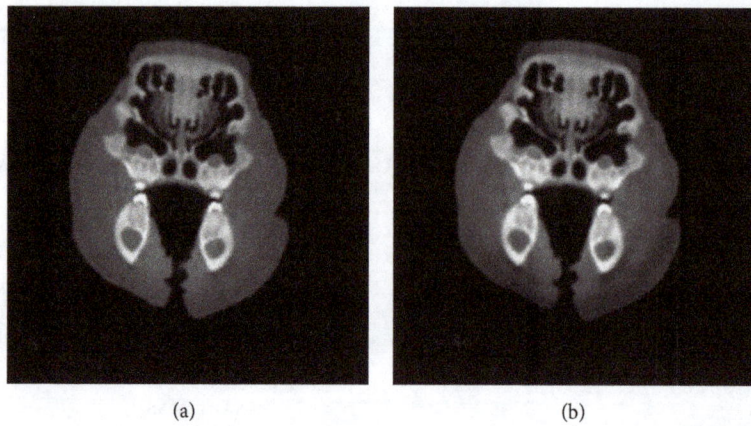

FIGURE 7: Transverse images of a pig's head with projections collected using the TBCT benchtop system and reconstructed using the (a) FDK algorithm and (b) SART algorithm with MAS scheme.

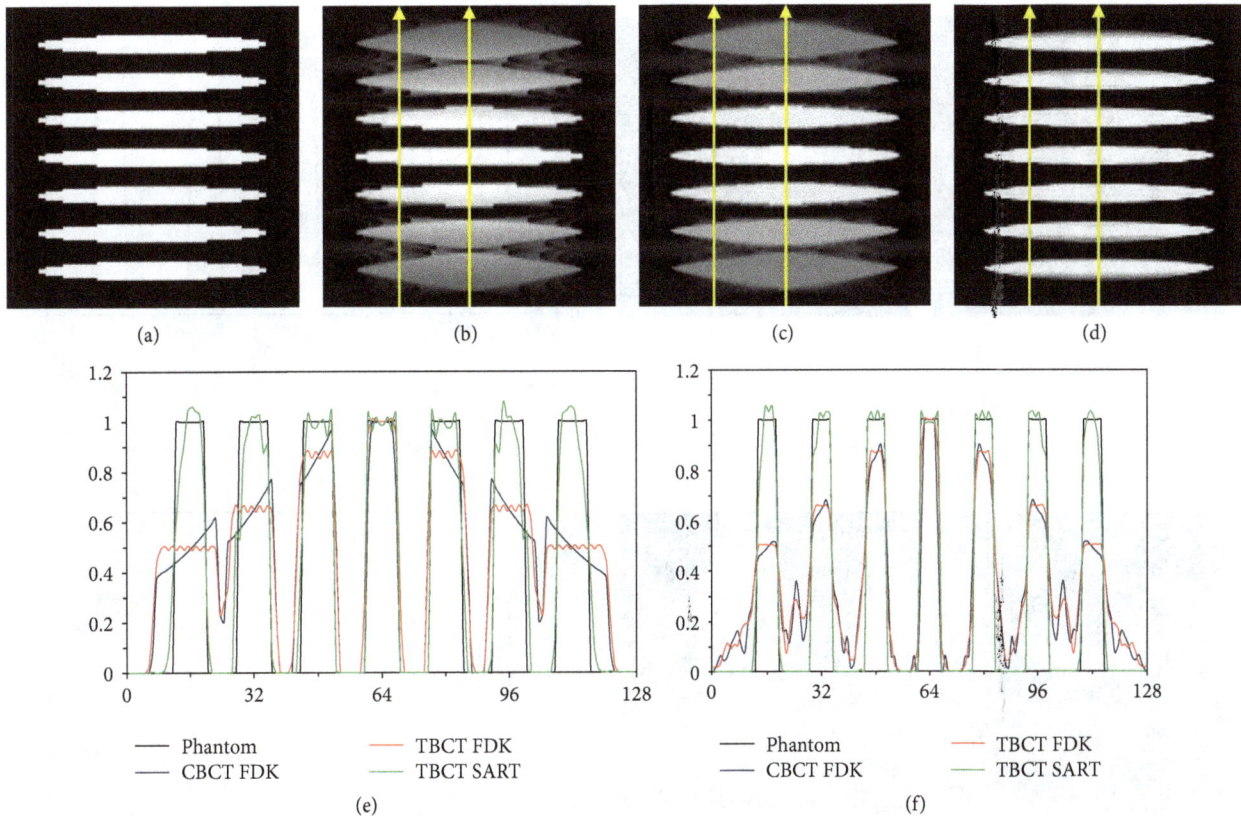

FIGURE 8: Comparison of reconstruction of a disk phantom with different methods. (a)–(d) Coronal views of original phantom, reconstructions using CBCT FDK, TBCT FDK, and TBCT SART methods, respectively. (e) and (f) are line profiles taken through the center and edges, respectively, of the images as indicated by the arrows.

the edges of the disk, though not to the extent experienced by the FDK reconstructions.

The sphere phantom was reconstructed using the FDK and SART with MAS algorithms that were modified for use with the TBCT system. The TBCT system dimensions that were used for the disk phantoms were also used here. Figure 9 shows the coronal views of the FDK and SART reconstructions. Line profiles were taken through the central column of spheres to verify that there is neither elongation nor decay in CT values for the spheres along the longitudinal axis. A slight elongation of the disks could still be observed in the FDK reconstruction but not in the reconstructed images produced by the SART algorithm. To check that the CT values were constant at the borders of the image, a line profile was also taken through a side column of spheres. The results were generally consistent with those obtained from the line profile through the central column, but the FDK reconstructions showed a slight drop in CT values toward the edges.

We further tested the reconstruction methods using a patient image that was originally reconstructed using a diagnostic CT scanner. We generated TBCT projection data using the system geometry parameters of our benchtop TBCT system. Because the inherent resolution of the original patient image would be different than that of the TBCT reconstruction due to the differences in the scanning geometry used to create our projections as opposed to the scanning

geometry used with the diagnostic CT scanner, we generated a projection set using a fan-beam geometry that had exactly the same system dimensions as the central plane of our TBCT system. The resulting fan-beam reconstruction had the same inherent resolution as our TBCT system and could therefore be used for comparison with the TBCT reconstructions. The projections were reconstructed using the fan-beam filtered backprojection (FBP) algorithm, the FDK algorithm modified for the TBCT geometry, and the SART with MAS algorithm for TBCT. The reconstructed images had dimensions $256 \times 256 \times 123$ with voxel dimensions of $2\,mm \times 2\,mm \times 3\,mm$. Figures 10(a) and 10(d) show the transverse and coronal images, respectively, of the FBP algorithms using the simulated helical CT data. The cone angle to the outermost slices was $25°$. Figures 10(b) and 10(e) show the transverse and coronal images, respectively, reconstructed using the modified FDK algorithm on the simulated TBCT data, and Figures 10(c) and 10(f) show the same two images after five iterations of the SART algorithm also using the simulated TBCT data. No elongation is apparent in the images produced using either the FDK or SART algorithms. The coronal images demonstrate that the TBCT reconstructions do not show any noticeable elongation for objects at higher cone angles during a patient scan. These results are consistent with the testing performed on the sphere phantom.

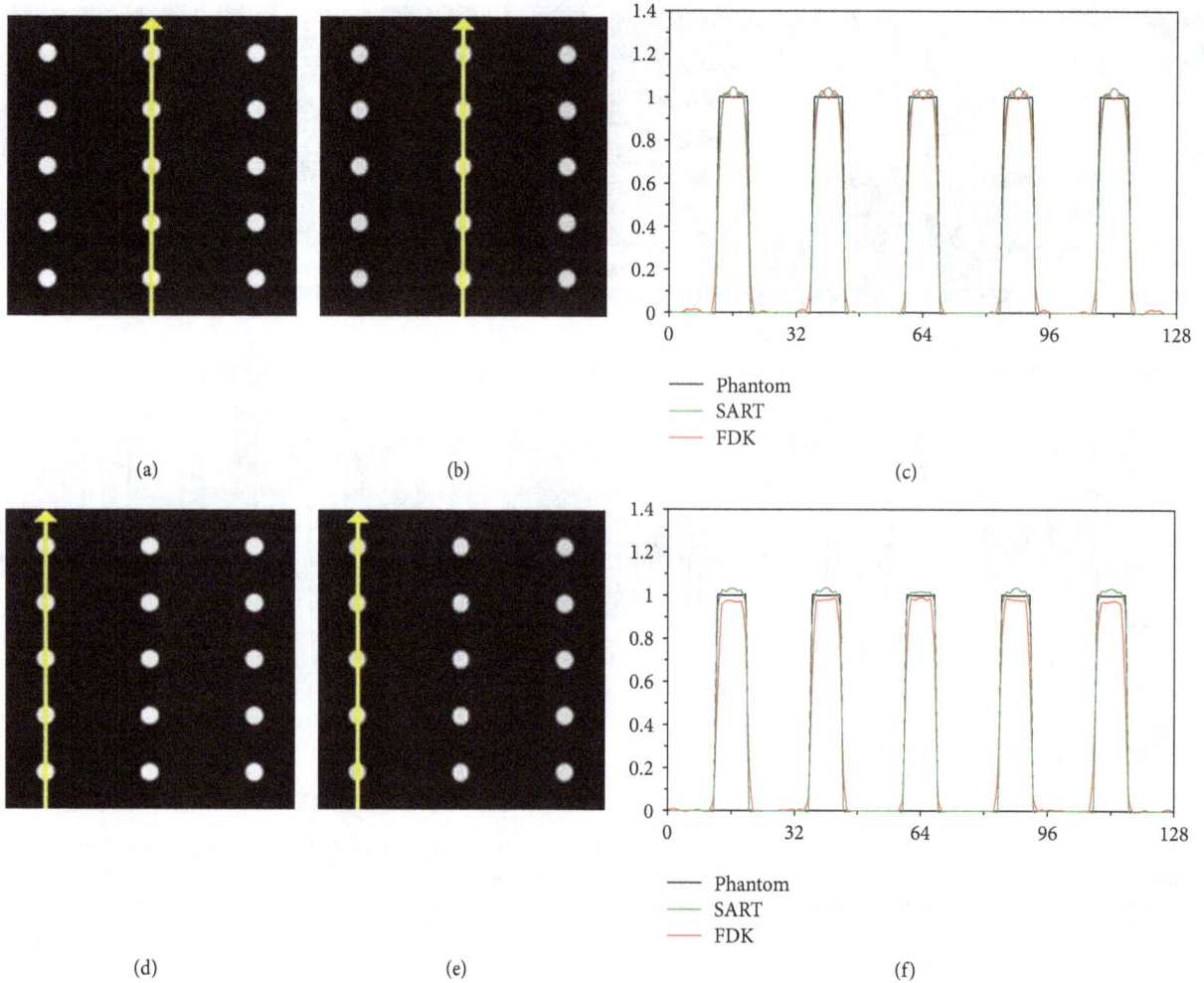

FIGURE 9: Coronal views of (a) SART and (b) FDK reconstructions with a (c) line profile taken through the center column. (d) SART and (e) FDK reconstructions with a (f) line profile taken through a side column.

3.3. Iterative Reconstruction for Dual Source-Dual Detector TBCT. The dual source-dual detector TBCT configuration is preferable for image-guided radiotherapy. However, for this configuration, the maximum cone angles are in the region of the central axis, and therefore, the large angle artifacts will be most significant at the center of the reconstructed image. Moreover, the detector and source arrays do not cover the full FOV so that the data is truncated both longitudinally and transversely. We used the Shepp-Logan phantom and clinical CT images to test the performance of the TBCT and SART algorithms that were modified for the dual source-dual detector TBCT geometry. The detector array was modified so that the projection data associated with each source array detector array pair had dimensions $75 \times 200 \times 5$. The size of the detectors was kept the same, and the reconstructed image dimensions were $256 \times 256 \times 128$ with an isotropic voxel length of 1 mm. We performed five iterations of the SART algorithm while using the MAS scheme and compared the results with those of the modified FDK algorithm. As seen in Figure 11, the image was reconstructed without the addition of significant artifacts that would have been caused by either longitudinal or transverse truncation.

To further evaluate the performance of the algorithms at large cone angles, we used the same disk and sphere phantoms defined above. The system parameters that were used to generate the data sets were kept constant. The reconstruction results are shown in Figure 12. As expected, the cone angle artifact in the FDK reconstruction increased towards the center of the image where the angle was the largest, while no artifact was observed in the SART reconstruction. There was a slight elongation of the disks that appeared around the central slice for both algorithms, but it was more pronounced in the FDK reconstruction. The reconstructions of the sphere phantom showed neither elongation nor cone artifacts when using the SART algorithm, but there was a slight elongation around all the spheres in the reconstructions produced by the FDK algorithm.

Similarly, a diagnostic CT image was then used to create the four simulated projection sets that would be produced by a dual source-dual detector TBCT system. As shown in Figure 13, there are no significant artifacts introduced into the image due to the transverse truncation. Because the inherent resolution of the patient image would again have been different due to the use of different scanning parameters,

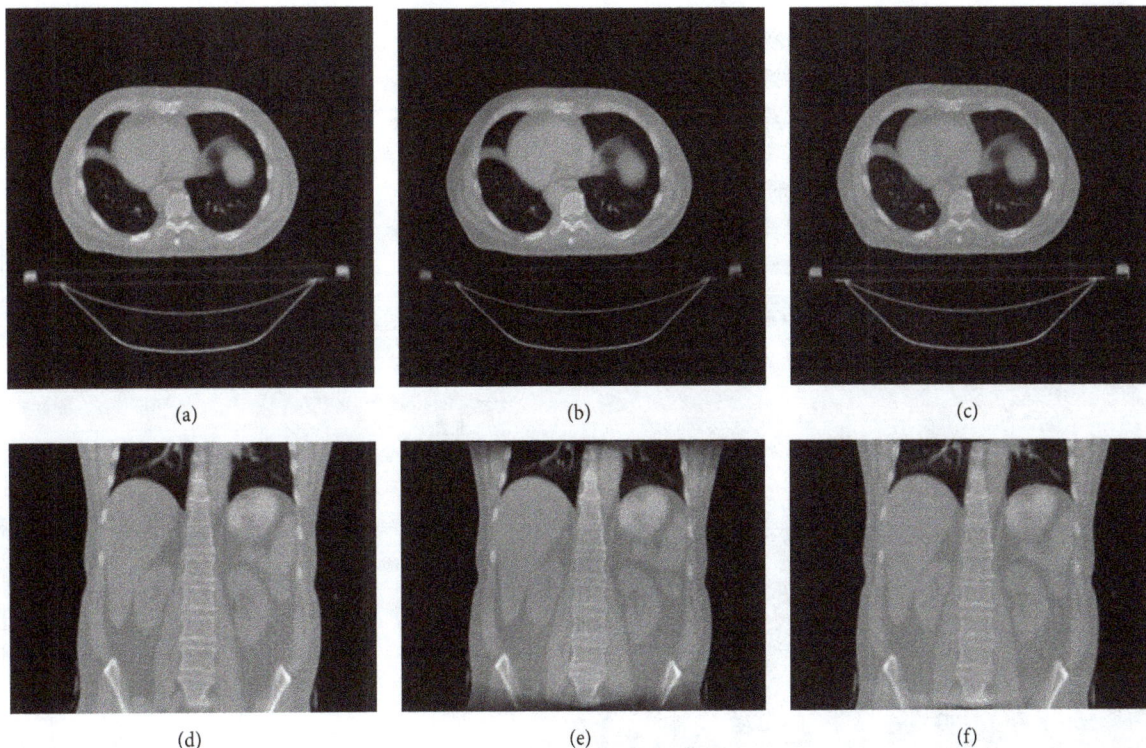

FIGURE 10: Reconstructed (top row) transverse images of a patient using the (a) fan-beam, (b) FDK, and (c) SART algorithms. Reconstructed (bottom row) coronal images using the (d) fan-beam, (e) FDK, and (f) SART algorithms.

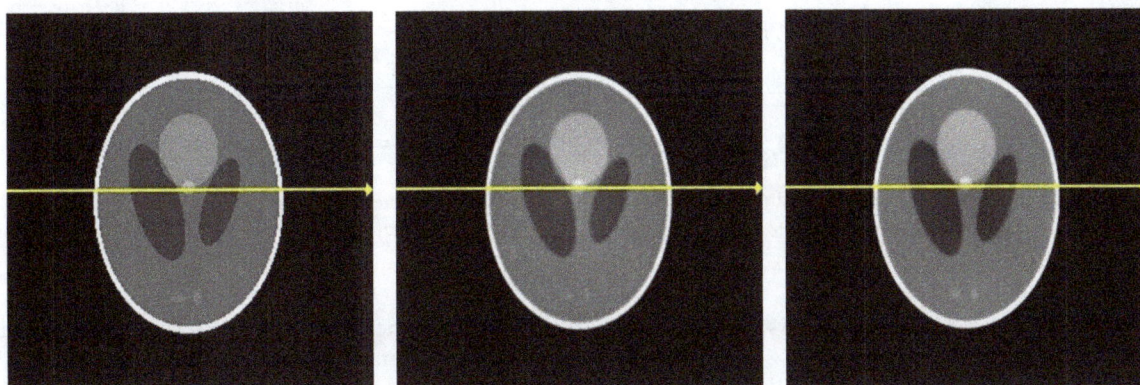

(a)

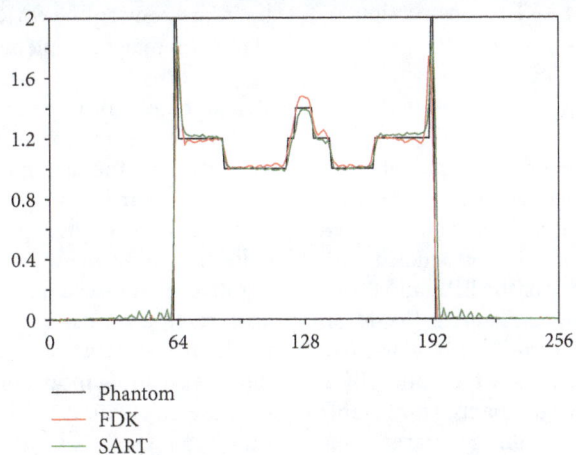

(b)

FIGURE 11: Reconstructions (a) of the (left) Shepp-Logan phantom using the (center) FDK filtered backprojection algorithm and the (right) SART algorithm with (b) a line profile taken through the reconstructions.

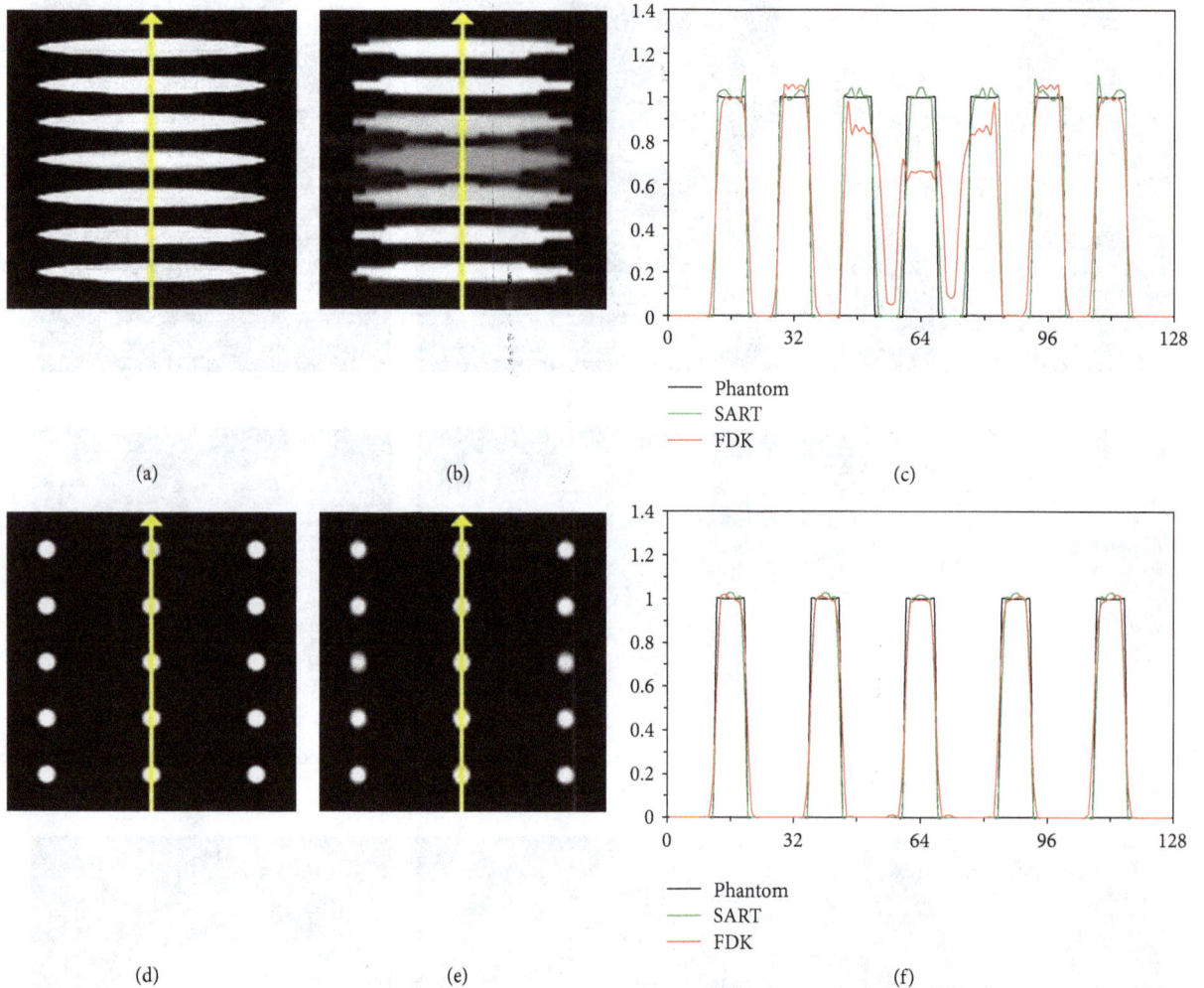

(a)

(b)

(c)

(d)

(e)

(f)

FIGURE 12: Transverse images reconstructed using the (a) FBP algorithm on data generated using fan-beam geometry and the (b) SART algorithm using the dual-source dual-detector geometry. Coronal images were also reconstructed using the (c) FBP and (d) SART algorithms.

we again used the same system parameters that were used for the central plane of our benchtop system to generate a fan-beam projection set. The spatial resolution of the image reconstructed using this new fan-beam projection set was comparable to that provided by the SART reconstruction.

4. Discussion and Conclusion

In this paper, the FDK and SART methods were implemented for the TBCT geometry. Data generated using numerical phantoms and clinical CT images as well as data collected using our TBCT benchtop system were reconstructed with these modified methods. The accuracy of the FDK and SART reconstructions was evaluated using the square Euclidean distance and the root mean square error FOMs. For small cone angles, the algebraic SART methods for both TBCT geometries were able to provide image quality comparable to that of the analytical FDK algorithm. For large cone angles, use of the algebraic image reconstruction algorithms significantly reduced the cone artifacts that were especially

prominent in the FDK phantom reconstructions. This was especially important for the dual source-dual detector TBCT geometry as the cone artifacts were most prominent in the center of the image for this geometry. The results given by implementing the SART method are promising, and the algorithm may be implemented in future TBCT systems.

The use of model-based statistical iterative image reconstruction methods, which can more accurately model the physics of the system and better take into account sources of noise and the statistical distribution of that noise, can potentially further improve the image quality. Because of their accurate modeling of the system geometry and data collection process, we expect that model-based statistical iterative image reconstruction methods can mitigate cone artifacts in a similar way as the SART method. Therefore, a model-based statistical reconstruction method that incorporates an accurate model of the system geometry and physics into the calculation of the system matrix is planned for a future study.

The use of the MAS ordering scheme improved the accuracy of the reconstruction during the first few iterations

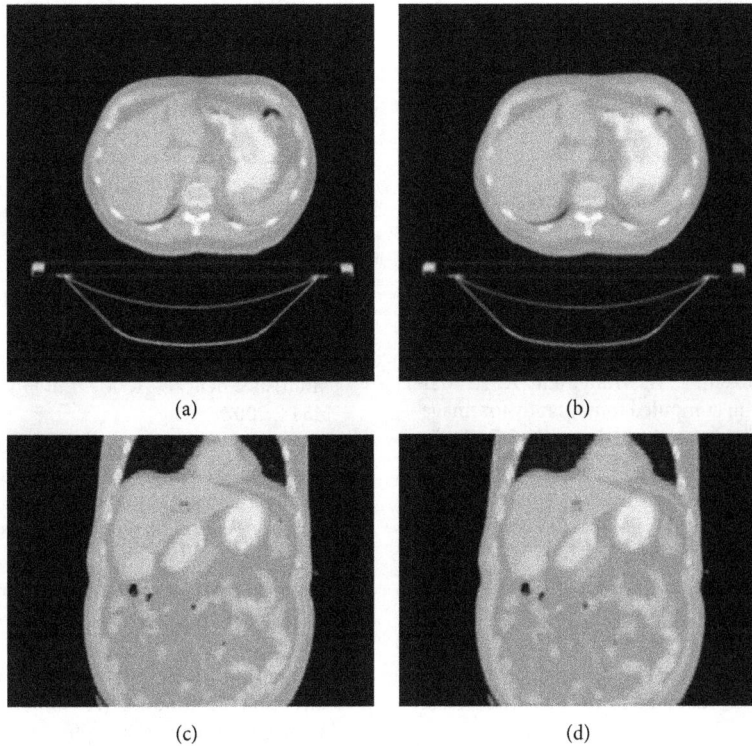

FIGURE 13: Transverse patient images reconstructed using the (a) FBP algorithm on data generated from fan beam geometry and the (b) SART algorithm from data generated using the dual source-dual detector geometry. Coronal images were also reconstructed using the (c) FBP and (d) SART algorithms.

of the SART method, particularly in the first iteration. After that, the reconstruction results both with and without using the MAS scheme were almost indistinguishable. One reason that the MAS scheme did not increase the convergence rate or accuracy after the initial iterations may be that the scheme was originally designed for a parallel-beam configuration. The most straightforward method that could be attempted to improve the performance of the MAS scheme would then be to rebin the fan-beam data in order to create a parallel beam projection data set. However, rebinning the data may unnecessarily complicate the calculation of the system matrix when we transition to model-based iterative reconstruction. Therefore, we kept the fan-beam geometry for this study.

The speed of the reconstruction method must improve for future implementation of the algorithm. The large computational burden required when employing iterative reconstruction algorithms is the main reason that it has taken so long for these methods to be implemented in the clinic. Using this algorithm, reconstructions would take as long as two hours to complete. However, the literature shows promising results from the implementation of iterative algorithms using graphics processing units (GPU). Acceleration in reconstruction times on the scale of one to two orders of magnitude have been reported [20, 28, 37, 38]. For these methods, though, the system matrix is much too large to hold in the GPU's memory and, therefore, must be calculated during runtime. The use of a spherical pixellation scheme has been used to take advantage of the symmetries of the circular scanning geometry of the system in order to reduce the storage requirement of the system matrix and to, therefore, improve the speed of reconstruction [39]. Therefore, the development of a cylindrical voxelization scheme in a separate study could potentially accelerate the reconstruction process on its own or, by reducing the size of the system matrix, make it feasible to implement the method on the GPU.

In conclusion, algebraic iterative reconstruction algorithms were successfully implemented for the TBCT system. The analytical and iterative reconstructions showed similar image quality for reconstructions at small cone angles, while the iterative methods were able to mitigate the cone artifacts that normally appear at large cone angles in analytical methods. The iterative algorithms were also able to accurately account for both longitudinal and transverse truncation of the projection data without introducing new artifacts into the image.

Conflict of Interests

Tiezhi Zhang and Joshua Kim have financial interests in TetraImaging Inc.

Acknowledgments

This work is supported in part by Oakland University and NIH SBIR Contract no. HHSN261201100045C.

References

[1] M. W. K. Kan, L. H. T. Leung, W. Wong, and N. Lam, "Radiation dose from cone beam computed tomography for image-guided radiation therapy," *International Journal of Radiation Oncology Biology Physics*, vol. 70, no. 1, pp. 272–279, 2008.

[2] J. A. Purdy, "Dose to normal tissues outside the radiation therapy patient's treated volume: a review of different radiation therapy techniques," *Health Physics*, vol. 95, no. 5, pp. 666–676, 2008.

[3] R. R. Allison, H. A. Gay, H. C. Mota, and C. H. Sibata, "Image-guided radiation therapy: current and future directions," *Future Oncology*, vol. 2, no. 4, pp. 477–492, 2006.

[4] D. A. Jaffray, J. H. Siewerdsen, J. W. Wong, and A. A. Martinez, "Flat-panel cone-beam computed tomography for image-guided radiation therapy," *International Journal of Radiation Oncology Biology Physics*, vol. 53, no. 5, pp. 1337–1349, 2002.

[5] H. Kanamori, N. Nakamori, K. Inoue, and E. Takenaka, "Effects of scattered X-rays on CT images," *Physics in Medicine and Biology*, vol. 30, no. 3, pp. 239–249, 1985.

[6] J. H. Siewerdsen and D. A. Jaffray, "Cone-beam computed tomography with a flat-panel imager: magnitude and effects of X-ray scatter," *Medical Physics*, vol. 28, no. 2, pp. 220–231, 2001.

[7] R. Ning, X. Tang, and D. Conover, "X-ray scatter correction algorithm for cone beam CT imaging," *Medical Physics*, vol. 31, no. 5, pp. 1195–1202, 2004.

[8] L. Zhu, Y. Xie, J. Wang, and L. Xing, "Scatter correction for cone-beam CT in radiation therapy," *Medical Physics*, vol. 36, no. 6, pp. 2258–2268, 2009.

[9] T. G. Flohr, S. Schaller, K. Stierstorfer, H. Bruder, B. M. Ohnesorge, and U. J. Schoepf, "Multi-detector row CT systems and image-reconstruction techniques," *Radiology*, vol. 235, no. 3, pp. 756–773, 2005.

[10] T. Zhang, Y. Chi, E. Meldolesi, and D. Yan, "Automatic delineation of on-line head-and-neck computed tomography images: toward on-line adaptive radiotherapy," *International Journal of Radiation Oncology Biology Physics*, vol. 68, no. 2, pp. 522–530, 2007.

[11] C. Maaß, F. Dennerlein, F. Noo, and M. Kachelrieß, "Comparing short scan CT reconstruction algorithms regarding cone-beam artifact performance," in *Proceedings of the Nuclear Science Symposium Conference Record (NSS/MIC '10)*, pp. 2188–2193, IEEE, November 2010.

[12] T. Zhang, D. Schulze, X. Xu, and J. Kim, "Tetrahedron beam computed tomography (TBCT): a new design of volumetric CT system," *Physics in Medicine and Biology*, vol. 54, no. 11, pp. 3365–3378, 2009.

[13] X. Xu, J. Kim, P. Laganis, D. Schulze, Y. Liang, and T. Zhang, "A tetrahedron beam computed tomography benchtop system with a multiple pixel field emission X-ray tube," *Medical Physics*, vol. 38, no. 10, pp. 5500–5509, 2011.

[14] H. K. Tuy, "Scatter correction for cone-beam CT in radiation therapy," *SIAM Journal on Applied Mathematics*, vol. 43, no. 3, pp. 546–552, 1983.

[15] X. Tang, J. Hsieh, A. Hagiwara, R. A. Nilsen, J. B. Thibault, and E. Drapkin, "A three-dimensional weighted cone beam filtered backprojection (CB-FBP) algorithm for image reconstruction in volumetric CT under a circular source trajectory," *Physics in Medicine and Biology*, vol. 50, no. 16, pp. 3889–3905, 2005.

[16] I. A. Feldkamp, L. C. Davis, and J. W. Kress, "Practical cone-beam algorithm," *Journal of the Optical Society of America A*, vol. 1, no. 6, pp. 612–619, 1984.

[17] A. K. Hara, R. G. Paden, A. C. Silva, J. L. Kujak, H. J. Lawder, and W. Pavlicek, "Iterative reconstruction technique for reducing body radiation dose at CT: Feasibility Study," *American Journal of Roentgenology*, vol. 193, no. 3, pp. 764–771, 2009.

[18] A. C. Martinsen, H. K. Saether, P. K. Hol, D. R. Olsen, and P. Skaane, "Iterative reconstruction reduces abdominal CT dose," *European Journal of Radiology*, vol. 81, no. 7, pp. 1483–1487, 2012.

[19] J. S. Liow, S. C. Strother, K. Rehm, and D. A. Rottenberg, "Improved resolution for PET volume imaging through three-dimensional iterative reconstruction," *Journal of Nuclear Medicine*, vol. 38, no. 10, pp. 1623–1631, 1997.

[20] J. B. Thibault, K. D. Sauer, C. A. Bouman, and J. Hsieh, "A three-dimensional statistical approach to improved image quality for multislice helical CT," *Medical Physics*, vol. 34, no. 11, pp. 4526–4544, 2007.

[21] K. Mueller and R. Yagel, "Rapid 3-D cone-beam reconstruction with the simultaneous algebraic reconstruction technique (SART) using 2-D texture mapping hardware," *IEEE Transactions on Medical Imaging*, vol. 19, no. 12, pp. 1227–1237, 2000.

[22] B. Chiang, S. Nakanishi, A. A. Zamyatin, and D. Shi, "Cone beam artifact reduction in circular computed tomography," in *Proceedings of the Nuclear Science Symposium and Medical Imaging Conference (NSS/MIC '11)*, pp. 4143–4144, IEEE, 2011.

[23] R. Gordon, R. Bender, and G. T. Herman, "Algebraic Reconstruction Techniques (ART) for three-dimensional electron microscopy and X-ray photography," *Journal of Theoretical Biology*, vol. 29, no. 3, pp. 471–481, 1970.

[24] A. H. Andersen and A. C. Kak, "Simultaneous algebraic reconstruction technique (SART): a superior implementation of the art algorithm," *Ultrasonic Imaging*, vol. 6, no. 1, pp. 81–94, 1984.

[25] B. De Man and S. Basu, "Distance-driven projection and backprojection in three dimensions," *Physics in Medicine and Biology*, vol. 49, no. 11, pp. 2463–2475, 2004.

[26] M. Jiang and G. Wang, "Convergence of the Simultaneous Algebraic Reconstruction Technique (SART)," *IEEE Transactions on Image Processing*, vol. 12, no. 8, pp. 957–961, 2003.

[27] H. Guan and R. Gordon, "A projection access order for speedy convergence of ART (algebraic reconstruction technique): a multilevel scheme for computed tomography," *Physics in Medicine and Biology*, vol. 39, no. 11, pp. 2005–2022, 1994.

[28] F. Xu, W. Xu, M. Jones et al., "On the efficiency of iterative ordered subset reconstruction algorithms for acceleration on GPUs," *Computer Methods and Programs in Biomedicine*, vol. 98, no. 3, pp. 261–270, 2010.

[29] W. M. Pang, J. Qin, Y. Lu, Y. Xie, C. K. Chui, and P. A. Heng, "Accelerating simultaneous algebraic reconstruction technique with motion compensation using CUDA-enabled GPU," *International Journal of Computer Assisted Radiology and Surgery*, vol. 6, no. 2, pp. 187–199, 2011.

[30] H. Guan and R. Gordon, "Computed tomography using algebraic reconstruction techniques (ARTs) with different projection access schemes: a comparison study under practical situations," *Physics in Medicine and Biology*, vol. 41, no. 9, pp. 1727–1743, 1996.

[31] A. Kak and M. Slaney, *Principles of Computerized Tomographic Imaging*, IEEE Press, 1988.

[32] H. Kudo, F. Noo, and M. Defrise, "Cone-beam filtered-backprojection algorithm for truncated helical data," *Physics in Medicine and Biology*, vol. 43, no. 10, pp. 2885–2909, 1998.

[33] A. H. Andersen, "Algebraic reconstruction in CT from limited views," *IEEE Transactions on Medical Imaging*, vol. 8, no. 1, pp. 50–55, 1989.

[34] W. Zbijewski and F. J. Beekman, "Characterization and suppression of edge and aliasing artefacts in iterative X-ray CT reconstruction," *Physics in Medicine and Biology*, vol. 49, no. 1, pp. 145–157, 2004.

[35] W. Zbijewski and F. J. Beekman, "Comparison of methods for suppressing edge and aliasing artefacts in iterative X-ray CT reconstruction," *Physics in Medicine and Biology*, vol. 51, no. 7, pp. 1877–1889, 2006.

[36] S. Matej and R. M. Lewitt, "Practical considerations for 3-D image reconstruction using spherically symmetric volume elements," *IEEE Transactions on Medical Imaging*, vol. 15, no. 1, pp. 68–78, 1996.

[37] F. Xu and K. Mueller, "Accelerating popular tomographic reconstruction algorithms on commodity PC graphics hardware," *IEEE Transactions on Nuclear Science*, vol. 52, no. 3, pp. 654–663, 2005.

[38] B. Keck, H. Hofmann, H. Scherl, M. Kowarschik, and J. Hornegger, "GPU-accelerated SART reconstruction using the CUDA programming environment," in *Medical Imaging 2009: Physics of Medical Imaging*, E. Samei and J. Hsieh, Eds., vol. 7258 of *Proceedings of SPIE*, February 2009.

[39] C. Mora, M. J. Rodríguez-Álvarez, and J. V. Romero, "New pixellation scheme for CT algebraic reconstruction to exploit matrix symmetries," *Computers and Mathematics with Applications*, vol. 56, no. 3, pp. 715–726, 2008.

11

Lung Segmentation in 4D CT Volumes Based on Robust Active Shape Model Matching

Gurman Gill[1,2] and Reinhard R. Beichel[1,2,3]

[1]*Department of Electrical and Computer Engineering, The University of Iowa, Iowa City, IA 52242, USA*
[2]*The Iowa Institute for Biomedical Imaging, The University of Iowa, Iowa City, IA 52242, USA*
[3]*Department of Internal Medicine, The University of Iowa, Iowa City, IA 52242, USA*

Correspondence should be addressed to Reinhard R. Beichel; reinhard-beichel@uiowa.edu

Academic Editor: Jyh-Cheng Chen

Dynamic and longitudinal lung CT imaging produce 4D lung image data sets, enabling applications like radiation treatment planning or assessment of response to treatment of lung diseases. In this paper, we present a 4D lung segmentation method that mutually utilizes all individual CT volumes to derive segmentations for each CT data set. Our approach is based on a 3D robust active shape model and extends it to fully utilize 4D lung image data sets. This yields an initial segmentation for the 4D volume, which is then refined by using a 4D optimal surface finding algorithm. The approach was evaluated on a diverse set of 152 CT scans of normal and diseased lungs, consisting of total lung capacity and functional residual capacity scan pairs. In addition, a comparison to a 3D segmentation method and a registration based 4D lung segmentation approach was performed. The proposed 4D method obtained an average Dice coefficient of 0.9773 ± 0.0254, which was statistically significantly better (p value $\ll 0.001$) than the 3D method (0.9659 ± 0.0517). Compared to the registration based 4D method, our method obtained better or similar performance, but was 58.6% faster. Also, the method can be easily expanded to process 4D CT data sets consisting of several volumes.

1. Introduction

Applications like lung cancer radiotherapy planning [1], assessment of lung diseases like COPD [2], or dynamic lung ventilation studies [3] require the acquisition and subsequent analysis of 4D lung CT scans (e.g., two lung scans at different respiratory states). Most quantitative analysis approaches utilize image registration methods [4, 5] for 4D analysis. In order to achieve accurate results and reduce computation time, registration is typically only performed within a lung mask. Thus, for such approaches, the segmentation of each lung CT volume acquired is a prerequisite. This can be accomplished by utilizing standard 3D lung segmentation methods like the ones proposed in [6–10], which assume a large density difference between air-filled lung parenchyma and surrounding objects/tissues. However, since 4D imaging is mainly performed for the assessment and/or treatment of lung diseases, such simple methods frequently fail to perform well. Recently, 3D segmentation methods have been developed to

deal with this issue, including approaches that utilize an atlas-based segmentation-by-registration scheme [11], an error-correcting hybrid system [12], a shape "break-and-repair" strategy [13], and a 3D robust active shape model (RASM) [14, 15]. However, none of these approaches takes advantage of 4D lung CT scans and thus requires lungs to be segmented individually. This can be problematic, especially when segmenting pairs of total lung capacity (TLC) and functional residual capacity (FRC) lung scans, because (diseased) lungs at FRC are typically more difficult to segment than lungs imaged at TLC. Consequently, algorithms that simultaneously segment lungs in all available CT volumes are more promising.

Work on 4D lung segmentation techniques is scant. Wilms et al. [16] adopted a 4D statistical shape model that was originally developed by Perperidis et al. [17] for segmentation of gated cardiac image sequences. A limitation of this approach is that it is based on standard least squares active shape model (ASM) matching, which is known to be affected by outliers [14, 18]. Consequently, disease induced changes of

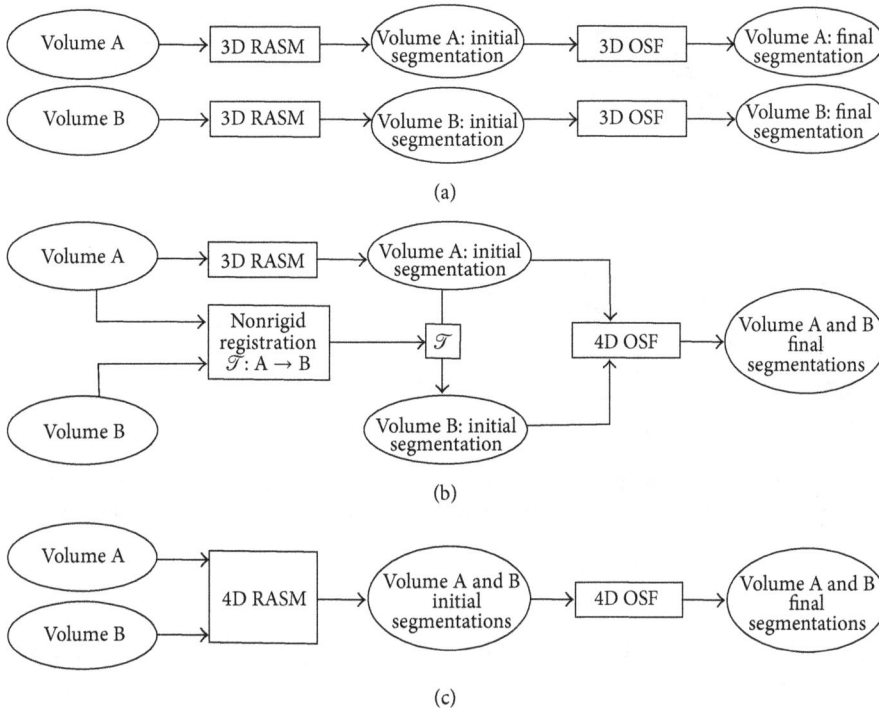

FIGURE 1: RASM-based approaches for segmenting lungs in a 4D CT volume (represented by 3D volumes A and B). (a) 3D segmentation method [14]. (b) Registration based 4D segmentation method [19]. (c) Proposed 4D segmentation approach with new 4D RASM (Section 3.1).

lung tissue (e.g., density) or artifacts resulting from sorting algorithm errors in case of free-breathing CT lung imaging can adversely impact model matching.

In our previous work, Sun et al. [19] introduced a 4D lung segmentation method based on 4D optimal surface finding (OSF). The approach requires a rough initial lung segmentation, which was obtained by applying a 3D RASM [14] to a TLC lung scan and transferring this segmentation by means of a nonrigid image registration to the corresponding FRC scan (Figure 1(b)). This approach has some potential shortcomings. First, the initial, rough segmentation step does not take full advantage of the available 4D CT data. Consequently, if the initial lung segmentation is inaccurate, the error is propagated to the other volume by the algorithm. Second, for many applications (e.g., segmentation of longitudinal TLC volumes), it is not obvious which volume should be utilized for 3D RASM segmentation to achieve good segmentation performance. Third, the registration step is quite time-consuming.

In this paper, we address these limitations by proposing a new 4D RASM model matching step that replaces the combination of single 3D RASM segmentation and subsequent registration to other volumes as proposed by Sun et al. [19]. In addition, we provide an extensive study, comparing the 3D base method published by Sun et al. [14] applied to each CT scan independently (Figure 1(a)), the registration based 4D version [19] (Figure 1(b)), and the proposed approach (Figure 1(c)) on a diverse set of 4D CT data, consisting of TLC and FRC scan pairs of normal and diseased lungs.

2. Prior Work

The proposed method extends our 3D RASM method [14] to mutual segmentation of lungs in 4D CT data. Thus, we briefly outline the RASM fitting process for a single 3D volume.

The RASM consists of a point distribution model (PDM) that captures the variation in lung shapes and a robust matching approach that iteratively fits the model to a lung CT scan to perform a segmentation. The PDM is constructed separately for left and right lungs from N lung volume training data sets that have m corresponding points (landmarks) [14]. An instance of a left or right lung shape is generated from the corresponding PDM by the linear model

$$\mathbf{x} = \bar{\mathbf{x}} + \mathscr{P}\mathbf{b}, \qquad (1)$$

where $\bar{\mathbf{x}}$ is the mean lung shape vector, $\mathscr{P}$ denotes the shape eigenvector matrix, and $\mathbf{b}$ represents the shape coefficients.

The matching process begins with automatically placing the mean lung shape $\bar{\mathbf{x}}$ in the target CT volume based on a ribs detection step [14]. The model shape points are then updated to $\mathbf{y}$ based on a gradient based cost function. For this purpose, a robust matching step is utilized to prevent that outliers are used during the model matching process. It is based on a robust PCA coefficient estimation method, which utilizes subsets of landmark points $\omega_{i,j}$ and a voting scheme [14]. During matching, for each of these subsets a reconstruction error $e_{\omega_{i,j}}$ is calculated, which is then being used to determine the inliers update points $\tilde{\mathbf{y}}$ of $\mathbf{y}$ (note the notation for specifying inliers using ~; e.g., $\tilde{\mathbf{y}}$ corresponds to the set $\mathbf{y}_{\{p_i=1\}}$ in [14] and

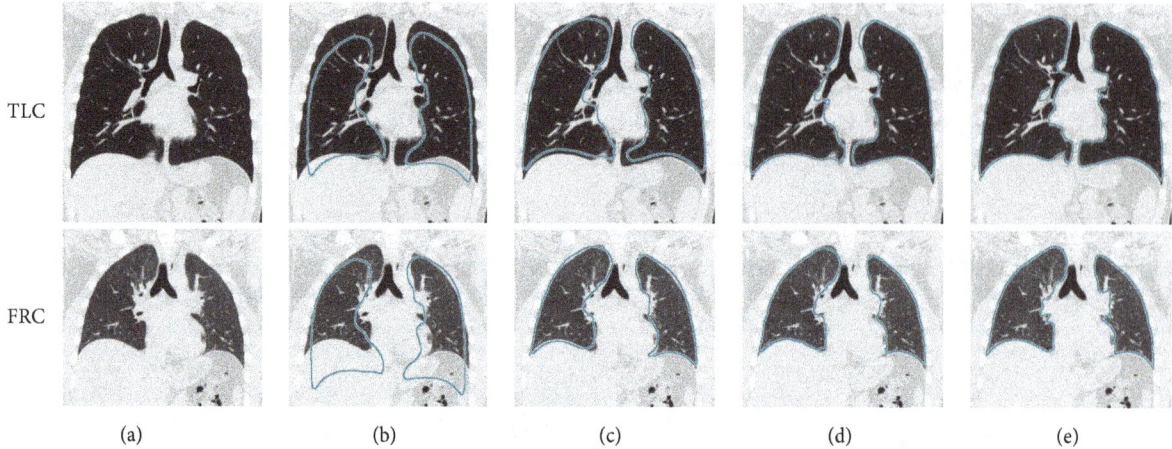

FIGURE 2: Illustration of intermediate and final results of the proposed 4D lung segmentation approach. (a) 4D CT data consisting of a TLC and FRC lung scan pair to be segmented. (b) Model initialization. (c-d) 4D RASM segmentation with (c) mutual segmentations and (d) result after the constrained adaptation step. (e) 4D OSF segmentation result.

is used here instead for the sake of clarity). Subsequently, $\tilde{\mathbf{y}}$ is utilized to update the shape coefficients by calculating

$$\mathbf{b} = \widetilde{\mathscr{P}}^T \left(\mathscr{T}\tilde{\mathbf{y}} - \tilde{\bar{\mathbf{x}}} \right), \qquad (2)$$

where $\mathscr{T}$ is the pose transformation matrix for mapping points from target image coordinate frame to model coordinate frame and $\tilde{\bar{\mathbf{x}}}$ denotes the points corresponding to inliers in the mean lung shape $\bar{\mathbf{x}}$. $\widetilde{\mathscr{P}}$ refers to the columns corresponding to inliers in the shape eigenvector matrix $\mathscr{P}$. A new instance of the model is calculated using (1), which is transformed to the image space by $\mathscr{T}^{-1}$. The model shape points are then iteratively updated until convergence.

Once the robust matching process is finished, the resulting RASM segmentation is used as an initial shape for a graph-based optimal surface finding (OSF) algorithm to further refine the segmentation [14] (Figure 1(a)).

3. Methods

Our method for generating a 4D lung segmentation (Figure 1(c)) is based on fitting a 3D RASM mutually to 4D volume data (Section 3.1), followed by a 4D OSF segmentation step (Section 3.2). The results of all the different processing stages are depicted in Figure 2. Below, we describe the segmentation process in detail for a TLC and FRC lung scan pair, but the approach would also work for other respiratory states or longitudinal scans and can be expanded to more than two lung volumes.

In addition to the main processing steps described in Sections 3.1 and 3.2, the following two preprocessing steps are performed. First, a modified system of the airway tree segmentation method [20] is utilized to extract the trachea and main bronchi, which are then dilated using a radius of 2 voxels. These locations are assigned a value of 50 HU in order to make them unattractive for RASM and OSF segmentation. Second, an overlap between left and right lung segmentations

is avoided by detecting the thin tissue layer between the lungs, as described by Gill et al. [21].

3.1. 4D RASM Segmentation. For model-based segmentation, a lung PDM is constructed from 75 TLC and 75 FRC normal lung CT scan pairs, which are not part of the image data utilized for method evaluation (Section 4.1). Note that model building is done separately for right and left lungs. Utilizing the right or left PDM, 4D RASM segmentation consists of the following main processing steps (Figure 3).

(a) Model Initialization. The mean lung model $\bar{\mathbf{x}}$ is placed independently in the target TLC and FRC volumes (Figure 2(b)). For this purpose, a ribs detection method [14] is applied on the respective volumes.

(b) Iterative Model Fitting. The matching steps (i) to (v) given below are repeated for 90 iterations, which are sufficient to achieve model convergence (Figure 2(c)). Alternatively, a convergence criterion could be used.

(i) *Updating Shape Points.* Utilizing a gray-value gradient based cost function [14] of TLC and FRC volumes, the model shape points are independently updated in the TLC and FRC volumes, resulting in $\mathbf{y}_{tlc}$ and $\mathbf{y}_{frc}$, respectively.

(ii) *Robustly Estimating Mutual Inlier Update Points.* Update point sets $\mathbf{y}_{tlc}$ and $\mathbf{y}_{frc}$ are used to calculate $e^{tlc}_{\omega_{i,j}}$ and $e^{frc}_{\omega_{i,j}}$, respectively, which is similar to that described in [14]. However, after this step, a mutual reconstruction error is calculated with

$$e^{mutual}_{\omega_{i,j}} = \frac{e^{tlc}_{\omega_{i,j}} + e^{frc}_{\omega_{i,j}}}{2} \qquad (3)$$

to enable mutual inlier estimation. Thus, $e^{mutual}_{\omega_{i,j}}$ is used in the voting scheme described in [14] instead

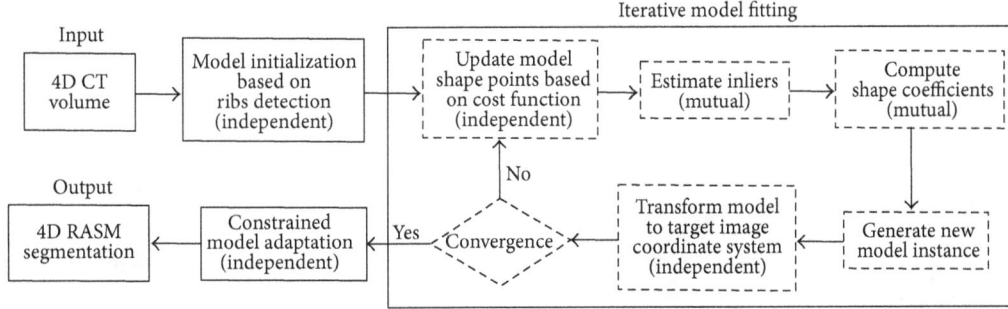

FIGURE 3: Flowchart showing the steps involved in fitting the model to 4D CT data. The independent and mutual steps are identified in the iterative model fitting process.

of individual reconstruction errors $e_{\omega_{i,j}}^{tlc}$ or $e_{\omega_{i,j}}^{frc}$. The outcomes of the voting process are inlier update point sets $\tilde{\mathbf{y}}_{tlc}$ and $\tilde{\mathbf{y}}_{frc}$. Note that, while $\tilde{\mathbf{y}}_{tlc}$ and $\tilde{\mathbf{y}}_{frc}$ are different, they have the same cardinality and correspond to the same landmark points of the lung PDM.

(iii) *Computing Mutual Shape Coefficients.* The inlier point sets $\tilde{\mathbf{y}}_{tlc}$ and $\tilde{\mathbf{y}}_{frc}$ are independently transformed to the model coordinate frame by using pose transformation matrices $\mathscr{T}_{tlc}$ and $\mathscr{T}_{frc}$, respectively. Each transformation is derived from a Procrustes analysis between inlier sets ($\tilde{\mathbf{y}}_{tlc}$ and $\tilde{\mathbf{y}}_{frc}$) and corresponding mean model ($\tilde{\bar{\mathbf{x}}}$) in model coordinate space. The shape coefficients $\mathbf{b}^{mutual}$ are computed using the average of the transformed inliers

$$\mathbf{b}^{mutual} = \tilde{\mathscr{P}}^T \left(\frac{\mathscr{T}_{tlc}\tilde{\mathbf{y}}_{tlc} + \mathscr{T}_{frc}\tilde{\mathbf{y}}_{frc}}{2} - \tilde{\bar{\mathbf{x}}} \right). \quad (4)$$

(iv) *Generating a New Model Instance.* A new instance of the model, which is used to represent the lung in TLC and FRC scans, is calculated using (1) and $\mathbf{b}^{mutual}$.

(v) *Transforming the Model.* The model is transformed back to TLC and FRC volumes using $\mathscr{T}_{tlc}^{-1}$ and $\mathscr{T}_{frc}^{-1}$, respectively.

(c) Constrained Model Adaptation. After the 4D fitting process converges, a single lung shape with individual transformation matrices $\mathscr{T}_{tlc}$ and $\mathscr{T}_{frc}$ results, which matches the lungs in TLC and FRC scans. However, the transformations only account for isotropic scaling. Thus, the fitted models will not be perfectly aligned with the image data, because the difference in TLC and FRC lung shapes cannot be explained by an isotropic scale factor. To obtain a better alignment, we subsequently allow the shape coefficients to individually adapt to the target images by continuing the RASM fitting process independently in both volumes for ten iterations (Figure 2(d)). Note that this adaptation is done in a constrained manner, only allowing a subset of model coefficients to change within certain limits to avoid major divergence of TLC and FRC models. The subset of model coefficients (sorted in decreasing order of their eigenvalues) is defined by the coefficients whose eigenvalues account for 80% of shape

variation. In our case, this resulted in a set of 22 coefficients out of 150, which were allowed to change by a maximum of 0.5 times the standard deviation σ in the respective eigenvalues. Thus, the final shape coefficients $\mathbf{b}^{adapted}$ after the individual adaptation step for the TLC or FRC volume are limited to

$$\mathbf{b}^{mutual}(l) \pm 0.5\sigma(l) \quad \text{if } l \leq 22$$
$$\mathbf{b}^{mutual}(l) \quad \text{otherwise.} \quad (5)$$

The parameters constraining the model were selected conservatively, and we found that small parameter variations have little impact on the overall lung segmentation.

3.2. 4D OSF Segmentation. After the initial model-based segmentations are created for TLC and FRC volumes, they are refined using the 4D OSF method [19], resulting in the final 4D lung segmentation (Figure 2(e)). For this purpose, the same parameter settings as proposed by Sun et al. [19] were utilized.

4. Evaluation

4.1. Image Data. For evaluation, 152 multidetector computed tomography (MDCT) thorax scans of lungs from 4 different sets S_{normal}, S_{asthma}, S_{COPD}, and S_{mix} with no significant abnormalities (normal), asthma (both severe and nonsevere), chronic obstructive pulmonary disease (COPD, GOLD 1 to 4), and a mixture of different lung diseases, respectively, were utilized. The total number of scans in sets S_{normal}, S_{asthma}, S_{COPD}, and S_{mix} were 40, 36, 36, and 40, respectively. All the four sets contained pairs of TLC (volume A) and FRC (volume B) images. The image sizes varied from $512 \times 512 \times 351$ to $512 \times 512 \times 781$ voxels with a mean size of $512 \times 512 \times 580$ voxels. The slice thickness of images ranged from 0.5 to 0.63 mm (mean: 0.52 mm) and the in-plane resolution from 0.49×0.49 to 0.91×0.91 mm (mean: 0.64×0.64 mm).

4.2. Experimental Setup. For all test data sets, an independent reference standard was generated. Manual segmentation of a whole lung is time-consuming, and due to the large number of 152 test CT scans, we utilize a sampling approach, which is similar to that utilized in [6, 11, 12], to reduce the substantial effort required for manual inspection and segmentation.

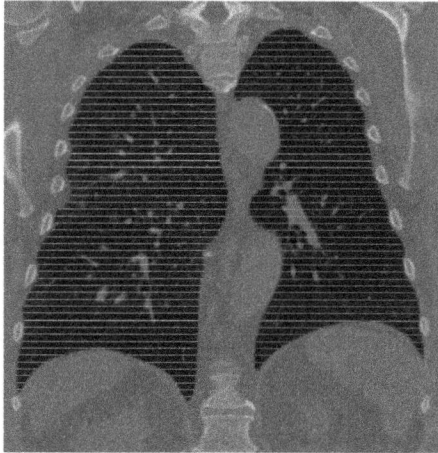

FIGURE 4: Example showing the location and density of axial reference segmentations in relation to lung anatomy.

Thus, for every tenth axial slice, a trained expert generated a reference segmentation under the supervision of a pulmonologist, resulting in a dense sampling of the lung volume with between 41 and 64 labeled slices for each data set (Figure 4). The same sampling approach was applied to the segmentation result to be evaluated. Based on the sampled volumes, the Dice coefficient D [22] was calculated. In addition, the mean unsigned distance error d [22] was computed with respect to the reference in all axial slices where a reference standard and segmentation result were both available. Subsequently, the average of all these locations was calculated per data set and reported.

In the following sections, the proposed method (Figure 1(c)) will be denoted by M_{4D}. In addition, two other methods will be utilized for comparison. M_{3D} will be utilized to denote the 3D approach proposed by Sun et al. [14] (Figure 1(a)). The 4D method of Sun et al. [19] (Figure 1(b)) was used in two variants; the variant where volume A (TLC) is registered to volume B (FRC) will be denoted by $M_{4DregAB}$, and the variant where volume B (FRC) is registered to volume A (TLC) will be denoted by $M_{4DregBA}$. Investigating these two variants allows us to assess and compare performance in situations with different but unknown respiratory state (e.g., longitudinal lung image data). For all methods utilized, the standard parameter setting as described in respective papers was used. Unless otherwise mentioned, all reported results refer to the final (OSF) segmentation.

A paired permutation test [23] was utilized for determining statistical significance, because it does not make assumptions about the distribution of the underlying data and a paired t-test or paired signed rank test was not applicable to our data.

5. Results

5.1. Segmentation Performance. Our novel 4D RASM matching approach (without final OSF segmentation step) showed an average Dice coefficient of 0.9468 ± 0.0318. In contrast, the standard 3D RASM approach resulted in an average

TABLE 1: Dice coefficient D for methods M_{3D} and M_{4D}. Statistically significant p values are marked with *.

Set	M_{3D}	M_{4D}	p value
S_{normal}	0.9822 ± 0.0129	**0.9850 ± 0.0058**	$\ll 0.001^*$
S_{asthma}	0.9667 ± 0.0437	**0.9789 ± 0.0108**	$\ll 0.001^*$
S_{COPD}	0.9685 ± 0.0514	**0.9839 ± 0.0068**	$\ll 0.001^*$
S_{mix}	0.9467 ± 0.0732	**0.9623 ± 0.0444**	0.012^*
TLC	0.9808 ± 0.0142	**0.9846 ± 0.0103**	$\ll 0.001^*$
FRC	0.9510 ± 0.0687	**0.9700 ± 0.0329**	$\ll 0.001^*$
ALL	0.9659 ± 0.0517	**0.9773 ± 0.0254**	$\ll 0.001^*$

TABLE 2: Mean unsigned distance error d in millimeters for methods M_{3D} and M_{4D}. Statistically significant p values are marked with *.

Set	M_{3D}	M_{4D}	p value
S_{normal}	1.20 ± 0.77	**0.89 ± 0.44**	$\ll 0.001^*$
S_{asthma}	1.68 ± 1.25	**1.14 ± 0.50**	$\ll 0.001^*$
S_{COPD}	1.66 ± 1.90	**1.00 ± 0.56**	$\ll 0.001^*$
S_{mix}	2.77 ± 4.42	**1.81 ± 1.45**	$\ll 0.001^*$
TLC	1.16 ± 0.68	**0.88 ± 0.53**	$\ll 0.001^*$
FRC	2.52 ± 3.50	**1.56 ± 1.11**	$\ll 0.001^*$
ALL	1.84 ± 2.61	**1.22 ± 0.93**	$\ll 0.001^*$

TABLE 3: Dice coefficient D for methods $M_{4DregAB}$ and M_{4D}. Statistically significant p values are marked with *.

Set	$M_{4DRegAB}$	M_{4D}	p value
TLC	0.9834 ± 0.0127	**0.9846 ± 0.0103**	$8.92e - 03^*$
FRC	**0.9718 ± 0.0233**	0.9700 ± 0.0329	$2.07e - 01$
ALL	**0.9776 ± 0.0196**	0.9773 ± 0.0254	$7.97e - 01$

TABLE 4: Dice coefficient D for methods $M_{4DregBA}$ and M_{4D}. Statistically significant p values are marked with *.

Set	$M_{4DregBA}$	M_{4D}	p value
TLC	0.9687 ± 0.0579	**0.9846 ± 0.0103**	$\ll 0.001^*$
FRC	0.9539 ± 0.0711	**0.9700 ± 0.0329**	$\ll 0.001^*$
ALL	0.9613 ± 0.0651	**0.9773 ± 0.0254**	$\ll 0.001^*$

Dice coefficient of 0.9391 ± 0.0525. The 4D RASM showed a statistically significant improvement (p value $\ll 0.001$) compared against 3D RASM.

Tables 1 and 2 summarize the resulting final (OSF) segmentation performance with corresponding p values, comparing results of M_{3D} and M_{4D}. In both tables, M_{4D} shows statistically significant improvement in each data set and for TLC and FRC scans. Figure 5 depicts some examples of segmentations (one from each test data set) obtained by methods M_{3D} and M_{4D}.

Tables 3 and 4 compare the final lung segmentation Dice coefficient of M_{4D} to $M_{4DregAB}$ and $M_{4DregBA}$, respectively. Overall, M_{4D} and $M_{4DregAB}$ were found to be equivalent (no statistically significant difference), but M_{4D} was found to be significantly better compared to $M_{4DregBA}$. Figure 6 provides a comparison of final Dice coefficients in form of box plots for

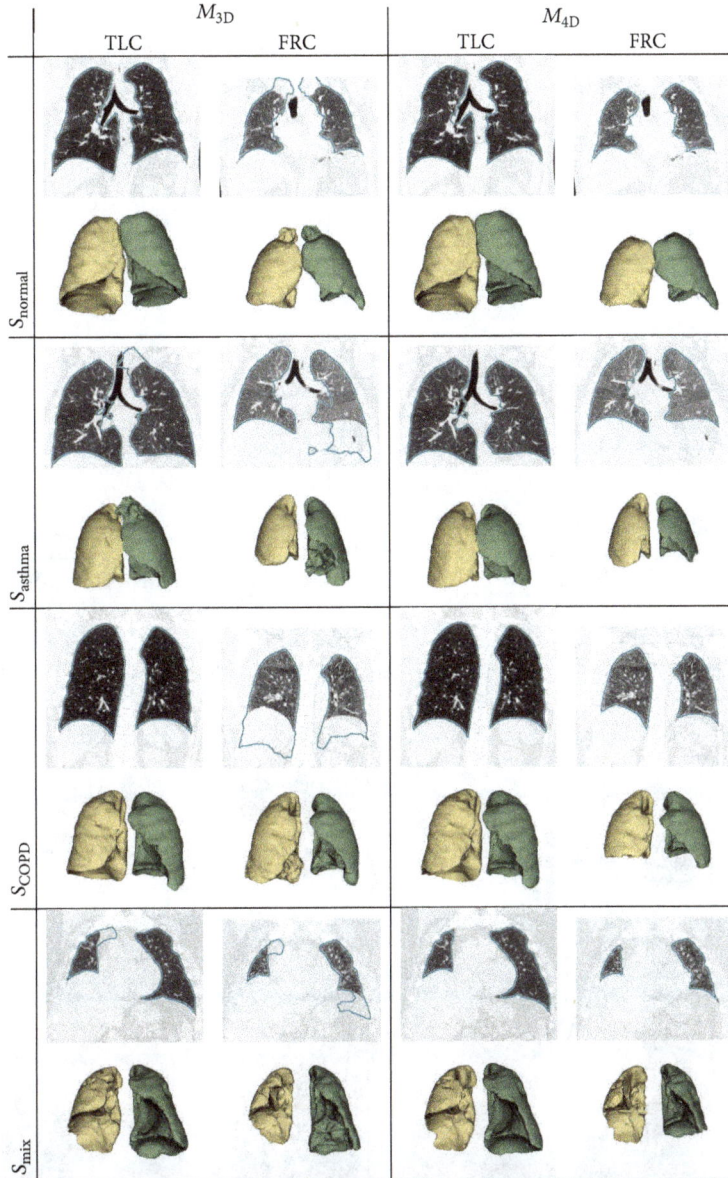

FIGURE 5: Comparison of segmentation results generated with methods M_{3D} and M_{4D}. Coronal CT cross sections with marked lung boundaries in combination with corresponding 3D lung mesh models are shown to enable locating and assessing segmentation errors as well as differences between results.

all methods and separated by respiratory state. A comparison of results generated with M_{4D}, $M_{4DregAB}$, and $M_{4DregBA}$ is shown in Figure 7.

5.2. Computing Time. Segmentation with M_{3D} took 13.21 minutes on average for TLC and FRC data sets combined (TLC: 6.73 minutes, FRC: 6.48 minutes). Method M_{4D} required 12.22 minutes per 4D case, on average. Compared to M_{3D}, the reduction in computing time was primarily achieved due to synergies of 4D processing. Approaches $M_{4DregAB}$ and $M_{4DregAB}$ took 29.49 minutes per 4D case, on average, where the registration procedure contributed to about 20 minutes of computing time.

6. Discussion

The main advantage of our 4D approach M_{4D} is that it utilizes both lung volumes acquired at different respirator states for segmentation during all main processing stages, which is in contrast to the standard M_{3D} method and 4D variants $M_{4DregAB}$ and $M_{4DregBA}$. The results presented in Section 5 clearly demonstrate this advantage.

6.1. Comparison of M_{4D} with M_{3D}. When compared to the 3D variant, statistically significant lung segmentation performance improvements, independent of test set, respiratory state, and performance metric, were observed

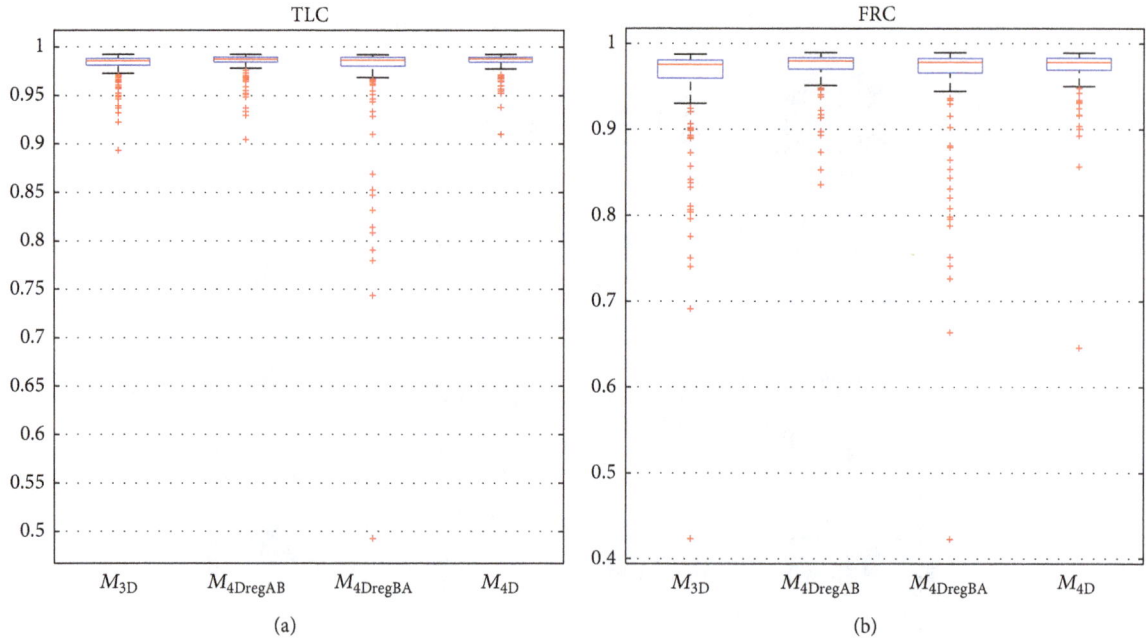

FIGURE 6: Box plots of Dice coefficients for methods M_{3D}, $M_{4DregAB}$, $M_{4DregBA}$, and M_{4D} on (a) TLC and (b) FRC lung scans.

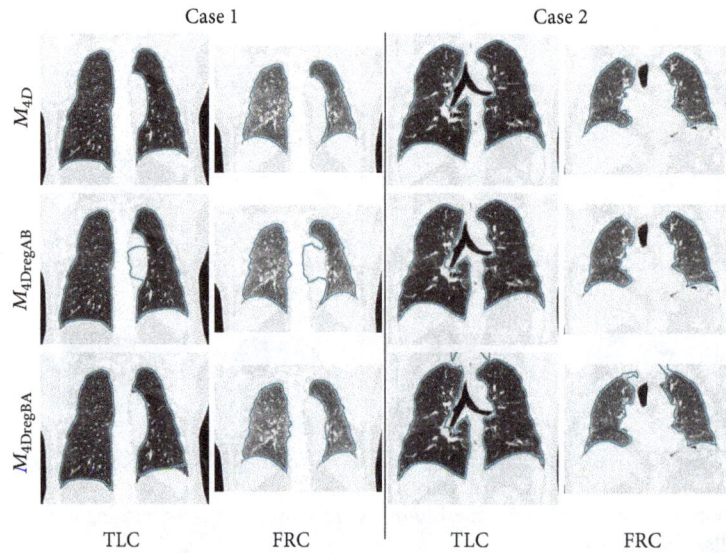

FIGURE 7: Examples of segmentation results generated with methods M_{4D}, $M_{4DregAB}$, and $M_{4DregBA}$.

(Tables 1 and 2). This is also clearly demonstrated by the examples shown in Figure 5. As shown in Tables 1 and 2, the observed gain in segmentation accuracy with M_{4D} was larger for cases with lung disease (test sets S_{asthma}, S_{COPD}, and S_{mix}) compared to normal cases (test set S_{normal}). The better segmentation performance of M_{4D} is expected, because it addresses several weaknesses of M_{3D} like problems with model initialization, which can cause the model to converge locally to other structures than lung boundaries. As Figure 6 as well as Tables 1 and 2 show, gains achieved with M_{4D} are higher for lungs imaged at FRC, which are generally more difficult to segment. Also, 4D processing

reduces the computing time by 7.5% compared to sequential 3D processing.

6.2. Comparison of M_{4D} with $M_{4DregAB}$ and $M_{4DregBA}$.
Overall, segmentation performance of M_{4D} and $M_{4DregAB}$ was found to be equivalent (Table 3), while the comparison between M_{4D} and $M_{4DregBA}$ (Table 4) showed a statistically significant improvement for our proposed M_{4D} approach. Also, compared to $M_{4DregAB}$ and $M_{4DregBA}$, our M_{4D} method showed a reduction in computing time by 58.6%. Thus, it is preferable to $M_{4DregAB}$ and $M_{4DregBA}$, especially when the exact respiratory states are unknown and picking a lung

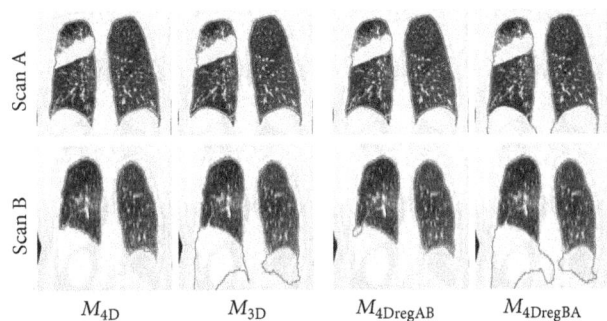

FIGURE 8: Comparison of results of methods M_{4D}, M_{3D}, $M_{4DregAB}$, and $M_{4DregBA}$ on a longitudinal CT volume pair. The time between scans A and B was 19 months, and the imaging protocol was quite different.

scan with lower lung volume (exhale) as starting point (Volume A in Figure 1(b)) could potentially adversely impact segmentation performance. Figure 7 depicts examples where either $M_{4DregAB}$ or $M_{4DregBA}$ produces a local segmentation error, but M_{4D} avoids such problems.

6.3. Possible Improvements and Extensions. As can be seen in Figure 6, the proposed approach reduces the number and/or severity of outlier cases. However, some room for improvement still exists, which we will address in future work. For example, a better FRC model initialization would help in further improving overall segmentation performance of 3D and 4D methods, but we expect that M_{4D} would still perform better, because it utilizes both scans for model matching, which offers increased robustness.

Our method can be expanded to handle processing of more than two lungs scans at the same time. This can be done by extending (3) and (4) accordingly. Another advantage is that M_{4D} does not require any prior knowledge of the breathing state of the lungs in individual CT scans, because it does not make any assumptions about respiratory state (e.g., breathing sequence). An example for processing longitudinal lung CT scans in the context of cancer treatment planning/assessment is provided in Figure 8. Note that, due to lung disease (cancer), patient compliance with the utilized imaging protocol (e.g., acquisition at TLC) cannot be assumed.

7. Conclusions

In this paper, we have presented a 4D lung segmentation approach that utilizes a new 4D robust active shape model matching method and provided an evaluation of this method on a diverse set of 76 TLC and FRC lung scan pairs. In addition, a detailed comparison with its 3D lung segmentation counterpart as well as two variants of 4D registration based lung segmentation methods was performed, demonstrating the advantages of our approach in terms of segmentation performance and/or computing time. By avoiding any assumptions about the respiratory state of the imaged lungs, our approach provides flexibility and is applicable to pairs of TLC and FRC scans, other dynamic 4D lung CT scans, and

longitudinal CT studies. Thus, the developed method is suited for applications like cancer treatment planning or assessment of other lung diseases like emphysema.

Conflict of Interests

The authors declare that there is no conflict of interests regarding the publication of this paper.

Acknowledgments

Gurman Gill contributed to the revision of this paper at Sonoma State University, CA. The authors thank Dr. Milan Sonka and Dr. Eric Hoffman at the University of Iowa for providing OSF code and image data, respectively. This work was supported in part by NIH Grant R01HL111453.

References

[1] R. W. M. Underberg, F. J. Lagerwaard, J. P. Cuijpers, B. J. Slotman, J. R. V. S. de Koste, and S. Senan, "Four-dimensional CT scans for treatment planning in stereotactic radiotherapy for stage I lung cancer," *International Journal of Radiation Oncology Biology Physics*, vol. 60, no. 4, pp. 1283–1290, 2004.

[2] M. O. Wielpütz, R. Eberhardt, M. Puderbach, O. Weinheimer, H.-U. Kauczor, and C. P. Heussel, "Simultaneous assessment of airway instability and respiratory dynamics with low-dose 4D-CT in chronic obstructive pulmonary disease: a technical note," *Respiration*, vol. 87, no. 4, pp. 294–300, 2014.

[3] T. Guerrero, K. Sanders, E. Castillo et al., "Dynamic ventilation imaging from four-dimensional computed tomography," *Physics in Medicine and Biology*, vol. 51, no. 4, pp. 777–791, 2006.

[4] S. Kabus, T. Klinder, K. Murphy, B. V. Ginneken, C. Lorenz, and J. P. W. Pluim, "Evaluation of 4D-CT lung registration," in *Medical Image Computing and Computer-Assisted Intervention—MICCAI 2009*, G.-Z. Yang, D. Hawkes, D. Rueckert, A. Noble, and C. Taylor, Eds., vol. 5761 of *Lecture Notes in Computer Science*, pp. 747–754, Springer, Berlin, Germany, 2009.

[5] J. Ehrhardt, R. Werner, A. Schmidt-Richberg, and H. Handels, "Statistical modeling of 4D respiratory lung motion using diffeomorphic image registration," *IEEE Transactions on Medical Imaging*, vol. 30, no. 2, pp. 251–265, 2011.

[6] S. Hu, E. A. Hoffman, and J. M. Reinhardt, "Automatic lung segmentation for accurate quantitation of volumetric X-ray CT images," *IEEE Transactions on Medical Imaging*, vol. 20, no. 6, pp. 490–498, 2001.

[7] J.-M. Kuhnigk, V. Dicken, S. Zidowitz et al., "New tools for computer assistance in thoracic CT. Part 1. Functional analysis of lungs, lung lobes, and bronchopulmonary segments," *Radiographics*, vol. 25, no. 2, pp. 525–536, 2005.

[8] P. Korfiatis, S. Skiadopoulos, P. Sakellaropoulos, C. Kalogeropoulou, and L. Costaridou, "Combining 2D wavelet edge highlighting and 3D thresholding for lung segmentation in thin-slice CT," *British Journal of Radiology*, vol. 80, no. 960, pp. 996–1004, 2007.

[9] S. G. Armato III and W. F. Sensakovic, "Automated lung segmentation for thoracic CT: impact on computer-aided diagnosis," *Academic Radiology*, vol. 11, no. 9, pp. 1011–1021, 2004.

[10] J. K. Leader, B. Zheng, R. M. Rogers et al., "Automated lung segmentation in X-ray computed tomography: development

and evaluation of a heuristic threshold-based schem," *Academic Radiology*, vol. 10, no. 11, pp. 1224–1236, 2003.

[11] I. Sluimer, M. Prokop, and B. van Ginneken, "Toward automated segmentation of the pathological lung in CT," *IEEE Transactions on Medical Imaging*, vol. 24, no. 8, pp. 1025–1038, 2005.

[12] E. M. van Rikxoort, B. de Hoop, M. A. Viergever, M. Prokop, and B. van Ginneken, "Automatic lung segmentation from thoracic computed tomography scans using a hybrid approach with error detection," *Medical Physics*, vol. 36, no. 7, pp. 2934–2947, 2009.

[13] J. Pu, D. S. Paik, X. Meng, J. Roos, and G. D. Rubin, "Shape 'break-and-repair' strategy and its application to automated medical image segmentation," *IEEE Transactions on Visualization and Computer Graphics*, vol. 17, no. 1, pp. 115–124, 2011.

[14] S. Sun, C. Bauer, and R. Beichel, "Automated 3D segmentation of lungs with lung cancer in CT data using a novel robust active shape model approach," *IEEE Transactions on Medical Imaging*, vol. 31, no. 2, pp. 449–460, 2012.

[15] G. Gill and R. R. Beichel, "Segmentation of lungs with interstitial lung disease in CT scans: a TV-L1 based texture analysis approach," in *Advances in Visual Computing*, vol. 8887 of *Lecture Notes in Computer Science*, pp. 511–520, Springer, 2014.

[16] M. Wilms, J. Ehrhardt, and H. Handels, "A 4d statistical shape model for automated segmentation of lungs with large tumors," in *Medical Image Computing and Computer-Assisted Intervention—MICCAI 2012: 15th International Conference, Nice, France, October 1–5, 2012, Proceedings, Part II*, vol. 7511 of *Lecture Notes in Computer Science*, pp. 347–354, Springer, Berlin, Germany, 2012.

[17] D. Perperidis, R. Mohiaddin, P. Edwards, and D. Rueckert, "Segmentation of cardiac MR and CT image sequences using model-based registration of a 4D statistical model," in *Medical Imaging 2007: Image Processing*, vol. 6512 of *Proceedings of SPIE*, p. 9, San Diego, Calif, USA, February 2007.

[18] K. Lekadir, R. Merrifield, and G.-Z. Yang, "Outlier detection and handling for robust 3-D active shape models search," *IEEE Transactions on Medical Imaging*, vol. 26, no. 2, pp. 212–222, 2007.

[19] S. Sun, M. Sonka, and R. R. Beichel, "Graph-based 4D lung segmentation in CT images with expert-guided computer-aided refinement," in *Proceedings of the IEEE 10th International Symposium on Biomedical Imaging (ISBI '13)*, pp. 1312–1315, San Francisco, Calif, USA, April 2013.

[20] C. Bauer, M. Eberlein, and R. R. Beichel, "Graph-based airway tree reconstruction from chest CT scans: evaluation of different features on five cohorts," *IEEE Transactions on Medical Imaging*, vol. 34, no. 5, pp. 1063–1076, 2015.

[21] G. Gill, C. Bauer, and R. R. Beichel, "A method for avoiding overlap of left and right lungs in shape model guided segmentation of lungs in CT volumes," *Medical Physics*, vol. 41, no. 10, Article ID 101908, 2014.

[22] M. Sonka, V. Hlavac, and R. Boyle, *Image Processing, Analysis, and Machine Vision*, Thompson Learning, Toronto, Canada, 2008.

[23] R. C. Blair and W. Karniski, "An alternative method for significance testing of waveform difference potentials," *Psychophysiology*, vol. 30, no. 5, pp. 518–524, 1993.

12

Automated Classification of Glandular Tissue by Statistical Proximity Sampling

Jimmy C. Azar, Martin Simonsson, Ewert Bengtsson, and Anders Hast

Centre for Image Analysis, Department of Information Technology, Uppsala University, 75105 Uppsala, Sweden

Correspondence should be addressed to Jimmy C. Azar; jimmy.azar@it.uu.se

Academic Editor: Yue Wang

Due to the complexity of biological tissue and variations in staining procedures, features that are based on the explicit extraction of properties from subglandular structures in tissue images may have difficulty generalizing well over an unrestricted set of images and staining variations. We circumvent this problem by an implicit representation that is both robust and highly descriptive, especially when combined with a multiple instance learning approach to image classification. The new feature method is able to describe tissue architecture based on glandular structure. It is based on statistically representing the relative distribution of tissue components around lumen regions, while preserving spatial and quantitative information, as a basis for diagnosing and analyzing different areas within an image. We demonstrate the efficacy of the method in extracting discriminative features for obtaining high classification rates for tubular formation in both healthy and cancerous tissue, which is an important component in Gleason and tubule-based Elston grading. The proposed method may be used for glandular classification, also in other tissue types, in addition to general applicability as a region-based feature descriptor in image analysis where the image represents a bag with a certain label (or grade) and the region-based feature vectors represent instances.

1. Introduction

There have been many attempts over the past decades for automating cancer grading in tissue, most notably in breast and prostate tissue, where the standard scoring systems in use are the Elston [1] and Gleason [2] grading systems, respectively. The first computerized grading of prostate tissue was published in 1978 [3]. More recently, high classification rates were obtained for the simple case of discriminating between low-grade and high-grade cancer in prostate tissue [4–7]. There have been attempts in [4, 5] at performing the classification task and extracting a large and diverse feature set including color, texture, morphometric, fractal, and wavelet features. Often this is followed by a feature reduction method such as sequential forward feature selection as in [4] or similar greedy algorithms, which, though being suboptimal approaches, are motivated by the fact that the feature set is large and a brute force or branch-and-bound method may become intractable or computationally inefficient.

Often a main factor that limits automated classification lies not in the choice of classifier but in the choice of feature set. The discriminative ability of a classifier is limited by the extent to which the classes themselves are separate in feature space. For well-represented classes, the intrinsic overlap and proximity of the classes in feature space determine the upper limit on the classification rate. The chosen features define the extent to which the classes overlap. The selection of a large number of different types of features is common in practice and is often an indication of lack of knowledge as to what features exactly have discriminative power; instead it reflects speculation over which features may prove useful or may have a contributing role [8]. However, choosing a plethora of features, whether informative or not, increases the dimensionality of the feature space and often exposes the classification task to the peaking phenomenon [9]. Furthermore, this shifts the burden of the problem toward feature selection or extraction which is often difficult to solve in a manner that is true to the final objective (i.e., the final classification rate), and this is due to computational limitations and the prevalence of either suboptimal criteria or criteria that are often not aligned with the final objective. It is therefore important to select a discriminative set of features that is able to separate among the different classes.

Automated tissue grading is very difficult for several reasons. One reason lies in the difficulty of translating the experience and observations of the human expert, that is, the trained pathologist, into well-defined features that can be extracted automatically from the image. Moreover, due to the complexity of the tissue structure and subjectivity of the grading process, especially among the intermediate grades, there is no clear consensus as to which features or combination of features is to be used consistently. Upon deeper examination, we find that experts' rules tend to eventually branch out into increasingly complicated conditions and exceptions. This leads to countless if-else situations where exceptions eventually outgrow the norm. There is therefore a problem in identifying features explicitly, and moreover even when such features have been suggested by pathologists, the complexity and variability of the images and tissue structures in addition to variables relating to stain absorption can still obstruct the extraction of such features in a reliable manner that allows for automation.

In general, there is a sensitive balance between overadapting to the complexity of the problem on the one hand and weakly accounting for it on the other hand such as the case when extracting global texture features without taking into account any knowledge of tissue architecture. Both of these extreme approaches may lead to inadequate results and an inability to generalize well. In the approach that we propose, we avoid the explicit extraction of structure properties (such as nuclei shape, glandular unit shape, and thickness of epithelium layer) beyond a rough decomposition of images into a few classes based on the staining. Yet, the method is still strongly founded on the architecture of glandular tissue (such as breast or prostate) and relies upon detecting glandular lumen and tissue components as a starting point. We use sequential region expansion to sample the space around lumen regions in the form of rings and preserve the statistics and component ratios within these rings in order to describe and represent these regions in an implicit manner. During the progression of cancer into advanced stages, when a glandular unit transforms into cribriform shape or splits into multiple lumen regions, such a phenomenon should be detected by the method due to the unusual presence of lumen and other structures in the outer sampling rings which reflects on the shape of the extracted profile curve and consequently on its classification and labeling.

As opposed to most local neighborhood sampling or *bag of features* methods that either are patch-based or result in orderless, histogram-based features [10, 11], the method we propose does the sampling around a given (lumen) region as opposed to a pixel, while preserving the region's boundary shape and encoding spatial distance from it. The contributions of our work can be stated as follows.

(1) We present a new approach to encode features in complex tissue images such as prostate and breast. The approach called *statistical proximity sampling* relies

on a method of boundary expansion around lumen regions; it uses rings or neighborhood strips around these regions while preserving the boundary shapes.

(2) The method is able to simultaneously encode the relative quantitative proportions of each tissue type around a lumen region as well as the spatial distribution of these proportions from the central lumen region, resulting in highly descriptive and discriminative features.

(3) Combining this neighborhood-based feature description with multiple-instance learning, we are able to represent complex images in an efficient and information-preserving manner, which is more consequential than representing an entire image with a single feature vector.

To highlight the context of our work, we briefly describe below the Elston and Gleason grading systems and how our method relates to some important aspects of these.

The Elston score is based on three different components. The first is tubular formation or "tubularity," where the presence of glandular tissue in the sample is given a score from 1 to 3, ranging, respectively, from healthy tissue (prevalently glandular) to solid tumors (scarcely glandular). The second component is nuclear pleomorphism and is concerned with nuclear size, shape, and chromatin texture; this attribute is also assigned a score from 1 to 3 depending on the morphological irregularities of nuclei. The third component of grading is mitotic activity which corresponds to growth rate and is determined by counting dividing cells, ranging from a low cell count (score 1) to a high cell count (score 3). The final, high-level Elston grade is then derived by summing up the individual scores from the three parts: a sum of 3–5 points is defined as Elston grade I, 6-7 as grade II, and 8-9 as grade III.

Analogously, Gleason grading for prostate is based on five patterns, which are highly dependent on tissue architecture and the description of glandular units. The patterns from 1 to 5 are described by how glands alter form while transitioning from small, well-defined, and closely packed units, corresponding to well-differentiated carcinoma (pattern 1), to larger glandular units with increased interglandular distances, corresponding to moderately differentiated carcinoma (pattern 2), until the glands are no longer recognizable and cells start to invade surrounding tissue in neoplastic clumps. In pattern 5, the tissue does not have any, or only a few, recognizable glands.

Thus, in conclusion, both Gleason grading and the first component of Elston grading are based on patterns that are defined by the amount and architecture of glandular units and tubules present in the tissue sample. The ability to identify tubules and glandular structures is an essential requirement for both grading systems. While there is a lot of work on identifying nuclear pleomorphism and mitotic count, as most recently in [12], our contribution in this paper is to propose a new effective way of extracting information concerning glandular architecture, which is directly related to the first component in Elston grading and is an essential part of Gleason grading. In particular, what we present in this paper

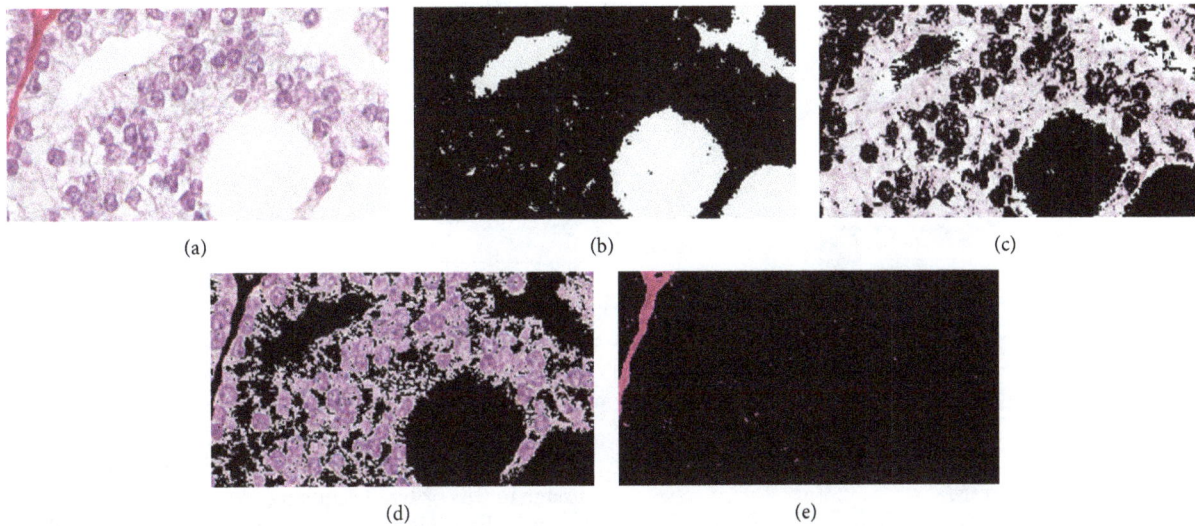

FIGURE 1: An image of prostate tissue (a) is decomposed into four classes: lumen, epithelium, nuclei, and stromal regions. The probability maps in this example were thresholded at a level of 10% for enhancing visibility.

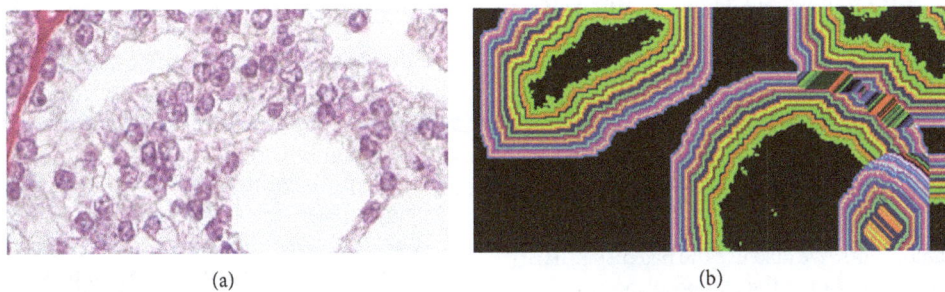

FIGURE 2: The sampling rings growing away from each lumen region for the example in Figure 1. Each ring is obtained by first dilating the lumen region and then subtracting it from the dilated version. This is done sequentially and the number of rings in this example is 30.

is a method that enables us to distinguish between images with tubular structures, denoted by $C1$, and images lacking tubular structures, denoted by $C0$, where these images are taken from both healthy and cancerous breast tissue, since we want to be able to identify tubules in both healthy and cancer tissue samples.

2. Materials and Methods

2.1. Statistical Proximity Sampling. The grading of cancerous tissue of glandular organs such as prostate and breast is to a large extent based on the tissue architecture around the glandular lumen regions. In previous work [13, 14], we have presented automated methods for color decomposition and pattern-based image segmentation that result in density or probability maps, one per stained tissue type. In the current work, we present a method that uses such types of maps as input for deriving a set of features based on statistically sampling the neighborhood of lumen regions. The purpose is to discriminate between tubule and nontubule regions in breast tissue sections.

Our method proceeds in the following manner.

(1) A tissue image is softly classified into a set of K probability maps using any method such as color decomposition (see [14]) or a pattern analysis approach (see [13]); an example is shown in Figure 1, where the K tissue types correspond to lumen, epithelium, nuclei, and stroma.

(2) Starting from the lumen regions, each region is separately dilated by a square structuring element in sequential unit steps forming a set of rings or annuli around the original lumen space (see Figure 2). These rings are regarded as neighborhood strips from which we will gather statistics on the quantity and location of surrounding tissue types. The boundary shape is preserved within a reasonable number of sampling rings.

(3) Within each ring, we compute the proportions of the different tissue types (lumen, epithelium, nuclei, and stroma) using the derived probability maps. Thus, for each ring, we obtain a vector of length K. For instance, a vector such as $[0.2, 0.4, 0.1, 0.3]$ in a given ring indicates that the relative proportions of lumen,

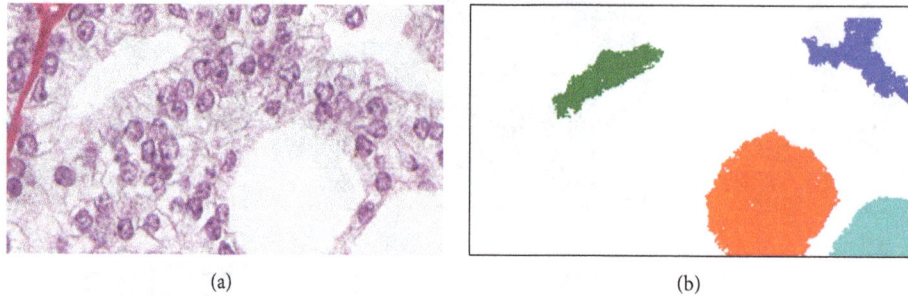

FIGURE 3: The lumen class from the original image shown in Figure 1 is extracted. The different regions are labeled according to their 4-connectivity. These regions form the basis and starting point of our algorithm for deriving features.

epithelium, nuclei, and stroma are 20%, 40%, 10%, and 30%, respectively.

(4) The vectors obtained in step (3) are stacked, forming a single vector of length $R \times K$, where R is the number of rings used, that is, neighborhood strips. Thus each lumen region from step (1) will be represented by such a feature vector of length $R \times K$. An example of these vectors is shown in Figure 4, where there are 4 lumen regions and consequently 4 such feature vectors plotted using different colors.

(5) We present each image as a bag or collection of feature vectors corresponding to lumen regions in the image. Thus, we use multiple-instance learning to represent an image using a collection of feature vectors and perform the classification of each image based on its contents. We also use the bag dissimilarity approach [15] to decouple the classification task from the multiple-instance formulation, allowing us to use any type of classifier without difficulty.

In step (2), it is possible to use dilations with larger steps or with a larger structuring element when deriving the rings. This would make the collected statistics less noisy but would also decrease the spatial resolution of the collected data (analogous to the effect of applying a moving average filter).

The method is designed to be applicable to any glandular tissue type. We have developed and tested it on breast and prostate tissue. We begin by explaining the method through an example for the case of prostate tissue. Figure 1 shows a cross-section of prostate tissue that has been stained with a Sirius-hematoxylin stain combination along with the resulting image decomposition into four probability maps which represent in this case the classes corresponding to lumen, epithelium, nuclei, and stromal regions. Note that the decomposition method used for prostate tissue follows from our previous work in [14]. The proximity sampling method takes as input the probability maps generated from the decomposition, regardless of which method was employed for the latter. The image selected for decomposition in Figure 1 is a cropped image of size 183×339 and was chosen to contain only a small number of lumen regions so that the number of feature profiles that follow remains tractable for display. The probability maps were automatically rearranged according to a descending order of mean intensity value. This

allows the automatic selection of the lumen class as the first image in this ordered sequence.

In what follows, we discuss in detail how the main feature vector of the statistical proximity sampling method is obtained. The method proceeds by statistically sampling the neighborhood around each lumen in terms of class component quantities. By sequential dilation of the lumen region and subtraction of the preceding area, we obtain concentric rings or annuli progressing spatially away from the lumen in either inward, outward, or both directions, extending the lumen shape (see Figure 2). Within each ring, the fraction of each class component, that is, lumen, epithelium, nuclei, and stroma, is computed as a ratio of the sum of class posterior probabilities within the ring to the total area of the ring. These are then concatenated into a vector with $K = 4$ parts, where K is the number of classes. The number of dilations or rings we have used in this case for illustration was 30. This creates a profile of how these class quantities are changing spatially as one moves away from the lumen within its neighborhood. As cancer progresses from benign to malignant, the different grades of cancer are expected to exhibit different patterns in terms of the quantities and order of these class components around the lumen which would result in different profile curves sampled from these rings. The features represent fractional values in the range $[0, 1]$. The shape of the curve captures spatial (order) information and represents statistical quantification of the classes.

Figure 3 shows lumen regions extracted from the corresponding posterior map and labeled according to their 4-connected neighborhood; that is, pixels that are adjacent diagonally are not considered neighbors. Figure 4 shows the profile curves obtained, one for each of the four lumen regions. The first 30 elements represent the changing amount of neighboring lumen within those rings; the second part consisting of another 30 elements represents that of epithelium, the third part that of nuclei, and the fourth that of stroma. To validate and understand what the curves represent, one should compare the profile of each lumen to its spatial neighborhood shown in Figure 3. The colors shown in Figure 4 have been set to match those lumen regions shown in Figure 3. For example, the cyan curve represents the cyan colored lumen region. From Figure 3, we notice that the sampling rings should contain a considerable fraction of lumen due to the large neighboring lumen region shown in

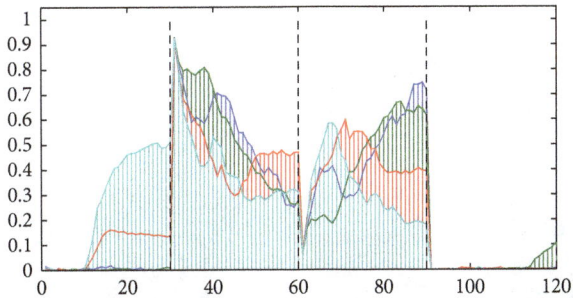

FIGURE 4: Feature vectors are shown, one for each of the four lumen regions illustrated in Figure 3. The vectors are divided into 4 parts delineated by black vertical lines: the first part depicts the first 30 elements representing the fraction of lumen within the 30 sampling rings, the second part depicts those for the epithelium component, the third part depicts those for the nuclei component, and the fourth part depicts those for the stromal component.

red color. Consequently, the first part of the cyan curve shows high values. Similar analysis follows for the other parts of the curve in which one can see how each class component varies as one moves away from the lumen region. The fourth part of the curve is particularly easy to notice since there is no stromal component close enough to the cyan luminal region.

Alternatively, in order to show how the different luminal regions compare to each other in terms of the spatial composition of their proximities, we replot the curves of Figure 4 such that the proportions of the four different tissue types (lumen, epithelium, nuclei, and stroma) across the rings are shown in a relative frequency pie chart for each luminal region separately. This is illustrated in Figure 5, where each subplot represents a luminal region indicated by the color of the central rectangle, and we note here that each of these exhibits a different profile.

We note that the previous example was based on the spectral decomposition of tissue that was specifically stained (using Sirius-hematoxylin) in order to express the different relevant tissue components (see [14]). However, in order to illustrate that the proposed concept is robust and generally applicable, we have also applied it to images of breast cancer tissues from the Human Protein Atlas database [16] which are stained using hematoxylin-eosin + DAB to visualize general background tissue structures and specific proteins. As an example, we show a cropped image region of size 362 × 450 selected from the case "Group R"—$C1$ in [13]. Figure 6 shows the decomposition of the image into four classes corresponding to lumen, stroma, nuclei, and DAB. Figure 7 shows four selected lumen regions from the posterior map of the lumen class in order to display their respective feature curves as based on the proximity sampling method described above. Finally, Figure 8 shows the profile curves for this example, where the number of sampling rings around each lumen was set to 10. In a similar manner to the previous example, several detailed conclusions may be drawn from these figures; however the most general one is that these feature curves capture the statistical distribution of the classes around each lumen region and may therefore be used to classify those regions.

2.2. Bag Dissimilarity for Classification. To test our method, we used a dataset consisting of images of breast tissue sections obtained from the Human Protein Atlas project [16], where every image has been assigned a malignancy grade by an expert. The assigned class labels denoted by $C0$ and $C1$ are associated with the tubule-based Elston grading, where the main factor is the absence ($C0$) or presence ($C1$) of milk ducts in the tissue. Sample images of the dataset are shown in Figure 9. Note that all microscopy images of the given dataset were acquired under the same magnification level of ×40. The dataset consists of tissue sections containing cells, glands, and luminal regions, and the proximity sampling method we have proposed applies in general also for images of tissue types that contain similar structures in living organisms.

In the dataset, an image may contain several lumen regions. A feature vector is derived for each of these lumen regions using the proximity sampling method described. The aim is to train a classifier on the labeled, that is, graded, images in order to predict the label of a new image automatically. Thus, there is an inherent relation between the formulation of this problem and multiple-instance learning [17]. In the context of the latter, the feature vectors derived from the lumen regions in an image may be regarded as "instances" or objects and the image itself as a "bag" or compound object consisting of one or more instances. The instances themselves are not labeled, but rather only the bag carries a label, which in this case is the tubule-based grade assigned by the pathologists. Also different bags may contain a different number of instances. Some of the instances in a bag may be less important in contributing to the bag label, whereas one or more may be key instances, belonging to the so-called "concept," that significantly define the bag label. For example, an image may contain one gland unit that characterizes a grade 3 cancer region, in addition to several noncontributing, background lumen regions. In such a case, one of the instances belongs to the "concept" that contributes to the grade 3 label.

The multiple-instance learning approach is more flexible than standard classification approaches in that the representation allows us to encode more information from a single image by considering it as a collection of feature vectors rather than encoding the entire image by a single feature vector. Images of real life objects (such as tissue sections) often contain a lot of important subregions with different characteristics and may be therefore too complex to be represented by a single feature vector [15]. The multiple-instance representation is highly informative in this situation since it encodes information from different regions in an image, each of which may contribute to the final grade or label of the image as a whole.

However, the classification task that ensues becomes more complex as a classifier is trained and optimized over the dataset. Therefore, in order not to add complexity to the construction of a classifier and preserve the flexibility of the task, we follow the bag dissimilarity approach described in [15], which does not attempt to locate a "concept" but rather uses a similarity measure across bags, which are seen as sets of instances. The dissimilarities computed between the bags become the new features, and this allows us to construct

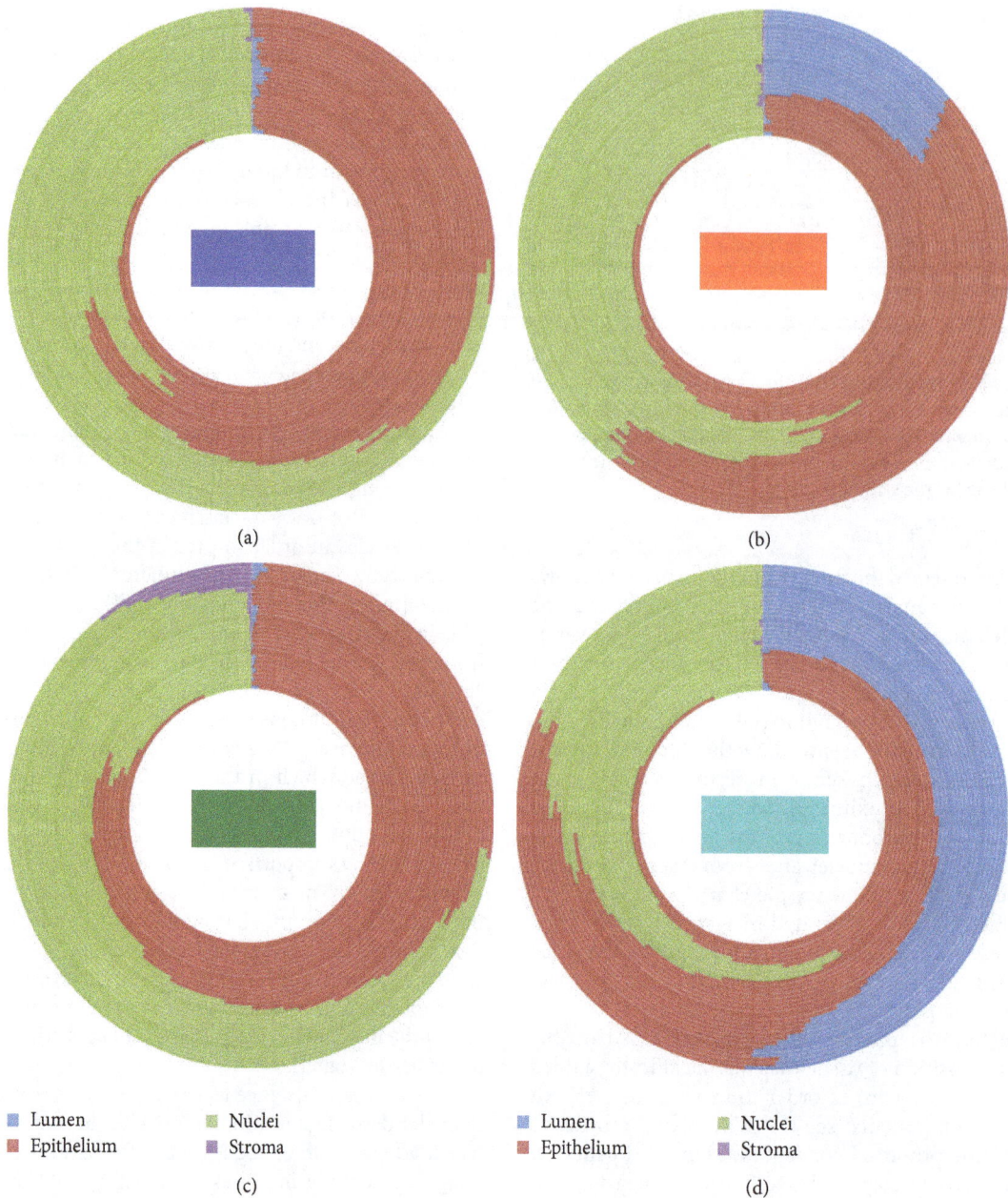

FIGURE 5: The four parts of each feature vector illustrated in Figure 4 are depicted in a relative frequency graph for each luminal region in this example. The color of the central rectangle in each subplot indicates the corresponding lumen region shown in Figure 3.

any classifier in this new feature space, thus decoupling the original multiple-instance problem from the classification task itself. Moreover, the bag dissimilarity approach allows us to consider multiclass data, that is, data with several grades, whereas in the traditional multiple-instance learning problem only two classes, namely, a positive and a negative class, are considered at any given time, and a one-against-one or one-against-all approach is often used in the classification of multiclass situations.

2.3. Additional Lumen Shape Features. Insofar, we have presented a new vectorial proximity-based feature for describing

tissue architecture around glands, and we proceed in the next section to demonstrate its usefulness as a feature descriptor. However, in order to evaluate whether more conventional scalar features add any information to the new feature, we have implemented four classical, well-known scalar features that are simple to compute from each lumen region. The first is the size of the region, while the other measures relate to its shape and are the bending energy, area-to-perimeter ratio, and convexity ratio. Bending energy [18] is defined around the lumen perimeter based on the chain code sequence and is given by $E_b = \sum_{p=1}^{P_f} \kappa^2(p)$, where $\kappa(p)$ is a smoothed

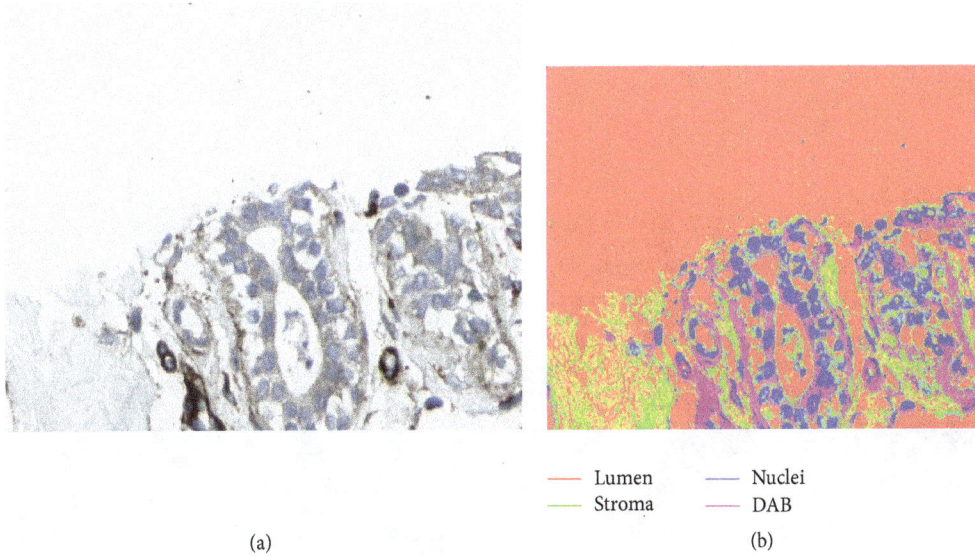

(a)   (b)

Lumen   Nuclei
Stroma   DAB

FIGURE 6: An image of breast tissue and its resulting decomposition into four classes: lumen, stroma, nuclei, and DAB regions.

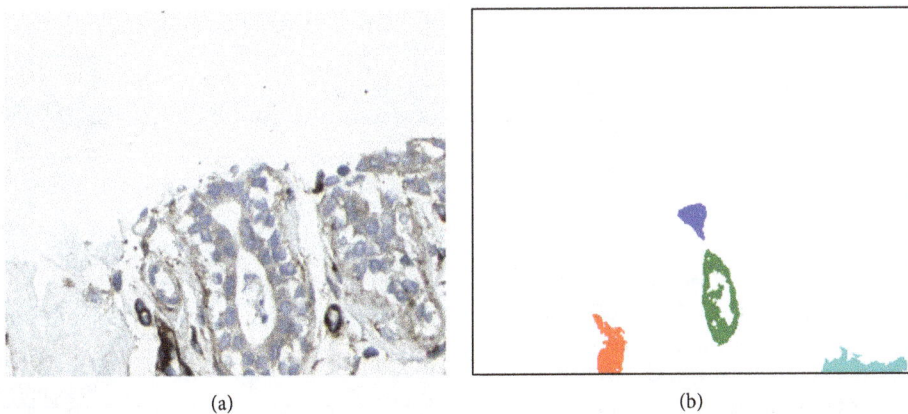

(a)   (b)

FIGURE 7: A few selected regions from the lumen class of the original image shown in Figure 6 are extracted. The different regions are labeled according to their 4-connectivity and shown using different colors.

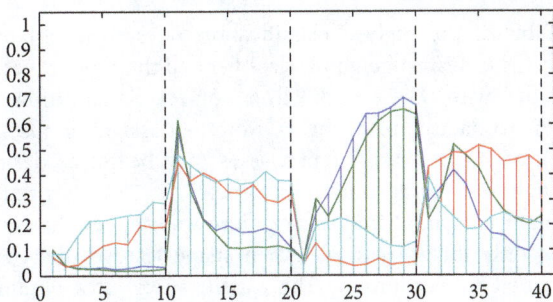

FIGURE 8: A feature vector is shown, one for each of the lumen regions illustrated in Figure 7. The vectors are divided into 4 parts delineated by black vertical lines: the first part depicts the first 10 elements representing the fraction of lumen within the 10 sampling rings, the second part depicts those for the stroma component, the third part depicts those for the nuclei component, and the fourth part depicts those for the DAB component.

version of the curvature signal $\theta(p) = \tan^{-1}((y_c(p) - y_c(p - 1))/(x_c(p) - x_c(p - 1)))$, where $(x_c(p - 1), y_c(p - 1))$ and $(x_c(p), y_c(p))$ are two consecutive points of the curvature. The minimum value is $2\pi/R$ and is attained for a circle of radius R. This feature is an indicator of convexity/concavity of the lumen boundary. The area-to-perimeter ratio is defined as $(4\pi A)/P^2$, where P is the perimeter and A the area of the lumen region. Convexity is defined as $A_{\text{lumen}}/A_{\text{convex hull}}$, where A_{lumen} is the area of the lumen region and $A_{\text{convex hull}}$ is the area covered by the convex hull encompassing the lumen region. This ratio is in the range $[0, 1]$ and is closer to 1 when the lumen shape is convex and closer to 0 when highly irregular such as the case of cribriform grade 3-4 glandular units in prostate tissue, for instance. These lumen shape features are then compared with the main proximity feature vector, and classification results are presented in Section 3.

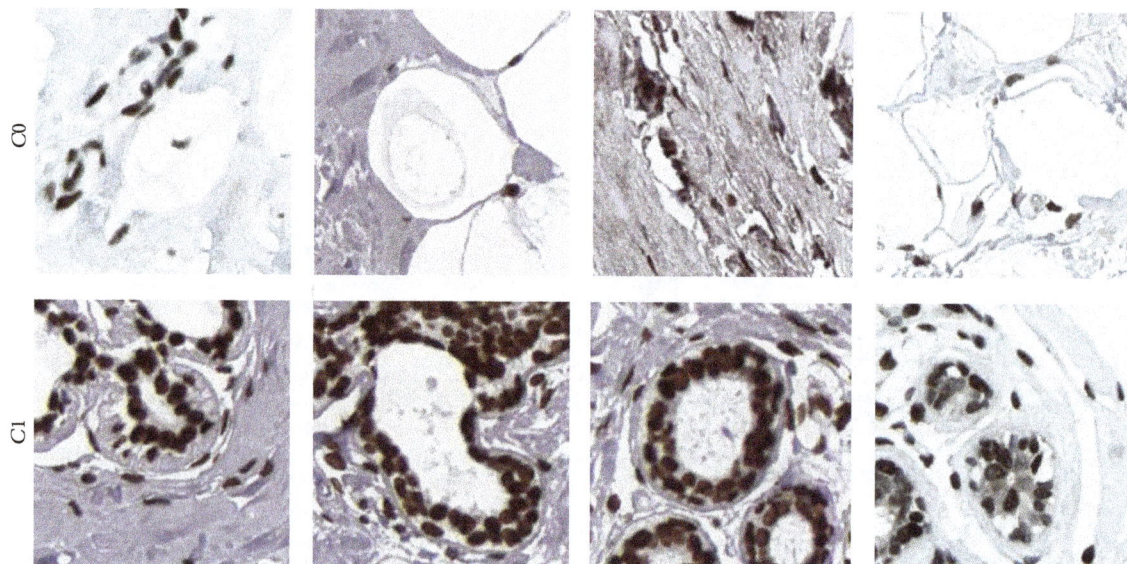

FIGURE 9: A few sample cases of the breast dataset consisting of images of breast tissue sections labeled as $C1$ and $C0$ based on the presence or absence of milk ducts, respectively.

TABLE 1: Summary statistics concerning the dataset used in this paper.

Dataset	Number of instances	Dimensionality	Number of bags	Number of instances per bag		
				Minimum	Median	Maximum
Breast	1309	40	104	1	10	37

3. Results and Discussion

For each image in the dataset, we have used our proximity-based feature method to obtain a set of descriptive features. Then we used multiple-instance learning to represent each image as a bag of instances and transform the feature space into a dissimilarity space by computing the distances among the different bags. The MIL toolbox and various classifiers were used for this purpose [19, 20]. Our dissimilarity matrix is computed among the bags based on the linear assignment distance measured between sets [15, 21]. The dataset is then randomly split into a training set and a test set, and cross-validation procedures are used throughout. The mean error and standard deviation are then reported for both datasets. The characteristics of our dataset are summarized in Table 1. Note that ten sampling rings were used for the statistical proximity sampling method throughout all cases resulting in 40-element feature vectors for the case of the breast dataset since the number of classes was four using the hematoxylin-eosin + DAB stain.

Figure 10 shows the classification rates and classifier learning curves using only the features derived by the statistical proximity sampling method. Note that the parameters for the support vector classifier and k-nearest neighbor classifier were optimized using leave-one-out cross-validation over a training set comprising randomly 25% of the original dataset. The 10-fold cross-validation rates for all classifiers over the remaining test set are then computed. The entire process is further repeated in 5 experiments. The results are presented

TABLE 2: Classification rates for the breast dataset using different classifiers. Classification was done using 10-fold cross-validation and results are reported as percentage of correct classification ± standard deviation.

Classifier	Classification rate Proximity features (Figure 10)
SVC	94.2 ± 2.0
KNN	93.4 ± 0.8
Logistic	80.5 ± 1.3
LDC	61.7 ± 1.2

in Table 2. The highest classification rates were obtained using the k-nearest neighbor classifier and the support vector classifier with 93.4% and 94.2% correct classification for the breast dataset, respectively. Note that assigning misclassification costs for different classes may be set as desired through the regularization parameter of SVC if needed. For comparison, a similar procedure was applied, however, using only the 4 classical lumen shape features that were described in Section 2.3. The classification rates obtained were much lower with the best performance at 62.69%.

3.1. Unsupervised Approach. Although we do not explore unsupervised methods for malignancy grading in this paper, we would like to highlight the possibility of applying a clustering-based approach coupled with an information criterion for classifying images. We demonstrate in what follows

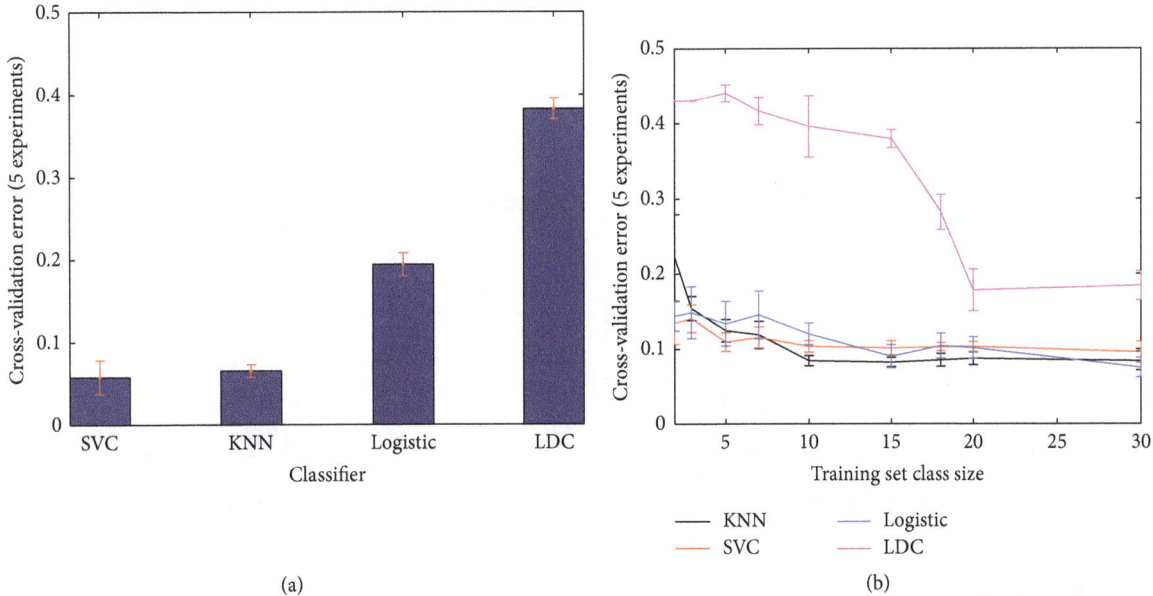

FIGURE 10: Classification results for the breast dataset, using only the features derived by statistical proximity sampling. Classifiers used are the linear support vector classifier (SVC), k-nearest neighbor classifier (KNN), the logistic classifier (Logistic), and normal-based linear discriminant classifier (LDC). (a) 10-fold cross-validation error. (b) Classifier learning curves. Error bars represent one standard deviation.

how clustering may be applied to classify instances in the absence of bag labels. In other words, we attempt to identify and locate key clusters or groups of instances forming main clusters. A bag label (i.e., image grade) may then be obtained using a voting scheme over the cluster labels of the instances that belong to it. To study whether there may be an inherent number of clusters in the data possibly due to a certain fixed number of neighborhood descriptions that tend to recur around lumen regions, we used the Bayesian information criterion (BIC). We clustered the breast dataset using the Gaussian mixture model (GMM) several times with a varying number of clusters k ranging from 1 to 10, and we computed the BIC values as defined by BIC $= -2\ln(L) + k\ln(n)$, where n is the number of objects in the data, L is the likelihood value of the mixture fit, and k is the number of clusters. Note that the mixture model was initialized randomly 10 times for each value of k. As the number of clusters increases, we expect the log-likelihood to increase monotonically; however the BIC measure also includes the model parameters into the tradeoff, which in this case is the number of clusters k. The optimal mixture model would have a high log-likelihood yet at a lowest possible complexity k. A plot of the BIC values versus the number of clusters is shown in Figure 11. We deduce in this case that for the breast dataset the optimal number of clusters at which the BIC curve attains a minimum is 2. This result does not necessarily imply that there are 2 clusters in the data in an absolute sense. When using the Akaike information criterion (AIC), we note in Figure 11 that the optimal number of clusters at which the curve attains a minimum becomes 4, since AIC in this case penalizes model complexity less heavily than BIC and thus results in the selection of a larger model. Conclusively, this might suggest that a model selection of 2, 3, or 4 classes in this case is a reasonable choice.

4. Conclusions

We have presented a general and simple method for statistically describing the distribution of glandular structures around lumen regions. The method makes use of sampling based on an iterative region expansion procedure that preserves the shape of the lumen areas. One advantage of this approach is that, by analyzing the neighborhoods of lumen regions and preserving the spatial and statistical information in these proximities, we avoid the need to extract explicit features concerning the underlying tissue structures themselves. The result is a set of feature vectors containing spatial and statistical information that may be used to describe regions in tissue images for a large variety of purposes, among which is tubule-based grading, as we have demonstrated in this paper. The input required for the method can be either a set of probability or binary maps derived from soft or crisp classification regardless of the supervised or unsupervised method (e.g., [13, 14]) used to generate these maps. The method is also robust and its dependence on the quality of these maps is minimal since the approach does not attempt to derive any precise cellular or subcellular features, which would require accurate image segmentation.

Due to the natural complexity of biological tissue and the grading process, we have avoided the single feature vector based representation used in standard pattern recognition. Automated grading was instead done using a bag dissimilarity approach while treating the problem in a similar manner to multiple-instance learning. Since images of tissue sections often contain various spatial subregions which may have completely different properties and characteristics, such an approach is more capable of encoding the diverse content and level of information represented in these images.

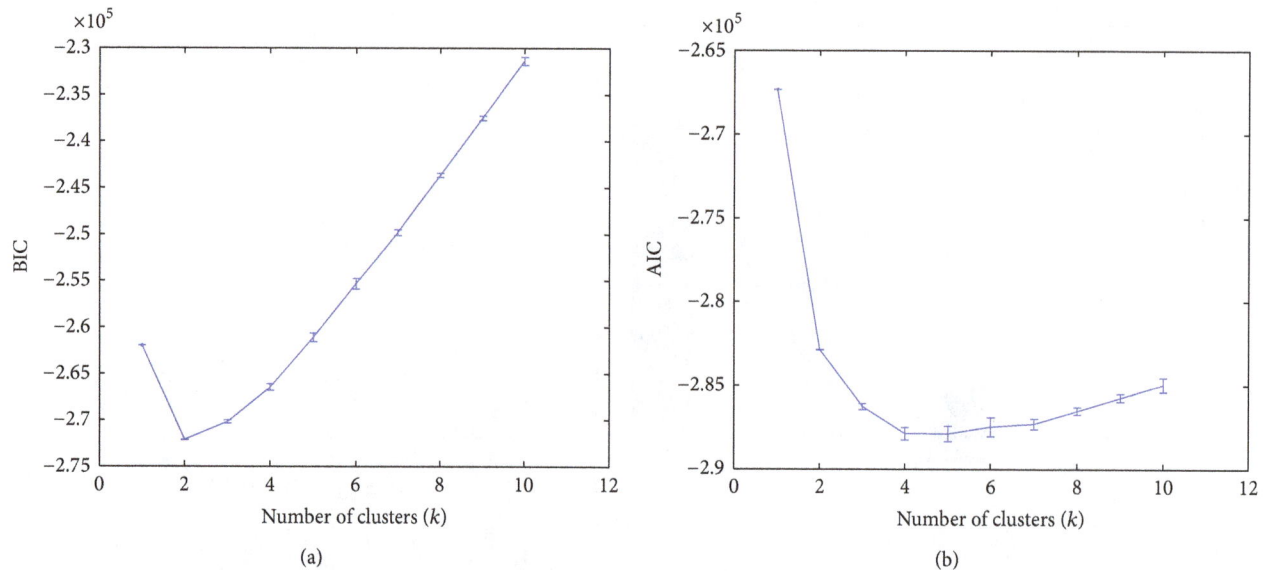

FIGURE 11: Optimal number of clusters using the Bayesian information criterion (BIC) and Akaike information criterion (AIC) over the breast dataset. The error bars represent the standard deviation at each value of "k."

Classification results using cross-validation have shown that the statistical proximity sampling method presented is able to provide a set of discriminative features for tubule-based cancer grading.

A possible drawback of the dissimilarity approach we have used in our classification is that although the classification task itself is accomplished and the diagnosis is automated, no single "concept" is identified during the process, as it remains hidden. However, alternative multiple-instance learning methods that are based on the notion of finding a "concept" may be used for this purpose if needed. The advantage of identifying a "concept" is that it becomes then possible to visually map the "concept" or its instances back to the corresponding regions in the image. This could be a basis for future work.

The results obtained for the HPA dataset in this paper are meant to illustrate the potential of our approach in feature extraction and grading and its prospect for further extended studies over large datasets and possible combination with complementary approaches that address other aspects of grading (such as nuclear pleomorphism and mitotic count), possibly leading to applications in the clinical context. A comprehensive automated system that would be able to eventually assign high-level grading akin to that by pathologists would undoubtedly have to incorporate, in addition to the work described in this paper, methods that are designed to address nuclear pleomorphism and mitotic count (as most recently in [12]). The final aim is to aid pathologists in the malignancy grading of cancer. As a first step towards that goal, we have in this paper addressed tubule-based grading, which contributes to one of the three components for malignancy grading under the Ellis-Elston system and which is also considered an important factor in Gleason grading.

Conflict of Interests

The authors declare that there is no conflict of interests regarding the publication of this paper.

References

[1] C. W. Elston and I. O. Ellis, "Pathological prognostic factors in breast cancer. I. The value of histological grade in breast cancer: experience from a large study with long-term follow-up," *Histopathology*, vol. 19, no. 5, pp. 403–410, 1991.

[2] J. I. Epstein, W. C. Allsbrook Jr., M. B. Amin et al., "The 2005 International Society of Urological Pathology (ISUP) consensus conference on Gleason grading of prostatic carcinoma," *The American Journal of Surgical Pathology*, vol. 29, no. 9, pp. 1228–1242, 2005.

[3] J. Prewitt and S. Wu, "An application of pattern recognition to epithelial tissues," in *Proceedings of the IEEE 2nd Annual Symposium on Computer Application in Medical Care*, pp. 15–25, November 1978.

[4] A. Tabesh, M. Teverovskiy, H.-Y. Pang et al., "Multifeature prostate cancer diagnosis and gleason grading of histological images," *IEEE Transactions on Medical Imaging*, vol. 26, no. 10, pp. 1366–1378, 2007.

[5] A. Tabesh, V. P. Kumar, H.-Y. Pang et al., "Automated prostate cancer diagnosis and Gleason grading of tissue microarrays," in *Medical Imaging 2005: Image Processing*, vol. 5747 of *Proceedings of SPIE*, pp. 58–70, San Diego, Calif, USA, 2005.

[6] S. Doyle, S. Agner, A. Madabhushi, M. D. Feldman, and J. E. Tomaszewski, "Automated grading of breast cancer histopathology using spectral clustering with textural and architectural image features," in *IEEE International Symposium on Biomedical Imaging: From Nano to Macro*, pp. 496–499, Paris, France, 2008.

[7] S. Naik, S. Doyle, S. Agner, A. Madabhushi, M. Feldman, and J. Tomaszewski, "Automated gland and nuclei segmentation for grading of prostate and breast cancer histopathology," in *Proceedings of the 5th IEEE International Symposium on Biomedical Imaging: From Nano to Macro (ISBI '08)*, pp. 284–287, Paris, France, May 2008.

[8] R. P. W. Duin, "Non-euclidean problems in pattern recognition related to human expert knowledge," in *Proceedings of the International Conference on Enterprise Information Systems (ICEIS '10), Funchal-Madeira, Portugal, June 2010*, vol. 73 of *Lecture Notes in Business Information Processing*, pp. 15–28, Springer, Berlin, Germany, 2011.

[9] S. Theodoridis and K. Koutroumbas, *Pattern Recognition*, Academic Press, New York, NY, USA, 4th edition, 2009.

[10] E. Nowak, F. Jurie, and B. Triggs, "Sampling strategies for bag-of-features image classification," in *Proceedings of the European Conference on Computer Vision*, vol. 3954 of *Lecture Notes in Computer Science*, pp. 490–503, Springer, Graz, Austria, May 2006.

[11] J. Zhang, M. Marszałek, S. Lazebnik, and C. Schmid, "Local features and kernels for classification of texture and object categories: a comprehensive study," *International Journal of Computer Vision*, vol. 73, no. 2, pp. 213–238, 2007.

[12] Mitos-Atypia-14, "Mitos & Atypia: detection of mitosis and evaluation of nuclear atypia score in breast cancer histological images," in *Proceedings of the 22nd International Conference on Pattern Recognition (ICPR '14)*, 2014, http://mitos-atypia-14.grand-challenge.org/.

[13] J. C. Azar, M. Simonsson, E. Bengtsson, and A. Hast, "Image segmentation and identification of paired antibodies in breast tissue," *Computational and Mathematical Methods in Medicine*, vol. 2014, Article ID 647273, 11 pages, 2014.

[14] M. Gavrilovic, J. C. Azar, J. Lindblad et al., "Blind color decomposition of histological images," *IEEE Transactions on Medical Imaging*, vol. 32, no. 6, pp. 983–994, 2013.

[15] D. M. J. Tax, M. Loog, R. P. W. Duin, V. Cheplygina, and W.-J. Lee, "Bag dissimilarities for multiple instance learning," in *Similarity-Based Pattern Recognition*, vol. 7005 of *Lecture Notes in Computer Science*, pp. 222–234, Springer, New York, NY, USA, 2011.

[16] HPA, *The Human Protein Atlas*, 2013, http://www.proteinatlas.org/.

[17] T. G. Dietterich, R. H. Lathrop, and T. Lozano-Pérez, "Solving the multiple instance problem with axis-parallel rectangles," *Artificial Intelligence*, vol. 89, no. 1-2, pp. 31–71, 1997.

[18] L. J. van Vliet and P. W. Verbeek, "Curvature and bending energy in digitized 2d and 3d images," in *Proceedings of the 8th Scandinavian Conference on Image Analysis*, vol. 2, pp. 1403–1410, Tromsø, Norway, 1993.

[19] D. M. J. Tax, "MIL, A Matlab Toolbox for Multiple Instance Learning, version 0.8.1," 2013, http://prlab.tudelft.nl/david-tax/mil.html.

[20] R. P. W. Duin, P. Juszczak, P. Paclík, E. Pękalska, D. DeRidder, and D. M. J. Tax, "A Matlab Toolbox for Pattern Recognition, PRTools4 version 4.2.5," 2013, http://www.37steps.com/.

[21] H. W. Kuhn, "The Hungarian method for the assignment problem," *Naval Research Logistics Quarterly*, vol. 2, no. 1-2, pp. 83–97, 1955.

13

Edge Detection in Digital Images Using Dispersive Phase Stretch Transform

Mohammad H. Asghari[1] and Bahram Jalali[1,2,3]

[1]*Department of Electrical Engineering, University of California, Los Angeles, Los Angeles, CA 90095, USA*
[2]*Department of Bioengineering, University of California, Los Angeles, Los Angeles, CA 90095, USA*
[3]*Department of Surgery, David Geffen School of Medicine, University of California, Los Angeles, Los Angeles, CA 90095, USA*

Correspondence should be addressed to Mohammad H. Asghari; asghari@ucla.edu

Academic Editor: Tiange Zhuang

We describe a new computational approach to edge detection and its application to biomedical images. Our digital algorithm transforms the image by emulating the propagation of light through a physical medium with specific warped diffractive property. We show that the output phase of the transform reveals transitions in image intensity and can be used for edge detection.

1. Introduction

Edge detection is the name for a set of mathematical methods for identifying patterns in digital images where brightness or color changes abruptly [1–3]. Applying an edge detection algorithm to an image can be used for object detection and classification. It also reduces the digital file size while preserving important information, albeit data compression is not the main objective in edge detection.

Many methods for edge detection have been proposed, but most of them can be grouped into two main categories: zero-crossing based and search-based. The zero-crossing based methods search for zero crossings in a Laplacian or second-order derivative computed from the image [1]. The search-based methods compute the edge strength, usually with a first-order derivative, and then search for local directional maxima of the gradient amplitude [2]. Detailed survey of available techniques for edge detection can be found in [3].

We employ a physics-inspired digital image transformation that emulates propagation of electromagnetic waves through a diffractive medium with a dielectric function that has warped dispersive (frequency dependent) property. We show that the phase of the transform has properties conducive for detection of edges and sharp transitions in the image. Our method emulates diffraction using an all-pass phase

filter with specific frequency dispersion dependencies. The output phase profile in spatial domain reveals variations in image intensity and when followed by thresholding and morphological postprocessing provides edge detection. We show how filters with linear and nonlinear phase derivatives can be used for edge detection and how the shape and magnitude of the phase function influence the edge image.

Earlier it was shown that the magnitude of the complex amplitude for a similarly transformed image exhibits reduction in space-bandwidth product and may be useful for data compression [4]. The present paper employs the phase of the transform for application to edge detection. Also, the details of the filter kernel are different in the two cases. Going further back, the concept of diffraction based image processing has its roots in the Photonic Time Stretch, a temporal signal processing technique that employs temporal dispersion to slow down, capture, and digitally process fast waveforms in real time [5]. Known as the time-stretch dispersive Fourier transform, this technique has led to the discovery of optical rogue waves and detection of cancer cells in blood with record sensitivity [6], as well as highest performance analog-to-digital conversion [7]. In this paper, we also demonstrate application of the proposed edge detection algorithm to some biomedical images.

Output phase image

Image → [Nonlinear phase dispersion] → Thresholding → [Morphological operations] → Detected edges

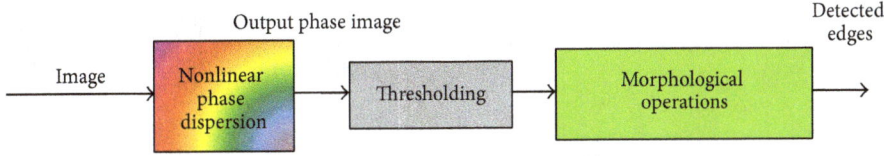

FIGURE 1: In the proposed method for edge detection, after the application of localization filter, a warped Phase Stretch Transform is performed on the image and the phase of the output image is thresholded and postprocessed by morphological operations to generate the image edges.

2. Technical Description

Different steps of the proposed method for edge detection are shown in Figure 1. In this method, the original image is first smoothed using a localization kernel and then is passed through a nonlinear frequency dependent (dispersive) phase operation, called Phase Stretch Transform (PST). PST applies a 2D phase function to the image in the frequency domain. The amount of phase applied to the image is frequency dependent; that is, a higher amount of phase is applied to higher frequency features of the image. Since image edges contain higher frequency features, PST emphasizes the edge information in the image by applying more phase to higher frequency features. Image edges can be extracted by thresholding the PST output phase image. After thresholding, the binary image is further processed by morphological operations to find the image edges.

In the remainder of this paper, we refer to this technique as the Phase Stretch Transform (PST). The image under analysis is represented by $B[n,m]$ where n and m are two-dimensional spatial variables. The PST in frequency domain can be described as follows:

$$A[n,m]$$
$$= \angle \left\langle IFFT2 \left\{ \widetilde{K}[p,q] \cdot \widetilde{L}[p,q] \cdot FFT2\{B[n,m]\} \right\} \right\rangle, \quad (1)$$

where $A[n,m]$ is the output phase image, $\angle\langle\cdot\rangle$ is the angle operator, $FFT2$ is the two-dimensional Fast Fourier Transform, $IFFT2$ is the two-dimensional Inverse Fast Fourier Transform, and p and q are two-dimensional frequency variables. The function $\widetilde{L}[p,q]$ is the frequency response of the localization kernel and the warped phase kernel $\widetilde{K}[p,q]$ is described by a nonlinear frequency dependent phase:

$$\widetilde{K}[p,q] = e^{j \cdot \varphi[p,q]}. \quad (2)$$

While arbitrary phase kernels can be considered for PST operation, here we study the phase kernels for which the kernel phase derivative $PD[p,q]$ is a linear or sublinear function with respect to frequency variables. A simple example of such phase derivative profiles (e.g., represented by least number of parameters) is the inverse tangent function which leads to the following PST kernel phase:

$$\varphi[p,q]$$
$$= \varphi_{\text{polar}}[r,\theta] = \varphi_{\text{polar}}[r]$$

$$= S$$

$$\cdot \frac{W \cdot r \cdot \tan^{-1}(W \cdot r) - (1/2) \cdot \ln\left(1 + (W \cdot r)^2\right)}{W \cdot r_{\text{max}} \cdot \tan^{-1}(W \cdot r_{\text{max}}) - (1/2) \cdot \ln\left(1 + (W \cdot r_{\text{max}})^2\right)}, \quad (3)$$

where $r = \sqrt{p^2 + q^2}$, $\theta = \tan^{-1}(q/p)$, $\tan^{-1}(\cdot)$ is the inverse tangent function, $\ln(\cdot)$ is the natural logarithm, and r_{max} is the maximum frequency r. S and W are real-valued numbers related to the strength (S) and warp (W) of the phase profile applied to the image. For simplicity, we have assumed that the PST kernel phase profile has circular symmetry with respect to frequency variables. For small warping factors $W \ll 1$, the phase profile $\varphi[p,q]$ becomes a quadratic phase and represents the case with linear phase derivative. The two parameters S and W along with the width of the localization kernel and the thresholding values are used to extract the edge information.

Application of PST to the image creates the phase image $A[n,m]$ which is further postprocessed. For edge detection, postprocessing includes cutting the negative phase values, thresholding, and morphological operations. Here we use one-level thresholding. Dependent on the application, the threshold can be set to allow more or less edges to be shown in the binary edge image. Morphological operations can be used to thin the edges, clean the phase image by removing the isolated pixels, or find prime lines representing edges. Frequency bandwidth (full width at half maximum) of the localization kernel is designed to reduce the noise in the proposed edge detection algorithm while preserving the vital edge information. In this paper we have used a Gaussian localization filter.

The parameters that are required to be designed for the proposed edge detection methods are

(1) S and W: Strength (S) and Warp (W)

 of the applied phase kernel

(2) Δf: Bandwidth of the localization kernel   (4)

(3) Thresh: Threshold value.

Figures 2(a) to 2(c) show typical phase derivative profiles that result in edge detection. The kernel applies a phase that increases with spatial frequency. Since edges contain higher frequencies, they are assigned a larger phase and therefore are spatially highlighted in the phase of the transformed image.

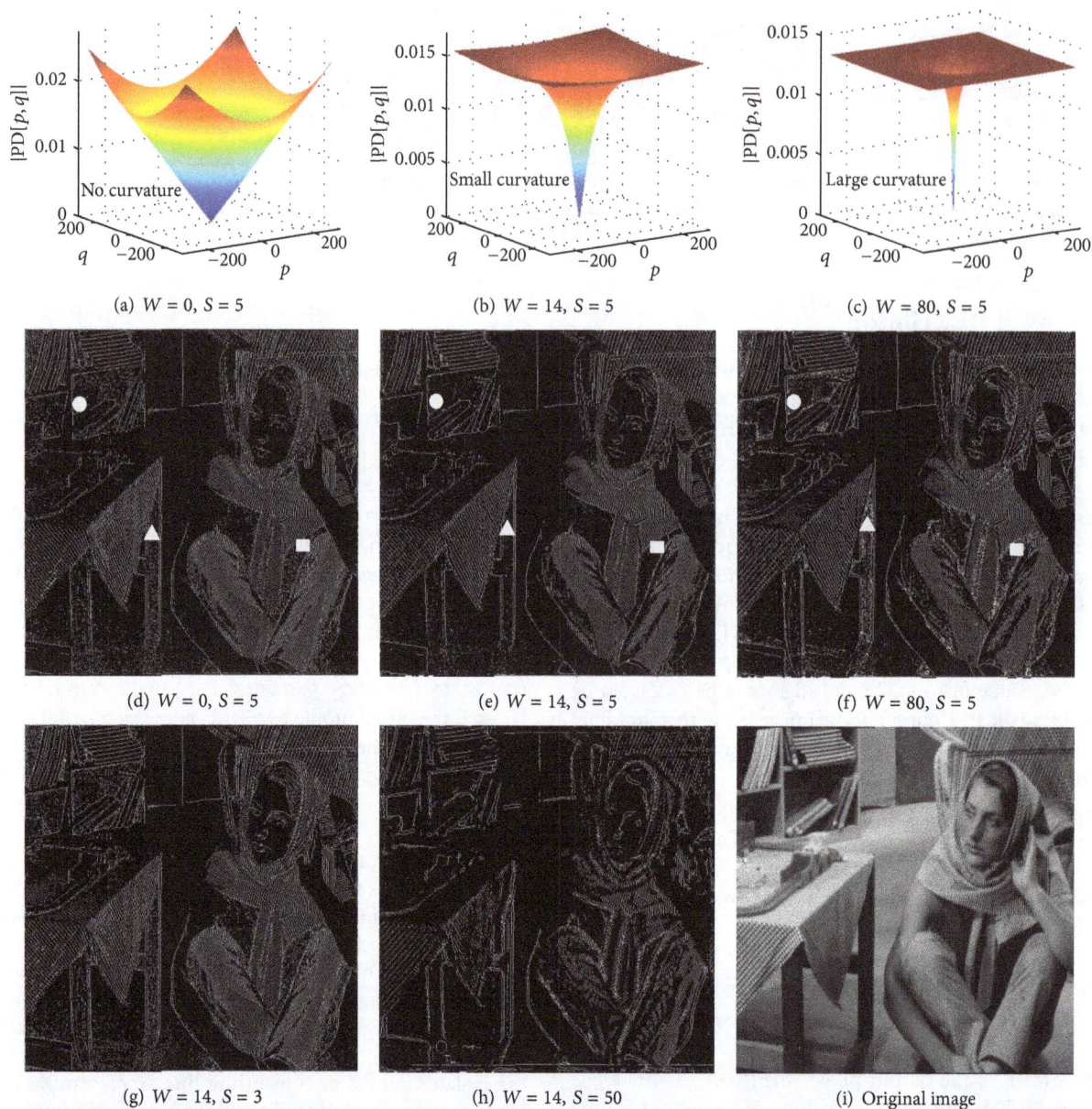

(a) $W = 0$, $S = 5$ (b) $W = 14$, $S = 5$ (c) $W = 80$, $S = 5$

(d) $W = 0$, $S = 5$ (e) $W = 14$, $S = 5$ (f) $W = 80$, $S = 5$

(g) $W = 14$, $S = 3$ (h) $W = 14$, $S = 50$ (i) Original image

FIGURE 2: Effect of warp (W) and the strength (S) of phase applied to a sample image (shown in (i)) on the edge detection performance in the proposed method. (a) to (f) Comparison of edge detection results with three different amounts of W in the phase applied to the image. Phase derivative profiles are shown in (a) to (c) and the corresponding edge detection results are shown in (d) to (f). As seen, edge detection with medium warp has better noise performance than the case with very large warp or the case with linear phase derivative; compare regions indicated with white triangular, circle, and rectangular markers. (e), (g), and (h) Comparison of edge detection performance for the case of $W = 14$ with three different amounts of S applied to the image. As seen, larger phase results in less edge noises but also less resolution to detect the edges. Thus, there is an optimum value for S and W parameters to reduce the edge noises while preserving the vital edge information.

Parameters of the kernel (S and W) control the edge detection process. In the proposed method, there is a trade-off between spatial resolution and noises of edge detection. A larger phase (larger S) results in better noise performance in edge detection but at the expense of lower spatial resolution. Also a larger warp (larger W) in the phase derivative results in a sharper edge but it also increases the edge noise. These parameters can be adjusted manually or optimized by iterative algorithms. They can be either globally fixed or locally optimized.

Figure 2 illustrates the effect of warp and the strength of applied phase on the edge detection performance. The test image used here is the "Barbara" image shown in Figure 2(i). Figures 2(d) to 2(f) compare the edge detection results with different amounts of warp (W) in the applied phase. Figures 2(a) to 2(c) show the phase derivative (group delay) profiles and Figures 2(d) to 2(f) show the corresponding edge images. In all cases, identical localization kernel bandwidth ($\Delta f = 2$), thresholding (Thresh = 0.047), and morphological operations are used. Three different amounts of warp are considered:

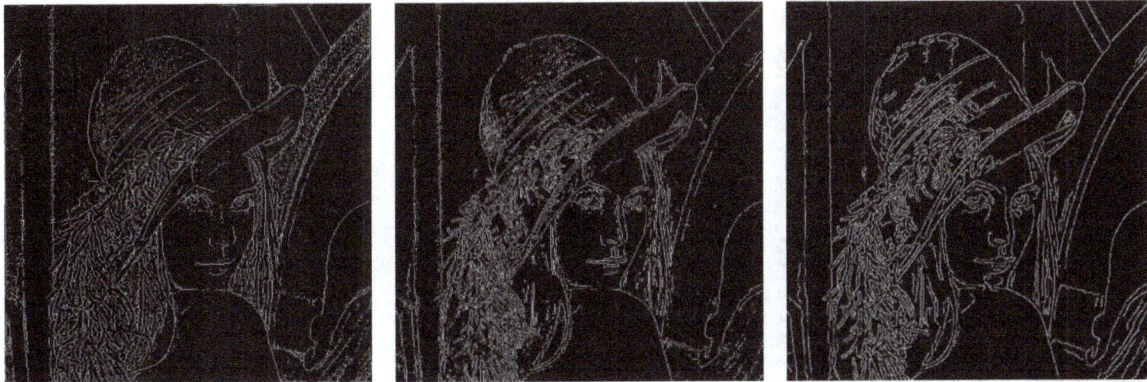

(a) Proposed method, phase strength (S) = 0.48, and warp (W) = 12.14

(b) Sobel: Thresh = 7.9

(c) Canny: sigma = 1.28; Thresh (min, max) = [0.024, 0.117]

FIGURE 3: Qualitative comparison of the performance of the proposed method for edge detection (a) to the Sobel (b) and Canny (c) methods. Image under analysis is the "Lena" image with 512×512 pixels. For the proposed method, designed parameters are phase strength $S = 0.48$, phase warp $W = 12.14$, localization kernel bandwidth $\Delta f = 0.21$, and binary threshold = 0.028. Designed threshold value for Sobel method is 7.9 and designed parameters for Canny method are sigma = 1.28, low threshold = 0.024, and high threshold = 0.117.

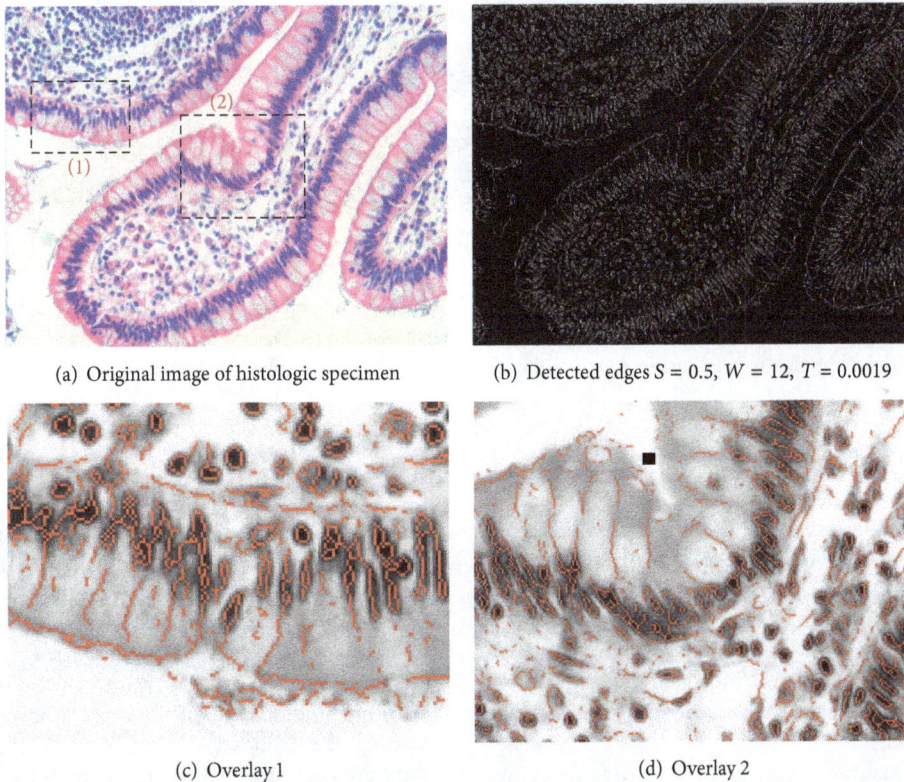

(a) Original image of histologic specimen

(b) Detected edges $S = 0.5$, $W = 12$, $T = 0.0019$

(c) Overlay 1

(d) Overlay 2

FIGURE 4: Edge detection of biomedical images based on Phase Stretch Transform (PST). In this example, image under analysis is histologic specimen of a tissue stained with hematoxylin and eosin. (a) Original image. (b) Detected edges using the proposed method. (c) and (d) Detected edges overlaid with the original image for the two boxes shown in (a). For the proposed method, designed parameters are phase strength $S = 0.5$, phase warp $W = 12$, localization kernel bandwidth $\Delta f = 0.21$, and binary threshold = 0.0019. Figure 4 shows accurate edge detection using the proposed method. We also note that the weak edges shown in (d) with black square are not extracted properly. This can be improved by using better thresholding and localization methods.

very small warp ($W = 0.001$) corresponding to linear phase derivative (Figures 2(a) and 2(d)), medium warp ($W = 14$) (Figures 2(b) and 2(e)), and large warp ($W = 80$) (Figures 2(c) and 2(f)). In this paper, all the S and W parameters are calculated assuming the spatial span of image is from −0.5 to 0.5 in each of the two dimensions. Compared regions are indicated with white triangular, circle, and rectangular markers. As seen, edge detection with medium warp has better noise performance than the case with very large warp or the case with linear phase derivative. Figures 2(e),

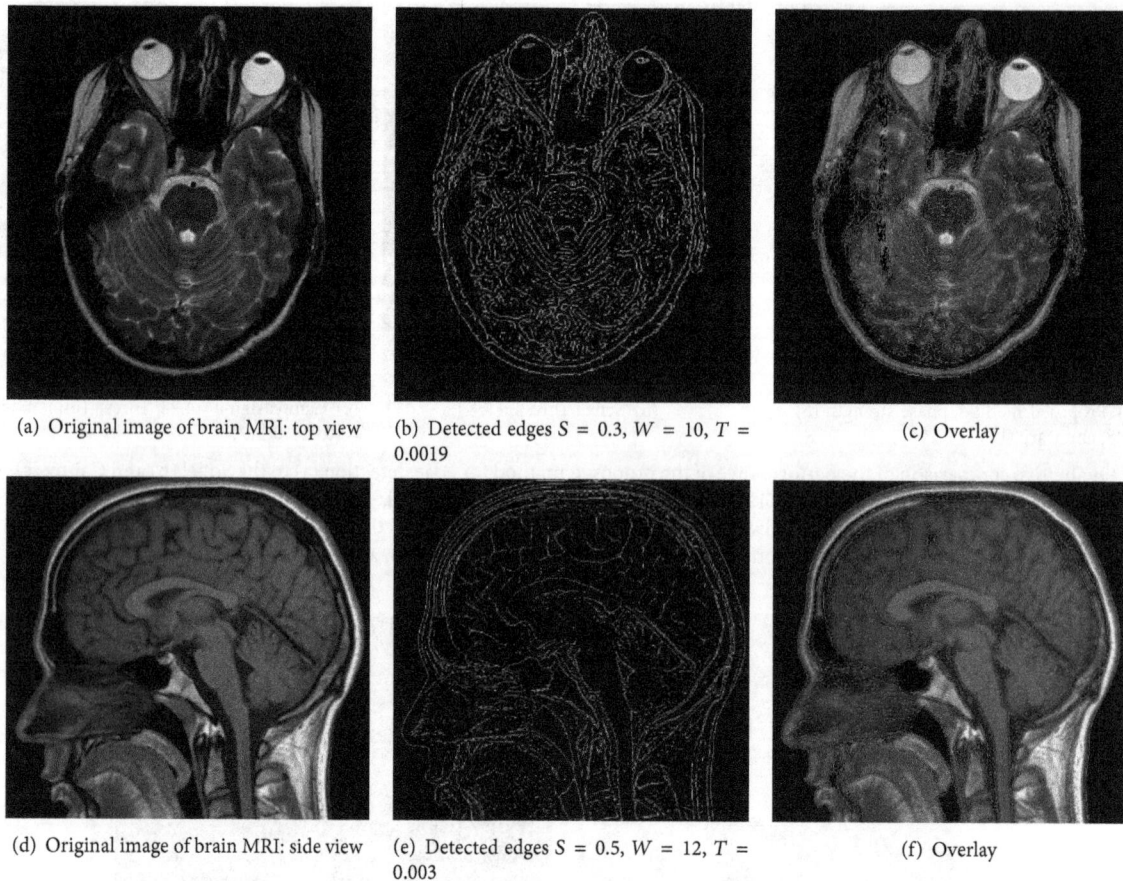

(a) Original image of brain MRI: top view   (b) Detected edges $S = 0.3$, $W = 10$, $T = 0.0019$ (c) Overlay

(d) Original image of brain MRI: side view   (e) Detected edges $S = 0.5$, $W = 12$, $T = 0.003$ (f) Overlay

FIGURE 5: Edge detection of biomedical images based on Phase Stretch Transform (PST). In the two examples presented here, images under analysis are top and side view brain MRI images. (a) and (d) Original images. (b) and (e) Detected edges using the proposed method. (c) and (f) Detected edges overlaid with the original image. As evident in the figure, in both examples, the image edges are accurately extracted using the proposed method.

2(g), and 2(h) compare the performance of edge detection for three different amounts of phase strength (S). In all cases, identical warp value of $W = 14$, localization kernel bandwidth ($\Delta f = 2$), thresholding (Thresh = 0.047), and morphological operations are used. As seen, larger phase strength results in less noise but also less resolution for edge detection. To summarize, Figure 2 indicates that value for S and W parameters can be used to tune and optimize the edge detection performance.

Here we show qualitative comparison of edge detection using the proposed method with the powerful and popular Canny and Sobel methods. We emphasize that these comparisons are not intended as quantitative benchmarks but rather as a qualitative validation of the functionality of the new method proposed here.

The image under analysis is a gray-scale Lena image with 512×512 pixels. Results of edge detection using the three methods are shown in Figure 3. Edge detection using the proposed method is shown in Figure 3(a). For the proposed method, designed parameters are phase strength $S = 0.48$, phase warp $W = 12.14$, localization kernel bandwidth $\Delta f = 0.21$, and binary threshold = 0.028. Morphological operations used for the result shown in Figure 3(a) include

edge thinning and isolated pixel removing. Edge detection using Sobel method with threshold value of 7.9 is shown in Figure 3(b). Edge detection using Canny method with sigma value of 1.28, low threshold values of 0.024, and high threshold value of 0.117 is shown in Figure 3(c). Sobel and Canny methods were implemented using the embedded functions in MATLAB software. All the three methods use postmorphological operations such as edge thinning and cleaning the isolated edge pixels. As evident in Figure 3, edges are accurately extracted with all three techniques. We note that, in a few regions (e.g., nose), Sobel and Canny provide more complete edge profile and have less edge noises. For the present technique, these issues can be improved by optimization of the PST kernel, localization kernel, and threshold settings.

3. Experimental Results

Here we show some examples of the proposed edge detection algorithm on biomedical images. In particular, we consider edge detection of histology and brain MRI images.

In the first example, the image under analysis is a histologic specimen of a tissue stained with hematoxylin and eosin with 800×600 pixels; see Figure 4(a). Edge detection using the proposed method is shown in Figure 4(b). For the proposed method, designed parameters are phase strength $S = 0.5$, phase warp $W = 12$, localization kernel bandwidth $\Delta f = 0.21$, and binary threshold = 0.0019. Morphological operations used for the result shown in Figure 4(b) include edge thinning and isolated pixel removing. We have also shown the detected edges overlaid with the gray-scale version of the original image in Figures 4(c) and 4(d). As evident in Figure 4, edges are accurately extracted using the proposed technique. We note that in a few regions with weaker edges (see Figure 4(d), the region around the black square) the edges are not extracted. For the present technique, these issues can be improved by optimization of the PST kernel, localization kernel, and threshold settings.

In the second example, the images under analysis are two gray-scale brain MRI images: (i) view from the top and (ii) view from the side. The top view brain MRI image has 500×500 pixels and is shown in Figure 5(a). The side view brain MRI image has 652×600 pixels and is shown in Figure 5(d). Edge detection using the proposed method for the two sample images is shown in Figures 5(b) and 5(e). We have also shown the detected edges overlaid with the gray-scale version of the original image in Figures 5(c) and 5(f). Designed edge detection parameters for the top view brain MRI image are phase strength $S = 0.3$, phase warp $W = 10$, localization kernel bandwidth $\Delta f = 0.21$, and binary threshold = 0.0019. For the side view brain MRI image case, the designed edge detection parameters are phase strength $S = 0.5$, phase warp $W = 12$, localization kernel bandwidth $\Delta f = 0.21$, and binary threshold = 0.003. In both cases, edge thinning and isolated pixel removing were used for morphological operations. Figure 5 proves that edges are accurately extracted using the proposed technique for the two examples of brain MRI images as well.

4. Conclusions

A new approach to edge detection in images has been introduced. It is based on a nonlinear dispersive phase operation applied to the image. The output phase of the transform reveals transitions in image intensity and can be used for edge detection and feature extraction. Examples of edge detection on biomedical images presented here show that the proposed edge detection algorithm has promising application in segmentation and analysis of biomedical images.

Conflict of Interests

The authors declare that there is no conflict of interests regarding the publication of this paper.

References

[1] D. Marr and E. Hildreth, "Theory of edge detection," *Proceedings of the Royal Society of London B*, vol. 207, no. 1167, pp. 187–217, 1980.

[2] J. Canny, "A computational approach to edge detection," *IEEE Transactions on Pattern Analysis and Machine Intelligence*, vol. 8, no. 6, pp. 679–698, 1986.

[3] N. Senthilkumaran and R. Rajesh, "Image segmentation—a survey of soft computing approaches," in *Proceedings of the International Conference on Advances in Recent Technologies in Communication and Computing*, pp. 844–846, October 2009.

[4] M. H. Asghari and B. Jalali, "Discrete anamorphic transform for image compression," *IEEE Signal Processing Letters*, vol. 21, no. 7, pp. 829–833, 2014.

[5] Y. Han and B. Jalali, "Photonic time-stretched analog-to-digital converter: fundamental concepts and practical considerations," *Journal of Lightwave Technology*, vol. 21, no. 12, pp. 3085–3103, 2003.

[6] K. Goda and B. Jalali, "Dispersive Fourier transformation for fast continuous single-shot measurements," *Nature Photonics*, vol. 7, no. 2, pp. 102–112, 2013.

[7] W. Ng, T. Rockwood, and A. Reamon, "Demonstration of channel-stitched photonic time-stretch analog-to-digital converter with ENOB $\geq$ 8 for a 10 GHz signal bandwidth," in *Proceedings of the Government Microcircuit Applications & Critical Technology Conference (GOMACTech '14)*, Paper 26.2, Charleston, SC, USA, March 2014.

14

Automated Diagnosis of Otitis Media: Vocabulary and Grammar

Anupama Kuruvilla,[1] **Nader Shaikh,**[2] **Alejandro Hoberman,**[2] **and Jelena Kovačević**[1,3]

[1] *Department of BME and Center for Bioimage Informatics, Carnegie Mellon University, Pittsburgh, PA 15213, USA*
[2] *Division of General Academic Pediatrics, Children's Hospital of Pittsburgh, University of Pittsburgh School of Medicine, Pittsburgh, PA 15213, USA*
[3] *Department of ECE Carnegie Mellon University, Pittsburgh, PA 15213, USA*

Correspondence should be addressed to Anupama Kuruvilla; anupamak@andrew.cmu.edu

Academic Editor: Fabrice Meriaudeau

We propose a novel automated algorithm for classifying diagnostic categories of otitis media: acute otitis media, otitis media with effusion, and no effusion. Acute otitis media represents a bacterial superinfection of the middle ear fluid, while otitis media with effusion represents a sterile effusion that tends to subside spontaneously. Diagnosing children with acute otitis media is difficult, often leading to overprescription of antibiotics as they are beneficial only for children with acute otitis media. This underscores the need for an accurate and automated diagnostic algorithm. To that end, we design a feature set understood by both otoscopists and engineers based on the actual visual cues used by otoscopists; we term this the *otitis media vocabulary*. We also design a process to combine the vocabulary terms based on the decision process used by otoscopists; we term this the *otitis media grammar*. The algorithm achieves 89.9% classification accuracy, outperforming both clinicians who did not receive special training and state-of-the-art classifiers.

1. Introduction

Otitis media is a general term for middle-ear inflammation and may be classified clinically as either *acute otitis media* (AOM) or *otitis media with effusion* (OME); AOM represents a bacterial superinfection of the middle ear fluid and OME represents a sterile effusion that tends to subside spontaneously. Although middle ear effusion is present in both cases, this clinical classification is important because antibiotics are generally beneficial only for AOM [1, 2]. However, proper diagnosis of AOM as well as distinction from both OME and no effusion (NOE) requires considerable training (see Figure 1, e.g., images).

AOM is a frequent condition affecting the majority of the pediatric population for which antibiotics are prescribed. It is the most common childhood infection, representing one of the most frequent reasons for visits to the pediatrician. The number of otitis media episodes has increased substantially in the past two decades, with approximately 25 million visits to office-based physicians in the US and a total of 20 million prescriptions for antimicrobials related to otitis media yearly

[3]. This results in significant social burden and indirect costs due to time lost from school and work, with an estimated annual medical expenditure of approximately 2$ billion [4].

The current standard of care in diagnosing AOM includes visual examination of the tympanic membrane with a range of available otoscopes: from simple hand-held ones with a halogen light source and low-power magnifying lens to more sophisticated, videootoscopes and otoendoscopes, which connect to a light source (halogen, xenon, or LED) and a computer and can record images or video. Single hand-held otoscopes do not permit acquisition of images and/or video and require diagnosis on the spot, while videootoscopes and otoendoscopes do; however, the clinician views the feed on a side screen while holding the device in the ear canal of an often-squirming young child.

Misdiagnosis. The inherent difficulties in distinguishing among the three diagnostic categories of otitis media, together with the above issues, make the diagnosis by non-expert otoscopists notoriously unreliable and lead to the following

(1) *Overprescription of Antibiotics.* AOM is frequently overdiagnosed; this happens when NOE or OME is diagnosed as AOM, resulting in unnecessary antibiotic prescriptions that lead to adverse effects and increased bacterial resistance [5]. Overdiagnosis is more common than underdiagnosis because doctors typically try to avoid the possibility of leaving an ill patient without treatment, leading to antibiotic prescriptions in uncertain cases.

(2) *Underprescription of Antibiotics.* Misdiagnosis of AOM as either NOE or OME leads to underdiagnosis. Most importantly, children's symptoms are left unaddressed. Occasionally, underdiagnosis can lead to an increase in serious complications such as perforation of the tympanic membrane and, very rarely, mastoiditis [6].

(3) *Increased Financial Costs and Burden.* There are direct and indirect financial costs associated with misdiagnoses such as medication costs, copayments, emergency department and primary care provider visits, missed work, and special day care arrangements.

For all the reasons above, accurate diagnosis is imperative to ensure that antimicrobial therapy is limited to the appropriate patients; this, in turn, increases the likelihood of achieving optimal outcomes and minimizing antibiotic resistance.

Goal. Currently, clinical diagnosis of otitis media is time consuming and subjective and shows limited intra and interobserver reproducibility, underscoring the critical need for an accurate classification algorithm.

We develop the first such algorithm as diagnostic aid to classify tympanic membrane images into one of the three stringent clinical diagnostic categories: AOM, OME, and NOE.

To our knowledge, the only related work in this area is [7] where the authors investigate the influence of color on the classification accuracies of individual classes and conclude that the color alone is not sufficient for accurate classification.

Guiding Principles. To achieve our goal, we adopt the guiding principles below, partly inspired by [8–12]. The authors performed extensive research on understanding how humans perceive and measure similarity of color patterns. To understand and describe the mechanism of human perception, a subjective experiment was conducted, leading to a set of basic categories—*vocabulary* used by humans in judging similarity of color patterns and their relative importance and relationships, as well as the hierarchy of rules—*grammar*. We aim here to find the corresponding vocabulary and grammar of otitis media.

(i) Vocabulary. We aim to design a feature set understood by both otoscopists and engineers based on the actual visual cues used by otoscopists; we term this the *otitis media vocabulary*.

To explore the diagnostic processes used, Dr. Shaikh et al. conducted a study to examine findings that the expert otoscopists use during their clinical diagnosis [13]. During the study, endoscopic still images of tympanic membranes of 783 children were obtained and examined by expert otoscopists. The examining otoscopist recorded information regarding a history of otalgia and findings concerning the following tympanic membrane characteristics: color (amber, blue, gray, pink, red, white, yellow), translucency (translucent, semiopaque, opaque), position (neutral, retracted, bulging), mobility (decreased, not decreased), and areas of marked redness, as distinct from mild or moderate redness (present, absent). A random sample of 135 (in ratio 2 : 2 : 1 of AOM : OME : NOE) of these images was sent for review to another group of 7 independent expert otoscopists, resulting in a dataset of 945 image evaluations. To control for differences in color rendition between computers, color-calibrated laptops were mailed to each expert. They were asked to independently describe tympanic membrane findings and assign a diagnosis of AOM/OME/NOE.

Just by evaluating still images, with no information about mobility or ear pain, the diagnosis (AOM versus no AOM) endorsed by the majority of experts was in agreement with the live diagnosis 88.9% of the time, underscoring the limited role that symptoms and mobility of the tympanic membrane have in the diagnosis of AOM. Live diagnosis refers to the diagnosis based on physical examination and evaluation of the child at the time of the encounter and is not based on images. Among both groups of otoscopists, bulging of the tympanic membrane was the finding judged best to differentiate AOM from OME: 96% of ears during live diagnosis and 93% of ear image evaluations were assigned a diagnosis of AOM. By members of the two groups who assigned the diagnosis of OME, bulging of the tympanic membrane was reported in 0% and 3% of ears during live diagnosis and ear image evaluations, respectively. Opacification of the tympanic membrane was the finding that best differentiated OME from NOE.

To design the otitis media vocabulary, we follow the guidelines in Table 1 that summarizes these otoscopic findings.

(ii) Grammar. We aim to design a rule-based decision process to combine the vocabulary terms based on the decision process used by otoscopists; we term this the otitis media grammar.

To design the grammar, we use the findings from [14], where the authors empirically examined the findings used by a group of expert otoscopists for diagnosing otitis media. In this study, relative importance of signs and symptoms in diagnosis of AOM was described and then used to develop a rule-based decision tree method to diagnose otitis media. At each visit of the patient, the otoscopist recorded the following tympanic membrane characteristics: color (amber, blue, gray, pink, white, yellow), degree of opacification (translucent, semi opaque, opaque), position (neutral, retracted, bulging), decreased mobility (yes, no), presence of air-fluid level(s) (yes, no), and presence of areas of marked redness (yes, no). A decision tree was then developed based on the recorded tympanic membrane characteristics using recursive partitioning to classify the cases into one of the three diagnostic categories. This manual decision tree uses two decisions to

TABLE 1: Guidelines for vocabulary design: Otoscopic findings associated with clinical diagnostic categories of tympanic membrane images [13].

	AOM	OME	NOE
Color	White, pale yellow, markedly red	White, amber, gray, blue	Gray, pink
Position	Distinctly full, bulging	Neutral, retracted	Neutral, retracted
Translucency	Opacified	Opacified, semiopacified	Translucent

discriminate among the diagnostic categories; first, bulging is used to distinguish AOM from OME and NOE, and if no bulging was present, opacification or air-fluid level is used to distinguish between OME and NOE (see Figure 2). For ease of reference, we name the diagnosis of AOM, NOE, and OME as Stages 1, 2, and 3, respectively.

To design the otitis media grammar, we follow the guidelines in Figure 2 that summarizes this decision process.

Validation. We will compare our algorithm designed following the above guiding principles to diagnoses provided by three general pediatricians as well as five automated classifiers, three of which we designed previously and two generic classifiers that are available in the literature. The ground truth is provided by a panel of three expert otoscopists.

2. Methods

A general classification algorithm consists of two parts: numerical feature extraction meant to discriminate among classes, and classification based on these features. In the otitis media classifier, we add a preprocessing step prior to feature extraction to minimize the impact of image artifacts.

2.1. Preprocessing. To compute features, image preprocessing is crucial because it is expected that some regions may not be relevant or can contain foreign objects that occlude the tympanic membrane. Moreover, we aim to eliminate or minimize the impact of image artifacts associated with otoscopic images, which fundamentally consist of specular highlights. These artifacts will affect feature computation and hence must be corrected. To that end, we start with an automated segmentation step to locate the tympanic membrane and apply a local illumination correction to mitigate the problem of specular highlights. If a captured image is deemed not fit for processing, the algorithm will reject the image and prompt the clinician to retake it.

2.1.1. Automated Segmentation of Tympanic Membrane. Segmentation is a crucial step to extract relevant regions on which reliable features for classification can be computed. We now briefly summarize an active-contour based segmentation algorithm [15] we adapted for our purposes. First, a so-called snake potential of the grayscale version of the input image is computed, followed by a set of forces that

outline the gradients and edges of the image. The active-contour algorithm [16] is then initialized by a circumference in the center of the image. The algorithm iteratively grows this contour and stops at a predefined convergence criterion, which leaves an outline that covers the relevant region in the image. This outline is used to generate the final mask that is applied to the input image to obtain the final result shown in Figure 3. We evaluated the performance of the algorithm on automatically segmented images against hand segmented images by expert otoscopists and found that we can automatically segment prior to classification without hurting the performance of the classifier. By adding this segmentation stage, the classification system becomes completely automated by not requiring the clinician to specify where the tympanic membrane is positioned.

2.1.2. Correction of Specular Highlights. One of the problems encountered is the presence of specular highlight regions caused by residual cerumen (wax) in the ear canal and wax on surface of the hair in the ear canal, which might remain after the examination. Cerumen reflects the light from the otoscope, which results in white regions in the image as shown in Figure 4 (top). These regions of local specular highlights have to be corrected.

Several methods [17–19] are shown to be robust in correcting local illumination changes. Most of these methods adjust the pixel intensity value of the image using a nonlinear mapping function for illumination correction based on the estimated local illumination at each pixel location and combining the adjusted illumination image with the reflectance image to generate an output image. The extent of possible image correction and editing ranges from replacement or mixing with another source image region to altering some aspects of the original image locally such as illumination or color. Since these methods can be used to locally modify image characteristics, our aim is to detect the specular highlights in the image and use these techniques to locally correct them. We use a simple thresholding scheme on image intensities to identify the specular highlight regions as shown in Figure 4 (middle row), followed by the Poisson image editing technique [19] to correct the identified regions in Figure 4 (bottom row).

2.1.3. Rejection of Unreliable Data. Some of the segmented images may contain large regions of white pixels due to overexposure. The above-mentioned techniques rely on using the neighboring pixels to approximate intensities in the region to be corrected and thus are effective when the region to be corrected is small. We empirically found that if the area of continuous white pixels is more than 15% of total pixels in the segmented tympanic membrane image, correcting such regions gives unreliable results and hence such an image should be rejected. Our aim is to use the rejection stage in the real application and prompt the clinician to retake the image until deemed suitable for processing.

2.2. Otitis Media Vocabulary. The expert otoscopist uses his specialized knowledge when discriminating between

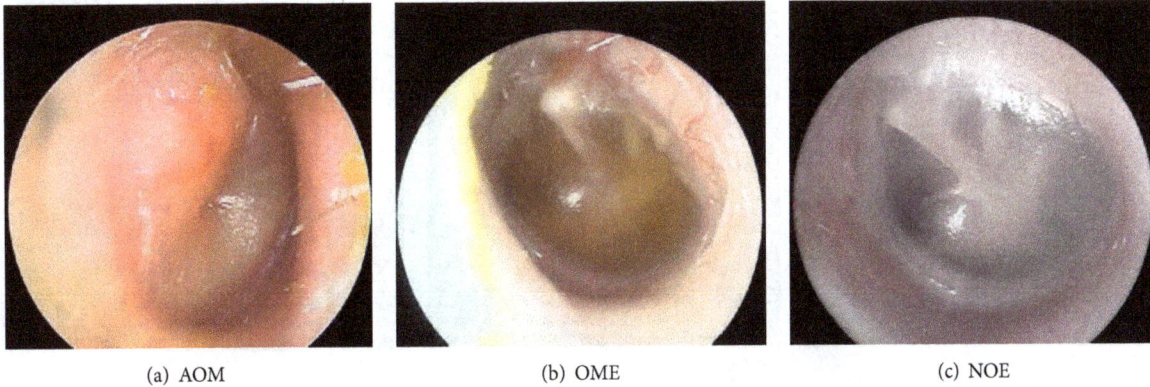

(a) AOM   (b) OME   (c) NOE

FIGURE 1: Sample (cropped) images from the three diagnostic categories of otitis media.

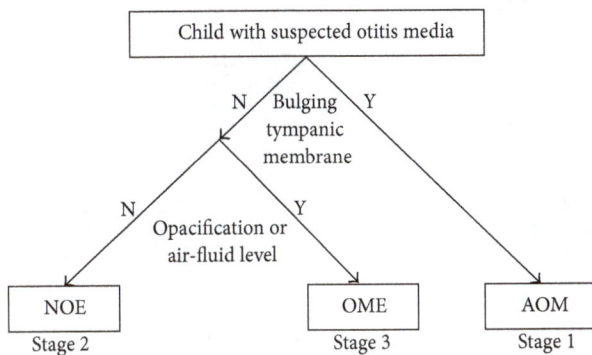

FIGURE 2: Guidelines for grammar design: decision tree for the diagnosis of otitis media [14].

the different diagnostic categories. The goal of our proposed methodology is to create a feature set—otitis media vocabulary, which will mimic the visual cues used by trained otoscopists.

2.2.1. Methodology.
To design the otitis media vocabulary we will follow the process outlined in [20], where a histopathology vocabulary was designed for automated identification and delineation of tissues in images of H&E-stained teratomas. Similar vocabulary features were used in [21] for automated detection of colitis.

Formulation of Initial Set of Descriptions. We obtain initial descriptions of those characteristics best describing a given diagnostic category from the summary of otoscopic findings in Table 1.

Computational Translation of Key Terms. From this set, the key terms, such as *bulging*, are translated into their computational synonyms, creating a computational vocabulary. In our case, we construct a feature called bulging, which measures the area of the bulged region in the tympanic membrane.

Computational Translation of Descriptions. Using the computational vocabulary, the entire otoscopist's descriptions, such as *bulging and white*, are translated.

Verification of Translated Descriptions. Based on these translated descriptions, and without access to the image, the otoscopist tries to identify the diagnostic category being described, emulating the overall system with translated descriptions as features and the otoscopist as the classifier.

Refinement of Insufficient Terms. If the otoscopist is unable to identify a diagnostic category based on translated descriptions, or if a particular translation is not understandable, then that translation is refined and presented again to the otoscopist for verification.

Otitis Media Vocabulary. If the otoscopist is able to identify a diagnostic category based on translated descriptions, then the discriminative power of the key terms and their corresponding computational interpretations are validated, and these terms can be included as otitis media vocabulary terms to create features.

This feedback loop is iterated until a sufficient set of terms have been collected to formulate the otitis media vocabulary:

bulging f_b

translucency f_t

central concavity f_c

amber level f_a

light f_ℓ

bubble presence f_{bp}

malleus presence f_m

grayscale variance f_v

2.2.2. Features.
We designed the vocabulary features, bulging, central concavity, malleus presence, translucency, amber level, and bubble presence based on otoscopic findings listed in Table 1. Supplementing the features designed based on otoscopic findings, we designed an additional two, light and grayscale variance, based on our observations and to catch classifier errors.

(1) The first three vocabulary features, *bulging, central concavity, and light*, describe the distinct characteristics associated with AOM and will be used to

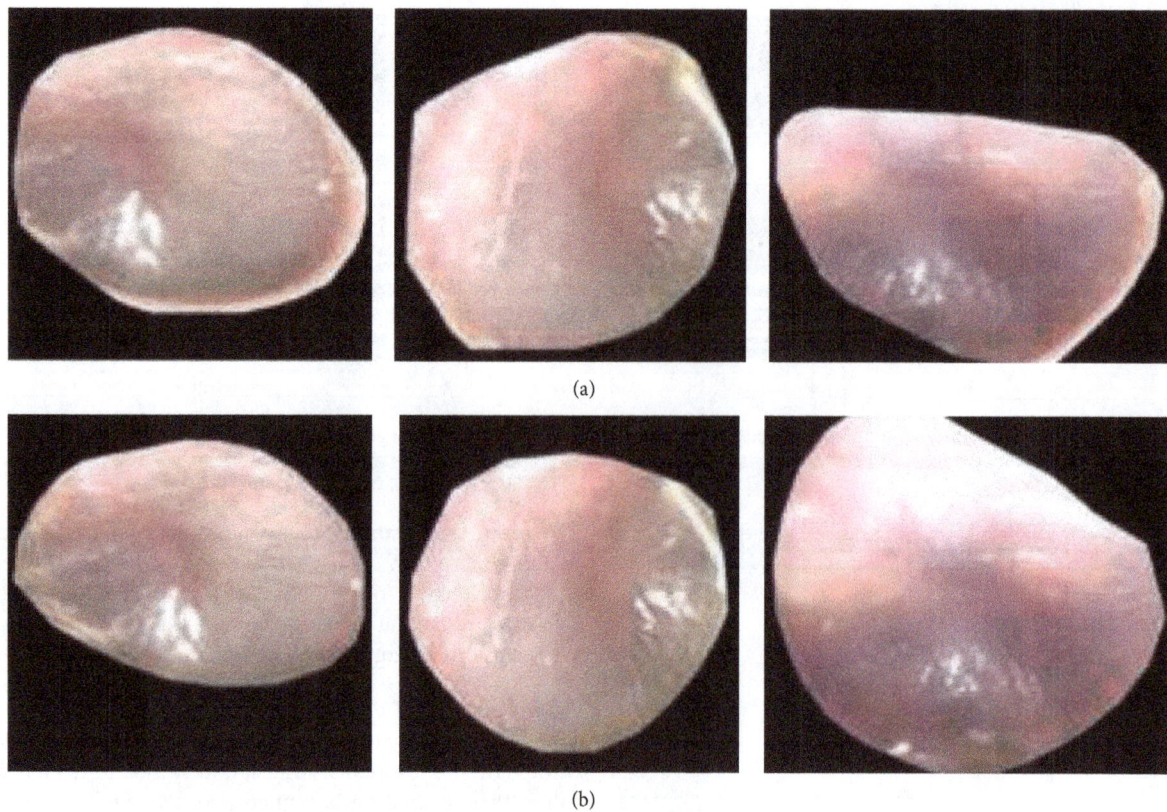

FIGURE 3: Comparison of automated segmentation (a) and hand segmentation by expert otoscopists (b).

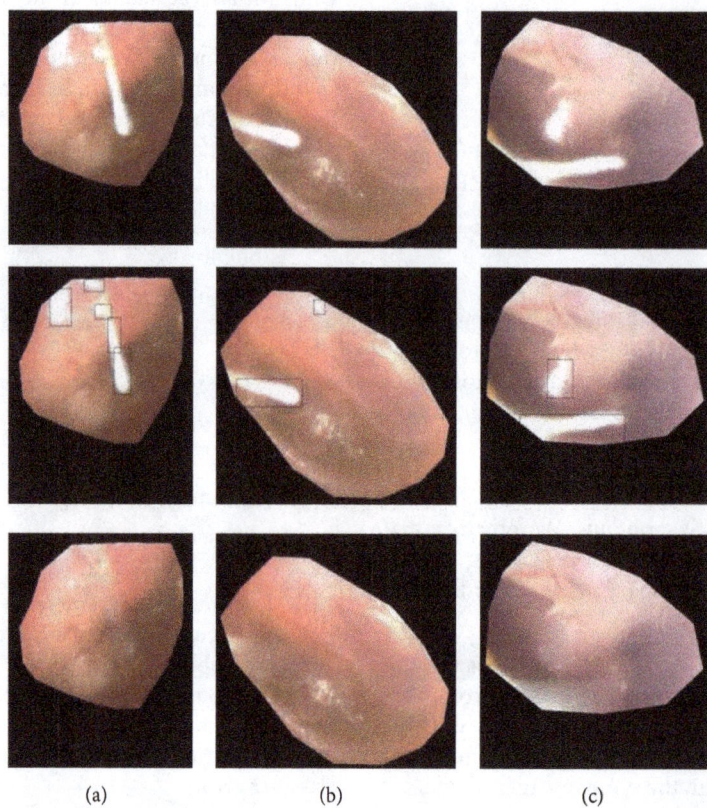

FIGURE 4: Correction of specular highlights for AOM (a), OME (b), and NOE (c). Input images are in the top row, identification of specular highlight regions in the middle row, and correction of the identified regions in the bottom row.

construct Stage 1 of the grammar to identify AOM, mimicking Stage 1 in Figure 2. The vocabulary feature bulging is the exact computational translation of *bulging tympanic membrane* in Figure 2.

(2) The next two vocabulary features, *malleus presence and translucency*, are indicative of NOE and will be used to construct Stage 2 of the grammar to identify NOE, mimicking Stage 2 in Figure 2. To describe *opacification* in Figure 2, we construct a vocabulary feature translucency, which detects the opposite.

(3) The final three vocabulary features, *amber level, bubble presence, and grayscale variance*, describe the characteristics of OME and will be used to construct Stage 3 of the grammar to identify OME, mimicking Stage 3 in Figure 2. The vocabulary feature bubble presence is the exact computational translation of *air-fluid level* in Figure 2.

We now explain each of the vocabulary features in detail.

Bulging. In [14], the authors showed that bulging of the tympanic membrane is crucial for diagnosing AOM. We will design a feature that calculates the percentage of bulged region in the tympanic membrane; we call it the *bulging* feature. The goal is to derive a 3D tympanic membrane shape from a 2D image, by expressing it in terms of depth at each pixel. For example, in AOM, we should be able to identify high-depth variation due to bulging of the tympanic membrane in contrast to low-depth variation in NOE due to tympanic membrane being neutral or retracted. The shape from shading technique [22] can be applied to recover a 3D shape from a single monocular image. The input is a grayscale version of the segmented original RGB image $X \in \mathbb{R}^{M \times N}$ as shown in Figure 5(a). The depth at each pixel can be calculated in an iterative manner using the image gradient and a linear approximation of the reflectance function of the image. Figure 5(b) shows the result of depth map X_d identifying the bulged regions in the tympanic membrane. The depth map X_d is then thresholded at T_d (here $T_d = 0.6$) to obtain a binary mask X_b of bulging regions in the tympanic membrane.

We then define the bulging feature as the mean of X_b,

$$f_b = E[X_b]. \quad (1)$$

Central Concavity. The tympanic membrane is attached firmly to the malleus that is one of the three middle ear bones called auditory ossicles. In the presence of an infection, the tympanic membrane begins to bulge in the periphery. The central region, however, remains attached to the malleus forming a concavity. We design a feature to identify the concave region located centrally in the tympanic membrane; we call it the *central concavity* feature. The input is a grayscale version (Figure 6(a)) of the segmented original RGB image $X \in \mathbb{R}^{M \times N}$ as in Figure 3. We use a sliding window to extract a local circular neighborhood, $X_R(m,n)$, of radius R ($R = 60$ in our experiments). That circular neighborhood is then

transformed into its polar coordinates to obtain $X_R(r, \theta)$, with $r \in \{1, 2, \ldots, R\}, \theta \in [0, 2\pi]$, and

$$r = \sqrt{(m-m_c)^2 + (n-n_c)^2}, \quad \theta = \arctan\frac{(n-n_c)}{(m-m_c)}, \quad (2)$$

where (m_c, n_c) are the center coordinates of the neighborhood X_R. In Figure 6(b), the resulting image has r as the horizontal axis and θ as the vertical one. The concave region changes from dark to bright from the center towards the periphery of the concavity; in polar coordinates this change from dark to bright occurs as the radius grows; see Figure 6(b). Defining the bright region $B = \{(r, \theta) \mid r > R'\}$ and the dark region $D = \{(r, \theta) \mid r \le R'\}$, and with $R' \in [(1/4)R, (3/4)R]$, we compute the ratio of the two means,

$$f_{c,R'} = \frac{E[X_R(r, \theta)|_{(r,\theta)\in B}]}{E[X_R(r, \theta)|_{(r,\theta)\in D}]}. \quad (3)$$

As the concave region is always centrally located, we experimentally determine a square neighborhood I (here 151×151) to compute the central concavity feature,

$$f_c = \max_{(m,n)\in I, R'} f_{c,R'}. \quad (4)$$

Light. Examination of the tympanic membrane is performed by an illuminated otoendoscope. The distinct bulging in AOM results in nonuniform illumination of the tympanic membrane, in contrast to the uniform illumination in NOE. Our aim is to construct a feature that will measure this nonuniformity as the ratio of the brightly lit to the darkly lit regions; we call it the *light* feature.

We start by performing contrast enhancement on the grayscale image in Figure 7(a) to make the nonuniform lighting prominent. The resulting image in Figure 7(b) is thresholded at T_ℓ (found experimentally) to obtain a mask of the brightly lit binary image X_{bl} in Figure 7(c).

To find the direction (θ_{max}) perpendicular to the maximum illumination gradient, we look at lines passing through (m_c, n_c) (the pixel coordinates at which f_c is obtained) at the angle θ with the horizontal axis. Defining the bright region $B = \{(m, n) \mid n \ge \tan(\theta)(m - m_c) + n_c\}$ and the dark region $D = \{(m, n) \mid n < \tan(\theta)(m - m_c) + n_c\}$, we compute the ratio of the two means,

$$r(\theta) = \frac{E[X_{bl}(m,n)|_{(m,n)\in B}]}{E[X_{bl}(m,n)|_{(m,n)\in D}]}. \quad (5)$$

Then, the direction perpendicular to the maximum illumination gradient is given by

$$\theta_{max} = \arg\max_\theta r(\theta) \quad (6)$$

and we define the light feature as

$$f_\ell = r(\theta_{max}). \quad (7)$$

Malleus Presence. In OME or in NOE, the tympanic membrane position is either neutral or retracted and makes the

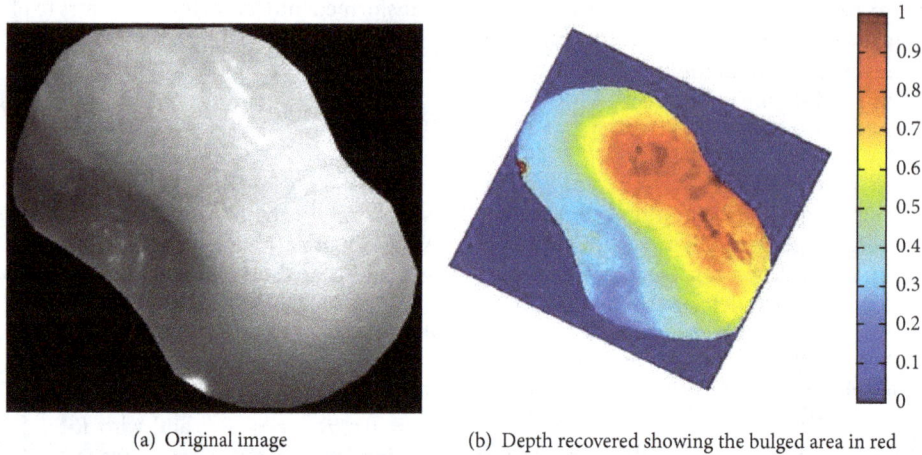

(a) Original image

(b) Depth recovered showing the bulged area in red

FIGURE 5: Computation of the bulging feature.

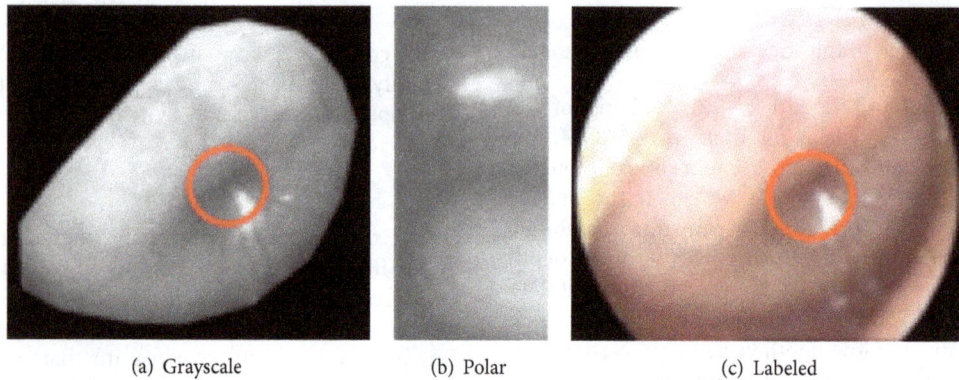

(a) Grayscale

(b) Polar

(c) Labeled

FIGURE 6: Computation of the central concavity feature.

short process of the malleus visible. We design a feature to detect the partial or complete appearance of the malleus that would help in distinguishing AOM from OME and NOE; we call it the *malleus presence* feature. To identify the presence of the malleus, we perform an ellipse fitting (shown as a red outline in Figure 8(a)) to identify the major axis. The image is then rotated to align the major axis with the horizontal axis. Mean-shift clustering [23] is then performed as shown in Figure 8(b), followed by Canny edge detection [24]. Hough transform [25] is applied on the obtained edges around the major axis (50-pixel neighborhood empirically obtained) to detect a straight line (shown in red Figure 8(c)) extending to the periphery that will indicate the visibility of the malleus. If such a line is detected then the feature malleus presence f_m is assigned a value of 1 and 0 otherwise.

Translucency. Translucency of the tympanic membrane is the main characteristic of NOE in contrast with opacity in AOM and semi-opacity in OME; it results in the clear visibility of the tympanic membrane, which is primarily gray. We design a feature to measure the grayness of the tympanic membrane; we call it the *translucency* feature. We do that by using a simple color-assignment technique. As these images were acquired under different lighting and viewing conditions, according

to [26], at least 3–6 images are needed to characterize a structure/region under all lighting and viewing conditions. We take the number of images to be $N_{tl} = 20$.

To determine gray-level clusters in translucent regions, we extract N_t pixels from translucent regions ($N_t = 100$) of N_{tl} RGB images by hand segmentation to obtain a total of $N_{tl}N_t$ pixels from images (here 2000). We then perform clustering of these $N_{tl}N_t$ pixels using k-means clustering to obtain K cluster centers $c_k \in \mathbb{R}^3$, $k = 1, 2, \ldots, K$, ($K = 10$) capturing variations of gray in the translucent regions.

To compute the translucency feature for a given image X, for each pixel (m, n), we compute K Euclidean distances of $X(m, n)$ to the cluster center c_k, $k = 1, 2, \ldots, K$,

$$d_k(m, n) = \sqrt{\sum_{i=1}^{3}(X_i(m, n) - c_{k,i})^2}, \quad (8)$$

with $i = 1, 2, 3$, denoting the color channel. If any of the computed K distances falls below a threshold $T_t = 10$ (found experimentally), the pixel is labeled as translucent and belongs to the region $R_t = \{(m, n) \mid \min_k d_k(m, n) < T_t\}$. The binary image X_t is then simply the characteristic function of the region R_t, $X_t = \chi_{R_t}$.

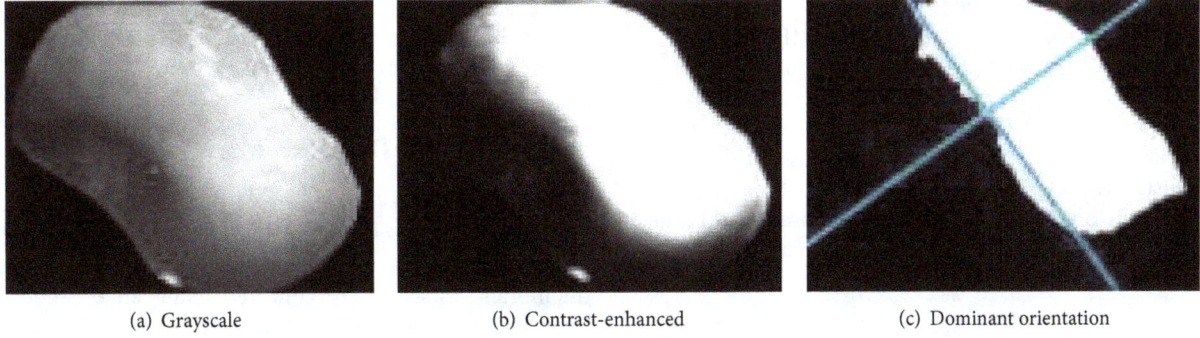

(a) Grayscale   (b) Contrast-enhanced   (c) Dominant orientation

FIGURE 7: Computation of the light feature.

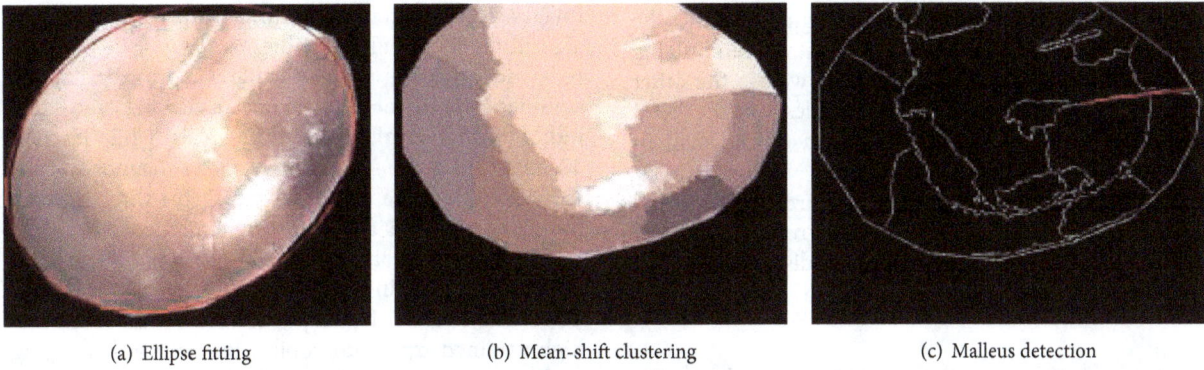

(a) Ellipse fitting   (b) Mean-shift clustering   (c) Malleus detection

FIGURE 8: Computation of the malleus presence feature.

We then define the translucency feature as the mean of X_t,

$$f_t = E\left[X_t\right]. \qquad (9)$$

Amber Level. We use the knowledge that OME is predominantly amber or pale yellow to distinguish it from AOM and NOE. We design a feature to measure the presence of amber in the tympanic membrane; we call it the *amber* feature. We apply a color-assignment technique similar to that used for computing X_t to obtain a binary image X_a, indicating amber and nonamber regions. We define the amber feature as the mean of X_a,

$$f_a = E\left[X_a\right]. \qquad (10)$$

Bubble Presence. The presence of visible air-fluid levels, or bubbles, behind the tympanic membrane is an indication of OME. We design a feature to detect the presence of bubbles in the tympanic membrane; we call it the *bubble presence* feature. The algorithm takes in red and green channels of the original RGB image and performs Canny edge detection [24], to place parallel boundaries on either sides of the real edge, creating a binary image X_{bp} in between. This is followed by filtering and morphological operations to enhance edge detection and obtain smooth boundaries. We then define the bubble feature as the mean of X_{bp},

$$f_{bp} = E\left[X_{bp}\right]. \qquad (11)$$

Grayscale Variance. Another discriminating feature is the variance of the intensities across the grayscale version of the image X_v. We define the feature *grayscale variance* as the variance of the pixel intensities in the image X_v,

$$f_v = \mathrm{var}\left(X_v\right); \qquad (12)$$

for example, OME has a more uniform appearance than AOM and NOE and has consequently a much lower variance that can be used to distinguish it from the rest.

2.3. Otitis Media Grammar. The modeling of human perception of otitis media diagnosis is new—starting with the vocabulary feature design and the set of rules considered as the basic grammar of the otoscopist's language. For the actual implementation of the grammar, it is important to understand the way these rules are applied. An important aspect of our work is to use feedback from expert otoscopists to improve classification performance by trying to mimic their diagnostic process.

In our previous work [27], we designed an initial grammar as a simple hierarchical classifier that uses two levels. At the first level, binary decisions were used to split the images into two superclasses; AOM/OME (acute infection/middle ear fluid infection) and NOE/OME (no infection/middle ear fluid infection). At the second level, these superclasses were split into individual diagnostic categories using a weighted combination (w_a, w_{bp}, w_t, w_v) of four features, amber level f_a, bubble presence f_{bp}, translucency f_t, and grayscale variance

f_v. The weighted combination $w_a f_a + w_{bp} f_{bp} + w_t f_t + w_v f_v$ was used to split superclasses into AOM/OME/NOE.

Here, we design the grammar to mimic the decision process used by expert otoscopists in Figure 2 exactly. The decision process will use a hierarchical rule-based classification scheme based on the domain knowledge of the expert otoscopists. The classification is done in three stages by distinguishing one diagnostic category at a time: AOM (Stage 1), NOE (Stage 2), and OME (Stage 3), respectively, which we now describe in more detail.

2.3.1. Stage 1: Identification of AOM. As the first stage, we detect the instances of AOM based on bulging, light, central concavity, and malleus presence features as shown in Figure 9. While ideally, if there is bulging present, the image should be classified as AOM as in Figure 2, our bulging feature alone cannot accomplish the task; we use the other features in the otitis media vocabulary that describe the AOM characteristics such as light, central concavity, and malleus presence to aid separation of AOM from NOE and OME. In some cases, OME images can exhibit partial bulging and therefore have a high possibility of being grouped as AOM. In such cases, we use low amber level to distinguish AOM from OME.

2.3.2. Stage 2: Identification of NOE. Low values of bulging, light, central concavity, and malleus presence features eliminate the possibility of AOM being the diagnosis. Such a situation results in either the diagnosis being NOE or OME (see Figure 10). In Stage 2, our goal is to distinguish NOE from OME. The translucency feature, which is the most distinguishing characteristic of NOE, can be used here to identify normal cases. A high value of translucency clearly indicates NOE and low values of those features characteristic of OME indicate NOE. Thus, in this stage, NOE is identified from the superclass NOE/OME by a high value of the translucency feature or low values of all the features characteristic of OME: amber level, bubble presence, and grayscale variance.

2.3.3. Stage 3: Identification of OME. Figure 11 shows the complete otitis media grammar. Most of the OME cases are identified from the superclass NOE/OME from Stage 2 as high values of amber level, bubble presence, and grayscale variance features. Some cases of OME can exhibit partial bulging resulting in high values of the bulging feature; in such cases, we can correctly detect OME if the values of light and central concavity features are low, and the value of amber level feature is high.

The threshold values for the features were calculated during the training phase of the algorithm. We performed a fivefold nested cross-validation. During each fold, the data was split into training and testing, and the training set was further split into two sets: learning and validation. We used misclassification rate on the validation set as the criterion to learn the threshold for each split. The threshold was fixed where we obtained the least misclassification rate during training and was used on the testing set.

The complete otitis media grammar we designed in Figure 11 thus follows the exact structure of the decision tree designed by expert otoscopists in Figure 2.

3. Results and Discussion

3.1. Ground Truth: Diagnosis by Expert Otoscopists. As part of a clinical trial evaluating the efficacy of antimicrobials in young children with acute otitis media, 826 tympanic membrane images were collected using an otoendoscope from children with AOM, OME, and NOE [28]. A panel of three expert otoscopists examined these images and provided labels. As these images pose challenges even for expert otoscopists, the agreement was rather poor in labeling the images. Having accurate ground-truth labels is crucial for algorithm development, and thus, we asked the panel to rediagnose the entire dataset while also providing a diagnosis confidence level for each image; levels between 80 and 100 indicated high confidence in diagnosis, while levels below 30 indicated almost no confidence in diagnosis. Based on these, we selected a subset for which the three experts gave the same diagnosis and expressed confidence of over 60 in that diagnosis; we use this set as our *ground truth* set. The number of images in this ground-truth set is 181; 63 AOM, 70 OME, and 48 NOE. It is important to note that even for these highly trained expert otoscopists, this set is a challenging one, as there were no acquisition guidelines, and thus, the images depict a diverse set of conditions.

3.2. Validation: Diagnosis by General Pediatricians. To validate the algorithm against a realistic diagnostic situation, we asked three general pediatricians to examine our ground-truth set of 181 tympanic membrane images provided by expert otoscopists. The experiment also required them to state their level of confidence in diagnosing each of the tympanic membrane images. In cases of diagnosis with high confidence, the examiner assigned only one diagnostic category to the image, whereas in cases where the confidence of diagnosis was either medium or low, the examiner was asked to also provide a second possible choice of diagnosis, resulting in two diagnoses of an image representing first and second diagnostic choices, respectively.

To evaluate how the group of three general pediatricians performed on the ground-truth dataset, Table 2 shows three confusion matrices: the first is the average diagnosis by the three pediatricians, while the other two are average diagnoses with high and medium/low confidence, respectively. The diagnostic accuracy that was obtained as an average of the accuracies from the three examining pediatricians was found to be 79.6% (91.7%, 75.7%, and 71.3%, resp.), well below that of expert otoscopists that we use as our ground truth of 100%.

In terms of misdiagnoses, NOE and OME are the categories with the highest level of misdiagnosis. The misdiagnosis of OME as AOM (15.7%) is clearly a cause of concern since it leads to the unnecessary prescription of antibiotics. Similarly, NOE is often misdiagnosed as OME (45.8%). It is surprising to note that only 50% cases of NOE were diagnosed with high confidence, of which 9 out of 24

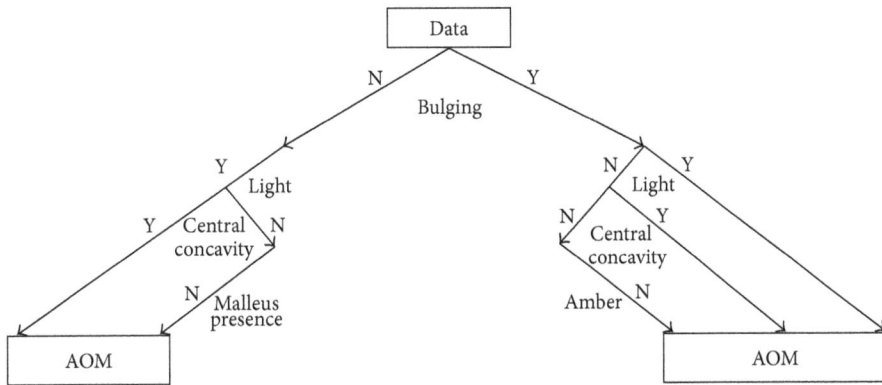

FIGURE 9: Stage 1: grammar for identifying AOM.

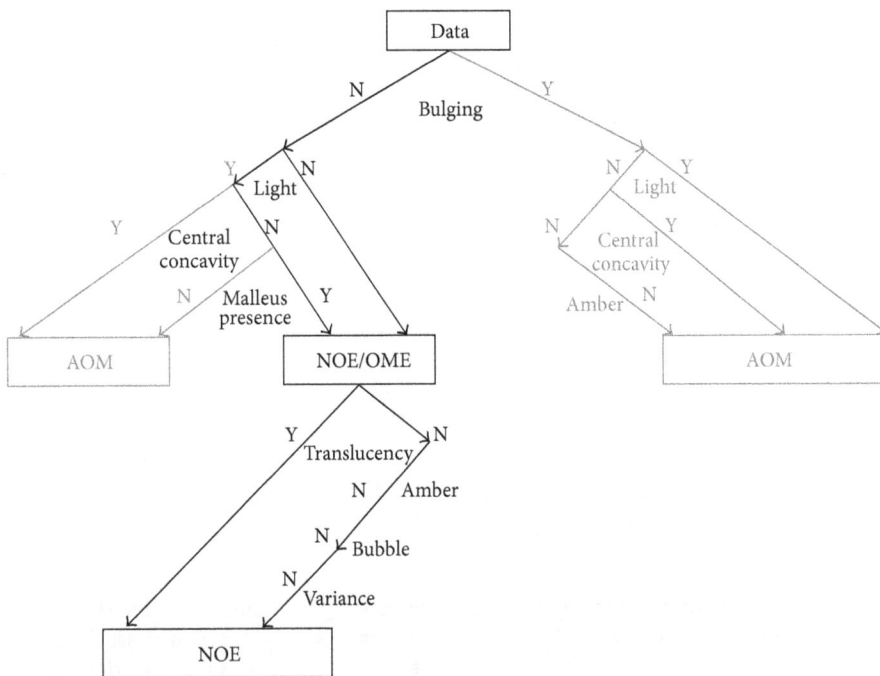

FIGURE 10: Stage 2: grammar for identifying NOE (black arrows/boxes denote those paths belonging to this stage; gray ones belong to Stage 1).

were misdiagnosed. In the remaining 50% of cases, 13 out of 24 (54.2%) were misdiagnosed as OME; such instances of misdiagnosis may lead to unnecessary treatment procedures.

3.3. Validation: Automated Classifiers.

To validate our algorithm, we also compare it to five automated classifiers, three of which we designed previously, correlation filter classification system, multiresolution classifier and SIFT and shape description using SVM classifier, and two that are available in the literature, WND-CHARM classifier and random forest classifier. We now briefly describe each of these. Note that for all the experiments, we used a 5-fold cross-validation setup.

3.3.1. Correlation Filter Classification System.

In this classifier, the image is first transformed into the polar domain. Overlapping concentric annular regions of different radii are extracted from the image. The center of the annular regions is assigned as the centroid of the segmented tympanic membrane image. During the training phase, templates of annular regions for each class are obtained. These templates are then used to assign a class label to the test images based on their similarity using normalized cross-correlation measure.

3.3.2. Multiresolution Classifier.

The multiresolution classifier, which was designed for biomedical applications [29], decomposes the image into subbands using a multiresolution decomposition (e.g., wavelets or wavelet packets), followed by feature extraction and classification in each subband using neural networks (any classifier can be used in each individual subband) and a global decision based on weighted individual subband decisions. We ran the multiresolution classifier with

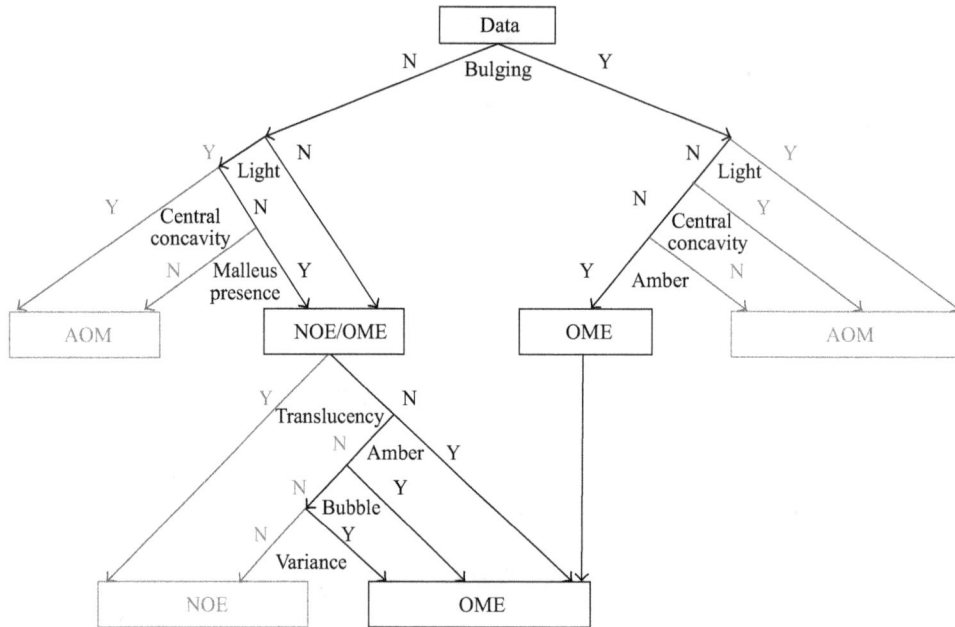

FIGURE 11: Stage 3: grammar for identifying OME (black arrows/boxes denote those paths belonging to this stage; gray ones belong to Stages 1 and 2).

TABLE 2: Diagnoses by three general pediatricians (columns) versus the ground truth of expert otoscopists (rows).

	Total			High confidence			Medium/low confidence		
	AOM	OME	NOE	AOM	OME	NOE	AOM	OME	NOE
AOM	62	1	0	60	0	0	2	1	0
OME	11	56	3	6	37	1	5	19	2
NOE	4	18	26	1	8	15	3	10	11
Accuracy	**79.6%**								

2 levels and 26 Haralick texture features on the grayscale image and each of the 20 subbands (546 in total).

3.3.3. SIFT and Shape Descriptors with SVM Classifier. In this classifier, we combined SIFT and shape features. SIFT features [30, 31] are first extracted from the images using the VLFeat library [32]. The shape descriptors were used as an attempt to detect bulging in the tympanic membrane. The main idea was to extract areas with bright and dark symmetry. On the segmented image, we applied phase symmetry detection algorithm described in [33]. Bright and dark regions were segmented using Otsu thresholding algorithm [34], resulting in two masks; one for the bright bulging regions and the other for the rest. Based on these masks the following features were computed: total area of bright regions, total area of dark regions, average symmetry measure in bright areas, number of dark regions, number of bright regions, and mean area of bright regions. All these features were normalized and we used a bag-of-words model. The classification was performed using support vector machine [35].

3.3.4. WND-CHARM Classifier. This is a universal classifier that extracts a large number (4,008) of generic image-level

features [36]. The computed features include polynomial decompositions, high contrast features, pixel statistics, and textures. These features are derived from the raw image, transforms of the image, and compound transforms of the image (transforms of transforms). The algorithm performs a feature selection during the training stage by assigning a weight to each feature depending on its ability to distinguish between the classes. These weighted features are then used to classify test images based on their similarity to the training classes using the nearest neighbor algorithm.

3.3.5. Random Forest Classifier. This is an ensemble classifier [37] that consists of many decision trees and outputs the class that is the result of the majority vote of the classes output by individual trees. Each split was based on the feature from the randomly selected subset of 5 features that gave the best performance. The number of trees in the forest is fixed as 500 since during multiple runs of random forest we observed that the out-of-bag error converged in the range of 475–500 trees. We used the implementation of random forest in [38].

3.4. Results. Table 3 compares the performance of the diagnosis by three general pediatricians (GP) as well as eight

TABLE 3: Classification accuracies (in %) on the ground-truth set of 181 tympanic membrane images. Each row corresponds to the class-wise classification accuracies and columns correspond to the diagnosis by three general pediatricians (GP) as well as the following algorithms: correlation filter classification system (CFC), WND-CHRM (WCM), multiresolution classifier (MRC), SIFT and shape descriptors with SVM classifier (SSC), random forest classifier (RF), our previous classifier from [27], and otitis media classifier (OMC).

	CFC	WCM	MRC	SSC	GP	RF	[27]	OMC
AOM	66.7	68.2	53.5	66.7	98.4	84.1	81.3	88.8
OME	57.1	60.8	66.3	81.0	80.0	81.4	85.7	82.6
NOE	62.5	63.4	75.1	60.0	54.2	66.6	81.4	85.4
Accuracy	61.8	64.1	64.1	70.2	79.6	80.1	84.0	**85.6**

TABLE 4: Classification accuracies (in %) on the ground-truth set of 170 tympanic membrane images out of 181 images after rejection. Each row corresponds to the class-wise classification accuracies and columns correspond to classification by the following algorithms: correlation filter classification system (CFC), WND-CHRM (WCM), multiresolution classifier (MRC), SIFT and shape descriptors with SVM classifier (SSC), random forest classifier (RF), and otitis media classifier with rejection (OMCR).

	CFC	WCM	MRC	SSC	RF	OMCR
AOM	65.6	65.5	61.0	76.2	80.3	90.0
OME	56.7	58.2	65.3	72.8	79.1	89.1
NOE	71.4	69.0	83.9	58.3	69.4	93.2
Accuracy	63.6	63.6	68.2	70.0	77.1	**89.9**

classifiers: correlation filter classification system (CFC), WND-CHRM (WCM), multiresolution classifier (MRC), SIFT and shape descriptors with SVM classifier (SSC), random forest classifier (RF), our previous classifier from [27], and otitis media classifier (OMC). Table 4 compares the results of the above-mentioned classifiers on the dataset of 170 images after automatic rejection of unreliable images. For ease of reference we name the otitis media classifier with rejection as OMCR. The otitis media classifier with rejection outperforms the other classifiers by a fair margin (12.8%). Random forest classifier shows the highest performance among the five compared algorithms but fails to outperform the otitis media classifiers. There are a couple of reasons for this poorer performance: since each image is assigned an output label based on majority vote of outputs from all the decision trees in the forest, the final output label can be a result contributed by poorly formed decision trees, and, a random forest classifier is known to exhibit better performance when the features used are uncorrelated which is not the case in this work, since more than one vocabulary feature is directly targeted to characterize a specific diagnostic category.

While the overall performance increases between the otitis media classifier presented in [27] and otitis media classifier using the new vocabulary and grammar might not seem substantial, the increase in classification accuracy of AOM cases is significant. This increase can be attributed to the new grammar presented in Figure 11, which includes

new vocabulary features; bulging and malleus presence. In [27], identifying AOM was solely based on central concavity and light features, which only indicate the presence of a bulge unlike the bulging feature that measures the total area of bulging in the tympanic membrane. The performance presented by otitis media classifier with rejection is a trade-off between misclassification and not classifying all the input data. A total of 11 (2 AOM, 3 OME, and 6 NOE) images were rejected using a simple rejection procedure explained earlier. We believe that this rejection step during preprocessing will ensure the collection of good-quality images that are suitable for processing and high-quality diagnosis.

Overall, the otitis media classifier performs better than the average of the three general pediatricians by a good margin (from 79.6% to 85.6%). Note that for the comparison to be fair, we did not compare the performance of the pediatricians to the otitis media classifier with rejection because they do not have an objective way of rejecting images of poor quality. At the same time, the rejection capability is a clear advantage of an automated algorithm and leads to improved performance (from 85.6% without rejection to 89.9% with rejection). Pediatricians performed well on diagnosing AOM but with a high possibility of overdiagnosing AOM. When comparing misdiagnoses of OME and NOE as AOM between pediatricians and the algorithm, 15.7% (11 out of 70) cases of OME and 8.3% (4 out of 48) cases of NOE were misdiagnosed as AOM by pediatricians compared to 10.0% (7 out of 70) cases of OME and 4.2% (2 out of 48) of NOE by the classifier, with a P value of 0.1309 for the two-tailed Fisher exact test. When comparing misdiagnoses of NOE and OME between pediatricians and the algorithm, 50.0% (24 out of 48) cases of NOE were misdiagnoses as OME by pediatricians compared to only 14.6% (7 out of 48) by the classifier, with a P value of 0.0016 for the two-tailed Fisher exact test. From these observations, we conclude that, on average, our algorithm outperforms general pediatricians.

The above discussion validates our methodology that a small number of targeted, physiologically meaningful features, vocabulary, together with a well-designed grammar that mimics the decision process of expert otoscopists, is what is needed to achieve accurate classification in this problem.

4. Conclusions and Future Work

We created an automated system for classifying the three diagnostic categories of otitis media. Our guiding principles were to design a *vocabulary* of features that mimics the actual visual cues used by expert otoscopists as well as a *grammar* to mimic their decision-making process. This automated algorithm that exhibits high levels of accuracy in identifying the diagnostic categories of otitis media is comparable to the diagnoses by expert otoscopists.

Results demonstrate that our simple and concise 8-feature otitis media vocabulary is effective on the problem, underscoring the importance of using targeted, physiologically meaningful features instead of a large number of general-purpose features. The classification process, grammar, is a hierarchical process mimicking the diagnostic process used by otoscopists. Increasing the accuracy from the current stage becomes harder, as we have reached a high accuracy range; we now discuss potential strategies for achieving that as directions for further work.

Images captured using a digital otoscope exhibit a large variability. Depending on the angle and amount of light incident on the membrane and the ear canal, we encounter different illumination problems related to brightness and contrast. In our current implementation, we only correct local illumination problems but have not solved for global illumination problems. Artifacts such as shading, shadows, and changes due to global variation in the intensity or color due to overexposure or underexposure will affect feature computation. Strategies for minimizing such artifacts are subject of future studies. In [39], the illumination field is estimated from an image and then compensated by using the estimated field and thus recovering the reflectance function. Global illumination correction can also be achieved as shown in [40] where the algorithm uses both illumination field and surface reflectance. The algorithm reports good performance in case of sufficient illumination variation as well as surface reflectance on natural scene images. These methods have also been applied in other image classification problems before feature extraction. We have not explored the issue of illumination normalization and plan to do so in future work.

Another problem we have observed has to do with the natural variability across the images, perceived as different orientations or poses of the tympanic membrane resulting from nonuniform positioning of the otoscope while capturing the image. If deemed necessary to deal with the variability of pose, we will investigate the use of active appearance models [41–43], which have been successfully used to register face images from an arbitrary pose to a frontal face or other specified profiles [44]. This preprocessing is implemented before feature extraction; it aligns new images to a universal template, with the aim of making feature extraction more stable. In other image recognition fields, such as in face recognition, the use of image preprocessing to align and normalize images is crucial for the overall performance of the system and might provide a performance boost in our case as well.

Finally, we believe that the performance of our system could be further improved by refining the otitis media grammar. Although the current grammar has a set of clear intuitive rules closely mimicking the expert otoscopists, we intend to use soft decision splits on each feature instead of hard binary decisions. Our current method does not use the relative importance of vocabulary feature in decision making. Future work includes investigating methods for refining the hierarchical decision process and using the relative importance of each of the vocabulary features in the classification process.

We expect to establish that the diagnostic categories of otitis media or its absence that are provided by our automated otitis media classification system are accurate representations of what expert otoscopists diagnose when examining the images of tympanic membranes. Should the otitis media classifier demonstrate good diagnostic capability, it can be employed as a clinical diagnostic aid to drastically decrease both underdiagnosis and overdiagnosis of AOM, assuring adequate antimicrobial use when AOM is present and reducing inappropriate use when AOM is absent, thus avoiding adverse side effects and the risk of contributing to bacterial resistance.

Acknowledgments

The authors gratefully acknowledge support from the NSF through Award 1017278, the NIH through Award 1DC010283, the NIH-NIAID through Award 3U01AI066007-02S1, and the CMU CIT Infrastructure Award. They also would like to thank Dr. Pablo Hennings Yeomans for his early work on this project and for implementing the segmentation algorithm, Dr. Pedro Quelhas for implementing the SIFT and shape descriptor classifier, Mr. Jian Li for his work on features, and Miss Lakshmi Dhevi Jayagobi for implementing the random forest classifier. they follow the principles of reproducible research. To that end, they created a reproducible research page at [45], where the code and necessary information needed to reproduce the results in this paper are available (except for data, which cannot be made public). Initial parts of this work were presented at ICIP 2012 [27].

References

[1] M. E. Pichichero, "Diagnostic accuracy of otitis media and tympanocentesis skills assessment among pediatricians," *European Journal of Clinical Microbiology and Infectious Diseases*, vol. 22, no. 9, pp. 519–524, 2003.

[2] C. M. Buchanan and D. D. Pothier, "Recognition of paediatric otopathology by general practitioners," *International Journal of Pediatric Otorhinolaryngology*, vol. 72, no. 5, pp. 669–673, 2008.

[3] D. W. Teele, J. O. Klein, and B. Rosner, "Epidemiology of otitis media during the first seven years of life in children in greater Boston: a prospective, cohort study," *Journal of Infectious Diseases*, vol. 160, no. 1, pp. 83–94, 1989.

[4] American Academy of Pediatrics, "Diagnosis and management of acute otitis media," *Pediatrics*, vol. 113, no. 5, pp. 1451–1465, 2004.

[5] E. Asher, E. Leibovitz, J. Press, D. Greenberg, N. Bilenko, and H. Reuveni, "Accuracy of acute otitis media diagnosis in community and hospital settings," *Acta Paediatrica, International Journal of Paediatrics*, vol. 94, no. 4, pp. 423–428, 2005.

[6] P. A. Tähtinen, M. K. Laine, P. Huovinen, J. Jalava, O. Ruuskanen, and A. Ruohola, "A placebo-controlled trial of antimicrobial treatment for acute otitis media," *The New England Journal of Medicine*, vol. 364, no. 2, pp. 116–126, 2011.

[7] C. Vertan, D. C. Gheorghe, and B. Ionescu, "Eardrum color content analysis in video-otoscopy images for the diagnosis support of pediatric otitis," in *Proceedings of the International Symposium on Signals, Circuits and Systems (ISSCS '11)*, pp. 129–132, rou, July 2011.

[8] A. Mojsilović, J. Kovačević, J. Hu, R. J. Safranek, and K. Ganapathy, "Matching and retrieval based on the vocabulary and grammar of color patterns," in *Proceedings of the IEEE International Conference Multimedia Computer Systems*, Florence, Italy, June 1999.

[9] A. Mojsilović, J. Kovačević, J. Hu, R. J. Safranek, and K. Ganapathy, "Matching and retrieval based on the vocabulary

and grammar of color patterns," in *Proceedings of the IEEE Transactions on Image Processing, Image Video Process Digita Libraries*, vol. 9, pp. 38–54, IEEE Signal Processing Society Young author Best Paper Award, 2000.

[10] A. Mojsilović, J. Kovačević, D. A. Kall, R. J. Safranek, and K. Ganapathy, "Vocabulary and grammar of color patterns," *IEEE Transactions on Image Processing*, vol. 9, no. 3, Article ID 417431, 2000.

[11] K. Ganapathy, J. Hu, J. Kovačević, A. Mojsilović, and R. J. Safranek, *Retrieval and Matching of Color Patterns Based on a Predetermined vocabulary and grammar*, US Patent, 2002.

[12] K. Ganapathy, J. Hu, J. Kovačević, A. Mojsilović, and R. J. Safranek, *Retrieval and Matching of Color Patterns Based on a Predetermined vocabulary And grammar: II*, US Patent, 2002.

[13] N. Shaikh, A. Hoberman, P. H. Kaleida et al., "Otoscopic signs of otitis media," *Pediatric Infectious Disease Journal*, vol. 30, no. 10, pp. 822–826, 2011.

[14] N. Shaikh, A. Hoberman, H. E. Rockette, and M. Kurs-Lasky, "Development of an Algorithm for the Diagnosis of Otitis Media," *Academic Pediatrics*, vol. 12, no. 3, pp. 214–218, 2012.

[15] M. Kass, A. Witkin, and D. Terzopoulos, "Snakes: active contour models," *International Journal of Computer Vision*, vol. 1, no. 4, pp. 321–331, 1988.

[16] C. Xu and J. L. Prince, "Snakes, shapes, and gradient vector flow," *IEEE Transactions on Image Processing*, vol. 7, no. 3, pp. 359–369, 1998.

[17] R. Bornard, E. Lecan, L. Laborelli, and J.-H. Chenot, "Missing data correction in still images and image sequences," in *Proceedings of the 10th International Conference of Multimedia*, pp. 355–361, Juan-les-Pins, December 2002.

[18] M. Varma and A. Zisserman, "Classifying images of materials: achieving viewpoint and illumination independence," in *Proceedings of the Eurographics Conference Computer Vision*, vol. 3, pp. 255–271, May 2002.

[19] P. Perez, M. Gangnet, and A. Blake, "Poisson image editing," *ACM Siggraph*, vol. 22, no. 3, pp. 313–318, 2003.

[20] R. Bhagavatula, M. Fickus, W. Kelly et al., "Automatic identification and delineation of germ layer components in H&E stained images of teratomas derived from human and nonhuman primate embryonic stem cells," in *Proceedings of the 7th IEEE International Symposium on Biomedical Imaging: From Nano to Macro (ISBI '10)*, pp. 1041–1044, Rotterdam, The Netherlands, April 2010.

[21] M. T. McCann, R. Bhagavatula, M. C. Fickus, J. A. Ozolek, and J. Kovačević, "Automated colitis detection from endoscopic biopsies as a tissue screening tool in diagnostic pathology," in *Proceedings of the IEEE International Conference on Image Processing*, pp. 2809–2812, Orlando, Fla, USA, 2012.

[22] T. Ping-Sing and M. Shah, "Shape from shading using linear approximation," *Image and Vision Computing*, vol. 12, no. 8, pp. 487–498, 1994.

[23] Y. Cheng, "Mean shift, mode seeking, and clustering," *IEEE Transactions on Pattern Analysis and Machine Intelligence*, vol. 17, no. 8, pp. 790–799, 1995.

[24] J. Canny, "A computational approach for edge detection," *IEEE Transactions on Pattern Analysis and Machine Intelligence*, vol. 8, no. 6, pp. 1293–1299, 1986.

[25] R. O. Duda and H. P. Hart, "Use of the Hough transformation to detect lines and curves in pictures," *Communications of the ACM*, vol. 15, no. 1, pp. 11–15, 1972.

[26] P. N. Belhumeur and D. J. Kriegman, "What is the set of images of an object under all possible lighting conditions?" in *Proceedings of the IEEE Computer Society Conference on Computer Vision and Pattern Recognition*, pp. 270–277, June 1996.

[27] A. Kuruvilla, J. Li, P. H. Yeomans et al., "Otitis media vocabulary and grammar," in *Proceedings of the IEEE International Conference on Image Processing*, pp. 2845–2848, Orlando, Fla, USA, September 2012.

[28] A. Hoberman, J. L. Paradise, H. E. Rockette et al., "Treatment of acute otitis media in children under 2 years of age," *The New England Journal of Medicine*, vol. 364, no. 2, pp. 105–115, 2011.

[29] A. Chebira, Y. Barbotin, C. Jackson et al., "A multiresolution approach to automated classification of protein subcellular location images," *BMC Bioinformatics*, vol. 8, article 210, 2007.

[30] D. G. Lowe, "Object recognition from local scale-invariant features," in *Proceedings of the 7th IEEE International Conference on Computer Vision (ICCV '99)*, pp. 1150–1157, September 1999.

[31] D. G. Lowe, "Distinctive image features from scale-invariant keypoints," *International Journal of Computer Vision*, vol. 60, no. 2, pp. 91–110, 2004.

[32] A. Vedaldi and B. Fulkerson, *VLFeat: An Open and Portable Library of Computer Vision Algorithms*, 2008.

[33] P. Kovesi, Matlab and octave functions for computer vision and image processing, http://www.csse.uwa.edu.au/~pk/research/matlabfns/.

[34] N. Otsu, "A threshold selection method from gray-level histograms," *IEEE Trans Syst Man Cybern*, vol. 9, no. 1, pp. 62–66, 1979.

[35] C. C. Chang and C. J. Lin, "LIBSVM: a library for support vector machines," *ACM Transactions on Intelligent Systems and Technology*, vol. 2, pp. 1–27, 2011.

[36] N. Orlov, L. Shamir, T. Macura, J. Johnston, D. M. Eckley, and I. G. Goldberg, "WND-CHARM: multi-purpose image classification using compound image transforms," *Pattern Recognition Letters*, vol. 29, no. 11, pp. 1684–1693, 2008.

[37] L. Breiman, "Random forests," *Machine Learning*, vol. 45, no. 1, pp. 5–32, 2001.

[38] A. Jaiantila, "Randomforest-matlab," https://code.google.com/p/randomforest-matlab/.

[39] R. Gross and V. Brajovic, "An image preprocessing algorithm for illumination invariant face recognition," in *Proceeding of the International Conference on Audio- and Video-Based Biometric Person Authentication*, pp. 10–18, Springer, Berlin, Germany, 2003.

[40] K. Barnard, G. Finlayson, and B. Funt, "Color constancy for scenes with varying illumination," *Computer Vision and Image Understanding*, vol. 65, no. 2, pp. 311–321, 1997.

[41] T. F. Cootes, G. J. Edwards, and C. J. Taylor, "Active appearance models," *IEEE Transactions on Pattern Analysis and Machine Intelligence*, vol. 23, pp. 681–685, 2001.

[42] J. Matthews and S. Baker, "Active appearance models revisited," *International Journal of Computer Vision*, vol. 60, no. 2, pp. 135–164, 2004.

[43] X. Yun, J. Tian, and J. Liu, "Active appearance models fitting with occlusion," in *Proceedings of the American Statistical Association Statistics and Computing*, pp. 137–144, 2007.

[44] S. Ting, B. C. Lovell, and C. Shaokang, "Face recognition robust to head pose from one sample image," in *Proceedings of the 18th International Conference on Pattern Recognition (ICPR '06)*, pp. 515–518, August 2006.

[45] A. Kuruvilla, N. Shaikh, A. Hoberman, and J. Kovačević, *Automated Diagnosis of Otitis Media: A Vocabulary and Grammar*, 2013, http://jelena.ece.cmu.edu/repository/rr/13_Kuruvilla-SHK/13_KuruvillaSHK.html.

15

Endoscopy-MR Image Fusion for Image Guided Procedures

Anwar Abdalbari,[1] Xishi Huang,[2] and Jing Ren[1]

[1] *Faculty of Engineering and Applied Science, University of Ontario Institute of Technology, 2000 Simcoe Street North, Oshawa, ON, Canada L1H 7K4*

[2] *Department of Medical Imaging, University of Toronto, Toronto, ON, Canada M5T 1W7*

Correspondence should be addressed to Jing Ren; jing.ren@uoit.ca

Academic Editor: Tiange Zhuang

Minimally invasive endoscope based abdominal procedures provide potential advantages over conventional open surgery such as reduced trauma, shorter hospital stay, and quick recovery. One major limitation of using this technique is the narrow view of the endoscope and the lack of proper 3D context of the surgical site. In this paper, we propose a rapid and accurate method to align intraoperative stereo endoscopic images of the surgical site with preoperative Magnetic Resonance (MR) images. Gridline light pattern is projected on the surgical site to facilitate the registration. The purpose of this surface-based registration is to provide 3D context of the surgical site to the endoscopic view. We have validated the proposed method on a liver phantom and achieved the surface registration error of 0.76 ± 0.11 mm.

1. Introduction

In this paper, we develop a new method for endoscopy-MR image fusion of the liver organ for minimally invasive endoscope based surgery. Image guidance is an essential tool in minimally invasive endoscope based abdominal procedures [1]. Effective image guidance can compensate the restricted perception during the operation, which is considered a major limitation in endoscopic procedures. Without image guidance, the surgeon cannot see through the surface of the operation site and may accidentally cause damages to the critical structures of the patient. A typical procedure in image guidance is to map pre-operative high quality MR images to intra-operative endoscopic video images, or the patient thereby provides a good quality context to the real-time endoscopic images. Thus, the surgeon will be able to visually access the operation site during the procedure. As a result, the damage to the critical organs or tissues will be substantially minimized.

Fusion of endoscopic video images with high quality MR images requires good match of these two modalities. In this paper, we adopt a surface based image fusion because the two modalities are different in acquisition and nature [2, 3]. In order to find the corresponding 3D surface model from endoscopic images, we utilize stereovision to snapshot the surgical site from two different angles and compute the 3D location by using triangulation [4]. Cameras are calibrated before triangulation is used [5, 6].

Although a liver phantom is used to validate the proposed technique, our method is not restricted to the liver surgery. The integrated image guidance can also be applied to other endoscopic procedures. This paper is organized as follows. Section 2 introduces the experimental setup and the camera calibration of the stereo endoscope. Section 3 discusses automatic surface reconstruction, and Section 4 presents surface based registration and experimental results of image fusion. Section 5 discusses the issues in this study. Section 6 presents the conclusion and future work.

2. Experimental Setup and Camera Calibration

Experimental setup is shown in Figure 1. In the experiments of this study, we use the following major components: a Visionsense VSII stereo endoscope, an Optoma PK301 Pocket Projector, a liver phantom, and a chessboard calibration pattern. Optoma PK301 Pocket Projector is a small size projector and can be easily mounted. The resolution of this

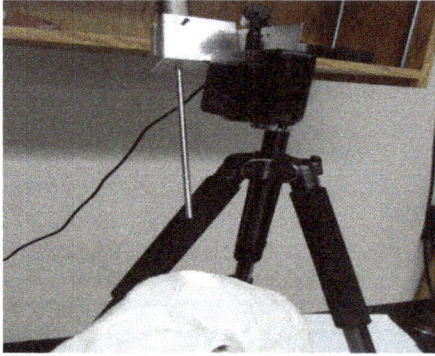

FIGURE 1: Experimental setup for stereo endoscope and liver phantom.

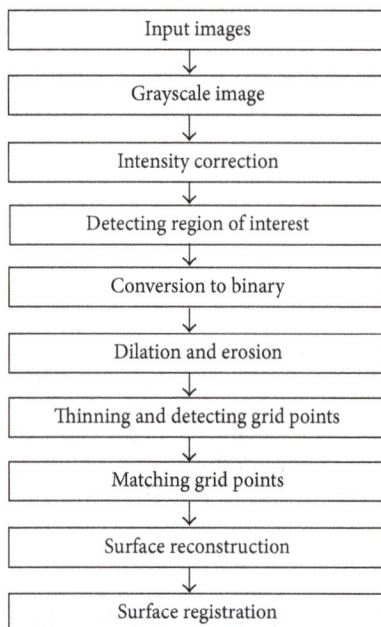

FIGURE 2: Flowchart for automatic fusion of intraoperative endoscopic images to preoperative images.

projector is 848 by 480. The liver phantom was printed using a 3D printer based on the liver model that was segmented from MR images of a human subject.

In this study, robust 3D surface reconstruction requires accurate camera calibration of the stereo endoscope. The calibration process aims to find intrinsic parameters and correct the optical distortion inherent in the endoscope and to compute extrinsic parameters to capture the spatial relationship between left and right cameras of the stereo endoscope. We have modified the Camera Calibration Toolbox for MATLAB [7] and performed calibration of the stereo endoscope using a chessboard calibration pattern.

3. Surface Reconstruction from Stereo Endoscope

In this section, we propose a novel approach to reconstruct the surface of the surgical site from two stereo endoscopic

images. The reconstruction procedure is shown in Figure 2. First, a gridline pattern is projected on the surgical site, and both left and right images are acquired at the same time. Second, the intersection points of the gridlines are automatically detected and matched in both images. Then we reconstruct the surface with the matched intersection points. We will describe major steps in detail in the following sections.

3.1. Conversion of Input Images to Grayscale Images.
In order to detect the intersections of the grid lines pattern of an image, we use the image of binary format as algorithm input. We first convert the color images acquired from the stereo endoscope to grayscale images (as shown in Figures 3 and 4). According to the thinning algorithm used in the proposed system, the gridlines of the light pattern should be bright to detect their intersections. The grayscale image is thus inverted to meet this constraint. In this process, the dark areas become bright and vice versa. Next, multiple steps are employed to obtain good binary images.

3.2. Intensity Correction.
The image intensity of the endoscopic images is not uniform given that variation in illumination and ambient lights exist. As a consequence, conventional threshold methods cannot be directly used to achieve good binary images which can successfully separates gridlines from the background. In this paper, we present an intensity correction technique to improve the image. The improvement aims to equalize the contrast between gridlines and background over the whole image. The new corrected pixel value is calculated by

$$I_{new} = 255 - \left(\frac{(I_{ave} - I_c)}{2} + 127 \right), \tag{1}$$

where I_c is the intensity value of the current pixel, I_{ave} is the avarage intensity of its neighbourhood pixels, and I_{new} is the new intensity value after correction.

Figure 5 shows the image after intensity correction, in which the contrast between the gridlines and background is more uniform compared with the image before correction in Figure 4(b). Figure 6 shows binary images by thresholding, which will be used for intersection detection. With intensity correction, all gridlines are clearly shown in the binary image, while without intensity correction, only a part of the gridlines is shown in the cluttered binary image. The intensity correction also significantly improves the detection and matching accuracy with the successful rate of 98% versus 57% without intensity correction (see Table 1).

3.3. Detection of Region of Interest.
In this paper, region of interest (ROI) is defined as the region which only covers the projected gridline light pattern in the endoscopic image. Automatic detection of ROI is critical for accurate detection and matching of intersection points in the gridline pattern. During the image preprocessing step, the area out of ROI should be cut out. ROI detection leads to automatic removal of unwanted areas. This step significantly improves the

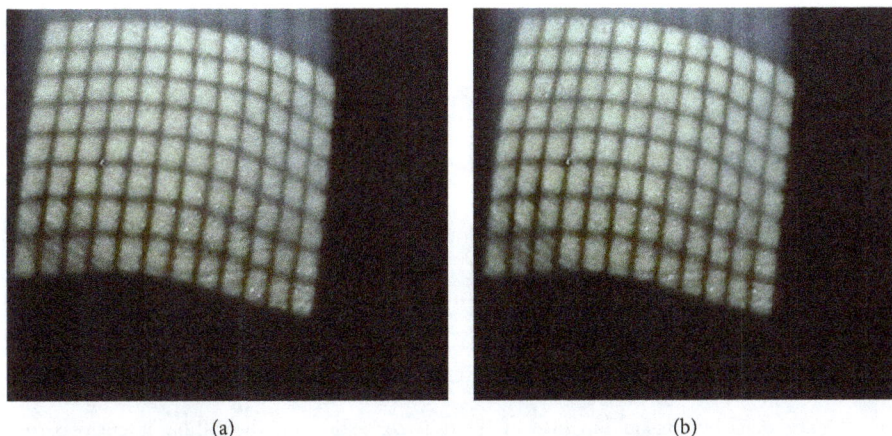

(a)   (b)

FIGURE 3: Original stereo endoscopic color images: (a) left image and (b) right image.

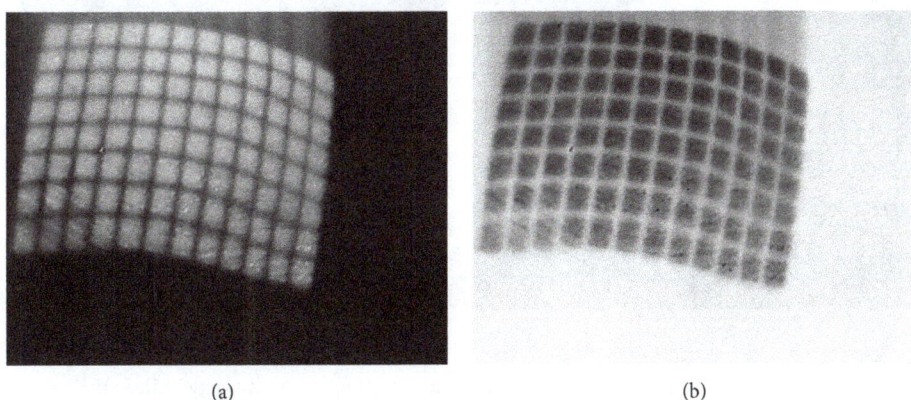

(a)   (b)

FIGURE 4: Left (a) grayscale image and (b) negative image.

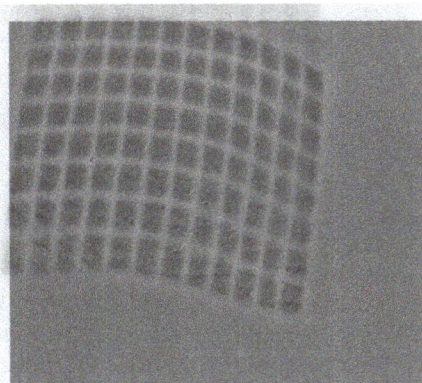

FIGURE 5: Intensity correction image.

correctness of gridline intersection detection as well as the processing speed.

The ROI detection process aims to generate a mask of the grid lines pattern. Following intensity correction, we threshold the images in order to convert the corrected grayscale image into a binary image for further processing. Next, the dilation and the erosion operations are performed.

Eventually, as the consequence of dilation and erosion processes, we obtain a binary mask image only covering the region of the projected gridline pattern. Then, we apply the mask image to the intensity corrected image to produce a cropped image within the desired ROI. The cropped image is then converted to a binary image by applying a threshold to it, which is used for feature detection. Figure 7(a) shows the detected ROI of the input image (ROI mask image), and Figure 7(b) shows the cropped image within ROI.

3.4. Image Dilation and Erosion. Because of the conversion to a binary image, some white pixels in the binary image are far away from the gridlines. Hence, these types of pixels could cause false positive pixels in the thinning process. By using dilation, we can expand the gridlines to fill the gaps between them and the protrusions pixels. Dilation process followed by erosion process is used to return the structure to its original state by removing the added structure of the gridlines. As a result, we have smoother gridlines without holes and protrusion pixels. Figure 8 shows the binary images before and after dilation and erosion process, respectively.

3.5. Thinning and Intersection Detection. In order to detect the intersections of the gridline pattern, we used a thinning

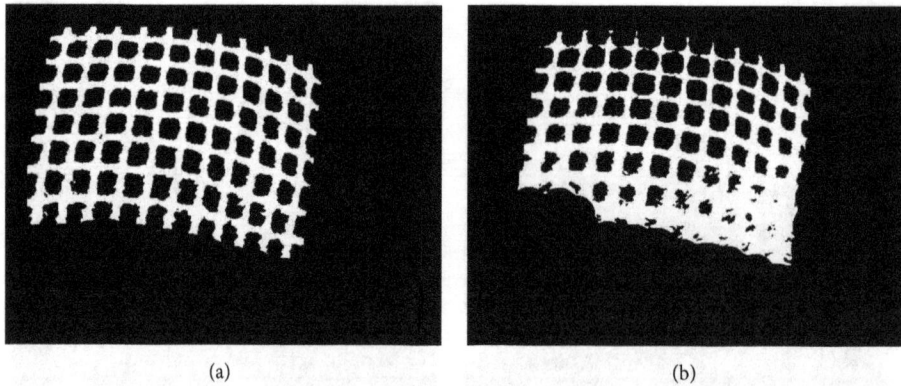

(a)   (b)

FIGURE 6: Binary image by thresholding (a) with intensity correction and (b) without intensity correction.

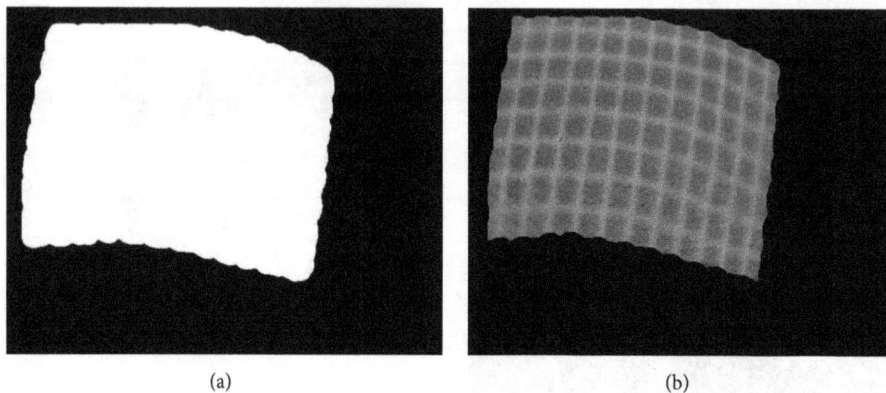

(a)   (b)

FIGURE 7: (a) Detected ROI mask image and (b) intensity correction image within ROI mask.

process applied to the above processed binary image. The thinning process generates an image with one pixel width; that is, it generates a skeleton image of the input binary image. Then we proceeded to detect the intersections of the image gridlines. This process was accomplished by applying a hybrid approach for cross-point detection called the combined cross-point number (CCN) method [6]. The CCN method uses two techniques to detect intersections of gridlines: simple cross-point number (SCN) and the modified cross-point number (MCN). The CCN algorithm is used to detect the intersection points of the gridlines.

In simple cross-point number, the image is iterated with a small window of size 3 by 3 pixels [6], as a result we have eight pixels surrounding the tested pixel. To test if the center pixel of the 3 by 3 window is a cross-point pixel, we iterate this window on the image and get the cross-point number (CPN) for the center pixel. The CPN is calculated by

$$\text{CPN}_{\text{SCN}} = \frac{1}{2}\sum_{n=1}^{8} |P_n - P_{n+1}|, \qquad (2)$$

where P_n is the pixel value of nth pixel of the 3 by 3 window and $P_8 = P_1$. A point is considered a cross point if its CPN is four.

In modified cross-point number method, the image is iterated by a window of size 5 by 5 pixels surrounding the center pixel. The CPN is calculated by

$$\text{CPN}_{\text{MCN}} = \frac{1}{2}\sum_{n=1}^{16} |P_n - P_{n+1}|, \qquad (3)$$

where $P_{17} = P_1$. The pixel is considered a cross-point pixel if $\text{CPN}_{\text{MCN}} \geq 4$. In the combined cross-point number both simple cross-point number and modified cross-point number methods are used. The simple cross-point number is used in the inner 3×3 neighbors of the center pixel, while the modified cross-point number is used in the outer 5×5 neighbors of the center pixel. Each pixel in the image has been tested against CPN using the modified cross-point number method, in which it is considered a cross point if and only if it satisfies $\text{CPN}_{\text{SCN}} \geq 4$ and $\text{CPN}_{\text{MCN}} \geq 4$. Because of the low quality of the images, we adjust the CPN of the combined CPN to be in the range of 3.0 and 4.0. Figure 9(a) shows the left skeleton image by thinning operation. Figure 9(b) shows the detected intersection points plotted on the left image. Figure 9(c) shows the detected intersection points and plotted on the right image. Notice that there are false positive points in both images, and as shown in Figure 10, these false points are eliminated by our method using the epipolar geometry matching constraint.

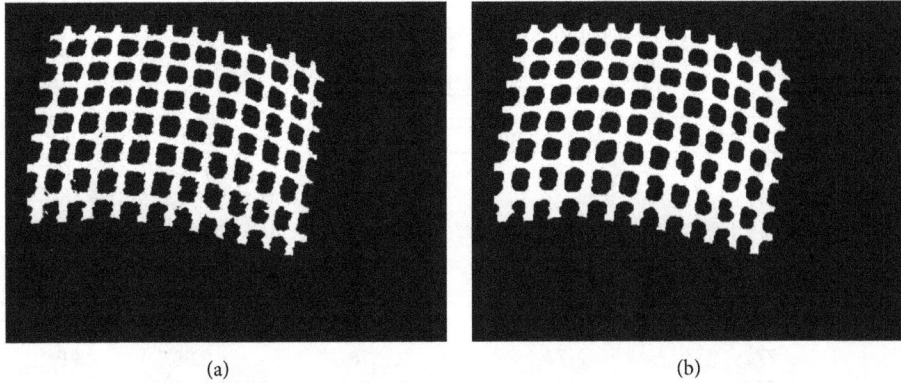

(a)

(b)

FIGURE 8: (a) Binary image before dilation and erosion (holes and spikes), (b) image after dilation and erosion process.

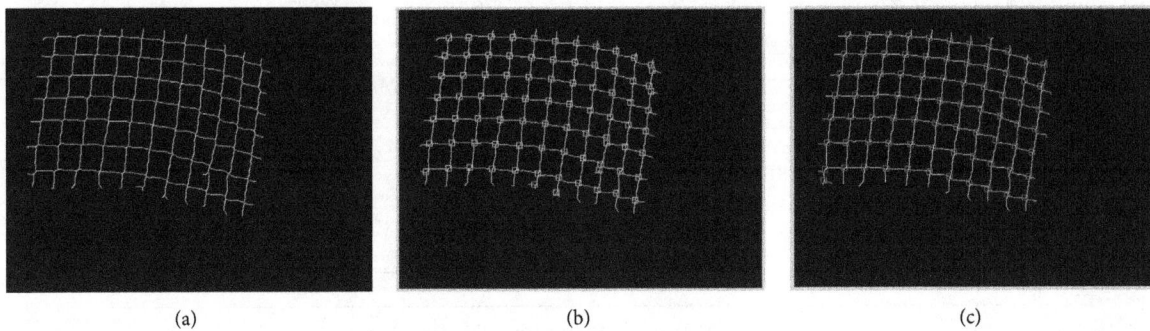

(a)

(b)

(c)

FIGURE 9: (a) An skeleton left image after thinning, (b) detected intersection points plotted on a left image, and (c) detected intersection points plotted on a right image.

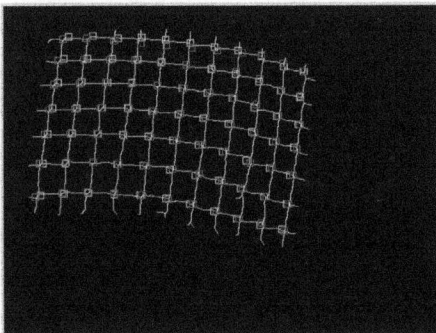

FIGURE 10: The matched points from both images.

3.6. Matching Grid Points.

In order to reconstruct the surface within the ROI using the triangulation technique, we need to find the corresponding intersection points in the left and right images. Since these grid points have similar features, these correspondence relationships cannot be effectively obtained using conventional feature matching methods such as Scale Invariant Feature Transform (SIFT) and Speeded Up Robust Features (SURF) based techniques. In this paper, we adopt the method of epipolar constraints [2]. The intersection points are matched column-by-column to achieve good matching in our study.

We have validated the proposed approach using 19 pairs of images acquired at different position and orientation of the stereo endoscope. Figure 10 shows the matched grid points superimposed in one image. Table 1 shows the actual number of points in each image, the number of the points detected, the number of correct points, the number of false positive points (FPP), and the number of false negative points (FNP). The average of sensitivity detection of the proposed method is 0.9822.

3.7. Points/Surface Reconstruction.

In general, a video image generated from the endoscope is a 2D projection of the 3D scene. This process can be represented using the pinhole camera model [8]. After we obtain the camera calibration parameters, we reconstruct a 3D point x from left and right image projections by using stereo triangulation. A smooth surface can be reconstructed by fitting these reconstructed 3D grid points as shown in Figure 11(a). This figure has demonstrated that the proposed method can achieve accurate surface reconstruction from the stereo endoscopic images.

In order to investigate the impact of the previous image processing procedures on the reconstructed surface, we have performed the following experiments. We use image intensity correction as an example to examine the effects in detail. We repeat the entire process of the surface reconstruction as shown in Figure 2, except that no intensity correction is performed. Figure 11(b) shows the reconstructed surface without intensity correction, and Figure 14 shows

TABLE 1: It shows the actual number of points in each image, the number of the points detected, the number of correct points, the number of false positive points (FPP), and the number of false negative points (FNP).

(a) With intensity correction

Image	Number of points	Detected points	Correct points	Sensitivity	FPP	FNP
Im1	77	73	73	0.9481	0	4
Im2	77	74	74	0.961	0	3
Im3	77	74	74	0.961	0	3
Im4	77	73	73	0.9481	0	4
Im5	77	76	76	0.987	0	1
Im6	77	78	77	1.0	1	0
Im7	77	77	76	0.987	1	1
Im8	77	76	76	0.987	0	1
Im9	77	76	76	0.987	0	1
Im10	77	76	76	0.987	0	1
Im11	77	76	76	0.987	0	1
Im12	77	76	76	0.987	0	1
Im13	77	77	77	1.0	0	0
Im14	77	76	76	0.987	0	1
Im15	77	77	77	1.0	0	0
Im16	77	76	76	0.987	0	1
Im17	77	76	76	0.987	0	1
Im18	77	76	76	0.987	0	1
Im19	77	76	76	0.987	0	1
Average				0.9822		

(b) Without intensity correction

Image	Number of points	Detected points	Correct points	Sensitivity	FPP	FNP
Im1	77	51	51	0.66	0	26
Im2	77	48	48	0.62	0	29
Im3	77	25	24	0.31	1	53
Im4	77	53	52	0.67	1	25
Im5	77	53	53	0.68	0	24
Im6	77	39	38	0.49	1	39
Im7	77	42	42	0.54	0	35
Im8	77	39	39	0.50	0	38
Im9	77	60	60	0.77	0	17
Im10	77	56	55	0.71	1	22
Im11	77	53	53	0.68	0	24
Im12	77	52	52	0.67	0	25
Im13	77	44	44	0.57	0	33
Im14	77	42	41	0.53	1	36
Im15	77	42	40	0.51	2	37
Im16	77	41	40	0.51	1	37
Im17	77	36	35	0.45	1	42
Im18	77	36	35	0.45	1	42
Im19	77	41	33	0.42	2	44
Average				0.5653		

the corresponding average registration error without intensity correction. Comparing Figures 11, 13, and 14, we can clearly see that intensity correction has significantly improved the reconstruction accuracy. With intensity correction, the average surface reconstruction error reduces from 1.86 mm to 0.76 mm. Similarly, the proposed automatic detection method for ROI improve the reconstruction accuracy as well.

In Table 2, we show how the average surface error is affected by previous image processing procedures.

4. Surface Based Registration

4.1. ICP Registration. The Iterative Closest Point (ICP) algorithm is widely employed to align two three-dimensional

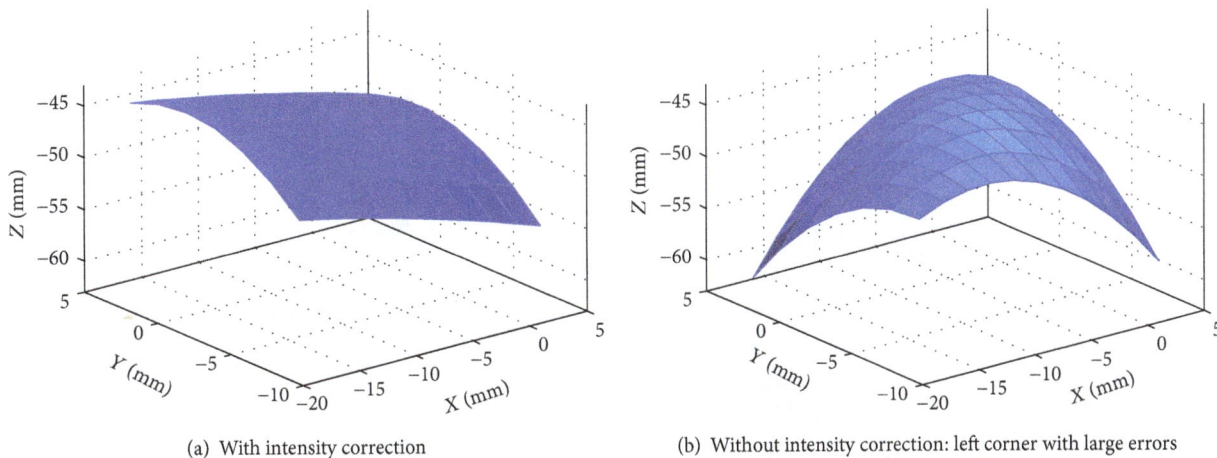

(a) With intensity correction

(b) Without intensity correction: left corner with large errors

FIGURE 11: Reconstructed surface from stereo endoscopic images.

TABLE 2: Average surface distance error (ASD) impacted by image processing procedures.

Case	Mean (mm)	Standard deviation (mm)
Proposed method	0.76	0.11
Without intensity correction	1.86	0.68
Without detection of ROI	1.24	0.73

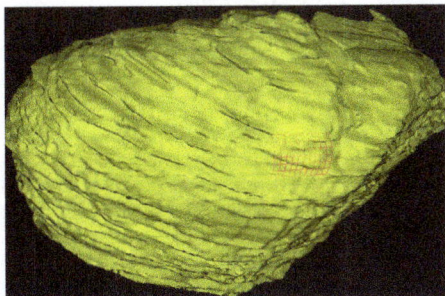

FIGURE 12: Overlay of 3D liver phantom surfaces after registration. Red mesh: reconstructed from endoscopic images, yellow surface: from MR images.

surfaces. The ICP algorithm was first proposed by Besl and McKay [9], which is an iterative two-step method. The first step is to establish point correspondences by finding the corresponding point closest to the second surface for each point in the first surface. The second step is to calculate a transformation based on these matched points, which produces incremental transformations whose composition is the registration results.

In this study, the ICP is employed to register the reconstructed surface from endoscopic images with the surface extracted from MR images. Figure 12 shows the overlay of 3D surfaces after surface registration.

4.2. Registration Accuracy. The projected gridline pattern used to test the proposed approach consists of seven rows

and eleven columns, and we have 77 intersection points to detect in each image. We used 19 pairs of left and right images acquired by the stereo endoscope at different poses for validation. After ICP surface registration, we calculated the average surface distance (ASD) between two corresponding surfaces as registration accuracy. The resulting ASD is 0.76 ± 0.11 mm (see Figure 13). Figure 14 shows the corresponding registration accuracy without intensity correction.

After surface based registration, we are able to fuse the reconstructed surface from stereo endoscopic images with pre-operative high quality MR images and the corresponding patient-specific models such as vessel centerlines as shown in Figure 15. This will enable surgeons to see through critical structures beyond the operational site surface.

5. Discussion

Developing a rapid and accurate approach to reconstruct the surface from stereo endoscopic images is a very challenging task especially for soft tissues with few features. Many techniques have been developed to acquire or reconstruct surgical surface such as using laser scanners and Time-of-Flight (ToF) cameras [10–12]. Hayashibe et al. used a laser-scan endoscope technique to reconstruct the shape and texture of the area of interest [13]. A laser scanner was proposed to acquire the liver surface for image-guided liver surgery, but it took about 5–20 seconds [10]. Therefore it is not suitable for free-breathing patients since average respiratory rates of children are 16–30 breaths per minute. ToF cameras produce a depth map that can be immediately used to generate a 3D surface model in real time, but current devices are too large for endoscopic procedures [11, 12]. For this study, we employed a small stereo endoscope with the diameter of 4.9 mm, which can be used with a typical 5 mm trocar in clinical practice. For proof of concept, we used a general purpose projector to project the light pattern of gridlines. In the future, this easy-to-implement light pattern can be generated by using a very small lithographic pattern generator with 10 μm thick lines at a distance of 50 μm [14], which can generate a pattern of 50 × 50 lines within the size of 3 mm × 3 mm.

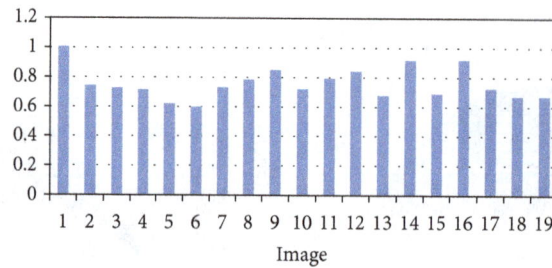

FIGURE 13: Surface registration accuracy wih intensity correction. Unit: mm.

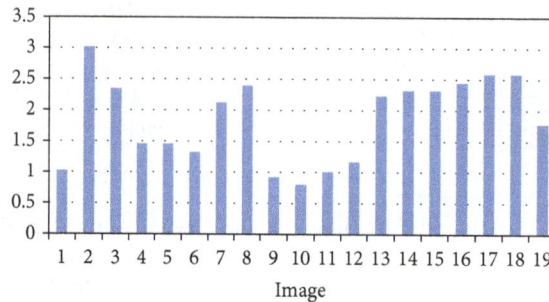

FIGURE 14: Surface registration accuracy without intensity correction. Unit: mm.

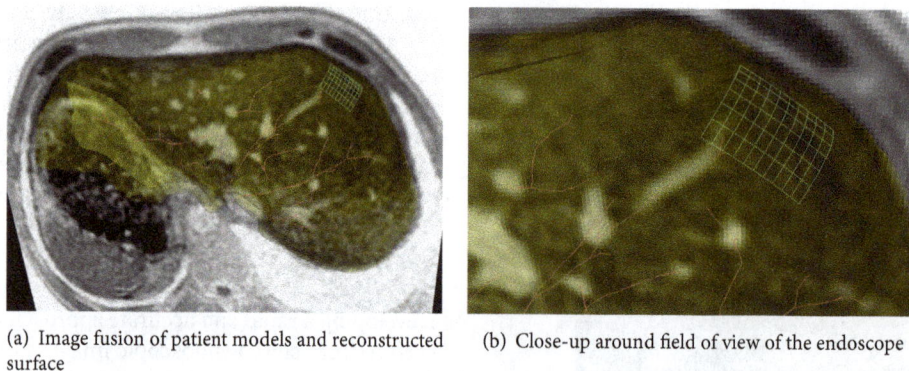

(a) Image fusion of patient models and reconstructed surface

(b) Close-up around field of view of the endoscope

FIGURE 15: Fusion of patient models and reconstructed surface from the stereo endoscope. Green mesh is the reconstructed surface from two endoscopic images, red curves are the centerlines of vessels, segmented surface from MR images is shown in semitransparent yellow, and background is one MR slice with bright vessels.

Many works [15–17], proposed to reconstruct the soft tissue structures of the abdomen using stereovision. However, it is difficult to find the correspondences between the two images, even when taking into account epipolar constraints. Moreover, 3D surface reconstruction for abdominal procedures is more challenging due to few or no features on the surface of some organs such as the liver. To tackle this, structured light based methods were presented in [18]. Traditionally, the structured light technique projects the coded pattern onto the object and substitutes one camera in the stereovision with a projector [19]. Consequently, the correspondence problem becomes a decoding problem, and we can determine the correspondences between the acquired image and the original known coded pattern. Many light patterns are proposed for 3D surface reconstruction in the

last decades [20, 21]. The design and realization of a new endoscopic device by means of a robust structured light coding are presented in [4]. However, the coded pattern employed in [4] is not commercially available and is not easy to be implemented for clinical use.

Since we mainly consider minimally invasive image guided procedures, one major criterion of selecting light patterns is easy implementation. In this study, we select the gridline light pattern, which can be easily generated by a commercial projector or a special device. However, this choice of light pattern poses a great challenge for matching feature points (i.e., intersections) of gridlines due to symmetry and similar features of gridline points. Conventional methods [22, 23] such as SIFT cannot be employed effectively for surface reconstruction in our study. Based on the specific characteristics of the gridline light pattern in this paper, we adopt a new method for robust feature detection and matching.

In this study, we have proposed to use dedicated gridline light patterns to create noninvasive artificial features on the tissue surface, which is then used to robustly reconstruct 3D surface from stereo endoscopic images. This is a robust 3D surface reconstruction technique for procedures involving soft tissue organs especially with few surface features. Another feature of the proposed system is the use of a stereo endoscope for 3D surface reconstruction. The major advantage of using stereo endoscope is that it can acquire two synchronized images simultaneously, which provides necessary information for 3D surface reconstruction and eliminates the challenging temporal synchronization problem inherently with mono endoscope for moving deformable targets. The stereo endoscope not only provides two synchronized images at the same time but also reduces intra-operative image acquisition time and eliminates unnecessary motion of mono endoscope to acquire two images at different poses which is required for robust 3D surface reconstruction.

Effective and good display of virtual reality (VR) is an important factor for clinicians to accept and support the multimodality image guidance system in the clinical environment. It is still an active research topic as to how to present and fuse real images with patient-specific preoperative images and models in an optimal way so that they register correctly in the physician's brain. Stereo display is one effective way to present the information to physicians. Some 3D video stereo monitors do not require a separate apparatus such as synch box, ZScreen, or active glasses. In order to effectively use our stereo endoscope, we still need 3D glasses in the current configuration; however, it would be more convenient for physicians to watch 3D video stereo monitor without glasses. Fused anatomy and models can provide physicians with more information where all supporting information becomes available. Multiple monitors can be used to display different information separately. For example, the first monitor can display real-time video stereo endoscopic images, while a second monitor is used to display the fused images/models. Thus in challenging scenarios, doctors can selectively watch different monitors to acquire needed information including surgical plans and other critical structures such as tumors and blood vessels without interference from unnecessary information.

6. Conclusion

In this study, we proposed a novel approach to match stereo endoscopic images and MR images. The proposed surface-based registration has proved to be an effective method for registering these images of different imaging mechanisms. Moreover, the light patterns of the gridlines facilitated the surface reconstruction of surgical sites with few surface features. In this paper, we validated the proposed method with static objects; however, our method has the potential to be extended to procedures involving moving organs.

We have demonstrated the effectiveness of our technique in registration of the reconstructed surface with the surface extracted from MR images of a liver phantom. We have shown that various image processing techniques we used before the image registration have a significant impact on the resulting registration accuracy. We have achieved a surface registration accuracy of 0.76 ± 0.11 mm. The proposed technique has the potential to be used in clinical practice to improve image guidance in endoscope based minimally invasive procedures. The fused image guidance may also be applied to the endoscopic procedures of other organs in the abdomen, chest cavity, and pelvis such as the kidneys and the lungs.

Future work includes integration of our method into the clinical image guidance system and further validation by animal study and clinical study.

Acknowledgments

The authors would like to thank Dr. James Drake, Thomas Looi, and other members at CIGITI in the Hospital for Sick Children for the valuable assistance and support.

References

[1] M. Baumhauer, M. Feuerstein, H.-P. Meinzer, and J. Rassweiler, "Navigation in endoscopic soft tissue surgery: perspectives and limitations," *Journal of Endourology*, vol. 22, no. 4, pp. 751–766, 2008.

[2] M. Sonka, V. Hlavac, and B. Roger, *Image Processing Analysis and Machine Vision*, 3rd edition, 2008.

[3] J. L. Prince and J. M. Links, *Medical Imaging Signals and Systems*, Printice Hall, Upper Saddle River, New Jersey, NJ, USA, 2006.

[4] X. Maurice, C. Albitar, C. Doignon, and M. De Mathelin, "A structured light-based laparoscope with real-time organs' surface reconstruction for minimally invasive surgery," in *Proceedings of the Annual International Conference of the IEEE Engineering in Medicine and Biology Society (EMBC '12)*, pp. 5769–55772, 2012.

[5] M. Feuerstein, T. Mussack, S. M. Heining, and N. Navab, "Intraoperative laparoscope augmentation for port placement and resection planning in minimally invasive liver resection," *IEEE Transactions on Medical Imaging*, vol. 27, no. 3, pp. 355–369, 2008.

[6] V. Bevilacqua, S. Cambo, L. Cariello, and G. Mastronardi, "A combined method to detect retinal fundus features," in *European Conference on Emergent Aspects In Clinical Data Analysis*, pp. 1–6, Pisa, Italy, 2005.

[7] J. Y. Bouguet, Camera Calibration Toolbox for Matlab, http://www.vision.caltech.edu/bouguetj, 2010.

[8] D. Dey, D. G. Gobbi, P. J. Slomka, K. J. M. Surry, and T. M. Peters, "Automatic fusion of freehand endoscopic brain images to three-dimensional surfaces: creating stereoscopic panoramas," *IEEE Transactions on Medical Imaging*, vol. 21, no. 1, pp. 23–30, 2002.

[9] P. J. Besl and N. D. McKay, "A method for registration of 3-D shapes," *IEEE Transactions on Pattern Analysis and Machine Intelligence*, vol. 14, no. 2, pp. 239–256, 1992.

[10] L. W. Clements, W. C. Chapman, B. M. Dawant, R. L. Galloway Jr., and M. I. Miga, "Robust surface registration using salient

anatomical features for image-guided liver surgery: algorithm and validation," *Medical Physics*, vol. 35, no. 6, pp. 2528–2540, 2008.

[11] L. Maier-Hein, M. Schmidt, A. M. Franz et al., "Accounting for anisotropic noise in fine registration of time-of-flight range data with high-resolution surface data," *Medical Image Computing and Computer-Assisted Intervention*, vol. 6361, no. 1, pp. 251–258, 2010.

[12] A. Groch, A. Seitel, S. Hempel et al., "3D surface reconstruction for laparo-scopic computer-assisted interventions: comparison of state-of-the-art methods," in *Proceedings of the Medical Imaging 2011: Visualization, Image-Guided Procedures, and Modeling*, vol. 7964, 2011.

[13] M. Hayashibe, N. Suzuki, and Y. Nakamura, "Laser-scan endoscope system for intraoperative geometry acquisition and surgical robot safety management," *Medical Image Analysis*, vol. 10, no. 4, pp. 509–519, 2006.

[14] M. Proesmans, L. J. Van Gool, and A. J. Oosterlinck, "Active acquisition of 3D shape for moving objects," in *Proceedings of the IEEE International Conference on Image Processing (ICIP '96)*, pp. 647–650, September 1996.

[15] M. Hu, G. Penney, P. Edwards, and D. Hawkes, "3D reconstruction of internal organ surfaces for minimal invasive surgery," in *International Conference on Medical Image Computing and Computer-Assisted Intervention*, pp. 68–77, Brisbane, Australia, 2007.

[16] W. W. Lau, N. A. Ramey, J. J. Corso, N. V. Thakor, and G. D. Hager, "Stereo-based endoscopie tracking of cardiac surface deformation," in *Proceedings of the 7th International Conference on Medical Image Computing and Computer-Assisted Intervention (MICCAI 2004)*, pp. 494–501, St Malo, France, September 2004.

[17] D. Stoyanov, A. Darzi, and G. Z. Yang, "Dense 3D depth recovery for soft tissue deformation during robotically assisted laparoscopic surgery," in *Proceedings of the 7th International Conference Medical Image Computing and Computer-Assisted Intervention (MICCAI '04)*, pp. 41–48, St Malo, France, September 2004.

[18] M. Hayashibe, N. Suzuki, and Y. Nakamura, "Laser-scan endoscope system for intraoperative geometry acquisition and surgical robot safety management," *Medical Image Analysis*, vol. 10, no. 4, pp. 509–519, 2006.

[19] J. Salvi, J. Pagès, and J. Batlle, "Pattern codification strategies in structured light systems," *Pattern Recognition*, vol. 37, no. 4, pp. 827–849, 2004.

[20] A. Bhatti, *Current Advancements in Stereo Vision*, InTech, 2012.

[21] J. Salvi, S. Fernandez, T. Pribanic, and X. Llado, "A state of the art in structured light patterns for surface profilometry," *Pattern Recognition*, vol. 43, no. 8, pp. 2666–2680, 2010.

[22] P. Mountney, D. Stoyanov, and G.-Z. Yang, "Three-dimensional tissue deformation recovery and tracking," *IEEE Signal Processing Magazine*, vol. 27, no. 4, pp. 14–24, 2010.

[23] D. G. Lowe, "Distinctive image features from scale-invariant keypoints," *International Journal of Computer Vision*, vol. 60, no. 2, pp. 91–110, 2004.

16

Classifying Dementia Using Local Binary Patterns from Different Regions in Magnetic Resonance Images

Ketil Oppedal,[1,2] Trygve Eftestøl,[1] Kjersti Engan,[1] Mona K. Beyer,[3,4] and Dag Aarsland[2,5]

[1]Department of Electrical Engineering and Computer Science, University of Stavanger, 4036 Stavanger, Norway
[2]Centre for Age-Related Medicine, Stavanger University Hospital, Stavanger, Norway
[3]Department of Radiology and Nuclear Medicine, Oslo University Hospital, Oslo, Norway
[4]Department of Life Sciences and Health, Faculty of Health Sciences, Oslo and Akershus University College of Applied Sciences, Oslo, Norway
[5]Alzheimer's Disease Research Centre, Karolinska Institutet (KI), Stockholm, Sweden

Correspondence should be addressed to Ketil Oppedal; ketil.oppedal@gmail.com

Academic Editor: Yantian Zhang

Dementia is an evolving challenge in society, and no disease-modifying treatment exists. Diagnosis can be demanding and MR imaging may aid as a noninvasive method to increase prediction accuracy. We explored the use of 2D local binary pattern (LBP) extracted from FLAIR and T1 MR images of the brain combined with a Random Forest classifier in an attempt to discern patients with Alzheimer's disease (AD), Lewy body dementia (LBD), and normal controls (NC). Analysis was conducted in areas with white matter lesions (WML) and all of white matter (WM). Results from 10-fold nested cross validation are reported as mean accuracy, precision, and recall with standard deviation in brackets. The best result we achieved was in the two-class problem NC versus AD + LBD with total accuracy of 0.98 (0.04). In the three-class problem AD versus LBD versus NC and the two-class problem AD versus LBD, we achieved 0.87 (0.08) and 0.74 (0.16), respectively. The performance using 3DT1 images was notably better than when using FLAIR images. The results from the WM region gave similar results as in the WML region. Our study demonstrates that LBP texture analysis in brain MR images can be successfully used for computer based dementia diagnosis.

1. Introduction

Dementia Is an Evolving Challenge. As a result of increasing age, dementia is an evolving challenge in society. The annual health care costs related to dementia were estimated to $604 billion worldwide in 2010 [1]. Alzheimer's disease (AD) is the most common neurodegenerative dementia and accounts for 50–60% of people with dementia [2]. The classical neuropathological signs of AD are amyloid plaques and neurofibrillary tangles [3]. No efficient disease-modifying treatment for AD exists today. Dementia with Lewy-bodies (DLB) together with dementia associated with Parkinson's disease (PDD) account for 15–20% of people with dementia [2]. The defining pathological feature for these patients is Lewy-body degeneration in brain stem, forebrain, and limbic and cortical structures, and the DLB and PDD are therefore often combined into a Lewy-body dementia group (LBD) [4, 5]. However, the relationship between localization and density of Lewy-bodies with clinical dementia symptoms is not strong [6], suggesting that other pathologies contribute as well, such as AD pathology and vascular brain changes seen as white matter hyperintensities (WML) or lacunar infarcts, which may contribute to the clinical presentation of LBD. For example, vascular changes in the basal ganglia are common in the elderly and may cause parkinsonism and cognitive impairment [7].

Early Diagnosis Is Important. AD and LBD are very complex diseases making them difficult to be prevented, delayed, or cured. Current therapy focuses on many approaches, for example, helping patients maintain an acceptable mental functioning, managing typical behavioural changes, and slowing symptom progression. Early intervention is important, and the ability to identify these types of dementia and healthy controls early in the disease course may be essential for successful patient care. Differentiating between

AD and LBD is also important since they differ in prognosis and response to drug treatment. Currently, the only available method to differentiate between AD and LBD is the dopamine transporter scan, which is expensive and not readily available at all centres.

Neuroimaging in Dementia. Neuroimaging is an important tool for studying dementia and cognitive deterioration. Several excellent reviews are available [8–10]. In [11], Malloy et al. review available methods for quantitative imaging of white matter anatomy and pathology as well as recent findings in ageing and dementia. They state that computer aided quantification offers better statistical power compared to visual rating scales and that diffusion imaging is able to detect abnormalities not recognised in conventional acquisition sequences. Early detection of disease and relevant functional connections between brain areas are important benefits.

Computer Aided Diagnosis in Dementia. Computer aided diagnosis (CAD) can be a helpful tool to pinpoint diagnosis early in the disease course in a cost-effective manner and unbiased to human inconsistencies [12]. Recent advances in the field have focused especially on AD and patients with mild cognitive impairment (MCI), which are considered a precursor to AD [13–16]. Less attention has been put into developing CAD systems for LBD. As mentioned above, LBD have high prevalence, and accurate clinical diagnosis depends on little available and expensive dopamine transporter scan and postmortem histology. Few papers report high accuracy discerning patients with AD and LBD or other dementias [17, 18]. A promising approach is reported in [19] where Lebedev et al. use sparse partial least squares (SPLS) classification of cortical thickness measurements reporting a sensitivity of 94.4 and a specificity of 88.89 discerning AD from LBD.

White Matter and White Matter Lesions in Dementia. White matter (WM) comprises approximately half the brain volume and provides connectivity between the two brain hemispheres as well as ensuring efficient transfer of neural activity complementing information processing in the gray matter (GM). WM neuropathology is often diffuse and affects many neuronal networks which can be disturbed simultaneously resulting in a multidomain syndrome. In [20], Filley emphasizes the contribution of white matter disease (WMD) in mild cognitive dysfunction, cognitive ageing, and dementia. Bartzokis [21] proposes a hypothesis for AD called the *"myelin model"* where axonal transport disruption, formation of axonal swellings, neuritic plaques, and proteinaceous deposits such as Aβ and tau are by-products of homeostatic myelin repair processes. Gunning-Dixon et al. [22] review results of MRI studies of white matter changes that occur with normal ageing and the relationship of age-associated changes in white matter to age-related declines in cognitive abilities.

White matter lesions or white matter hyperintensities (WML) are among the neuroimaging expressions of cerebral small-vessel disease and are associated with various disturbances with poor prognosis [23]. WML are localized areas of increased signal intensities in the white matter of the brain visible on T2-weighted MR images. The underlying pathology of WML is heterogeneous, ranging from mild demyelination to incomplete subcortical infarctions. They are typically seen around the ventricles (periventricular WML), but also as focal lesions in the deep white matter. In the elderly, WML usually represent small-vessel cerebrovascular disease (CVD) [24]. WML becomes more abundant with increasing age in healthy subjects [25], but they are also found to be associated with AD [26] and other dementias [27, 28]. Clinical symptoms associated with WML include gait disturbances [29], depression [27, 30], and cognitive impairment [31], although the exact mechanisms are not fully understood. In [32], Tuladhar et al. concludes that cortical changes mediated by WML and vascular risk factors might lead to cognitive decline and dementia. Muñoz Maniega et al. [33] write that age-related deterioration of normal appearing white matter (NAWM) is strongly associated with the severity of WML, indicating that WML is important in dementia research. Fujishima et al. conclude in [34] that mild cognitive impairment, poor episodic memory, and late-life depression are associated with cerebral cortical thinning and WML.

Texture Analysis in Neuroimaging. Harrison [35] extensively reviews the use of texture analysis in a clinical context, analysing MR images in non-Hodgkin lymphoma, mild traumatic brain injury, and multiple sclerosis. She concludes that "non visible lesions and physiological changes as well as visible focal lesions of different aetiologies could be detected and characterized by texture analysis of routine clinical 1.5 Tesla scans." The application of texture analysis in a machine learning (ML) environment has shown success in discerning different dementias from each other and from healthy controls. Freeborough and Fox reported a classification rate of 91% discerning AD from healthy controls using measures from a spatial gray-level dependent method applied in a stepwise discriminant analysis approach in [36]. de Olivieira et al. [37] found statistical significant differences in gray level cooccurrence matrix measurements in subjects with mild AD, amnestic mild cognitive impairment (aMCI), and healthy controls. Zhang et al. [38] performed 3D texture analysis in MR images of the hippocampus and entorhinal cortex in AD patients and achieved a classification accuracy between 64.3% and 96.4%. Sivapriya et al. showed in [39] that texture analysis in brain MRI gave high classification accuracy in AD. As of the authors knowledge, the only paper considering texture analysis as an approach to distinguish AD, LBD, and NC is [40], where Kodama and Kawase performed discriminant analysis on features extracted from a cooccurrence matrix and a run-length matrix with an accuracy of 91.7%, 70.0%, and 88.0%, respectively.

Local binary pattern (LBP) was introduced by Ojala et al. [41, 42] as a texture descriptor. It is a simple yet very efficient texture operator which labels the pixels of an image by thresholding the neighbourhood of each pixel and considers the result as a binary number. Unay et al. [43] showed that the rotation invariant LBP is invariant to some common MRI artefacts which makes it a robust texture feature when used in brain MR image analysis.

Aims. We have earlier shown that there were no differences in WML volume between patients with AD and LBD or between a combined dementia group (AD + LBD) and healthy controls in the DemVest study [44]. Now we want to test if the WML regions inherit textural information in an extent that can be used to classify dementia patients from normal controls and AD from LBD. As the detection of textural information in WML might not be dependent on an exact delineation of WML, we also want to test if a comparable classification accuracy can be achieved using all of WM as ROI, since WM segmentation is more available and only a 3DT1 MR image is needed which is commonly acquired in a clinical setting.

Earlier we have shown that using LBP texture analysis in WML regions in FLAIR MR images in a machine learning (ML) context can discern patients with dementia from healthy controls with high accuracy [45]. We want to test different types of LBP calculations together with a contrast measure (C) calculated from FLAIR and 3DT1 MR images from a cohort study (the DemWest and ParkWest study) and on a subset containing data from one scanner only.

Because of the challenging situation with imbalanced data having different numbers of subjects in the represented groups in the abovementioned cohorts, we want to test how the use of resampling of instances affects classification results.

Organisation of Paper. The paper is organised as follows: Section 2 describes the data material, Section 3 describes the image preprocessing procedures followed by Section 4 which describes the image processing methods and Section 5 describing the experimental setup. Section 6 reveals the results. Section 7 discusses the results and ends the paper with a conclusion.

2. Material

2.1. Subjects. MR images of dementia subjects included in this study were drawn from the DemWest cohort, Stavanger, Norway, and MR images of the healthy controls from the ParkWest cohort, Stavanger, Norway. Inclusion and exclusion criteria can be found in [2] and [46], respectively. The dementia and healthy control subjects were matched for sex, age, and years of education.

The Regional Committee for Medical Research Ethics, Western Norway, approved the study. All participants signed informed consent to participate in the study after the study procedures had been explained in detail to the patient and a caregiver, usually the spouse or offspring.

2.2. MRI. The dementia patients were scanned at three different sites: Stavanger University Hospital, Stavanger, Norway, Haugesund Hospital, Haugesund, Norway, and Haraldsplass Deaconess Hospital, Bergen, Norway. A 1.5 T scanner was used in all three centres (Philips Intera in Stavanger and Haugesund and GE Signa Excite in Bergen), using the same scanner in each centre during the entire study period and a common study imaging protocol.

The NCs were scanned at four different sites. They were scanned on the same scanners as the patients in Stavanger and Haugesund. Additionally MR images of NC subjects were acquired from Sørlandet Hospital Arendal, Arendal, Norway (1.0T Philips Intera), and Unilabs, Bergen, Norway (1.5T Siemens Symphony).

After visual inspection, some patient scans were excluded due to either insufficient image quality, not having both FLAIR and T1 images for the patient, or movement and other artefacts.

A total of 73 mild dementia subjects, 57 with AD and 16 with LBD, had MRI scans of sufficient quality and were included in this study as well as 36 healthy controls. In [44], further clinical details as well as MR imaging parameters can be found.

To ensure high reliability between scans acquired at different centres and at different time points, three volunteers were scanned at all centres using the same scanners and protocols. Details of the procedure can be found in [44]. Cronbachs alpha between MR scanners at different centres was calculated based on total brain volume and was reported to be 0.958. Cronbachs alpha between two time points varied between 0.982 and 0.995, indicating excellent reliabilities both between centres and between different time points. Similar results were reported for the MR images of the NCs from the ParkWest study.

3. Image Preprocessing

3.1. Region of Interest Extraction. Two common approaches for MR image segmentation of the brain are tissue classification and template registration. In the tissue classification approach, voxels are assigned to a class based on the class voxel intensity distribution. In the template registration approach, a template image with predefined classes is warped to the actual MR image. In our study, WM partitions were segmented using the common functions in SPM8 on the T1 images. The procedure unifies a tissue segmentation approach with a template registration method; see [47] for further details.

WML segmentation was performed according to a method developed and previously published by Firbank et al. in Newcastle, England [48]. The method is based on determining a threshold value from the image gray scale intensity values and then classifying the hyperintense voxels as WML. Briefly, the nonbrain regions were removed from the T1 image, using the segmentation routines in the software package SPM5 [49]. After transforming to the image space of the FLAIR image, the segmented T1 image was used as a mask for scull stripping of the FLAIR image. Then the WML were segmented automatically on a slice-by-slice basis from the FLAIR images with the images in native space. A scale factor determined experimentally was multiplied by the mode of the histogram of pixel intensities for each image slice and used as a threshold value for WML segmentation. To explore the regional distribution of WML throughout the brain, a region of interest (ROI) template in standard MNI space [50] was used. This ROI template was transformed from MNI space to the image space (FLAIR) of each subject by use of the normalization routines in SPM5, and the volumes of WML in each ROI were calculated. The ROI map was based on the Brodmann template. Further details can be found in [51].

Because of the variability in MR image quality acquired from the different centres participating in this study, a scale factor that gave an overestimation of the lesion load in every subject was selected, and manual editing was then done to correct this by removing excess pixels using FSLView [52], a medical image-editing program being a part of the FSL software bundle. A medical doctor did the manual editing after training by a consultant radiologist who is experienced at evaluation of WML. We performed inter- and intrarater reliability testing between the two raters to ensure good quality. They both edited the same 10 data sets twice: once in the beginning to ensure good interrater reliability and a second time at the end to ensure that similar reliability still persisted and to evaluate intrarater reliability. Intraclass correlation coefficient (ICC) was 0.998 for interrater reliability and 0.964 for intrarater reliability.

4. Image Processing Methods

4.1. LBP. Ojala et al. [41, 42] introduced LBP as a texture operator. Since its discriminative power is high and at the same time computationally simple, LBP is a popular texture descriptor used in various applications and unifies traditionally divergent statistical and structural models of texture analysis. Adding an image contrast measure (C) calculating the local variance in the pixel neighbourhood, as well as varying the texture neighbourhood, enhances the discriminative power of the LBP feature even further. In [43], Unay et al. demonstrated that the rotation invariant LBP is invariant to some common MRI artefacts, that is, the bias field.

The derivation of the gray scale and rotation invariant texture operator LBP starts by defining texture T in a local neighbourhood of a monochrome texture image as the joint distribution of the gray levels of P ($P > 1$) image pixels:

$$T = t\left(g_c, g_0, \ldots, g_{P-1}\right),\qquad(1)$$

where gray value g_c corresponds to the gray value of the center pixel of the local neighbourhood and g_p ($p = 0, \ldots, P-1$) corresponds to the gray value of P equally spaced pixels on a circle of radius R ($R > 0$) that form a circularly symmetric neighbour set. When the coordinates of g_c are $(0,0)$, the coordinates of g_p are given by $(-R\sin(2\pi p/P), R\cos(2\pi p/P))$ and the gray values of neighbours which do not fall exactly in the center of pixels are estimated by interpolation.

To achieve gray-scale invariance, the gray value of the center pixel (g_c) is subtracted from the gray values of the circular symmetric neighbourhood g_p ($p = 0, \ldots, P-1$), giving

$$T = t\left(g_c, g_0 - g_c, g_1 - g_c, \ldots, g_{P-1} - g_c\right).\qquad(2)$$

By assuming that differences $g_p - g_c$ are independent of g_c and thereby factorizing, we get

$$T \approx t\left(g_c\right) t\left(g_0 - g_c, g_1 - g_c, \ldots, g_{P-1} - g_c\right).\qquad(3)$$

The distribution $t(g_c)$ describes the overall luminance of the image and is unrelated to local image texture and is removed. The approximated distribution

$$T \approx t\left(g_0 - g_c, g_1 - g_c, \ldots, g_{P-1} - g_c\right)\qquad(4)$$

conveys many of the textural characteristics from the original.

By considering just the signs of the differences instead of their exact values, invariance with respect to gray-scale shifts is achieved:

$$T \approx t\left(s\left(g_0 - g_c\right), s\left(g_1 - g_c\right), \ldots, s\left(g_{P-1} - g_c\right)\right),\qquad(5)$$

where

$$s(x) = \begin{cases} 1, & x \geq 0 \\ 0, & x < 0. \end{cases}\qquad(6)$$

Each sign $s(g_p - g_c)$ is assigned a binomial factor 2^p, such that T is transformed into a unique $\mathrm{LBP}_{P,R}$ number that characterizes the spatial structure of the local image texture:

$$\mathrm{LBP}_{P,R} = \sum_{p=0}^{P-1} s\left(g_p - g_c\right) 2^P.\qquad(7)$$

See also Figure 1.

To assign a unique identifier to each rotation invariant local binary pattern, $\mathrm{LBP}_{P,R}^{ri}$ is defined as

$$\mathrm{LBP}_{P,R}^{ri} = \min\left\{\mathrm{ROR}\left(\mathrm{LBP}_{P,R}, i\right) \mid i = 0, 1, \ldots, P-1\right\},\qquad(8)$$

where $\mathrm{ROR}(x, i)$ performs a circular bitwise right shift on the P-bit number x i times.

Certain local binary patterns are fundamental properties of texture. "Uniform" patterns are circular structures that contain very few spatial transitions. They function as templates for microstructures such as bright spot, flat area, dark spot, and edges of varying positive and negative curvature. The uniformity relates to the number of spatial transitions (i.e., bitwise 0/1 changes) in the LBP pattern; for example, 00000000_2 and 11111111_2 have a uniformity value $U(\text{"pattern"})$ of 0 and 00000011_2 and 10000111_2 of 1 and 2, respectively. Patterns that have a U value of at most 2 are designated as "uniform." A gray-scale, rotation invariant, and uniform LBP texture operator are defined as follows:

$$\mathrm{LBP}_{P,R}^{riu2} = \begin{cases} \displaystyle\sum_{p=0}^{P-1} s\left(g_p - g_c\right), & \text{if } U\left(\mathrm{LBP}_{P,R}\right) \leq 2, \\ P + 1, & \text{otherwise,} \end{cases}\qquad(9)$$

where

$$U\left(\mathrm{LBP}_{P,R}\right) = \left|s\left(g_{P-1} - g_c\right) - s\left(g_0 - g_c\right)\right| + \sum_{p=1}^{P-1}\left|s\left(g_p - g_c\right) - s\left(g_{p-1} - g_c\right)\right|.\qquad(10)$$

Superscript *riu2* reflects the use of rotation invariant "uniform" patterns that have a U value of at most 2. By definition, exactly $P + 1$ "uniform" binary patterns can occur in a circularly symmetric neighbour set of P pixels whereas the "nonuniform" patterns are grouped under a miscellaneous label ($P + 1$).

4.2. Contrast. The $\mathrm{LBP}_{P,R}^{ri}$ and $\mathrm{LBP}_{P,R}^{riu2}$ operators are excellent measures of spatial patterns but discard contrast. If gray-scale invariance is not required, the contrast (C) of local image

The value of the LBP code of a pixel (x_c, y_c) is given by

$$LBP_{P,R} = \sum_{p=0}^{P-1} s(g_p - g_c)2^p \qquad\qquad s(x) = \begin{cases} 1, & \text{if } x \geqslant 0; \\ 0, & \text{otherwise.} \end{cases}$$

Sample   Threshold

$$x = 1*2^0 + 1*2^1 + 0*2^2 + 0*2^3 + 0*2^4 + 1*2^5 + 0*2^6 + 1*2^7 = 163$$

Multiply by powers of two and sum

(a)

(b)

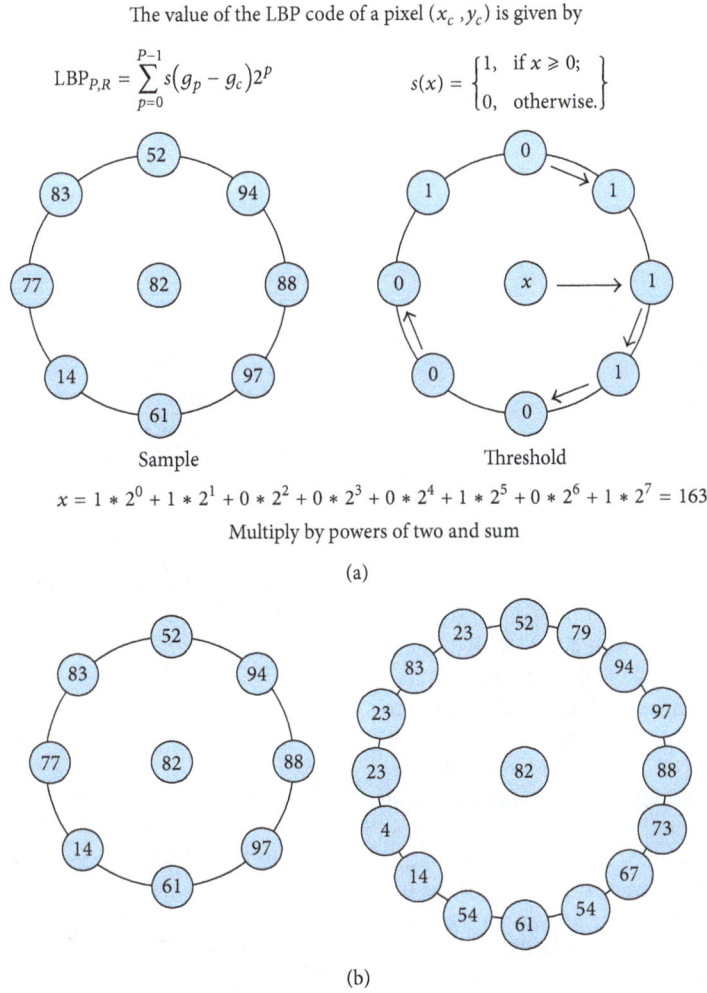

FIGURE 1: (a) Demonstrates LBP thresholding. A neighbour to a center pixel is set to one if it has equal or higher pixel value and zero if it has lower pixel value. In an anticlockwise manner, every neighbour is multiplied by powers of two and summed as demonstrated in (9). (b) demonstrates how the radius and number of samples can be varied in the choice of neighbourhood. (b) Left figure with small radius and 8 samples. Right figure with large radius and 16 samples.

texture can be measured with a rotation invariant measure of local variance defined as

$$VAR_{P,R} = \frac{1}{P}\sum_{p=0}^{P-1}(g_p - \mu)^2, \quad \text{where } \mu = \frac{1}{P}\sum_{p=0}^{P-1}g_p, \qquad (11)$$

which is invariant against shifts in gray-scale.

The LBP and C values are calculated for every voxel in the specified region of interest creating an LBP- and a C-valued image. Typically, the LBP and C values are collected and represented as a histogram for each instance in the data set. The histogram can be used as a vector of features. Other approaches include calculating new features from the histogram.

5. Proposed Method and Experimental Setup

5.1. Overview of Proposed Method. A computer based system for classification of AD, LBD, and healthy controls based on texture analysis was applied. Firstly, the two regions of

interest, WML and WM, were extracted from the MR images. The WM regions were segmented using common functions in SPM8 and the WML were segmented from the FLAIR images using the thresholding technique proposed by Firbank et al. [48], as briefly described in Section 3.1. See also Block 1 in Figure 2.

Secondly, rotation invariant 2D LBP and contrast were extracted voxel-wise for the two different ROIs using different combinations of neighbourhood radii and number of samples. The 2D LBP and contrast texture analysis were done both on the FLAIR and the T1 MR images (see Section 4.1 for information concerning the calculation of the LBP texture feature and Section 4.2 for the contrast measure and Block 2 of Figure 2). Statistical features were calculated from all the LBP and C values in each ROI were then calculated.

Eventually, a combined feature selection and classification procedure were applied using a Random Forest [53] classifier together with a nested cross validation procedure [54]. See Block 3 in Figure 2.

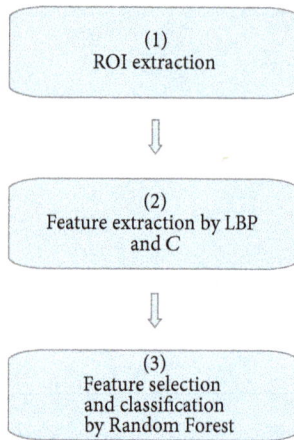

FIGURE 2: Overview of proposed method. See Section 5.1 for details.

TABLE 1

	Actual positive	Actual negative
Predicted positive	TP	FP
Predicted negative	FN	TN

5.2. Texture Feature Extraction. For the 2D texture analysis approach, the LBP values as well as the C measure were calculated from every voxel in the selected ROI and MR image type for all subjects in the data set using Matlab [55]. Three different combinations of neighbourhood radius (R) and number of samples (P), namely, $R = 1$ and $P = 8$, $R = 2$ and $P = 12$, and $R = 4$ and $P = 16$, were used. Mean, standard deviation, variation, median, interquartile range, entropy, skewness, and kurtosis of the ROI-wise collected LBP and C values were calculated to be used as a descriptor of the distributions of the LBP and C values. These features were subjected to further selection and classification resulting in 8 features for each of the three combinations of R and P for both LBP and C resulting in a total of 48 features for each subject. See Figure 3 for an example of the FLAIR and T1 MR images and the WML segmentation results. See also Figure 4 for an example of LBP- and C-valued images based on the FLAIR and T1 MR images.

5.3. Feature Selection and Classification. A challenge in the developed machine learning task was the high number of features calculated compared to the size of the data set. Since the data were collected in a cohort study and thereby inexpedient to expand, a method for feature subset selection was needed. A method combining feature selection and classification using two nested cross validation loops together with a Random Forest classifier was chosen: an inner CV scheme for classification parameter and feature selection and an outer CV scheme for final model testing; see Figure 5 for details. Such an approach prevents the improper procedure of using the complete data set for supervised feature selection ahead of using cross validation for performance evaluation. The latter approach would give an overly optimistic result.

Image data were selected with stratification during bootstrap rounds in the cross validation procedure, meaning that the relative representation of instances in each class was kept intact.

Feature selection and classification were done using a 10-tree Random Forest classifier and 10-fold nested cross validation for performance evaluation. Search method was *best first*, start set with *no attributes*, search direction *forward*,

stale search *after five node expansions*, subset evaluation *f-measure*, and number of folds for accuracy estimation was *10*.

Pretesting was done using different classifiers, including support vector machines, Random Forests, and a Bayesian network classifier. The Random Forest classifier outperformed the other classifiers, and thus all experiments presented in this work are conducted using Random Forest classifiers.

To give a fairly acceptable graphic display of the selected features, the feature and model parameter selection were eventually performed on the complete data set and a matrix of scatter plots displaying the five selected features pairwise against each other was made; see Figure 6. Note that this was only done for the sake of practical graphical display and as an example of which features that typically would be selected.

Random Forest is a classifier based on ensembles of decision trees developed by Breiman [53]. Many decision trees are built using bootstrap aggregation (bagging) and randomized feature subset sampling where the mode of the classes output by individual trees is voted for.

Three separate tests were explored: a three-class approach classifying NC versus AD versus LBD, a two-class approach classifying a NC versus a combined dementia group (AD + LBD), and another two-class approach classifying AD versus LBD.

5.4. Classification Accuracy. Precision for a class is the fraction of instances that are correctly classified to all instances that are classified as this class and is also known as positive predictive value. Recall for a class is the fraction of instances that are correctly classified to all the instances that really belong to this class and is also known as true positive rate or sensitivity.

In the context of a two-class problem where one class is the positive class and the other is the negative class, the true positives (TP) are the instances that are correctly classified as belonging to the positive class and the false positives (FP) are the instances that are classified as the positive class but really belong to the negative class. The true negatives (TN) and false negatives (FN) can be explained similarly. An overview of results can be presented as a confusion matrix, see Table 1.

Precision is then defined as Precision = TP/(TP+FP) and recall is defined as Recall = TP/(TP + FN). Total accuracy (T), precision (P), and recall (R) were calculated for each of the ten folds in the cross validation procedure resulting in ten values for each ($T_1, T_2, \ldots, T_{10}$), ($P_1, P_2, \ldots, P_{10}$), and ($R_1, R_2, \ldots, R_{10}$). Empirical mean over the ten values was calculated using the equation below:

$$m_x = \frac{1}{n}\sum_{k=1}^{n} x_k, \quad \text{where } 0 \le x_k \le 1, \ 0 \le m_x \le 1, \quad (12)$$

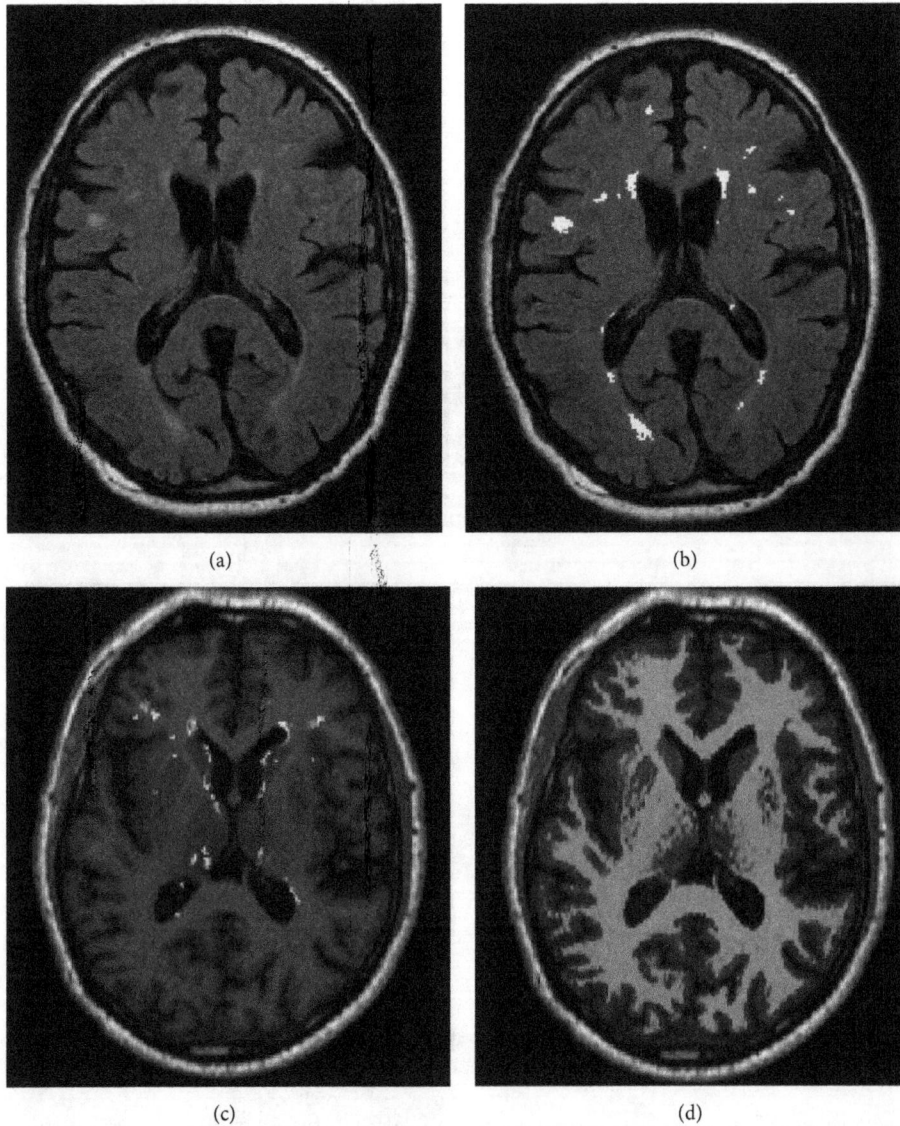

FIGURE 3: Overview of MR images and the ROIs used for feature extraction. (a) in the top left corner shows an example of an axial FLAIR MR image. The white matter lesions are possible to see as hyperintense areas. (b) in the top right shows the segmented voxels labelled as WML overlayed on the FLAIR MR image seen in (a). (c) in the bottom left corner shows the segmented WML voxels, found from the corresponding FLAIR, overlayed on the T1 MR image. (d) in the bottom right corner shows the segmented WM voxels overlayed on the T1 MR image.

where x is either T, P, or R and $n = 10$. The empirical standard deviation was calculated as below:

$$s_x = \left(\frac{1}{n-1} \sum_{k=1}^{n} \left(x_k - m_{x,k} \right)^2 \right)^{1/2}$$

$$\text{where } 0 \le x_k \le 1, \quad 0 \le s_x \le 1,$$

(13)

where x is either T, P, or R, $n = 10$, and m_x is defined as in (12). T, P, and R are reported as $m(s)$ over 10-fold CV.

5.5. Imbalanced Data Set. The data set used in this study was drawn from a cohort. A common drawback is the problem of imbalanced data, meaning that the data set contains groups of different sizes. Typically, machine learning algorithms will perform poorly under such circumstances. As a measure to prevent such a problem, a resampling technique was used to even out the sizes of the groups.

All tests were done using the Synthetic Minority Over-sampling Technique (SMOTE) [56, 57] to resample data, such that all classes had the same number of instances and are similar to the largest class in the original data. Similar tests were done without resampling as well, and, in all of the cases, the classification accuracy for the LBD class improved using SMOTE at the expense of classification accuracy for the other classes. Total accuracy was either improved or at

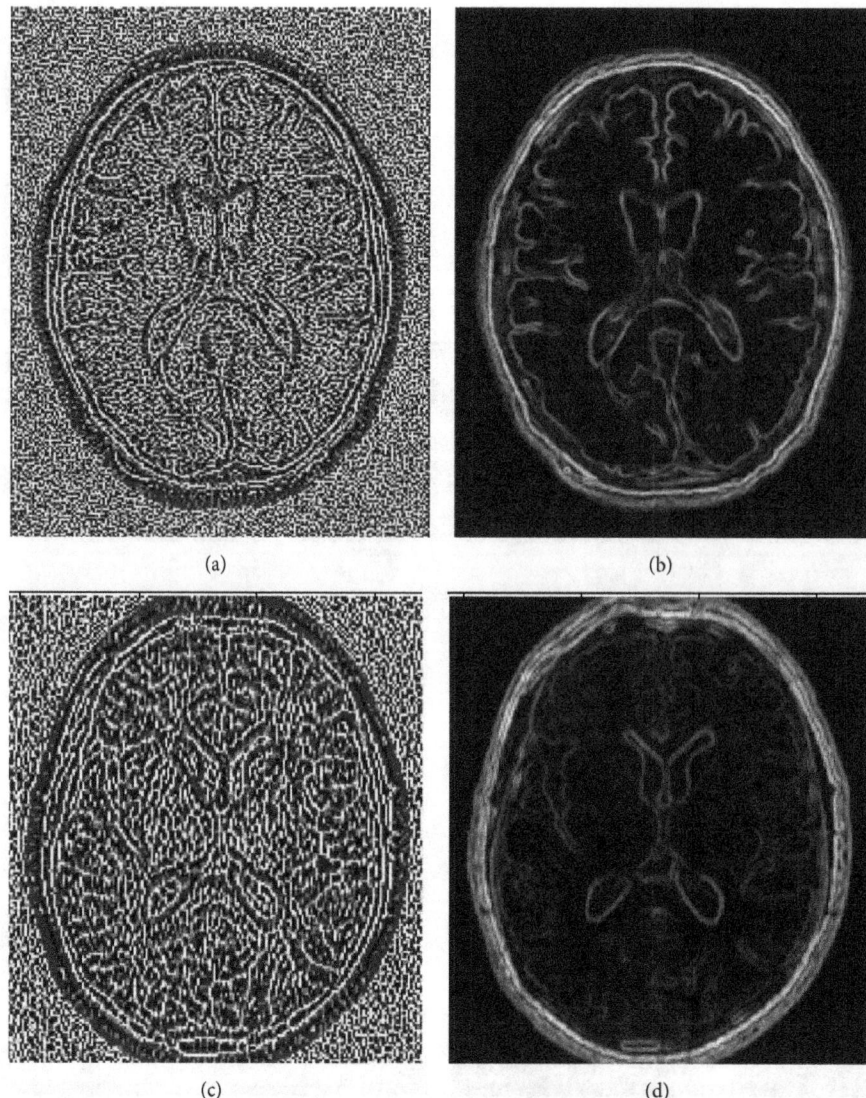

FIGURE 4: Overview of LBP texture- and contrast-valued images based on the FLAIR and T1 images. (a) in the top left corner shows an example of an LBP-valued image calculated from a FLAIR MR image. (b) in the top right corner shows a contrast-valued image calculated from FLAIR MRI. (c) in the bottom left corner shows an LBP-valued image calculated from a T1 image. (d) in the bottom right corner shows a contrast-valued image calculated from a T1 MR image.

least preserved. In conclusion, balancing out the number of instances in each class in the data set balanced out the classification performance for each class as well.

6. Results

6.1. Three-Class Problem: NC versus AD versus LBD. Results for the three-class problem with class 0 being NC, class 1 being AD, and class 2 being LBD are shown in detail in Table 2. T is the total accuracy for all three classes. $P0$ is the precision for the NC group, $P1$ is the precision for the AD group, $P2$ is the precision for the LBD group, $R0$ is the recall for the NC group, $R1$ is the recall for the AD group, and $R2$ is the recall for the LBD group.

The first test named FLAIR-WML$_{ri}$ indicates that the FLAIR MR image was used for calculation of LBP and C, that

WML was the ROI, and that the rotational invariant variant of the LBP feature was used. The second test named T1WML$_{ri}$ indicates that the T1 MR images were used for calculation of LBP and C, that WML was the ROI, and that the rotational invariant variant of the LBP feature was used. The third test named T1WM$_{ri}$ indicates that the T1 MR images were used for calculation of the LBP and C, that the WM was the ROI, and that the rotational invariant variant of the LBP feature was used.

The total accuracy showed great variation throughout the different tests ranging from 0.6 (0.13) to 0.87 (0.08). The performance increased considerably when calculating the LBP and C features from the T1 MR image as compared to the FLAIR MR image. The classification performance proved best in the T1 case and when WML was used as ROI.

For comments on the T1WML$_{svg,ri}$ test, see Section 6.4.

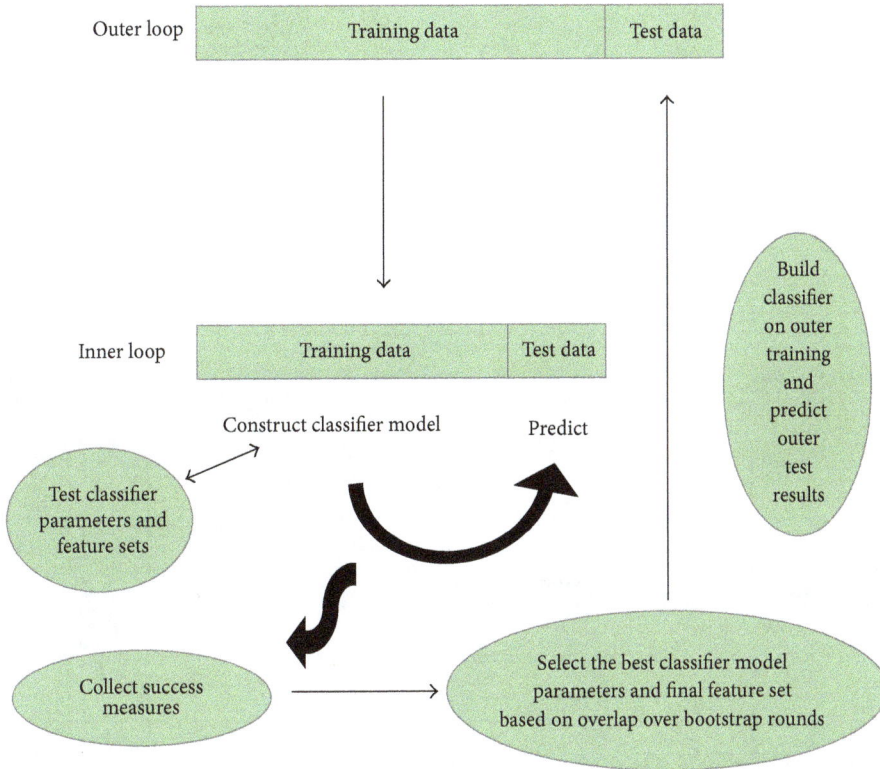

FIGURE 5: Nested cross validation: in the inner loop, the performance of different sets of classifier parameters and features is estimated based on a bootstrap cross validation. The optimal classifier parameters and features are selected based on the performance evaluation over several bootstrap rounds. In the outer loop, model performance of the optimized classifier parameters and features is evaluated on the hold-out test set in the outer loop. The outer loop is repeated several times, every time with potentially different classifier parameters and features.

TABLE 2: Results are reported as mean with standard deviation in brackets, $m(s)$, over 10-fold cross validation, classifying NC versus AD versus LBD. T = total accuracy, R = recall, and P = precision. 0 for class NC, 1 for class AD, and 2 for class LBD. ROI is either WM for white matter or WML for white matter lesion area.

Test	T	$P0$ $R0$	$P1$ $R1$	$P2$ $R2$
FLAIR-WML$_{ri}$	0.60 (0.13)	0.71 (0.28) 0.48 (0.25)	0.61 (0.14) 0.77 (0.28)	0.33 (0.41) 0.20 (0.35)
T1WML$_{ri}$	0.82 (0.12)	0.96 (0.10) 0.98 (0.08)	0.80 (0.11) 0.88 (0.18)	0.58 (0.49) 0.25 (0.35)
T1WML$_{ri}^{SMOTE}$	**0.87 (0.08)**	0.97 (0.07) 1.00 (0.00)	0.81 (0.17) 0.82 (0.16)	0.85 (0.11) 0.78 (0.20)
T1WM$_{ri}$	0.82 (0.09)	0.96 (0.08) 1.00 (0.00)	0.81 (0.11) 0.88 (0.16)	0.42 (0.49) 0.20 (0.35)
T1WM$_{ri}^{SMOTE}$	0.75 (0.13)	0.90 (0.12) 1.00 (0.00)	0.66 (0.16) 0.72 (0.19)	0.70 (0.21) 0.55 (0.22)
T1WML$_{svg,ri}^{SMOTE}$	0.91 (0.15)	1.00 (0.00) 1.00 (0.00)	1.00 (0.00) 0.77 (0.42)	0.87 (0.22) 1.00 (0.00)

6.2. Two-Class Problem: NC versus AD + LBD. Results for the two-class problem with class 0 being NC and class 1 being AD and LBD together are shown in detail in Table 3. T is the total accuracy for the two classes. $P0$ is the precision for the NC group and $P1$ is the precision for the combined AD and LBD group; $R0$ is the recall for the NC group and $R1$ is the recall for the combined AD and LBD group.

In addition to the abovementioned tests, another test named T1WML$_{riu2}$ was applied to assess whether the classification performance would differ when rotational invariant LBP were calculated alone or in combination with selection of uniform LBP values only.

Total accuracy is generally higher in the T1 case (ranging from 0.97 (0.04) to 0.98 (0.04)) compared to the FLAIR case

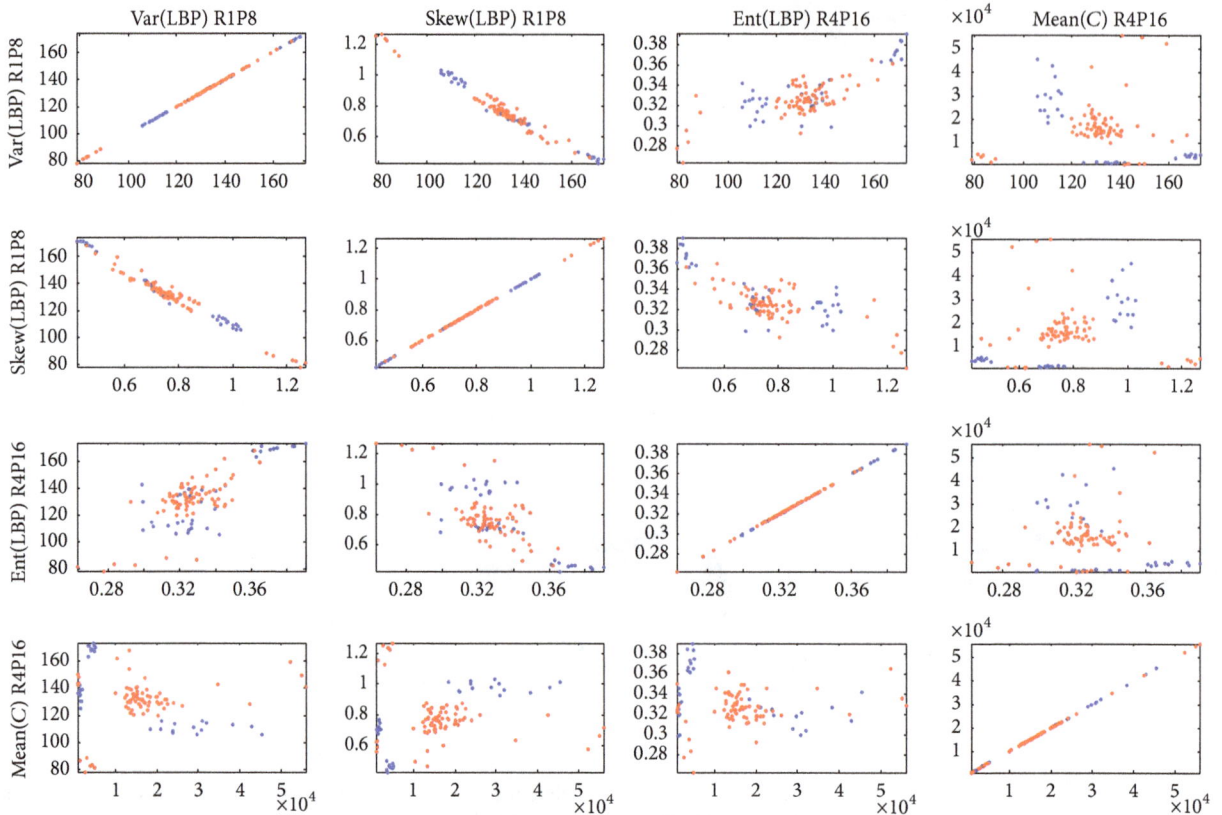

FIGURE 6: Matrix of scatter plots displaying the five selected features pairwise against each other. Blue depicts normal controls and red depicts dementia.

TABLE 3: Results are reported as mean with standard deviation in brackets, $m(s)$, over 10-fold cross validation, classifying NC versus AD + LBD. T = total accuracy, R = recall, and P = precision. 0 for class NC and 1 for class AD + LBD. ROI is either WM for white matter or WML for white matter lesion area.

Test	T	$P0$ $R0$	$P1$ $R1$
FLAIR-WML$_{ri}$	0.80 (0.12)	0.69 (0.20) 0.72 (0.23)	0.87 (0.11) 0.84 (0.12)
T1WML$_{ri}$	**0.98 (0.04)**	0.98 (0.06) 0.98 (0.08)	0.99 (0.04) 0.99 (0.05)
T1WM$_{ri}$	0.97 (0.04)	0.96 (0.08) 0.98 (0.08)	0.99 (0.04) 0.97 (0.06)
T1WML$_{riu2}$	0.98 (0.04)	0.96 (0.08) 1.00 (0.00)	1.00 (0.00) 0.97 (0.06)
T1WML$_{svg,ri}$	1.00 (0.00)	1.00 (0.00) 1.00 (0.00)	1.00 (0.00) 1.00 (0.00)

(0.80 (0.12)) but approximately similar to the two different ROIs when T1 MR images are used. Precision for class 0 is higher in the case of LBP and C calculated in the WML area of the T1 image (0.98 (0.06)) as compared to all of the WM area (0.96 (0.08)). Recall for class 0 is similar for both ROIs. This is also the case for precision for class 1 (0.99 (0.04)), but recall for class 1 is higher when LBP and C are calculated in

the WML region 0.99 (0.05) as compared to the WM region (0.97 (0.06)).

When the rotational invariant calculation of LBP is combined with selection of the uniform values only, the $P0$ and $R1$ are similar to the ri-case. The $riu2$-case had marginally higher values for total accuracy, $P1$, and $R0$.

For comments on the T1WML$_{svg,ri}$ test, see Section 6.4.

6.3. Two-Class Problem: AD versus LBD. Results for the two-class problem with class 1 being AD and class 2 being LBD are shown in detail in Table 4.

Classification performance was highest in the T1 case when WM was used as ROI.

6.4. Stavanger Data Only. In both the three-class problem and the two-class problem, NC versus AD + LBD, a fifth test was run, named T1WML$_{svg,ri}$, which indicates that the T1 MR images were used for calculation of the LBP and C, that the WM was the ROI, and that only data from the MR scanner located at Stavanger University Hospital were used. This experiment was done to assess the robustness of the method. The rotational invariant variant of the LBP feature was used in this test. An even better performance was reached in both cases. In the three-class problem, a total accuracy of 0.91 (0.15) was achieved and all of the cases in the data set were classified correctly in the two-class problem. An implication of this is that between-centre noise falsely reduces classification

TABLE 4: Results are reported as mean with standard deviation in brackets, $m(s)$, over 10-fold cross validation, classifying AD versus LBD. T = total accuracy, R = recall, and P = precision. 1 for class AD and 2 for class LBD. ROI is either WM for white matter or WML for white matter lesion area.

Test	T	P1 R1	P2 R2
FLAIR-WML$_{ri}$	0.73 (0.15)	0.78 (0.11) 0.91 (0.12)	0.20 (0.45) 0.10 (0.32)
T1WML$_{ri}$	0.66 (0.17)	0.74 (0.10) 0.84 (0.18)	0.00 (0.00) 0.00 (0.00)
T1WML$_{ri}^{SMOTE}$	0.73 (0.16)	0.72 (0.18) 0.75 (0.20)	0.76 (0.17) 0.71 (0.19)
T1WM$_{ri}$	0.74 (0.16)	0.80 (0.09) 0.75 (0.20)	0.45 (0.51) 0.71 (0.19)
T1WM$_{ri}^{SMOTE}$	0.68 (0.14)	0.67 (0.14) 0.69 (0.29)	0.75 (0.21) 0.68 (0.14)

accuracy and that the developed method shows even higher performance when all data come from the same scanner.

7. Discussion

Our results improved doing LBP texture analysis in 3DT1 image rather than the FLAIR image, indicating that there exists more textural information in the 3DT1 image compared to the FLAIR image relevant to our problem formulation. In the three-class problem as well as in the two-class problem NC versus AD + LBD, our results indicate that there exists similar amount of relevant textural information regarding dementia classification using all of WM as ROI compared to using only WML. This could be a benefit. WML segmentation is unsatisfactorily developed and very often demanding manual outlining is required as well as a FLAIR MR image, where WML is hyperintense, while WM segmentation is readily available from many well known and freely downloadable software packages needing only a 3DT1 MR image which is a common part of a clinical MR protocol. In addition, recent focus on diffusion tensor imaging (DTI) in vascular disease [58], amnestic mild cognitive impairment (aMCI) [59], and dementia [60–62] strengthens the view that age-related changes in WM play an important role in the development of dementia. DTI is, nevertheless, not sufficiently available and at the same time is costly making other approaches for WM analysis, like ours, a valuable addition.

In the two-class problem, AD versus LBD, we did not reach a comparable classification result compared to the AD + LBD versus NC case. There probably exist several explanations for that, one of the most obvious being the small sample size in the LBD class compared to the other classes. The LBD subjects are mainly classified as AD subjects indicating that the two groups experience similarities concerning our methods. Even though the two groups show different neurological etiologies, they do not differ equally regarding vascular changes. Having few subjects in the LBD group, the calculated texture features may not represent the group with

proper specificity or generality. Another explanation could be related to the common basis for neurodegenerative dementias pointed out by Bartzokis in [21] or Schneider's observations about mixed brain pathologies in dementia [63].

In the three-class problem, NC versus AD versus LBD, the accuracy for the LBD class is improved showing a precision of 0.85 (0.11) and recall of 0.78 (0.20). When doing the same test on the data from Stavanger only, even better results were achieved with a precision of 0.87 (0.22) and a recall of 1.00 (0.00) for the LBD class. Vemuri et al. [18] used atrophy maps and a k-means clustering approach to diagnose AD with a sensitivity of 90.7% and a specificity of 84%, LBD with a sensitivity of 78.6% and specificity of 98.8%, and FTLD with a sensitivity of 84.4% and a specificity of 93.8%. A strength of their study was that they only used MR images of later histologically confirmed LBD patients. They also report sensitivity and specificity for the respective clinical diagnoses. AD with a sensitivity of 89.5% and a specificity of 82.1%, LBD with a sensitivity of 70.0% and specificity of 100.0%, and FTLD with a sensitivity of 83.0% and a specificity of 95.6%. Compared to the reported sensitivity and specificity for clinical diagnosis, our method shows substantial higher accuracy for LBD and comparable accuracy for AD. A limitation is the use of different measures of goodness to the classification results and that different data is used. In Kodama and Kawase [40], a classification accuracy of 70% for the LBD group from AD and NC is reported. Burton et al. report a sensitivity of 91% and a specificity of 94% using calculations of medial temporal lobe atrophy assessing diagnostic specificity of AD in a sample of patients with AD, LBD, and vascular cognitive impairment but do not report results for the LBD group [17]. In [19], Lebedev et al. use sparse partial least squares (SPLS) classification of cortical thickness measurements reporting a sensitivity of 94.4 and a specificity of 88.89 discerning AD from LBD.

To verify that the classification results are not driven by differences in the local variation of signal intensities (the C values) between centres used during collection of MR data in the study, the test T1WML$_{svg,ri}$ was conducted on the Stavanger data only. The results showed an increase in classification performance, which gives us reason to believe that the results reflect real diagnostic differences.

LBP is based on local gradients and is therefore prone to noise and could be a limitation to our approach. LBP values calculated in a noisy neighbourhood would be recognised by many transitions between 0s and 1s. We performed a test, the T1WML$_{riu2}$ test, where only rotational invariant and uniform LBP values, showing a maximum of two transitions between 0s and 1s, are collected. The result showed identical results as the T1WML$_{ri}$ test indicating that noise does not constitute a severe problem in our method. Even though noise reduction procedures can be useful in the application of, for example, segmentation, a noise reduction approach could remove relevant textures. The contrast measure is invariant to shifts in gray-scale but not invariant to scaling. We do not use any normalization of the images prior to the feature calculation. Thus, one could argue that different patients are scaled differently making the contrast measure less trustworthy. On the other hand, if a normalization is done, for example, based on a maximum intensity value, this could indeed change the local subtle textures and affect the contrast measures, possibly in a negative way. In the present work, we have investigated the discriminating power of the features calculated without any smoothing or normalization, since the effect of such operators is not clear for this application. In future work, we want to investigate the use of different preprocessing steps, using both denoising and normalization, and compare the discrimination power of the features with and without preprocessing. The improvement in results when using data from one centre only (Stavanger) indicates lack of robustness which can be related to the facts mentioned above.

As mentioned in Section 2.2, Cronbach's alpha was calculated using total brain volume to ensure that our data material was consistent even though it was collected from different centres spanning a time scale. Texture features can be exposed to noise and a limitation to our study is the lack of using texture features for the reliability analysis.

Another limitation to our study is the lack of clinical interpretation of texture features which is difficult in our case, since brain regional information is lost in the process of feature calculation.

7.1. Conclusion. This study demonstrates that LBP texture features combined with the contrast measure C calculated from brain MR images are potent features used in a machine learning context for computer based dementia diagnosis. The results discerning AD + LBD from NC are especially promising, potentially adding value to the clinical diagnose. In the three-class problem, the classification performance exceeded the accuracy of clinical diagnosis for the LBD group, at the same time keeping the classification accuracy for the AD group comparable to the clinical diagnoses. A lower accuracy was achieved when classifying AD from LBD in the two-class problem, AD versus LBD. We considered it good news that the results using WM as ROI gave almost equally good classification performance as WML, since the WM segmentation routine is much more accessible compared to WML segmentation. The performance using 3DT1 images for texture analysis was notably better than when using FLAIR images, which is an advantage, since most common MR protocols include a 3DT1 image.

For future work we will look into texture features calculated in a 3D neighbourhood. 3D texture features have shown to be an important step towards better discrimination in machine learning systems when the images are intrinsic three-dimensional like many MR sequences are [64]. In addition, we will perform correlation analysis between texture features and cognition, since that could improve the clinical value of our work.

Conflict of Interests

Author "D. Aarsland" received honoraria from Novartis, Lundbeck, GSK, Merck Serono, DiaGenic, GE Health, and Orion Pharmaceuticals and has provided research support for Merck Serono, Lundbeck, and Novartis. No other author has anything to disclose.

Acknowledgments

The authors want to thank principal investigators of the ParkWest [46] cohort JP Larsen and OB Tysnes for giving access to MR images of the normal controls in the study. We also want to thank The Western Norway Regional Health Authority for providing funding by grant 911546.

References

[1] A. Wimo and M. Prince, *World Alzheimer Report 2010: The Global Economic Impact of Dementia*, Alzheimer's Disease International, 2010, http://www.alz.co.uk/research/files/World-AlzheimerReport2010.pdf.

[2] D. Aarsland, A. Rongve, S. P. Nore et al., "Frequency and case identification of dementia with Lewy bodies using the revised consensus criteria," *Dementia and Geriatric Cognitive Disorders*, vol. 26, no. 5, pp. 445–452, 2008.

[3] D. P. Perl, "Neuropathology of Alzheimer's disease," *The Mount Sinai Journal of Medicine*, vol. 77, no. 1, pp. 32–42, 2010.

[4] D. Aarsland, C. G. Ballard, and G. Halliday, "Are Parkinson's disease with dementia and dementia with Lewy bodies the same entity?" *Journal of Geriatric Psychiatry and Neurology*, vol. 17, no. 3, pp. 137–145, 2004.

[5] C. F. Lippa, J. E. Duda, M. Grossman et al., "DLB and PDD boundary issues: diagnosis, treatment, molecular pathology, and biomarkers," *Neurology*, vol. 68, no. 11, pp. 812–819, 2007.

[6] I. G. McKeith, D. W. Dickson, J. Lowe et al., "Diagnosis and management of dementia with Lewy bodies: third report of the DLB consortium," *Neurology*, vol. 65, no. 12, pp. 1863–1872, 2005.

[7] B. Thanvi, N. Lo, and T. Robinson, "Vascular parkinsonism—an important cause of parkinsonism in older people," *Age and Ageing*, vol. 34, no. 2, pp. 114–119, 2005.

[8] M. Filippi and F. Agosta, "Structural and functional network connectivity breakdown in Alzheimer's disease studied with magnetic resonance imaging techniques," *Journal of Alzheimer's Disease*, vol. 24, no. 3, pp. 455–474, 2011.

[9] J. A. Bertelson and B. Ajtai, "Neuroimaging of dementia," *Neurologic Clinics*, vol. 32, no. 1, pp. 59–93, 2014.

[10] D. Wang, S. C. Hui, L. Shi et al., "Application of multimodal MR imaging on studying Alzheimer's disease: a survey," *Current Alzheimer Research*, vol. 10, no. 8, pp. 877–892, 2013.

[11] P. Malloy, S. Correia, G. Stebbins, and D. H. Laidlaw, "Neuroimaging of white matter in aging and dementia," *The Clinical Neuropsychologist*, vol. 21, no. 1, pp. 73–109, 2007.

[12] J. Stoitsis, I. Valavanis, S. G. Mougiakakou, S. Golemati, A. Nikita, and K. S. Nikita, "Computer aided diagnosis based on medical image processing and artificial intelligence methods," *Nuclear Instruments and Methods in Physics Research Section A: Accelerators, Spectrometers, Detectors and Associated Equipment*, vol. 569, no. 2, pp. 591–595, 2006.

[13] K. R. Gray, P. Aljabar, R. A. Heckemann, A. Hammers, and D. Rueckert, "Random forest-based similarity measures for multimodal classification of Alzheimer's disease," *NeuroImage*, vol. 65, pp. 167–175, 2013.

[14] M. Liu, D. Zhang, and D. Shen, "Ensemble sparse classification of Alzheimer's disease," *NeuroImage*, vol. 60, no. 2, pp. 1106–1116, 2012.

[15] R. Cuingnet, E. Gerardin, J. Tessieras et al., "Automatic classification of patients with Alzheimer's disease from structural

MRI: a comparison of ten methods using the ADNI database," *NeuroImage*, vol. 56, no. 2, pp. 766–781, 2011.

[16] S. Klöppel, C. M. Stonnington, J. Barnes et al., "Accuracy of dementia diagnosis—a direct comparison between radiologists and a computerized method," *Brain*, vol. 131, no. 11, pp. 2969–2974, 2008.

[17] E. J. Burton, R. Barber, E. B. Mukaetova-Ladinska et al., "Medial temporal lobe atrophy on MRI differentiates Alzheimer's disease from dementia with Lewy bodies and vascular cognitive impairment: a prospective study with pathological verification of diagnosis," *Brain*, vol. 132, no. 1, pp. 195–203, 2009.

[18] P. Vemuri, G. Simon, K. Kantarci et al., "Antemortem differential diagnosis of dementia pathology using structural MRI: differential-STAND," *NeuroImage*, vol. 55, no. 2, pp. 522–531, 2011.

[19] A. V. Lebedev, E. Westman, M. K. Beyer et al., "Multivariate classification of patients with Alzheimer's and dementia with Lewy bodies using high-dimensional cortical thickness measurements: an MRI surface-based morphometric study," *Journal of Neurology*, vol. 260, no. 4, pp. 1104–1115, 2013.

[20] C. M. Filley, "White matter dementia," *Therapeutic Advances in Neurological Disorders*, vol. 5, no. 5, pp. 267–277, 2012.

[21] G. Bartzokis, "Alzheimer's disease as homeostatic responses to age-related myelin breakdown," *Neurobiology of Aging*, vol. 32, no. 8, pp. 1341–1371, 2011.

[22] F. M. Gunning-Dixon, A. M. Brickman, J. C. Cheng, and G. S. Alexopoulos, "Aging of cerebral white matter: a review of MRI findings," *International Journal of Geriatric Psychiatry*, vol. 24, no. 2, pp. 109–117, 2009.

[23] A. Poggesi, L. Pantoni, D. Inzitari et al., "2001–2011: a decade of The Ladis (Leukoaraiosis and Disability) study: what have we learned about white matter changes and small-vessel disease?" *Cerebrovascular Diseases*, vol. 32, no. 6, pp. 577–588, 2011.

[24] V. G. Young, G. M. Halliday, and J. J. Kril, "Neuropathologic correlates of white matter hyperintensities," *Neurology*, vol. 71, no. 11, pp. 804–811, 2008.

[25] F.-E. de Leeuw, J. C. de Groot, E. Achten et al., "Prevalence of cerebral white matter lesions in elderly people: a population based magnetic resonance imaging study. The Rotterdam Scan Study," *Journal of Neurology, Neurosurgery & Psychiatry*, vol. 70, no. 1, pp. 9–14, 2001.

[26] M. Yoshita, E. Fletcher, D. Harvey et al., "Extent and distribution of white matter hyperintensities in normal aging, MCI, and AD," *Neurology*, vol. 67, no. 12, pp. 2192–2198, 2006.

[27] R. Barber, P. Scheltens, A. Gholkar et al., "White matter lesions on magnetic resonance imaging in dementia with Lewy bodies, Alzheimer's disease, vascular dementia, and normal aging," *Journal of Neurology Neurosurgery and Psychiatry*, vol. 67, no. 1, pp. 66–72, 1999.

[28] N. D. Prins, E. J. van Dijk, T. den Heijer et al., "Cerebral white matter lesions and the risk of dementia," *Archives of Neurology*, vol. 61, no. 10, pp. 1531–1534, 2004.

[29] H. Baezner, C. Blahak, A. Poggesi et al., "Association of gait and balance disorders with age-related white matter changes: the LADIS Study," *Neurology*, vol. 70, no. 12, pp. 935–942, 2008.

[30] H. Soennesyn, K. Oppedal, O. J. Greve et al., "White matter hyperintensities and the course of depressive symptoms in elderly people with mild dementia," *Dementia and Geriatric Cognitive Disorders Extra*, vol. 2, no. 1, pp. 97–111, 2012.

[31] N. D. Prins, E. J. van Dijk, T. den Heijer et al., "Cerebral small-vessel disease and decline in information processing speed,

executive function and memory," *Brain*, vol. 128, no. 9, pp. 2034–2041, 2005.

[32] A. M. Tuladhar, A. T. Reid, E. Shumskaya et al., "Relationship between white matter hyperintensities, cortical thickness, and cognition," *Stroke*, vol. 46, no. 2, pp. 425–432, 2015.

[33] S. Muñoz Maniega, M. C. Valdés Hernández, and J. D. Clayden, "White matter hyperintensities and normal-appearing white matter integrity in the aging brain," *Neurobiology of Aging*, vol. 36, no. 2, pp. 909–918, 2015.

[34] M. Fujishima, N. Maikusa, K. Nakamura, M. Nakatsuka, H. Matsuda, and K. Meguro, "Mild cognitive impairment, poor episodic memory, and late-life depression are associated with cerebral cortical thinning and increased white matter hyperintensities," *Frontiers in Aging Neuroscience*, vol. 6, 2014.

[35] L. Harrison, *Clinical applicability of mri texture analysis [Ph.D. thesis]*, University of Tampere, Tampere, Finland, 2011, http://tampub.uta.fi/bitstream/handle/10024/66779/978-951-44-8527-5.pdf?sequence=1.

[36] P. A. Freeborough and N. C. Fox, "MR image texture analysis applied to the diagnosis and tracking of alzheimer's disease," *IEEE Transactions on Medical Imaging*, vol. 17, no. 3, pp. 475–479, 1998.

[37] M. S. de Oliveira, M. L. F. Balthazar, A. D'Abreu et al., "MR imaging texture analysis of the corpus callosum and thalamus in amnestic mild cognitive impairment and mild Alzheimer disease," *The American Journal of Neuroradiology*, vol. 32, no. 1, pp. 60–66, 2011.

[38] J. Zhang, C. Yu, G. Jiang, W. Liu, and L. Tong, "3D texture analysis on MRI images of Alzheimer's disease," *Brain Imaging and Behavior*, vol. 6, no. 1, pp. 61–69, 2012.

[39] T. R. Sivapriya, V. Saravanan, and P. R. J. Thangaiah, "Texture analysis of brain MRI and classification with BPN for the diagnosis of dementia," *Communications in Computer and Information Science*, vol. 204, pp. 553–563, 2011.

[40] N. Kodama and Y. Kawase, "Computerized method for classification between dementia with Lewy bodies and Alzheimer's disease by use of texture analysis on brain MRI," in *Proceedings of the World Congress on Medical Physics and Biomedical Engineering*, pp. 319–321, Munich, Germany, September 2009.

[41] T. Ojala, M. Pietikainen, and D. Harwood, "Performance evaluation of texture measures with classification based on kullback discrimination of distributions," in *Proceedings of the 12th International Conference on Pattern Recognition*, vol. 1, pp. 582–585, Jerusalem, Israel, 1994.

[42] T. Ojala, M. Pietikäinen, and D. Harwood, "A comparative study of texture measures with classification based on feature distributions," *Pattern Recognition*, vol. 29, no. 1, pp. 51–59, 1996.

[43] D. Unay, A. Ekin, M. Cetin, R. Jasinschi, and A. Ercil, "Robustness of local binary patterns in brain MR image analysis," in *Proceedings of the 29th Annual International Conference of the IEEE Engineering in Medicine and Biology Society (EMBS '07)*, pp. 2098–2101, Lyon, France, August 2007.

[44] K. Oppedal, D. Aarsland, M. J. Firbank et al., "White matter hyperintensities in mild Lewy body dementia," *Dementia and Geriatric Cognitive Disorders Extra*, vol. 2, no. 1, pp. 481–495, 2012.

[45] K. Oppedal, K. Engan, D. Aarsland, M. Beyer, O. B. Tysnes, and T. Eftestøl, "Using local binary pattern to classify dementia in MRI," in *Proceedings of the 9th IEEE International Symposium on Biomedical Imaging: From Nano to Macro (ISBI '12)*, pp. 594–597, May 2012.

[46] G. Alves, B. Müller, K. Herlofson et al., "Incidence of Parkinson's disease in Norway: the Norwegian ParkWest study," *Journal of Neurology, Neurosurgery and Psychiatry*, vol. 80, no. 8, pp. 851–857, 2009.

[47] J. Ashburner and K. J. Friston, "Unified segmentation," *NeuroImage*, vol. 26, no. 3, pp. 839–851, 2005.

[48] M. J. Firbank, A. J. Lloyd, N. Ferrier, and J. T. O'Brien, "A volumetric study of MRI signal hyperintensities in late-life depression," *The American Journal of Geriatric Psychiatry*, vol. 12, no. 6, pp. 606–612, 2004.

[49] SPM5, *Statistical Parametric Mapping*, 2005, http://www.fil.ion .ucl.ac.uk/spm/

[50] MNI. Montreal Neurological Institute, 1995, http://www.nil .wustl.edu/labs/kevin/man/answers/mnispace.html.

[51] M. J. Firbank, T. Minett, and J. T. O'Brien, "Changes in DWI and MRS associated with white matter hyperintensities in elderly subjects," *Neurology*, vol. 61, no. 7, pp. 950–954, 2003.

[52] FSLView v.3.1, "FMRIB Software Libary v4.0," August 2007, http://fsl.fmrib.ox.ac.uk/fsl/fslview/.

[53] L. Breiman, "Random forests," Tech. Rep., Statistics Department, University of California, Berkely, Calif, USA, 2001, http:// oz.berkeley.edu/users/breiman/randomforest2001.pdf.

[54] T. Hastie, R. Tibshirani, and J. Friedman, *The Elements of Statistical Learning*, vol. 2, Springer, 2009.

[55] Matlab R2012b, "Mathworks," October 2012, http://www.math-works.se/index.html.

[56] N. V. Chawla, K. W. Bowyer, L. O. Hall, and W. P. Kegelmeyer, "SMOTE: synthetic minority over-sampling technique," *Journal of Artificial Intelligence Research*, vol. 16, pp. 321–357, 2002.

[57] H. He and E. A. Garcia, "Learning from imbalanced data," *IEEE Transactions on Knowledge and Data Engineering*, vol. 21, no. 9, pp. 1263–1284, 2009.

[58] G. S. Alves, F. K. Sudo, C. E. D. O. Alves et al., "Diffusion tensor imaging studies in vascular disease: a review of the literature," *Dementia e Neuropsychologia*, vol. 6, no. 3, pp. 158–163, 2012.

[59] M. Dyrba, M. Ewers, M. Wegrzyn et al., "Predicting prodromal Alzheimer's disease in people with mild cognitive impairment using multicenter diffusion-tensor imaging data and machine learning algorithms," *Alzheimer's & Dementia*, vol. 9, no. 4, p. 426, 2013.

[60] M. Naik, A. Lundervold, H. Nygaard, and J.-T. Geitung, "Diffusion tensor imaging (DTI) in dementia patients with frontal lobe symptoms," *Acta Radiologica*, vol. 51, no. 6, pp. 662–668, 2010.

[61] M. J. Firbank, A. M. Blamire, A. Teodorczuk, E. Teper, D. Mitra, and J. T. O'Brien, "Diffusion tensor imaging in Alzheimer's disease and dementia with Lewy bodies," *Psychiatry Research: Neuroimaging*, vol. 194, no. 2, pp. 176–183, 2011.

[62] R. Watson, A. M. Blamire, S. J. Colloby et al., "Characterizing dementia with Lewy bodies by means of diffusion tensor imaging," *Neurology*, vol. 79, no. 9, pp. 906–914, 2012.

[63] J. A. Schneider, Z. Arvanitakis, W. Bang, and D. A. Bennett, "Mixed brain pathologies account for most dementia cases in community-dwelling older persons," *Neurology*, vol. 69, no. 24, pp. 2197–2204, 2007.

[64] V. A. Kovalev, F. Kruggel, H. J. Gertz, and D. Y. von Cramon, "Three-dimensional texture analysis of MRI brain datasets," *IEEE Transactions on Medical Imaging*, vol. 20, no. 5, pp. 424–433, 2001.

Automated Segmentation and Object Classification of CT Images: Application to *In Vivo* Molecular Imaging of Avian Embryos

Alexander Heidrich,[1] **Jana Schmidt,**[2] **Johannes Zimmermann,**[3] **and Hans Peter Saluz**[1,4]

[1] *Department of Cell and Molecular Biology, Leibniz Institute for Natural Product Research and Infection Biology,*
Hans Knöll Institute, Beutenberg Straße 11a, 07745 Jena, Germany
[2] *Institut für Informatik/I12, Technische Universität München, Boltzmannstrraße 3, 85748 Garching bei München, Germany*
[3] *Definiens AG, Bernhard-Wicki-Straße 5, 80636 München, Germany*
[4] *Friedrich Schiller University of Jena, Fürstengraben 1, 07743 Jena, Germany*

Correspondence should be addressed to Hans Peter Saluz; hanspeter.saluz@hki-jena.de

Academic Editor: Jie Tian

Background. Although chick embryogenesis has been studied extensively, there has been growing interest in the investigation of skeletogenesis. In addition to improved poultry health and minimized economic loss, a greater understanding of skeletal abnormalities can also have implications for human medicine. True *in vivo* studies require noninvasive imaging techniques such as high-resolution microCT. However, the manual analysis of acquired images is both time consuming and subjective. *Methods.* We have developed a system for automated image segmentation that entails object-based image analysis followed by the classification of the extracted image objects. For image segmentation, a rule set was developed using Definiens image analysis software. The classification engine was implemented using the WEKA machine learning tool. *Results.* Our system reduces analysis time and observer bias while maintaining high accuracy. Applying the system to the quantification of long bone growth has allowed us to present the first true *in ovo* data for bone length growth recorded in the same chick embryos. *Conclusions.* The procedures developed represent an innovative approach for the automated segmentation, classification, quantification, and visualization of microCT images. MicroCT offers the possibility of performing longitudinal studies and thereby provides unique insights into the morpho- and embryogenesis of live chick embryos.

1. Background

The *in ovo* chick embryo is a highly versatile model organism with a long history of use in biological and biomedical research [1, 2]. The embryonated chicken egg is favored in embryogenic studies [3, 4] because it allows for easier access and manipulation and is more economical.

Understanding the mechanisms of bone development is highly relevant for poultry farming, where skeletal deformities in long bones can have a substantial economic impact. Insights gained from the chick embryo model also allow for a greater understanding of human bone development and metabolism as well as associated diseases [5–8].

Several imaging modalities may be considered for the *in ovo* observation of the live avian embryo: fluorescence microscopy [9], magnetic resonance tomography (MRT) [10], ultrasound [11], and computed tomography (CT) [12]. Both MRT and CT are noninvasive; they do not entail damaging the egg shell. Both imaging modalities provide three-dimensional information at high spatial resolutions, thereby allowing for longitudinal studies and the study of long-term processes (e.g., bone growth and ossification) in the same chick embryo *in ovo*. However, only CT provides sufficient bone contrast.

Unfortunately, the overabundance of generated image data makes the manual analysis of resulting images a time-consuming and tedious task. Furthermore, the visual interpretation of images is error prone and highly subjective. Therefore, automated image analysis systems are highly desirable. The most important tasks of such systems are the automatic detection, segmentation, quantification, and classification of biological structures from various 2D, 3D, and 4D images.

As it mimics human visual perception, the object-oriented image analysis approach based on the Cognition Network Technology (CNT) offers key advantages over pixel-based approaches. Instead of solely relying on pixel information, CNT emulates the segmentation, description, and identification of image objects through context sensitive associations [13]. Based on CNT, rule-based solutions can be created for virtually any question related to image analysis. For rule set creation, a flexible programming language called Cognition Network Language (CNL) has been constructed. Recently, CNT and CNL have been used to solve image analysis tasks in such fields as infection, cell and developmental biology [14–16] and in clinical and preclinical radiology [17, 18].

The extracted image objects and associated properties can be used to train a model for machine learning, which can then be used to automatically classify anatomical units (i.e., bones) in unknown image datasets. As they work on nonlinear problems and can achieve high precision—even with small training sets, support vector machines (SVM) have proven advantageous for object-based image analysis (OBIA) [19].

We demonstrate how automated image analysis and machine learning techniques can be combined to segment microCT images and extract object information for the *in ovo* classification of bones in live chick embryos.

Using CNT, a rule set that reliably segments *in ovo* microCT images of chick embryos, including those at different stages of incubation, can be created in CNL. The bone objects of interest could be extracted, and their features were used to train an SVM that classifies long bones with high accuracy. To present a potential application of our workflow, we studied long bone growth of chick embryos *in ovo* from day 13 to day 15 of incubation based on daily microCT measurements.

2. Methods

2.1. Image Data. In the present study, *in ovo* microCT images of chick embryos from day 13 to day 19 of incubation (d13–d19, Hamburger-Hamilton (HH) stages 39–45) were used. The database for machine learning consisted of 27 microCT images ($n = 4$ for d13–d18 and $n = 3$ for d19, Group 1). The database for analyzing long bone growth from d13–d15 consisted of 12 microCT images acquired from the same four eggs. One microCT scan was performed daily over three consecutive days (Group 2).

The microCT images were acquired during a previous study [20] in which the bone metabolism of live chick embryos at different days of incubation was investigated using single and repeated 3D and 4D ^{18}F-fluoride microPET. The microCT images were used for the attenuation correction of microPET data.

2.2. Embryonated Chicken Eggs. Fertilized *Gallus gallus domesticus* (white leghorn chicken) eggs were obtained from a local breeder (Geflügel GmbH Borna, Germany) and incubated in a forced-air egg incubator (Grumbach BSS300 MP GTFS incubator; Grumbach Brutgeräte GmbH, Germany) at $37.7 \pm 0.2°C$ and a relative humidity of $60 \pm 2\%$. During incubation, eggs were candled and checked daily for viability. Motile embryos were considered healthy. As an additional measure, the Buddy Digital Egg Monitor (Avitronics, UK) was used to confirm a stable heartbeat.

Prior to microPET measurements, a blood vessel of the chorioallantoic membrane was catheterized through a small hole in the shell for injection of the radiotracer (^{18}F]NaF). To ensure the normal development of the experimental chick embryos, the beak length (from where the parasphenoid articulates with the palatine to the tip of the upper bill) was measured on microCT images and compared with controls.

2.3. Imaging System and Imaging Protocols. All microCT scans were performed with a Siemens Inveon Small Animal microPET/CT scanner (Siemens Medical Solutions, Siemens Healthcare Molecular Imaging, USA). The final microCT scans were assembled from two consecutive microCT scans (X-ray tube voltage: 80 kV, X-ray tube current: 500 μA) at two animal bed positions. The X-ray detector was operated in a four-by-four pixel binning mode, and 361 projections were acquired per bed position over a 360° rotation of the gantry. Projection slices were sent to a server running the Cobra software (Exxim Computing Corp., USA), where they were reconstructed into images. During reconstruction, the image data were calibrated to Hounsfield Units (HU) and beam hardening correction, as well as a medium noise and ring artifact reduction, was applied. The final microCT images consisted of 604 slices, each 256×256 pixels, and isotropic voxel dimensions of 0.216032 mm. For further processing, the image files were converted from a proprietary format into DICOM format using the Siemens Inveon Research Workplace Software (IRW, version 3.0; Siemens Medical Solutions, Siemens Healthcare Molecular Imaging, USA).

2.4. Automated Image Segmentation and Feature Extraction. The rule set for automated image segmentation and feature extraction of bone objects was developed with Definiens Developer XD 2 (Definiens AG, Germany) on a computer (Intel Xeon X5650, 2.66 GHz, 24 GB RAM) running Windows XP Professional x64 Edition (Version 2003, Service Pack 2). The rule set is described in detail in the results section.

2.5. Data Preparation for Automated Classification. For each egg of Group 1, the image object data extracted during the automated image segmentation step were annotated and classified according to the following categories: humerus, radius, ulna, carpometacarpus, femur, tibiotarsus, and tarsometatarsus. Only clearly discernable bones were classified. All remaining image objects, including those representing clotted or blurred bones or bones that appeared anatomically incorrect (e.g., because of image artifacts), were classified as not of interest (NOI). Finally, all annotated data were combined into a single file that was used to train and test the automated classification process.

For Group 2, the image object data were left unannotated and were further processed as individual files.

2.6. Workflow for Long Bone Classification. The automatic long bone classification system was built using the Waikato Environment for Knowledge Analysis (WEKA) machine learning tool [21]. It provides a support vector machine (SVM) implementation based on the sequential minimal optimization (SMO) method [22]. In general, an SVM is a classifier that can separate instances belonging to two classes in a nonlinear space. This is achieved by the kernel trick, which transforms the initial nonlinear problem into a linear one by adjusting the input space. Another key feature of SVMs is that they separate the instances so that a maximal margin between the two classes is achieved. This margin is then expressed by support vectors that define the separating hyperplane. The best parameters, C (the number of support vectors) and γ (the variance of the kernel function) for the SVM, were found using a Java implementation of a grid search method [23]. To use such an SVM, it must be trained on a dataset, which results in the specific vectors for the hyperplane. The SVM can then be applied on a test set to classify the long bones. The SVM was trained using the annotated data from the Group 1 eggs. Before training, all input data were standardized. To obtain probability estimates of the classification results, logistic regression models were fitted to the outputs of the SVM.

The accuracy of the trained model was evaluated using 10-fold cross-validation, whereby a set of instances (10 percent of the whole set) are systematically excluded from the training and subsequently used as test set. This is done 10 times with nonoverlapping test sets. To judge the quality of the SVM per bone class, the F-measure gives a good overview, because it combines recall and precision rates [24].

The trained SVM was evaluated based on the classification accuracy for the unlabeled data from Group 2 eggs. For this test, an additional constraint was implemented; each chick embryo could only have two long bones of each kind. Hence, if more than two bones were assigned the same classification, only the two with the highest probability were retained. The superfluous objects were classified as NOI. For assessing classification accuracy, the results were reviewed and the classification error was calculated. For the subsequent analysis of long bone growth, misclassifications were corrected.

2.7. The In Ovo Analysis of Long Bone Growth of Chick Embryos from d13 to d15. The image object feature *length* was used for the analysis of long bone growth. The feature is derived

from the three eigenvalues of a rectangular 3D space with the same volume as the image object and the same proportions of eigenvalues as the image object. The length of an image object is the largest of the eigenvalues.

3. Results

3.1. Rule Set for Automated Image Segmentation and Feature Extraction. The image segmentation and feature extraction process is divided into three steps (Figure 1), which are outlined next: egg detection, shell segmentation, and bone segmentation.

3.1.1. Egg Detection. Each input microCT image comprised the egg, the animal bed, and the background (i.e., air) (Figure 2(a)). Images occasionally contained anesthetic equipment (i.e., tubing or nozzles), which had to be removed. The first step of image processing involves separating the background from the rest of the image content. Therefore, a large Gaussian blur (kernel size: $51 \times 51 \times 99$) was applied. The resulting layer was min-max normalized, and every pixel with a value less than or equal to 0.1 was discarded as background (Figure 2(b)). All other pixels were kept as image objects.

To exclude additional periphery, only the largest image object (i.e., the egg and the complete animal bed object) was retained. Next, this *Coarse Egg (Complete)/Bed (Complete)* object needed to be segmented into its two components. Since the carbon fiber bed and the interior of the egg have similar pixel values, this separation cannot be performed based solely on these values. Therefore, a modeling approach that exploits morphological differences between the animal bed and the egg was developed. This approach is based on the knowledge that the egg is axially aligned in the field of view (FOV) of the microCT scanner and that in an axial view an egg is much rounder than the animal bed.

To separate the egg from the bed, the *Coarse Egg/Bed (Complete)* object was first split into a series of 2D slices (Figure 2(c)). On each slice, all parts of this object below a certain degree of roundness (calculated as the quotient of the radius of the largest enclosed ellipse divided by the radius of the smallest enclosing ellipse) were reclassified as *Temporary* objects (Figure 2 c_1). Using a pixel-based grow operation, the remaining round objects (Figure 2 c_2) were first expanded along the z-axis (i.e., from the blunt to the pointed end of the egg) and then along the x- and y-axes into the *Temporary* objects.

During the growth process, a stringent surface tension criterion was applied to prevent the new object from growing back into the initial *Coarse Egg/Bed (Complete)* object. The result of this step was the *Coarse Egg/Bed (Parts)* object (Figure 2(d)). The remaining *Temporary* objects were reclassified as background. Consequently, the background consisted only of air and the animal bed, a fact that could then be used to help remove the remaining part of the bed from the *Coarse Egg/Bed (Parts)* object. The strategy was to model the animal bed by segmenting the background into bed and air and then expand the bed through the *Coarse Egg/Bed (Parts)* object using the grow operation.

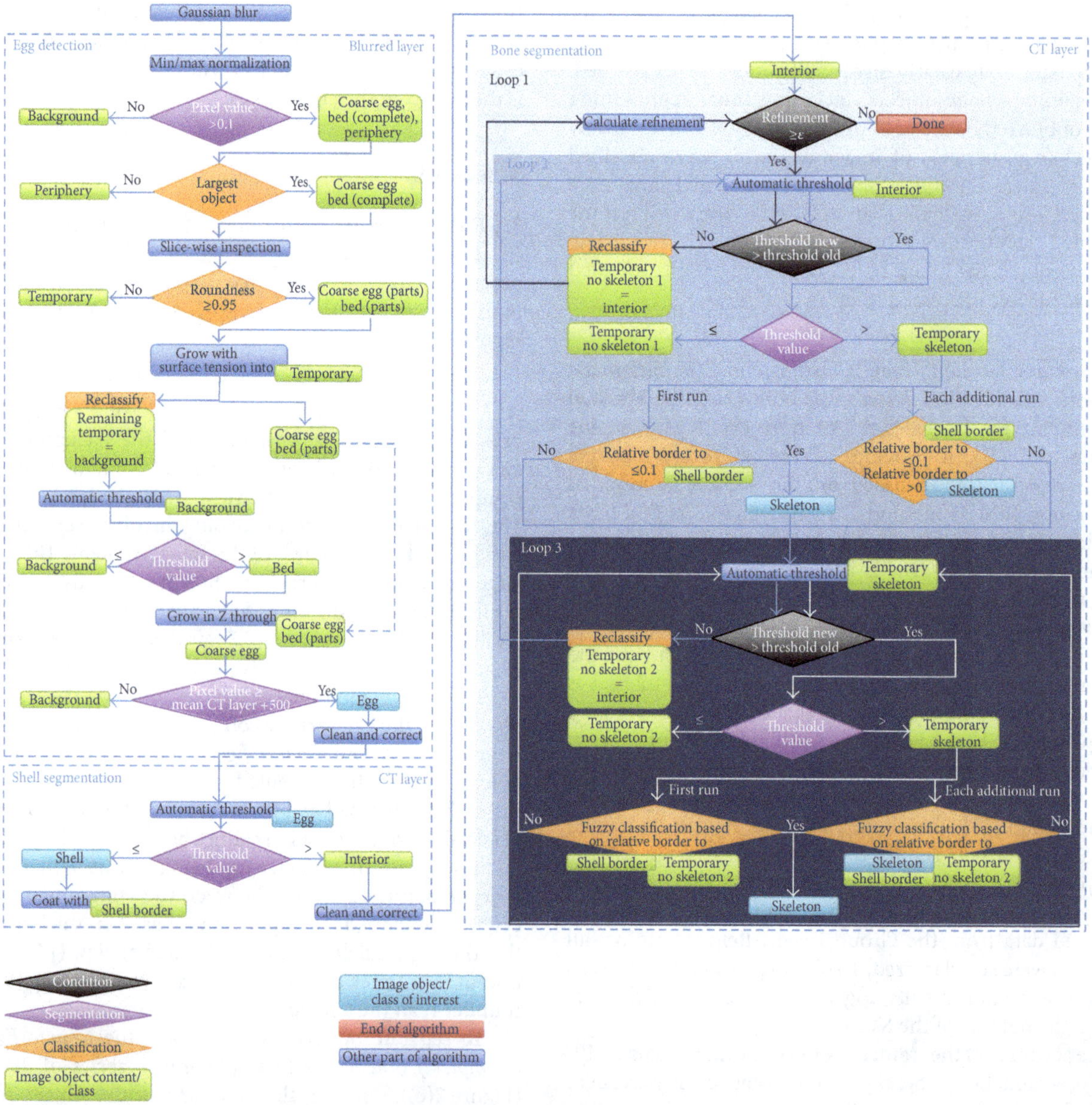

FIGURE 1: Graphical representation of the complete automated image segmentation procedure. A larger reproduction is provided in the Supplementary Material as Supplemental Figure S1 (see Supplementary material available online at http://dx.doi.org/10.1155/2013/508474).

To separate the two image parts of the background, a threshold was calculated by using the *automatic threshold* function (AT) on the original unfiltered CT layer. Based on a combination of histogram and homogeneity measurements, this function calculates a pixel value such that intensity differences and heterogeneity increase to a maximum between the resulting pixel subsets. In this case, the respective subsets were the animal bed and air. The background was segmented using the calculated threshold. All pixels with values above the threshold were then classified as *Bed*. This image object was then expanded along the z-axis through the *Coarse Egg/Bed (Parts)* object. As a result, all affected pixels, and thus the animal bed, were reclassified as *Background* and removed from this object (Figure 2(e)) resulting in the *Coarse Egg* object.

The last step of the egg detection step was to refine the remaining *Coarse Egg* object into its final shape. The object consisting of air and the actual egg was separated into these two components by applying another segmentation process that used a fixed intensity threshold (mean pixel value of the egg object + 500) on the unfiltered image layer. The resulting object was further smoothed into the final egg object using three expansion and reduction steps (i.e., grow and shrink operations) (Figure 2(f)).

3.1.2. Shell Segmentation. The aim of this step was to separate the eggshell from the egg interior. Here, the AT function could be reapplied, because the shell and the interior form two well-separated pixel subsets. The subsequent segmentation using the calculated threshold value resulted in a *Shell*

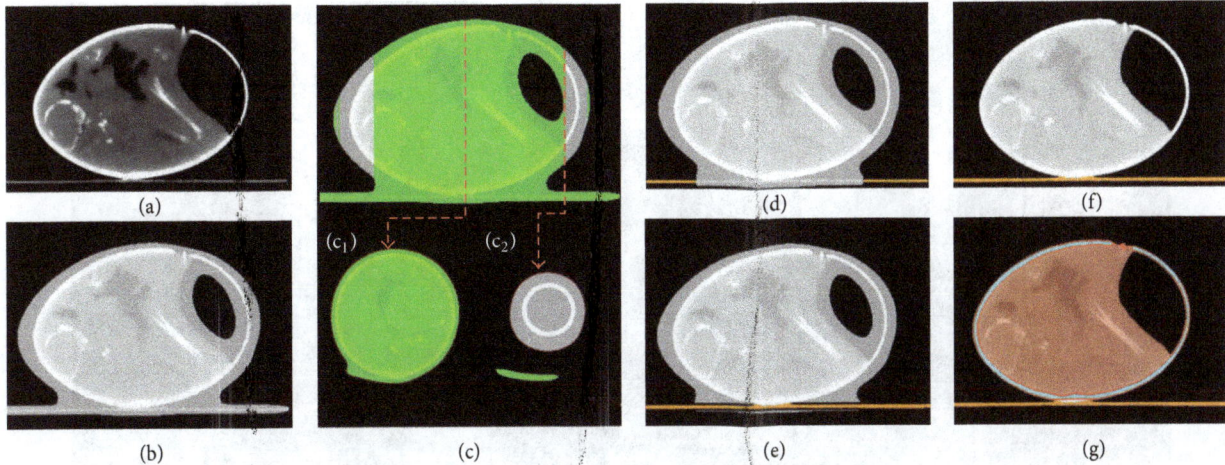

FIGURE 2: Steps of *Egg Detection* and *Shell Segmentation*. (a) input image; (b) initial segmentation after coarse Gaussian blur; (c) slicewise inspection and search for round image objects; (c_1) example of an image object (green) below the defined threshold for roundness; (c_2) example of image objects above (white) and below (green) the defined threshold for roundness; (d) parts of the animal bed (orange) were removed by retaining only the round (white) image objects from the previous step and reexpanding them by applying a stringent surface tension criterion to prevent expansion too far back into the animal be; (e) the animal bed was separated from the background and expanded along the z-axis through the *Coarse Egg/Bed (Parts)* (white) object; (f) the *Coarse Egg* (white) object was segmented using a fixed threshold and further smoothed by three consecutive expansion and reduction operations; (g) using an automatically calculated threshold, the refined *Egg* object was segmented into *Shell* (light blue) and *Interior* (light red). The *Shell* object was surrounded by two additional layers of pixels (*Shell Border, red*).

object and an object representing the *Interior* of the egg (Figure 2(g)). Additionally, the *Shell* object was surrounded by two layers of pixels classified as *Shell Border*.

3.1.3. Bone Segmentation.

In this step, the skeleton was separated from the rest of the egg interior. Because calcified bones have considerably high pixel values that form a pixel subset distinct from the egg interior, the AT function could also be applied extensively in this step. The AT function extends enough robustness to the entire rule set so that bones and bony structures are correctly segmented for eggs from d13 to d19. However, some additional measures needed to be taken for the correct segmentation of bones located close to the shell. Here, the AT function fails to directly calculate the best separating threshold, and consequently, initial segmentation often leads to large image objects that are attached to the shell and which need to be further treated.

A possible solution that provides robustness, as well as a high segmentation quality, was implemented in three nested loops that perform repeated automatic threshold calculation, image segmentation, and segmentation refinements (Figure 1).

The outer loop was used for global refinement and to control if the segmentation steps performed in the two inner loops contributed a substantial amount of new pixels to new or existing *Skeleton* image objects. The complete bone segmentation step was terminated when the last round of segmentation and classification performed by the two inner loops did not increase the number of pixels classified as *Skeleton* by 0.005% or greater.

In the first inner loop, a threshold was calculated, and the *Interior* was segmented into *Temporary Skeleton* and

Temporary No Skeleton 1 using that threshold. Following segmentation, only resulting *Temporary Skeleton* image objects were further processed. If it was the first run of the outer loop, all *Temporary Skeleton* image objects with a relative border to *Shell Border* smaller than or equal to 0.1 were classified as *Skeleton*. In all subsequent runs of the outer loop, a second condition was introduced; new *Temporary Skeleton* image objects also needed to share a relative border with existing *Skeleton* objects in order to also be classified as *Skeleton*.

All remaining *Temporary Skeleton* that could not be classified as *Skeleton* because they did not satisfy the border conditions were then fed into the second inner loop for the refinement of segmentation and the extraction of additional *Skeleton* image objects. The second inner loop had the same basic functional principle as the first inner loop. Using an automatically calculated threshold, the *Temporary Skeleton* image objects were further segmented into *Temporary Skeleton* and *Temporary No Skeleton 2* objects. However, unlike the first inner loop, the classification of the *Temporary Skeleton* objects was now performed using the relative border to the *Shell Border* and to *Temporary No Skeleton 2* as measurements combined in a fuzzy set with a linear or sigmoidal membership function. The second inner loop was exited when the AT function could not calculate a new threshold (i.e., the best separating value was reached). All remaining *Temporary No Skeleton 2* objects were then reclassified as *Interior* and fed back into the first inner loop.

The first inner loop was exited when a better separating threshold could not be calculated. The number of pixels added to existing *Skeleton* image objects or representing new *Skeleton* image objects was then calculated in order

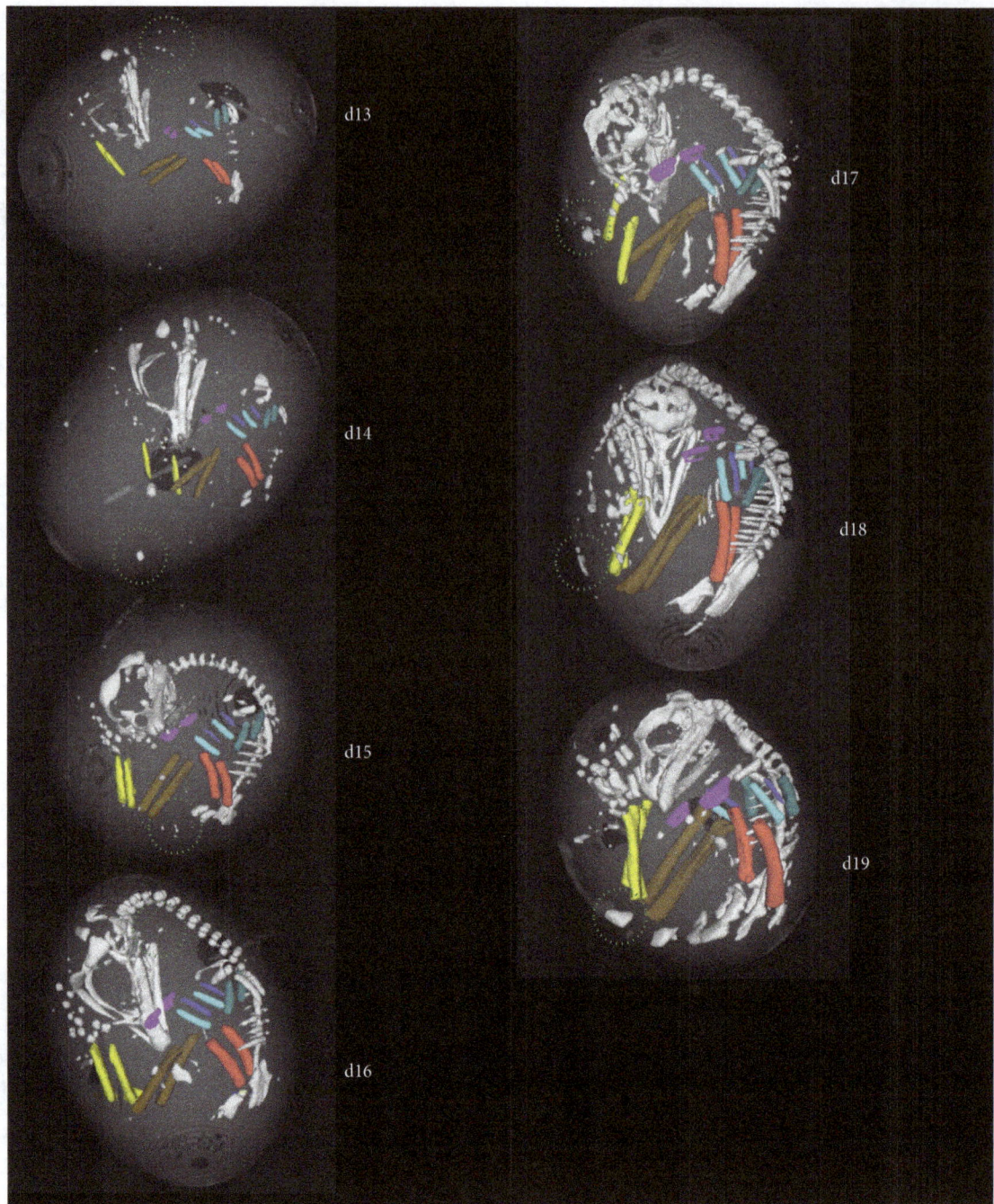

	Tarsometatarsus		Carpometacarpus
	Femur		Ulna
	Tibiotarsus		Radius
	Artifact		Humerus

FIGURE 3: Segmentation and classification of microCT images of Group 1 chick embryos from d13 to d19. The bone names and their corresponding colors are presented. Image artifacts are circled in green.

to confirm if the termination condition of the outer loop was satisfied. If the refinement was above the threshold, the *Temporary No Skeleton 2* objects were combined, reclassified as *Interior,* and subjected to another round of bone segmentation. Otherwise, after satisfying the termination condition of the outer loop, the final result of the bone segmentation step was a set of *Skeleton* image objects representing the chick embryo skeleton and a number of image artifacts (Figure 3). For each of these image objects, the following feature values were calculated and exported into a CSV file: day of incubation, asymmetry, border length, compactness, elliptical fit, length, thickness, width, length/thickness, length/width,

TABLE 1: Classification accuracy of the SVM after 10-fold cross-validation on the training data from Group 1 eggs.

Classes	True positive rate	False positive rate	Precision	Recall	F-measure	ROC-area
Humerus	0.941	0.003	0.842	0.941	0.889	0.999
Radius	0.929	0.001	0.929	0.929	0.929	0.996
Ulna	0.918	0.001	0.938	0.918	0.928	0.979
Carpometacarpus	0.865	0.002	0.900	0.865	0.882	0.988
Femur	1.000	0.001	0.962	1.000	0.981	1.000
Tibiotarsus	0.925	0.000	0.980	0.925	0.951	0.999
Tarsometatarsus	0.941	0.001	0.960	0.941	0.950	0.991
Not of interest (NOI)	0.994	0.043	0.994	0.994	0.994	0.996
Weighted avg.	**0.986**	**0.038**	**0.987**	**0.986**	**0.986**	**0.996**

TABLE 2: Confusion matrix of the SVM after 10-fold cross-validation on the training data from Group 1 eggs.

Classes	Classified as							
	a	b	c	d	e	f	g	h
a = humerus	48	0	0	0	0	0	0	3
b = radius	0	39	1	0	0	0	0	2
c = ulna	1	0	45	0	0	0	0	3
d = carpometacarpus	1	0	1	45	0	0	0	5
e = femur	0	0	0	0	51	0	0	0
f = tibiotarsus	0	0	0	0	1	49	2	1
g = tarsometatarsus	0	0	0	0	1	1	48	1
h = not of interest (NOI)	7	3	1	5	0	0	0	2586

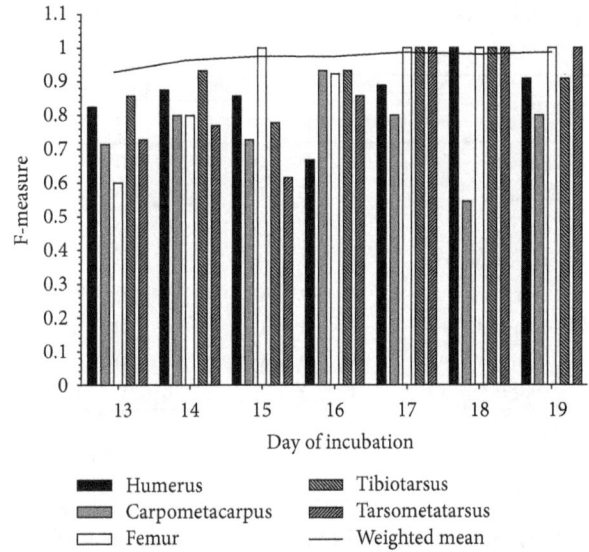

FIGURE 4: Bar chart of the classification accuracy of SVMs trained for single days of incubation. To evaluate the classification performance for a single day of incubation, an SVM was trained on all objects but the image objects belonging to the corresponding day. The resulting SVM was then applied to these excluded objects. The overall classification accuracy increases with the day of incubation.

volume in relation to the total volume of all extracted bone objects, radius of largest enclosed ellipse, radius of smallest enclosing ellipse, rectangular fit, roundness, shape index, mean of the CT image layer, standard deviation of the CT image layer, skewness of the CT image layer, minimal pixel value of the CT image layer, maximal pixel value of the CT image layer, number of other bone objects within a range of 50 pixels, distance to the nearest *Skeleton* object, and distance to *Shell*.

The typical run time of the rule set was between 6 and 15 min depending on the number of bones, bony objects, and artifacts in the image.

3.2. Training the SVM for Long Bone Classification. A total of 2951 annotated object instances extracted from the images of Group 1 were used for training the SVM. The grid search yielded an optimal setting of 1.25 for the C and 0.1125 for γ. After 10-fold cross-validation, the model proved to be highly accurate (Table 1) and was able to correctly classify 98.6% of the instances. The femur can be most accurately identified (F-measure 0.981), while the correct annotation of bones of the carpometacarpus is slightly more challenging (F-measure 0.882). The largest class (NOI) can also be readily separated from the other bone types. This is integral to the automated annotation of datasets not having bone name labels (unlabeled dataset). The highest numbers of false positives (15) and false negatives (16) were, however, identified during classification of the NOI objects (Table 2).

To evaluate the classification performance for a single day of incubation, an SVM that leaves out bones for that specific day, was trained on all remaining objects. The resulting SVM was then applied to the image objects of the excluded day of incubation. In general, the classification accuracy increases with the day of incubation (Figure 4). Bones become more calcified the longer the egg is incubated, thus allowing for improved differentiation. However, the classification accuracy is dependent on bone type. While the femur can easily be identified, annotation of the carpometacarpus can be problematic. Nevertheless, the intrinsic information from the other days facilitates accurate annotation. Hence, this model can also be used to transfer knowledge between different days of incubation.

The performance of the trained SVM model was evaluated on an unlabeled test set. The SVM correctly classified 98.6% of the 1203 object instances that were extracted from the microCT images of Group 2 eggs. The best classification

TABLE 3: Classification accuracy of the SVM on the test data from Group 2 eggs.

Classes	True positive rate	False positive rate	Precision	Recall	F-measure	ROC-area
Humerus	0.875	0.000	1.000	0.875	0.933	0.966
Radius	0.938	0.002	0.882	0.938	0.909	0.999
Ulna	0.864	0.002	0.905	0.864	0.884	0.999
Carpometacarpus	0.875	0.000	1.000	0.875	0.933	0.965
Femur	0.958	0.000	1.000	0.958	0.979	0.975
Tibiotarsus	0.875	0.000	1.000	0.875	0.933	0.978
Tarsometatarsus	0.905	0.001	0.950	0.905	0.927	0.980
Not of interest (NOI)	0.999	0.077	0.989	0.999	0.994	0.989
Weighted avg.	**0.986**	**0.068**	**0.986**	**0.986**	**0.988**	**0.989**

TABLE 4: Confusion matrix of the SVM on the test data from the Group 2 eggs.

Classes	Classified as							
	a	b	c	d	e	f	g	h
a = humerus	21	0	0	0	0	0	0	3
b = radius	0	15	0	0	0	0	0	1
c = ulna	0	2	19	0	0	0	0	1
d = carpometacarpus	0	0	1	21	0	0	0	2
e = femur	0	0	0	0	23	0	0	1
f = tibiotarsus	0	0	0	0	0	21	1	2
g = tarsometatarsus	0	0	0	0	0	0	19	2
h = not of interest (NOI)	0	0	1	0	0	0	0	1047

TABLE 5: Bone growth rates of the Group 2 chick embryos.

Classes	d13 to d14 (mm/day)	d14 to d15 (mm/day)
Humerus	1.186	0.626
Radius	1.245	0.504
Ulna	1.323	0.534
Carpometacarpus	0.802	0.529
Femur	1.625	1.174
Tibiotarsus	2.491	2.688
Tarsometatarsus	1.473	2.902

reliability (F-measure 0.979) was again obtained for the femur (Table 3). In contrast to Group 1, the ulna (F-measure 0.884), not the carpometacarpus (F-measure 0.933), was the bone with the lowest classification reliability. Interestingly, for the femur, the *Precision* is higher for the test set than for the training set (i.e., the application of the model to unknown datasets is highly confident). As with Group 1, the NOI objects from Group 2 also yielded the highest number of false positives (i.e., 12). A maximum of three false negatives were identified during classification of the humerus, radius, carpometacarpus, and tibiotarsus (Table 4).

3.3. In Ovo Measurement of Long Bone Growth of Chick Embryos from d13 to d15. Crural bones are much longer (Figure 5) and have a much higher rate of growth than aral bones (Table 5). The highest increase in length (2.902 mm/day) was recorded for the tarsometatarsus from d14 to d15, while for the same interval, the radius had the smallest increase (0.504 mm/day).

4. Discussion

Noninvasive microCT offers quantitative imaging with high spatial resolution as well as the possibility of repeatedly imaging and measuring the same chick embryo *in ovo*. The excellent bone contrast can be used to investigate bone-related questions, for example, bone formation (in conjunction with

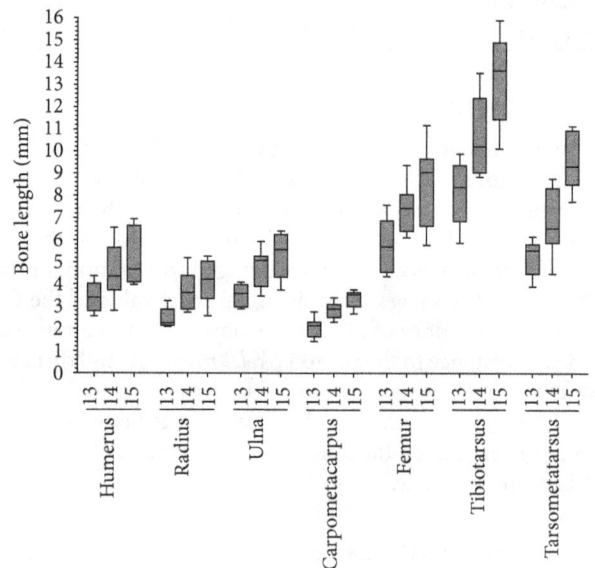

FIGURE 5: Box and whisker plot of long bone lengths of chick embryos from Group 2. The numerical values are presented in Supplemental Table S1.

automated image segmentation methods [25]) and tumor-induced bone destruction [26]. To our knowledge, these techniques had not yet been applied to the *in ovo* quantification of bone growth of live chick embryos. We developed an approach for the automated segmentation of *in ovo* microCT images from live chick embryos using OBIA, followed by automated classification of the extracted image objects. As automated routines heavily reduce processing time, more images can be analyzed within the same timespan. Moreover, such systems minimize observer bias. The Definiens Developer XD rule set for automated image segmentation was developed using only one egg at d18. However, it proved to be robust enough to successfully segment the skeleton from the rest of the egg and its periphery on microCT images for eggs from d13 to d19 without having to adjust parameters for incubation day. Thus, the approach could effectively manage variations in bone size and calcification. In addition for determining feature values for single bones, the segmentation and classification results could be also used to provide an excellent 3D *in ovo* visualization of the developing chick embryo (Figure 3).

The high classification accuracy using an SVM greatly facilitates the classification of objects extracted from microCT images, although bones with a low classification probability should be reviewed to avoid corruption of length measurements. An iterative approach comprising repeated classification and feature value calculation could, however, refine the existing classification and enable the classification of previously unclassified objects. In the first step, only objects with high classification probabilities would be classified. Based on this initial classification, new feature values (e.g., distances) could be calculated for unclassified objects in a subsequent step. In turn, these values could be used to train a new and extended classifier.

Long bone growth during chick embryogenesis has been extensively studied under normal conditions [27–29] as well as under various environmental influences such as insecticides [30], increased temperature [31], and acceleration [32]. However, none of these studies provided *in vivo* data; the chick embryos were sacrificed, removed from the egg, and fixed. Bone lengths were either measured while bones were still attached to the limb or after they were dissected from adherent tissue.

Therefore, the long bone length measurements presented in this study represent the first true *in vivo* data. While our results deviate from those of the aforementioned *ex ovo* and *ex vivo* measurements, there were also discrepancies among those studies. For example, for d15 we measured a mean femur length of 8.574 mm, Alfonso-Torres et al. [28] reported a length of 14.51 mm (by polynomial regression), and Hammond et. al reported a length of 11.25 mm (Figure 4(b) in [31]). In addition to human bias, these apparent differences may arise from variations in breeder age [28] and incubation temperature [31] as well as bone shrinkage resulting from fixation or preparation [33]. Our methodology imposes additional constraints that should be considered when comparing our measured lengths to those of classical studies. As CT has poor cartilage contrast, only areas of sufficiently mineralized bone can be imaged and measured. The image analysis software also calculates lengths differently than direct measurement (i.e., via a ruler or calipers).

We present an innovative approach for the automated segmentation, classification, quantification, and visualization of microCT images. MicroCT offers the possibility to perform longitudinal studies and thereby provides unique insights into the morpho- and embryogenesis of the live chick embryo. By using OBIA, image parts (e.g., bones) may

be extracted from an image in order to calculate various morphometric feature values. These can subsequently be used to train a classifier that can identify image objects based on these unique values. Despite a high classification accuracy, some misclassifications must still be manually corrected in order to yield statistically valid results. Human expertise is therefore still required for the interpretation and validation of results. Nevertheless, automated systems can greatly expedite image analysis and reduce observer bias.

Conflict of Interests

Johannes Zimmermann is a paid employee of Definiens AG. All other authors declare that they have no conflict of interests.

Authors' Contributions

Alexander Heidrich conceived the study, carried out CT measurements, participated in rule set development, and drafted the paper. Jana Schmidt performed data analysis and helped drafting the paper. Johannes Zimmermann participated in rule set development and helped drafting the paper. Hans Peter Saluz participated in the design of the study and helped drafting the paper. All authors read and approved the final paper.

Acknowledgments

This work was funded by the German Federal Ministry of Education and Health (BMBF; Grant Nos. 0314108 and 01KI1011D). The authors are indebted to Brent Sørensen for proofreading the paper. They also thank Vera Mittenzwei-Klujewa for excellent technical assistance as well as Andreas Hapfelmeier and Günter Schmidt for their valuable comments and advice.

References

[1] H. Rashidi and V. Sottile, "The chick embryo: hatching a model for contemporary biomedical research," *BioEssays*, vol. 31, no. 4, pp. 459–465, 2009.

[2] C. D. Stern, "The chick: a great model system becomes even greater," *Developmental Cell*, vol. 8, no. 1, pp. 9–17, 2005.

[3] C. D. Stern, "The chick embryo—past, present and future as a model system in developmental biology," *Mechanisms of Development*, vol. 121, no. 9, pp. 1011–1013, 2004.

[4] D. K. Darnell and G. C. Schoenwolf, "The chick embryo as a model system for analyzing mechanisms of development," *Methods in Molecular Biology*, vol. 135, pp. 25–29, 2000.

[5] E. V. Schmidt and R. E. Smith, "Skeletal hyperostoses. Viral induction of avian osteopetrosis," *American Journal of Pathology*, vol. 106, no. 2, pp. 297–299, 1982.

[6] M. F. Holick, "Perspective on the impact of weightlessness on calcium and bone metabolism," *Bone*, vol. 22, no. 5, pp. 105S–111S, 1998.

[7] M. E. Cook, "Skeletal deformities and their causes: introduction," *Poultry Science*, vol. 79, no. 7, pp. 982–984, 2000.

[8] N. C. Nowlan, J. Sharpe, K. A. Roddy, P. J. Prendergast, and P. Murphy, "Mechanobiology of embryonic skeletal development: insights from animal models," *Birth Defects Research Part C*, vol. 90, no. 3, pp. 203–213, 2010.

[9] P. M. Kulesa, C. M. Bailey, C. Cooper, and S. E. Fraser, "*In ovo* live imaging of avian embryos," *Cold Spring Harbor Protocols*, vol. 5, no. 6, 2010.

[10] Z. Zhou, J. Xu, Z. S. Delproposto et al., "Feasibility of *in ovo* diffusion tractography in the chick embryo using a dual-cooling technique," *Journal of Magnetic Resonance Imaging*, vol. 36, pp. 993–1001, 2012.

[11] M. A. Schellpfeffer and G. L. Kolesari, "Microbubble contrast imaging of the cardiovascular system of the chick embyro," *Ultrasound in Medicine and Biology*, vol. 38, no. 3, pp. 504–510, 2012.

[12] A. L. Henning, M. X. Jiang, H. C. Yalcin, and J. T. Butcher, "Quantitative three-dimensional imaging of live avian embryonic morphogenesis via micro-computed tomography," *Developmental Dynamics*, vol. 240, no. 8, pp. 1949–1957, 2011.

[13] M. Baatz, J. Zimmermann, and C. G. Blackmore, "Automated analysis and detailed quantification of biomedical images using definiens cognition network technology," *Combinatorial Chemistry and High Throughput Screening*, vol. 12, no. 9, pp. 908–916, 2009.

[14] F. Mech, A. Thywißen, R. Guthke, A. A. Brakhage, and M. T. Figge, "Automated image analysis of the host-pathogen interaction between phagocytes and aspergillus fumigatus," *PLoS ONE*, vol. 6, no. 5, Article ID e19591, 2011.

[15] J. Cunningham, V. Estrella, M. Lloyd, R. Gillies, B. R. Frieden, and R. Gatenby, "Intracellular electric field and pH optimize protein localization and movement," *PloS ONE*, vol. 7, Article ID e36894, 2012.

[16] A. Vogt, A. Cholewinski, X. Shen et al., "Automated image-based phenotypic analysis in zebrafish embryos," *Developmental Dynamics*, vol. 238, no. 3, pp. 656–663, 2009.

[17] R. Schönmeyer, M. Athelogou, H. Sittek et al., "Cognition Network Technology prototype of a CAD system for mammography to assist radiologists by finding similar cases in a reference database," *International Journal of Computer Assisted Radiology and Surgery*, vol. 6, no. 1, pp. 127–134, 2011.

[18] H. Weber, A. Rauch, S. Adamski et al., "Automated rodent in situ muscle contraction assay and myofiber organization analysis in sarcopenia animal models," *Journal of Applied Physiology*, vol. 112, no. 12, pp. 2087–2098, 2012.

[19] A. Tzotsos, K. Karantzalos, and D. Argialas, "Object-based image analysis through nonlinear scale-space filtering," *ISPRS Journal of Photogrammetry and Remote Sensing*, vol. 66, no. 1, pp. 2–16, 2011.

[20] L. Würbach, A. Heidrich, T. Opfermann, P. Gebhardt, and H. P. Saluz, "Insights into bone metabolism of avian embryos *in ovo* via 3D and 4D18F-fluoride positron emission tomography," *Molecular Imaging and Biology*, vol. 14, pp. 688–698, 2012.

[21] M. Hall, E. Frank, G. Holmes, and B. Pfahringer, "The WEKA data mining software: an update," *SIGKDD Explorations*, vol. 11, pp. 10–18, 2009.

[22] J. C. Platt, "Fast training of support vector machines using sequential minimal optimization," in *Advances in Kernel Methods Support Vector Learning*, B. Scholkopf, C. J. C. Burges, and A. J. Smola, Eds., pp. 185–208, MIT Press, Cambridge, Mass, USA, 1998.

[23] N. Thai-Nghe, Z. Gantner, and L. Schmidt-Thieme, "Cost-sensitive learning methods for imbalanced data," in *Proceedings of the International Joint Conference on Neural Networks (IJCNN '10)*, pp. 1–8, July 2010.

[24] D. Powers, "Evaluation: from precision, recall and F-measure to ROC, informedness, markedness & correlation," *Journal of Machine Learning Technologies*, vol. 2, pp. 37–63, 2011.

[25] S. J. Polak, S. Candido, S. K. L. Levengood, and A. J. Wagoner Johnson, "Automated segmentation of micro-CT images of bone formation in calcium phosphate scaffolds," *Computerized Medical Imaging and Graphics*, vol. 36, no. 1, pp. 54–65, 2012.

[26] L. C. Johnson, R. W. Johnson, S. A. Munoz, G. R. Mundy, T. E. Peterson, and J. A. Sterling, "Longitudinal live animal micro-CT allows for quantitative analysis of tumor-induced bone destruction," *Bone*, vol. 48, no. 1, pp. 141–151, 2011.

[27] L. E. Church and L. C. Johnson, "Growth of long bones in the chicken. Rates of growth in length and diameter of the humerus, tibia, and metatarsus," *The American Journal of Anatomy*, vol. 114, pp. 521–538, 1964.

[28] K. A. Alfonso-Torres, L. H. Gargaglioni, J. M. Pizauro, D. E. Faria Filho, R. L. Furlan, and M. Macari, "Breeder age and bone development in broiler chicken embryos," *Arquivo Brasileiro de Medicina Veterinaria e Zootecnia*, vol. 61, no. 1, pp. 219–226, 2009.

[29] C. W. Archer, A. Hornbruch, and L. Wolpert, "Growth and morphogenesis of the fibula in the chick embryo," *Journal of Embryology and Experimental Morphology*, vol. 75, pp. 101–116, 1983.

[30] M. Misawa, J. Doull, and E. M. Uyeki, "Teratogenic effects of cholinergic insecticides in chick embryos. III. Development of cartilage and bone," *Journal of Toxicology and Environmental Health*, vol. 10, no. 4-5, pp. 551–563, 1982.

[31] C. L. Hammond, B. H. Simbi, and N. C. Stickland, "*In ovo* temperature manipulation influences embryonic motility and growth of limb tissues in the chick (*Gallus gallus*)," *Journal of Experimental Biology*, vol. 210, no. 15, pp. 2667–2675, 2007.

[32] D. R. Redden, "Chronic acceleration effects on bone development in the chick embryo," *The American Journal of Physiology*, vol. 218, no. 1, pp. 310–313, 1970.

[33] D. Summerbell, "A descriptive study of the rate of elongation and differentiation of the skeleton of the developing chick wing," *Journal of Embryology and Experimental Morphology*, vol. 35, no. 2, pp. 241–260, 1976.

Respiratory Motion Compensation Using Diaphragm Tracking for Cone-Beam C-Arm CT: A Simulation and a Phantom Study

Marco Bögel,[1] **Hannes G. Hofmann,**[1] **Joachim Hornegger,**[1] **Rebecca Fahrig,**[2] **Stefan Britzen,**[3] **and Andreas Maier**[3]

[1] *Pattern Recognition Lab, Friedrich-Alexander-University Erlangen-Nuremberg, 91058 Erlangen, Germany*
[2] *Department of Radiology, Lucas MRS Center, Stanford University, Palo Alto, CA 94304, USA*
[3] *Siemens AG, Healthcare Sector, 91301 Forchheim, Germany*

Correspondence should be addressed to Andreas Maier; andreas.maier@cs.fau.de

Academic Editor: Michael W. Vannier

Long acquisition times lead to image artifacts in thoracic C-arm CT. Motion blur caused by respiratory motion leads to decreased image quality in many clinical applications. We introduce an image-based method to estimate and compensate respiratory motion in C-arm CT based on diaphragm motion. In order to estimate respiratory motion, we track the contour of the diaphragm in the projection image sequence. Using a motion corrected triangulation approach on the diaphragm vertex, we are able to estimate a motion signal. The estimated motion signal is used to compensate for respiratory motion in the target region, for example, heart or lungs. First, we evaluated our approach in a simulation study using XCAT. As ground truth data was available, a quantitative evaluation was performed. We observed an improvement of about 14% using the structural similarity index. In a real phantom study, using the artiCHEST phantom, we investigated the visibility of bronchial tubes in a porcine lung. Compared to an uncompensated scan, the visibility of bronchial structures is improved drastically. Preliminary results indicate that this kind of motion compensation can deliver a first step in reconstruction image quality improvement. Compared to ground truth data, image quality is still considerably reduced.

1. Introduction

C-arm CT has enabled reconstruction of 3D images during medical procedures, for example, cardiac interventions. However, the rather long acquisition time of several seconds may lead to motion artifacts, such as motion blur and streaks. These artifacts are very problematic in many clinical applications. The commonly used technique to reduce the influence of respiratory motion during cardiac procedures is the so-called single breath-hold scan. This approach requires the patient to hold his breath for the duration of the scan. Unfortunately, this technique does not guarantee perfect results. Jahnke et al. have measured residual respiratory motion in almost half of their test group containing 210 people [1]. We have two main applications in the focus of our work. One is the improvement of cardiac C-arm CT. While compensation of the motion of the heart has been

investigated intensively in the literature [2–4], the problem of respiratory motion during cardiac C-arm CT is much less frequently addressed. Residual respiratory motion during the cardiac scan causes a considerable reduction in image quality.

Motion artifacts are also very problematic in pulmonary procedures. In order to analyze the malignancy of a pulmonary tumor, a sample has to be extracted. A bronchoscope is inserted through the patient's nose and has to be navigated through the bronchial tree towards the tumor. This procedure requires an accurate plan of the bronchial tree. However, most tumors are only accessible through bronchi with diameters of less than 2 mm. Therefore, we require accurate imaging without motion blur, otherwise the small bronchi are not visible. Respiratory motion can be reduced with a jet ventilator that inflates the lung with oxygen. There are two downsides to this approach. The efficiency of this approach depends on the amount of pressure that is used. While too small pressure results in residual motion, too high pressure may cause rupture and pneumothorax in consequence. Additionally, natural reflexes of the human body may also cause residual motion. Therefore, it is necessary to develop new methods to estimate and compensate respiratory motion in C-arm CT. There are many different ways to acquire respiratory signals. Most are based on additional equipment, for example, Time-of-Flight or stereo vision cameras [5]. Other techniques try to extract the respiratory signal directly from the projection images. Using an image-based approach the extracted respiration signal is perfectly synchronized with the projection images. Image-based respiratory motion extraction often relies on tracking of fiducial markers in the projection images [6, 7]. Wang et al. have shown that the motion of the diaphragm is highly correlated to respiration-induced motion of the heart [8]. Sonke et al. propose to extract a 1D respiration signal by projecting diaphragm-like features on the superior-inferior axis and selecting the features with the highest temporal change [9]. However, the downside of this approach is that the extracted signal is not the real respiration signal. Due to perspective projection, the projected amplitude depends on the C-arm rotation angle. Kavanagh et al. recently proposed a similar approach analyzing the intensity values between projections that works without any external or internal oscillating structures [10]. Another recent approach by Chen and Siochi tracks the diaphragm using a combination of Hough Transform and Active Contours and an interpolated ray-tracing algorithm to estimate a respiration signal [11]. Vergalasova et al. proposed a Fourier Transform based approach that also works without any markers [12].

In this paper, we propose to estimate respiratory motion by tracking the diaphragm in the projection image sequence. The tracked position of the diaphragm top is used to compute a 1D respiration signal, which is then incorporated into the reconstruction algorithm to compensate for respiratory motion in the volume of interest.

2. Materials and Methods

The proposed method is composed of three major steps that are each discussed in the following sections. In the first step, the contour of the diaphragm is tracked throughout the entire projection image sequence. Based on this tracking, we are able to obtain the 2D projection of the diaphragm top for each image. In the second step, a motion corrected triangulation approach is used to compute the 3D position of the diaphragm top for each projection. Assuming superior-inferior respiratory motion, the 1D respiration signal is extracted. In the final step, the respiration signal is used to compensate for respiratory motion during reconstruction.

2.1. Diaphragm Tracking. We introduced a model-based tracking method that is able to accurately track the contour of a user-selected hemidiaphragm in a set of rotational projection images [13]. Compared to other tracking-based methods, for example, fiducial markers, the shape we want to track is not unique. The diaphragm appears as two similar

shaped hemidiaphragms. Therefore, it is necessary for the user to select the one to be tracked. The user selects a point roughly located at the top of the desired contour. Subsequently, we define a rectangular Region of Interest (ROI) symmetrically around the selection. We propose an ROI of size 250×55 for projection images of size 640×480. The image is then preprocessed using a gaussian low-pass filter and the Canny edge detector.

In the next step, the Random Sample Consensus (RANSAC) [14] is used to fit a parabolic curve to the obtained set of edge points. RANSAC can deal with datasets with large percentages of gross errors and is thus the ideal choice to fit a model to our very noisy set of points. The aim of this method is to model the diaphragm as a quadratic function $v = au^2 + bu + c$, where u and v are the detector coordinates. The parabolic model is a good fit for the top of the diaphragm, in which we are interested in. The asymmetry in lower parts of the diaphragm does not affect our model, as our ROI limits the estimation to the top region. The parabolic model allows for very fast model estimation, as well as a simple extraction of the diaphragm vertex. RANSAC has to estimate the three parameters a, b, and c. In the first step, three random points are selected. The model estimation is then formulated as the following optimization problem:

$$\sum_{i=1}^{3} \left(a \cdot u_i^2 + b \cdot u_i + c - v_i \right)^2 \longrightarrow \min. \tag{1}$$

A total of N models are estimated, each based on different randomly selected points, and evaluated to determine the best one. A model's quality is defined by the number of inliers. An inlier is a point that lies within a predefined distance to the model. Since an accurate model is desired, we only consider points with a one pixel distance to the model inliers. Subsequently, out of the N estimated models we choose the one with the highest number of inliers. Assuming small motion between subsequent frames, the contour is tracked by calculating the current contour's vertex and using it as the start point in the subsequent frame.

One additional important optimization is made. Instead of continuing to use the rectangular ROI, we restrict it to a parabolic ROI based on the model from the previous frame. The parabolic region should be of sufficient height to contain the current diaphragm. In our experiments we used a parabolic region of 21 pixels height, centered around the previous model. This approach decreases the number of points we have to consider in the model estimation drastically.

To guarantee accurate tracking in projections where both hemidiaphragms are visible in the ROI, we propose additional constraints based on the small motion assumption and prior knowledge: (i) the horizontal motion of the contour is limited by the average motion in previous frames, (ii) deformation of the contour (defined by the change of model parameter a) is limited to 5% compared to the previous model, and (iii) the direction of horizontal motion can be derived from patient position and C-arm rotation. Suppose acquisition starts from the right lateral view. Rotating towards the frontal view, the contour of the right hemidiaphragm

```
(1)  for each projections i ∈ [1, N_p] do
(2)     for each voxel (x, y, z) do
(3)        Project voxel (x, y, z) onto detector plane
(4)        if point on detector plane then
(5)           Get update value
(6)        else
(7)           Next voxel
(8)        end if
(9)        z_corr ← z + r̂_i
(10)       if (x, y, z_corr) in volume then
(11)          Update voxel (x, y, z_corr)
(12)       end if
(13)    end for
(14) end for
```

ALGORITHM 1: Motion compensated reconstruction. Respiratory motion is compensated in lines (9)–(11).

will move to the left, whereas the contour of the left hemidiaphragm moves to the right. From the frontal position to the left lateral position this motion is reversed. We can now enforce the model to move in one direction until the turning point and then move in the opposite direction. However, since the diaphragm is deforming during respiration, it is better to loosen this constraint, by allowing free motion around the turning point. Allowing free motion in the frontal views is not problematic as the hemidiaphragms do not overlap or interfere in these views.

2.2. Triangulation and Signal Extraction.

The result of the diaphragm tracking is a parabolic model of the hemidiaphragm for each image. Our approach relies on the assumption that the projection of the 3D diaphragm top coincides with the top of the 2D diaphragm contour. However, this assumption is quite restrictive. Based on this assumption, we are able to reconstruct the 3D position using multiview triangulation. We use triangulation to acquire a motion signal in millimeter that we can use for motion compensated reconstruction. However, triangulation algorithms are designed for static scenes and yield inaccurate results when used for dynamic scenes. For triangulation of dynamic scenes we propose the following four step process:

(1) select a pair of images,

(2) rectification of the image planes [15],

(3) motion correction,

(4) triangulation [16].

First, we select two images with the contour vertices $\tilde{\mathbf{g}} = (\tilde{g}_u, \tilde{g}_v, 1)^T$ and $\tilde{\mathbf{g}}' = (\tilde{g}'_u, \tilde{g}'_v, 1)^T$. Ideally, the selected images should be acquired from orthogonal views, as using nonorthogonal images results in lower triangulation accuracy. The second step is essential for the subsequent motion correction. The rectification algorithm by Fusiello et al. projects the two projection images onto a common image plane, so that their epipolar lines become parallel and horizontal [15]. Subsequently, the transformed images have one very important feature: assuming no motion, the projections

of a specific point have the same vertical coordinate in both image planes. Thus, after transforming the detected point correspondences, any residual difference in their vertical coordinates must be caused by respiratory motion during image acquisition. Therefore, we can eliminate the respiratory motion of this image pair in the third step. We choose the first point $\tilde{\mathbf{g}}$ as the reference and the corresponding point in the second image is set to

$$\tilde{\mathbf{g}}' = \left(\tilde{g}'_u, \tilde{g}_v, 1\right)^T. \tag{2}$$

Finally, we use the transformed and motion corrected point correspondences to triangulate the corresponding 3D point. In this work a simple iterative Linear-Eigen approach, as proposed by Hartley and Sturm [16], has yielded excellent results.

After we triangulate a 3D point corresponding to each image, we can now compute the respiration signal. Since respiratory motion is generally considered as a mainly translational motion along the superior-inferior axis, we compute the 1D respiration signal $\hat{\mathbf{r}}$ as

$$\hat{r}_i = z_{\text{ref}} - z_i, \tag{3}$$

with z_{ref} as the z-coordinate of the reference point and z_i as the z-coordinate of the triangulated point corresponding to a projection image i. Finally, the resulting signal is smoothed using a gaussian low-pass filter.

2.3. Motion Compensated Reconstruction.

The signal is now included in the reconstruction process. Schäfer et al. recently introduced a motion compensated backprojection algorithm for cone-beam CT [17]. As we only utilize a rigid 1D motion vector field, we use a simplified version of their approach. Algorithm 1 shows the motion compensated pixel-driven reconstruction algorithm. For each projection, each voxel is projected on the detector to get the update value. Instead of regularly updating the volume, we first compensate for respiratory motion by shifting the voxel back to its reference position using the estimated signal. Then, we update the corrected voxel. Therefore, we are able to obtain a reconstruction at the reference time we selected for the respiration signal. So far, the proposed method assumes a constant shift when compensating the respiratory motion of the heart.

3. Results and Discussion

The proposed methods were evaluated on the simulated XCAT software phantom [18, 19] and the artiCHEST phantom (PROdesign GmbH, Germany), a porcine lung phantom that allows simulation of respiratory motion. Note that a fraction of the experimental results were already published in two short conference abstracts [13, 20].

3.1. XCAT Software Phantom.

The first evaluation of this work was carried out on the XCAT software phantom [18, 19]. The purpose of this evaluation is to compensate respiratory motion of the heart. The XCAT phantom was created with respiratory motion only. We simulated an acquisition time of

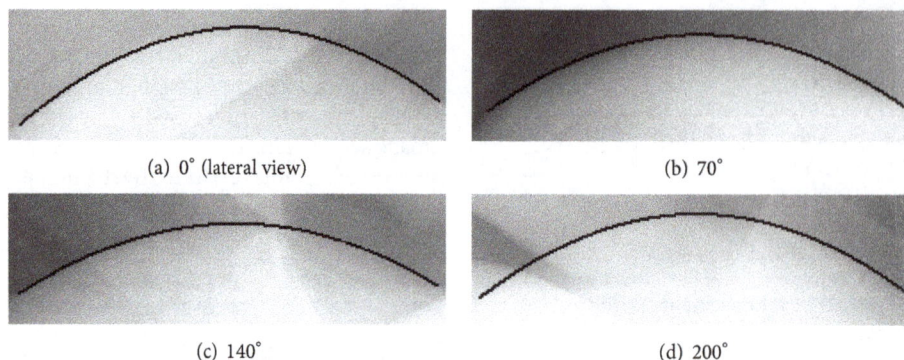

(a) 0° (lateral view)

(b) 70°

(c) 140°

(d) 200°

Figure 1: Diaphragm tracking on simulated XCAT data. Images (a)–(d) show projection images acquired from different angles.

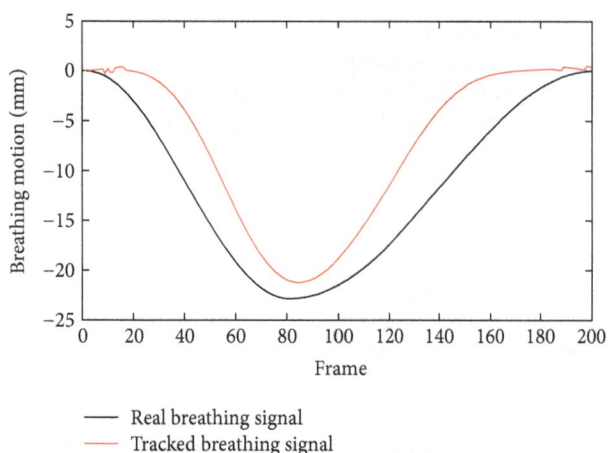

—— Real breathing signal
—— Tracked breathing signal

Figure 2: Comparison of the extracted diaphragm motion signal and the actual respiration signal of the simulated XCAT phantom. The amplitude of the signal cannot be estimated accurately, as the projections of the diaphragm top do not coincide with the 2D contour.

Table 1: Triangulation errors (in mm) based on projections of the real diaphragm top. Angular offset of the triangulated image pair in brackets.

	Mean 3D	Std. Dev. 3D	Mean Z	Std. Dev. Z
Rect. Iter. (90°)	0.20	0.06	0.10	0.06
Rect. Iter. (30°)	0.32	0.15	0.10	0.06
Rect. Iter. (10°)	0.89	0.60	0.11	0.08
Iterative (90°)	2.22	0.97	2.22	0.96

four seconds with one full respiration cycle. The simulated motion model was rigid; both heart and diaphragm moved about 2.3 cm along the superior-inferior axis; the rest of the scene was static. A detector of size 640 × 480 px was simulated with a resolution of 0.616 mm/px. 200 projections were acquired with an average angular increment of 1.0°. As ground truth, we used the reconstruction of an XCAT dataset that was simulated without respiratory motion.

The diaphragm tracking method was evaluated on the left and right hemidiaphragms in XCAT projection data [13]. We were able to track the vertex of the diaphragm contour with sub-pixel accuracy. We observed a Euclidean distance of the right vertex to the correct vertex of 0.45 ± 0.56 pixels and 0.75 ± 0.84 pixels for the left vertex, respectively [13]. Figure 1 shows the estimated parabolic model of the diaphragm from four different views of the XCAT phantom.

Figure 2 shows the extracted signal based on triangulation of the diaphragm tracking results. As previously noted, our approach depends on the assumption that the projection of the diaphragm top lies on the 2D contour. However, this is

a strong assumption that is not always fulfilled. In fact, the correct projection of the diaphragm top is often located below the contour, due to perspective projection. This results in inaccuracies in the estimated amplitude of the signal, caused by triangulation with false point correspondences. As shown earlier, we have a deterministic error in the reconstruction of the height of the diaphragm top caused by the perspective projection in the cone-beam data. However, this is only a limitation of the current triangulation approach and not a limitation of the method in general. Thus, we expect to get results that are similar to the correct correspondence case once we have solved this problem. In order to assess the accuracy of the triangulation approaches without the effect of false point correspondences, we tested the methods using the projections of the diaphragm top of the same XCAT simulation with respiratory motion as input for the rectified triangulation algorithm. Therefore, we can test the performance of our algorithm assuming a correct tracking. We triangulated the 3D position of the diaphragm top for each projection image using a second image with a certain angular offset (10°–90°). The triangulated 3D point was compared to the actual 3D position of the diaphragm top at the time the projection was acquired. As results in Table 1 show, our rectified iterative approach provides submillimeter accuracy even for image pairs with low angular offset, whereas the average error of the standard triangulation approach without rectification and motion correction is about 10% of the total respiratory motion. These results indicate that we are able to reconstruct an accurate respiration signal, given the correct positions of the diaphragm top in the 2D projection images. Our methods were tested on an Intel Xeon X5450 CPU. Even though it is not yet optimized and only implemented in Java,

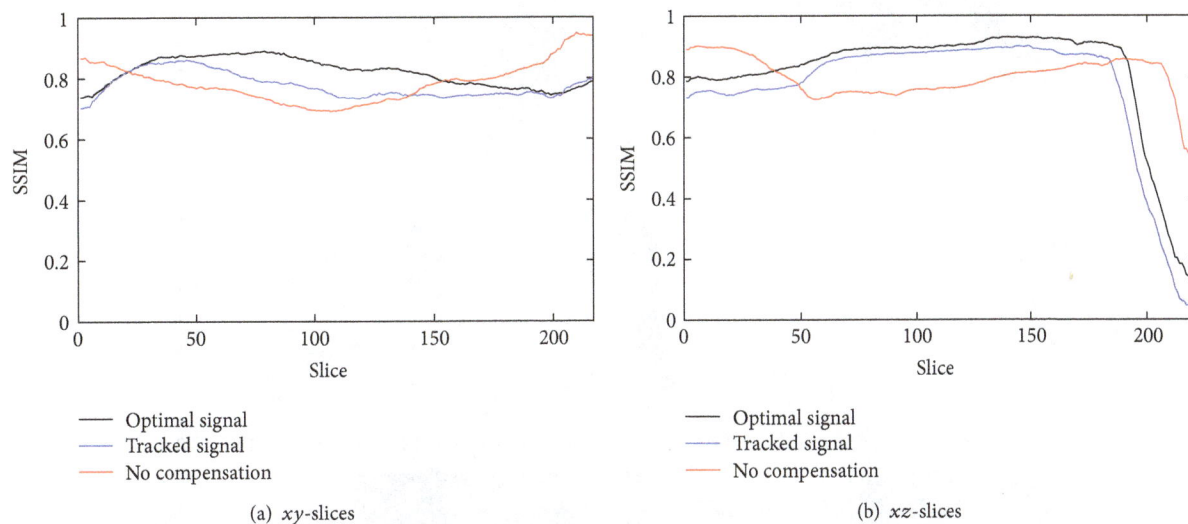

(a) xy-slices

(b) xz-slices

FIGURE 3: Structural similarity index of the heart volume for xy- and xz-slices. The uncompensated reconstruction shows better results in the beginning and the end, as the heart is only of small size in these slices.

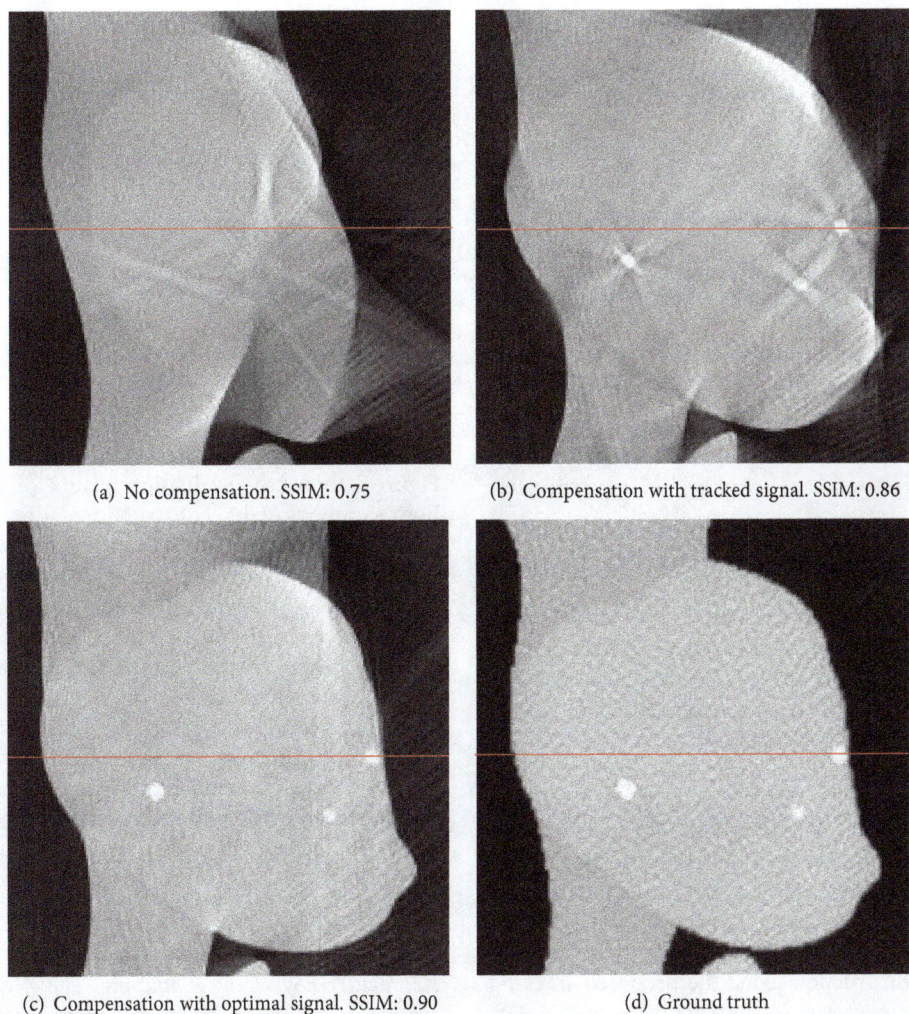

(a) No compensation. SSIM: 0.75

(b) Compensation with tracked signal. SSIM: 0.86

(c) Compensation with optimal signal. SSIM: 0.90

(d) Ground truth

FIGURE 4: Comparison of xy-slice 70 of compensated and uncompensated volumes (cf. Figure 3(a)). Simulated high-contrast heart lesions further illustrate the improved image quality. Line profiles were taken at the position of the red lines.

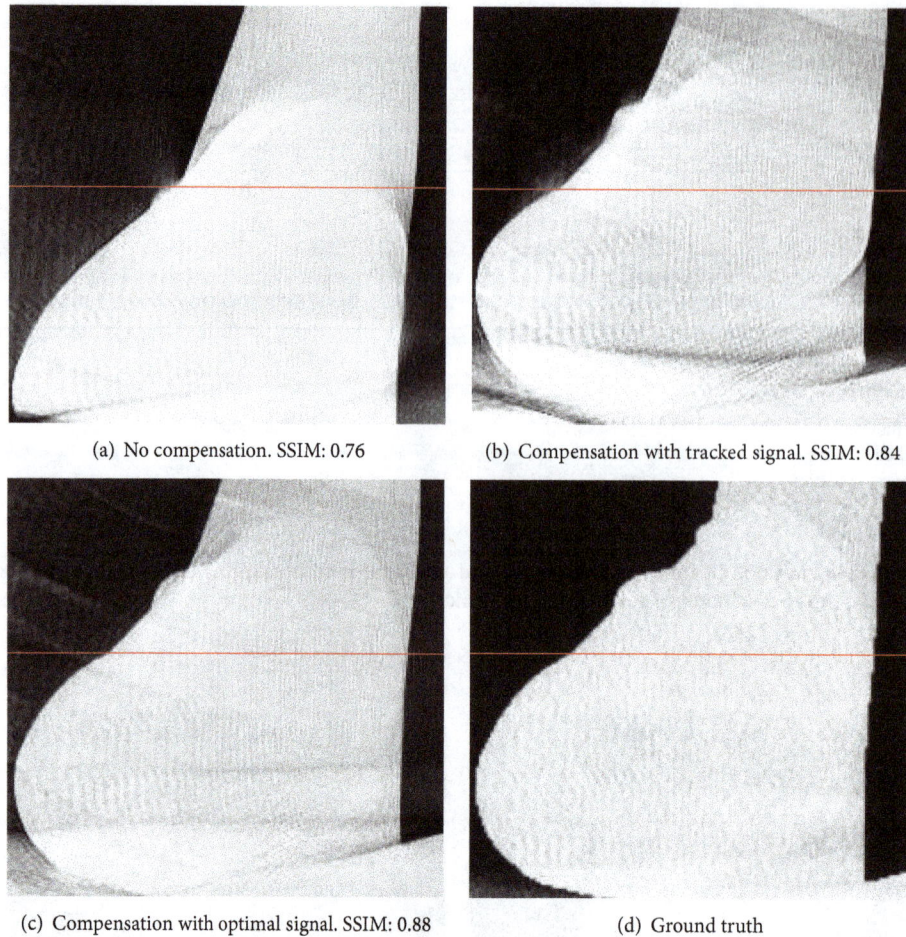

(a) No compensation. SSIM: 0.76

(b) Compensation with tracked signal. SSIM: 0.84

(c) Compensation with optimal signal. SSIM: 0.88

(d) Ground truth

FIGURE 5: Comparison of xz-slice 60 of compensated and uncompensated volumes (cf. Figure 3(b)). Line profiles were taken at the position of the red lines.

our proposed method is very efficient, yielding a computation time of the diaphragm tracking combined with triangulation of approximately 10 seconds, using 20000 RANSAC iterations per frame. This corresponds to a runtime of approximately 50 ms per frame.

For the evaluation of reconstruction quality we used the structural similarity index (SSIM) by Wang et al. [21]. SSIM was designed to improve on other methods such as mean squared error or peak signal-to-noise ratio. SSIM is a more accurate measure in terms of the perception of the human eye. SSIM measures the similarity of two images based on change in structural information, while traditional approaches are based on perceived errors. Two images are compared and a value between −1.0 and 1.0 is returned, where a value of 1.0 can only be reached when comparing identical images. In order to reduce the influence of the static background on the quality evaluation, the reconstructed volume was cropped to the bounding box that contains the heart. In total, we evaluated the quality of three different reconstructions: (i) a compensated reconstruction using the proposed tracking methods, (ii) a compensated reconstruction with the correct 2D projections of the diaphragm top (simulating an optimal diaphragm tracking), and (iii) an uncompensated

reconstruction. For motion compensation we directly used the computed respiration signal, as the simulated motion in the XCAT phantom is constant for any given voxel. Figure 3 shows the evaluation results for xy- and xz-slices. Both compensated reconstructions show highly improved image quality. As expected, the diaphragm tracking approach produces images slightly below the quality of the optimal reconstruction. However, it shows considerable improvement when compared to the uncompensated reconstruction. The uncompensated reconstruction seems to be superior in the first and last slices. The heart is only of small size in these slices. Therefore, the static background has a larger influence on the evaluation. Compensation blurs the static background which leads to a reduced SSIM, whereas it is perfectly reconstructed without motion compensation. Figures 4 and 5 show the results for two example slices. The red lines indicate the positions of the line profiles that are presented in Figures 6 and 7.

3.2. artiCHEST Lung Phantom. The second part of our evaluation will be focused on a pulmonary application. For this purpose we used the artiCHEST phantom (PROdesign GmbH, Germany). This phantom consists of a box with

(a) No compensation. SSIM: 0.75

(b) Compensation with tracked signal. SSIM: 0.86

(c) Compensation with optimal signal. SSIM: 0.90

(d) Ground truth

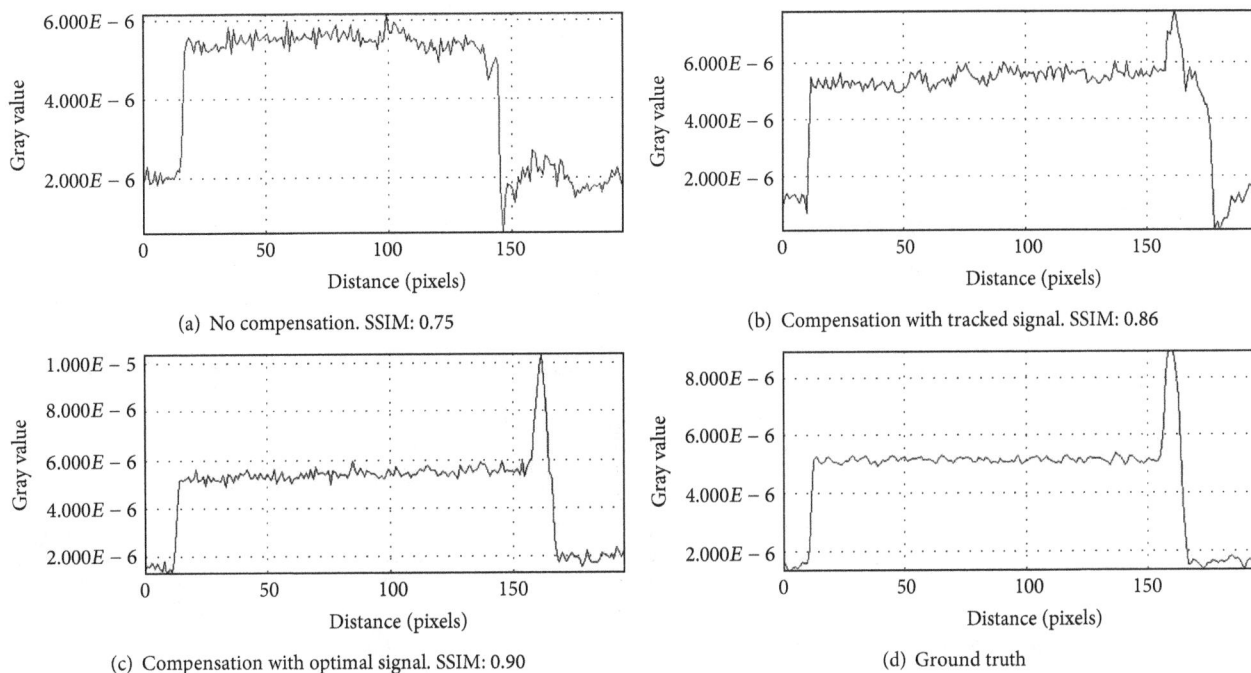

FIGURE 6: Line profiles of xy-slice 70 of compensated and uncompensated volumes (cf. Figure 3(a)). Line profiles were taken at the position of the red lines in Figure 4.

an artificial diaphragm. Inside the box a porcine lung is mounted that can be inflated and deflated by a computer controlled pump. In this manner, we can simulate previously configured respiration pattern. In our experiments, we set the respiration pattern to be sinusoidal with a maximum amplitude of about 1 cm. The borders of the box are filled with water. Figure 8 shows the test setup. Since the phantom consists only of one centric diaphragm, we had to simplify the diaphragm tracking approach. We only used the standard approach, without any additional motion constraints since the diaphragm remains relatively static in the center of the projections. While previously in the XCAT phantom only a constant motion was simulated, the motion simulated in this lung phantom is closer to reality. The motion is approximately linear; less motion is observed at the top of the lungs compared to the region close to the diaphragm. As no ground truth data was available to evaluate the tracking performance, tracking quality could only be inspected visually. Tracking performance appeared as robust as in the case of the simulated XCAT phantom. Figure 9 shows a cutout of an exemplary frame with the tracked parabola.

In the previous XCAT phantom test, the correlation of diaphragm and heart motion was already known. As previously noted, the relation of diaphragm and lung motion is typically linear. In order to approximate the linear scaling factor of our test lung, we acquired 11 static C-arm CT scans uniformly distributed along the simulated respiratory curve. Subsequently, we manually measured the position of the diaphragm top in each of these volumes to determine an optimal scaling for the z-coordinate correction; that is, we assume correct results in the triangulation in the following.

In order to approximate respiratory motion of the lung, we tested a simple linear motion model. While this model is obviously very simple, it already provides visible improvement to image quality. For clinical cases a simple model like this might only work in case of abdominal breathing. Compensation of thoracic breathing motion without prior knowledge is still an unsolved field of research. In this model, we estimated the slope of the linear function as

$$m = \frac{r_i}{(z_{max} - z_{dia})}, \qquad (4)$$

where r_i is the scaled diaphragm motion, z_{dia} is the z-coordinate of the diaphragm top in the current projection we are backprojecting, and z_{max} is the z-coordinate of a manually chosen point at which we assume the motion to be zero. In our case we used the topmost point of the lung.

Figure 10 shows a slice of a static reconstruction of the lung phantom without any motion present. In the lower part of the image the porcine heart is located. The heart has to be included in the phantom, as it provides stability. Unfortunately, this also means that the heart and its surrounding vessels and airways remain very static, due to the heart's mass and its location at the phantom border. The bright circular object in the center is a plastic tube that was included to simulate the spine and the metal artifacts to the left of the tube are caused by a pair of scissors that was included to mimic interventional constraints. Therefore, a meaningful evaluation can only be done in the center of the slice, which is depicted by the red bounding box in the image.

(a) No compensation. SSIM: 0.76

(b) Compensation with tracked signal. SSIM: 0.84

(c) Compensation with optimal signal. SSIM: 0.88

(d) Ground truth

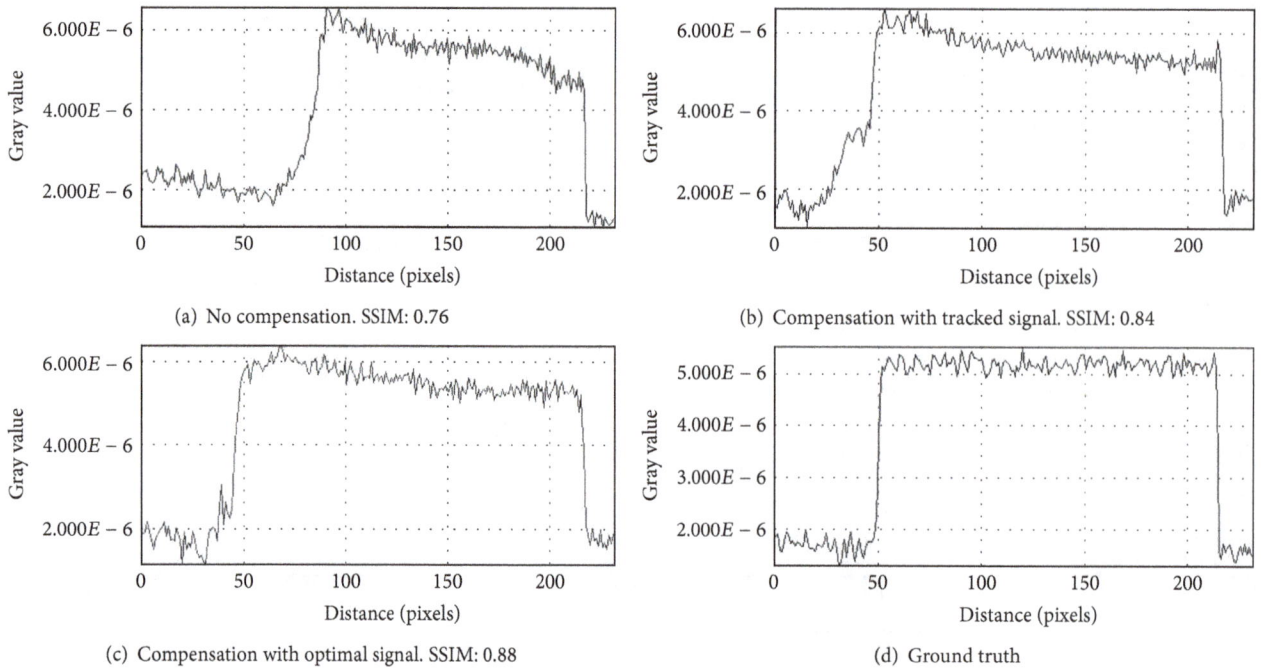

FIGURE 7: Line profiles of xz-slice 60 of compensated and uncompensated volumes (cf. Figure 3(b)). Line profiles were taken at the position of the red lines in Figure 5.

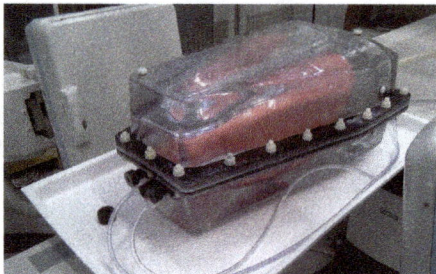

FIGURE 8: Illustration of the artiCHEST lung phantom. The box contains a porcine lung mounted on an artificial diaphragm and is filled with water.

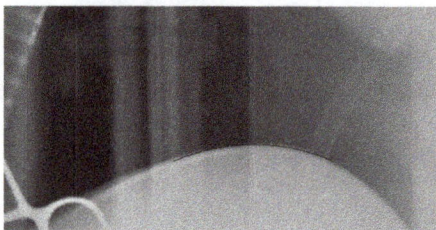

FIGURE 9: Zoomed in view of the diaphragm and the tracked function in a projection image.

The motion model was tested on two 20s C-arm CT scans. During the first scan approximately two full respiration cycles were simulated with a reduced amplitude of the simulated respiratory motion of 50%. For the second scan, the amplitude of the simulated respiratory motion was increased to 100%. Figure 11 depicts the red region of interest

that was introduced in Figure 10 for this first case. For comparison, an uncompensated reconstruction and a static reconstruction of the phantom are shown. The compensated reconstruction shows improved image quality compared to the uncompensated reconstruction. The airways are severely distorted in the uncompensated volume, while after motion compensation the contours of the airways are clearly visible and at the correct positions. Figure 12 shows the same slice for the second case with the full respiratory amplitude. While in the uncompensated image the airways are not visible at all, the compensation is able to restore the image partly. Compared to the static reconstruction, image quality is slightly degraded; however, this is still a notable improvement compared to the uncompensated reconstruction.

4. Conclusions

We have shown for two exemplary applications that our respiratory motion compensated reconstruction already shows promising image quality improvement with the current simple motion model assumptions. As shown in the simulated phantom data, the diaphragm tracking is already able to improve image quality considerably from an SSIM of about 0.7 to an SSIM of 0.85. Compensation with an ideal triangulation result could improve image quality further to 0.9. Thus, future work must focus on the improvement of the diaphragm triangulation. At present, we only use the topmost point of the tracked contour to reconstruct the diaphragm top. However, as the topmost vertex point is not necessarily projected onto the diaphragm contour in the projection, the triangulation with the topmost point of the tracked contour may be erroneous. We expect improved

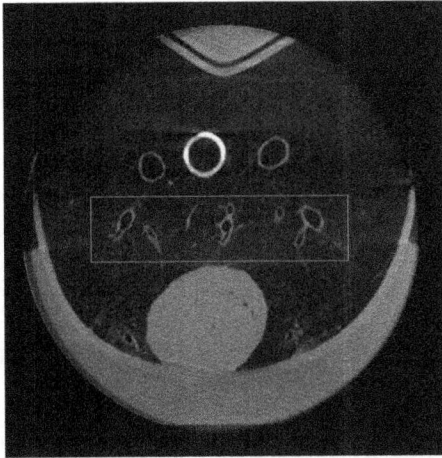

FIGURE 10: A slice of a static reconstruction of the artiCHEST phantom. At the bottom there is a porcine heart; the white circle is a plastic tube representing the spine. The red bounding box shows the region of interest for further evaluation.

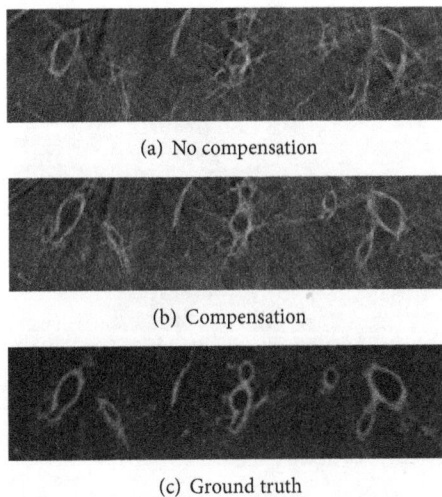

(a) No compensation

(b) Compensation

(c) Ground truth

FIGURE 11: Detailed view of compensated and not compensated slices of a 20s scan with 2 respiration cycles of only 50% respiratory amplitude.

(a) No compensation

(b) Compensation

(c) Ground truth

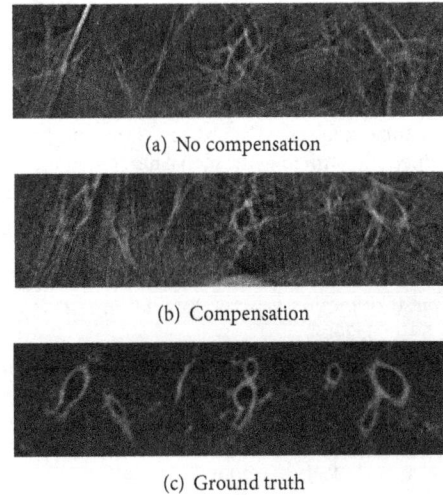

FIGURE 12: Detailed view of compensated and not compensated slices of a 20s scan with 2 full respiration cycles.

reconstruction results if not only the topmost point but the complete diaphragm surface is reconstructed. In this manner, perspective projection problems are modelled correctly and more accurate results will be obtained.

Another major issue of our current approach is the linear motion model. It yielded already an improved reconstruction. However, compared to ground truth data, image quality was still reduced. With this respect, we regard our approach as an initial guess that can be computed in a straight forward manner, as we only require the diaphragm to be tracked in the projection data. Application of the motion correction is straightforward and yields an improved reconstruction. In this respect, our method is comparable to ECG-gating in motion compensation of the heart. The method works rather well, if the model assumptions are met (in ECG gating, this is a regular heart beat). As soon as the observed data violates these assumptions, image quality is degraded. As shown by various authors, this does not mean that ECG gating is not of any clinical applicability, although most cardiac patients do not have a regular heart beat. Instead, the method is applied in many advanced cardiac motion compensation scenarios as an initial guess that is then used in an additional method to improve image quality further. Thus, we believe that our method will be applicable as well as an initial estimate for such advanced methods in respiratory motion compensation.

In addition, our method is not limited to only cardiac or pulmonary C-arm CT. The approach can also be applied in other applications where respiratory motion is present, for example, liver C-arm CT, as long as the diaphragm is visible and a sufficient motion model can be given.

Acknowledgments

The authors acknowledge the support by Deutsche Forschungsgemeinschaf and Friedrich-Alexander-Universität Erlangen-Nürnberg within the funding programme Open Access Publishing. This study was neither funded by PROdesign GmbH nor XCAT. The authors of this paper do not have any financial affiliation to PROdesign GmbH nor XCAT.

References

[1] C. Jahnke, I. Paetsch, S. Achenbach et al., "Coronary MR imaging: breath-hold capability and patterns, coronary artery rest periods, and β-blocker use," *Radiology*, vol. 239, no. 1, pp. 71–78, 2006.

[2] C. Blondel, G. Malandain, R. Vaillant, and N. Ayache, "Reconstruction of coronary arteries from a single rotational X-ray projection sequence," *IEEE Transactions on Medical Imaging*, vol. 25, no. 5, pp. 653–663, 2006.

[3] M. Prümmer, J. Hornegger, G. Lauritsch, L. Wigström, E. Girard-Hughes, and R. Fahrig, "Cardiac c-arm CT: a unified

framework for motion estimation and dynamic CT," *IEEE Transactions on Medical Imaging*, vol. 28, no. 11, pp. 1836–1849, 2009.

[4] K. Taguchi, W. P. Segars, G. S. K. Fung, and B. M. W. Tsui, "Toward time resolved 4D cardiac CT imaging with patient dose reduction; estimating the global heart motion," in *Proceedings of the Medical Imaging 2006: Physics of Medical Imaging (SPIE '06)*, vol. 6142, pp. 61 420J-1–61 420J-9, San Diego, CA, USA, February 2006.

[5] C. Schaller, J. Penne, and J. Hornegger, "Time-of-flight sensor for respiratory motion gating," *Medical Physics*, vol. 35, no. 7, pp. 3090–3093, 2008.

[6] S. Wiesner and Z. Yaniv, "Respiratory signal generation for retrospective gating of cone-beam CT images," in *Proceedings of the Medical Imaging 2008: Visualization, Image-Guided Procedures, and Modeling (SPIE '08)*, vol. 6918, pp. 691 817-1–691 817-12, San Diego, CA, USA, February 2008.

[7] T. E. Marchant, G. J. Price, B. J. Matuszewski, and C. J. Moore, "Reduction of motion artefacts in on-board cone beam CT by warping of projection images," *British Journal of Radiology*, vol. 84, no. 999, pp. 251–264, 2011.

[8] Y. Wang, S. J. Riederer, and R. L. Ehman, "Respiratory motion of the heart: kinematics and the implications for the spatial resolution in coronary imaging," *Magnetic Resonance in Medicine*, vol. 33, no. 5, pp. 713–719, 1995.

[9] J.-J. Sonke, L. Zijp, P. Remeijer, and M. van Herk, "Respiratory correlated cone beam CT," *Medical Physics*, vol. 32, no. 4, pp. 1176–1186, 2005.

[10] A. Kavanagh, P. M. Evans, V. N. Hansen, and S. Webb, "Obtaining breathing patterns from any sequential thoracic X-ray image set," *Physics in Medicine and Biology*, vol. 54, no. 16, pp. 4879–4888, 2009.

[11] M. Chen and R. A. Siochi, "Diaphragm motion quantification in megavoltage cone-beam CT projection images," *Medical Physics*, vol. 37, no. 5, pp. 2312–2320, 2010.

[12] I. Vergalasova, J. Cai, and F.-F. Yin, "A novel technique for markerless, self-sorted 4D-CBCT: feasibility study," *Medical Physics*, vol. 39, no. 3, pp. 1442–1451, 2012.

[13] M. Bögel, A. Maier, H. G. Hofmann, J. Hornegger, and R. Fahrig, "Diaphragm tracking in cardiac C-Arm projection data," in *Proceedings of the Bildverarbeitung fur die Medizin (BVM '12)*, pp. 33–38, Berlin, Germany, 2012.

[14] M. A. Fischler and R. C. Bolles, "Random sample consensus: a paradigm for model fitting 350 with applications to image analysis and automated cartography," *Communications of the ACM*, vol. 24, no. 6, pp. 381–395, 1981.

[15] A. Fusiello, E. Trucco, and A. Verri, "A compact algorithm for rectification of stereo pairs," *Machine Vision and Applications*, vol. 12, no. 1, pp. 16–22, 2000.

[16] R. I. Hartley and P. Sturm, "Triangulation," *Computer Vision and Image Understanding*, vol. 68, no. 2, pp. 146–157, 1997.

[17] D. Schäfer, J. Borgert, V. Rasche, and M. Grass, "Motion-compensated and gated cone beam filtered back-projection for 3-D rotational X-ray angiography," *IEEE Transactions on Medical Imaging*, vol. 25, no. 7, pp. 898–906, 2006.

[18] W. P. Segars, M. Mahesh, T. J. Beck, E. C. Frey, and B. M. W. Tsui, "Realistic CT simulation using the 4D XCAT phantom," *Medical Physics*, vol. 35, no. 8, pp. 3800–3808, 2008.

[19] A. Maier, H. G. Hofmann, C. Schwemmer, J. Hornegger, A. Keil, and R. Fahrig, "Fast simulation of X-ray projections of spline-based surfaces using an append buffer," *Physics in Medicine & Biology*, vol. 57, no. 19, pp. 6193–6210, 2012.

[20] M. Bögel, A. Maier, H. G. Hofmann, J. Hornegger, and R. Fahrig, "Diaphragm tracking for respiratory motion compensated cardiac C-Arm CT," in *Proceedings of the second international conference on image formation in x-ray computed tomography*, pp. 13–16, Salt Lake City, UT, USA, 2012.

[21] Z. Wang, A. C. Bovik, H. R. Sheikh, and E. P. Simoncelli, "Image quality assessment: from error visibility to structural similarity," *IEEE Transactions on Image Processing*, vol. 13, no. 4, pp. 600–612, 2004.

19

Insight into the Molecular Imaging of Alzheimer's Disease

Abishek Arora[1] and Neeta Bhagat[2]

[1]Amity Institute of Biotechnology, Amity University Uttar Pradesh, Noida 201303, India
[2]Amity Institute of Biotechnology, Amity University Uttar Pradesh, Room No. 312, J3 Block, III Floor, Noida 201303, India

Correspondence should be addressed to Neeta Bhagat; nbhagat@amity.edu

Academic Editor: Jyh-Cheng Chen

Alzheimer's disease is a complex neurodegenerative disease affecting millions of individuals worldwide. Earlier it was diagnosed only via clinical assessments and confirmed by postmortem brain histopathology. The development of validated biomarkers for Alzheimer's disease has given impetus to improve diagnostics and accelerate the development of new therapies. Functional imaging like positron emission tomography (PET), single photon emission computed tomography (SPECT), functional magnetic resonance imaging (fMRI), and proton magnetic resonance spectroscopy provides a means of detecting and characterising the regional changes in brain blood flow, metabolism, and receptor binding sites that are associated with Alzheimer's disease. Multimodal neuroimaging techniques have indicated changes in brain structure and metabolic activity, and an array of neurochemical variations that are associated with neurodegenerative diseases. Radiotracer-based PET and SPECT potentially provide sensitive, accurate methods for the early detection of disease. This paper presents a review of neuroimaging modalities like PET, SPECT, and selected imaging biomarkers/tracers used for the early diagnosis of AD. Neuroimaging with such biomarkers and tracers could achieve a much higher diagnostic accuracy for AD and related disorders in the future.

1. Introduction

A range of syndromes result in the destruction and loss of cells of the nervous system giving rise to various insidious but lethal neuropathies like Parkinsonism, Alzheimer's disease, Dementias, and Multiple Sclerosis. Such conditions are encompassed as neurodegenerative disorders [1]. The manifestation of such syndromes results in the degeneration of neurons, which ultimately culminates in the irreversible loss of neural function in the affected region of the brain [2, 3]. Neurodegenerative diseases induce characteristic impairments in the brain of the affected individual. These help in the characterisation and identification of specific neuropathies [4].

Advancements in the fields of clinical neuroscience have helped us in developing a deeper understanding of the induction as well as progression of neurodegenerative diseases [5]. The aggregation of misfolded proteins in various regions of the brain has been implicated in a majority of such neuropathies [6]. Despite various advancements in diagnostic techniques and the detailed study of molecules and subcellular process underlying such conditions, the neurological disorders are not well understood.

Conventionally, neurodegenerative disorders and allied syndromes were conclusively characterised at a late stage or via postmortem analysis [7]. The use of noninvasive techniques in medicine over the previous decade is popular owing to their ease of execution and increased patient well-being [8]. Molecular imaging has provided an alternative noninvasive tool for the diagnosis of neurological syndromes with high specificity in comparison to previous modalities [9]. The key advantage of molecular imaging modalities is due to its ability to elucidate sophisticated biological phenomenon at the cellular and molecular level, linking investigations to specific pathologies [10]. Also, molecular imaging makes it possible to provide information about changes before the pathological manifestation, which aids in the early diagnosis of neurological syndromes thereby allowing the timely implementation of appropriate therapeutic strategies [11].

There are various imaging modalities like magnetic resonance imaging (MRI) and Computerised Tomography (CT); however PET and SPECT are latest molecular imaging techniques that are extensively used in the diagnosis of neurological disorders [9, 12]. The molecular imaging procedure involves an imaging device and an imaging agent, or probe.

A variety of molecular probes are used to visualize the cellular activity and chemical processes involved in metabolism, oxygen distribution, or blood flow. Radiotracer atom or isotopes are also used for imaging the body. The imaging agent is introduced into the body, it accumulates at the target site, and its distribution is scanned, thus providing information about the changes taking place in the tissues and organs [13]. Commonly probes are used in the range of pico- to femtomoles per gram.

In the past decade, PET and SPECT were used to elucidate the neurochemical changes such as the role of neurotransmitters including dopamine, serotonin, and acetylcholine in neurodegenerative disorders. Recent technological advancements have enabled the use of these two techniques to probe a wide variety of intra- and extracellular proteins with impaired function and expression related to brain diseases. These advancements have enabled PET and SPECT to have applications from neurochemical imaging to molecular imaging, thereby elucidating various molecular pathophysiological processes of brain diseases.

The complete mechanism of neurodegenerative conditions has not yet been fully elucidated. Intense research in this field has identified as many as 500 novel molecular targets [14]. Novel molecular imaging agents like small molecules peptides, hormones, antibodies, aptamers, affibodies, transporter substrate nanoparticles, drugs, and oligonucleotides are used for the localization of such targets [15]. The use of novel compounds in PET and SPECT methods helps in diagnosing and understanding the pathophysiology involved in specific molecular changes that occur during the early stages of neurodegenerative disorders. In the present review, the applications of two imaging modalities, namely PET and SPECT, have been discussed in the molecular imaging of AD.

2. Pathophysiology and Biomarkers of Alzheimer Disease (AD)

Alzheimer's disease is an age-dependent neurodegenerative disorder that involves multiple molecular mechanisms. AD manifests as significant cognitive deficits, behavioural changes, sleep disorders, and loss of functional autonomy. The number of patients suffering from AD is growing rapidly worldwide. AD represents the foremost cause of Dementia and has become a major public health issue.

AD is a complex disorder which has many different pathophysiological features like impairment of cognitive domains, a characteristic pathological cortical and hippocampal atrophy, histological feature of senile plaques comprising of amyloid deposits and neurofibrillary tangles consisting of intraneuronal tau fibrillary tangles, and a resultant decrease in neurons. It is also accompanied by biochemical

changes like abnormalities of cholesterol metabolism, inflammation, oxidative damage, and lysosomal dysfunction. Clinical diagnosis of AD remains difficult in initial stages. Current methods for diagnosing AD involve a detailed history and neuropsychological testing to establish the presence of Dementia. Other investigations must then be conducted to distinguish AD from other forms of Dementias such as Vascular Dementia (VaD), Frontotemporal Dementia (FTD), and Lewy Body Disease (LBD) [16, 17].

In AD, it is currently not possible to directly measure the number of remaining cortical neurons *in vivo* and, therefore, alternative approaches are required. Clinical assessments in AD using scales to measure cognitive impairment, disability, quality of life, or global disease severity are tarnished by symptomatic effects of therapy and are unable to differentiate this effect from disease-modification, at least in the short term. There is a dire need of AD biomarkers for both an early and accurate diagnosis and prediction of disease progression. Many candidate biomarkers for disease progression in AD have also been studied.

Several proteins like total tau (t-tau) and phosphorylated tau (p-tau) are "AD Signatures" which show marked increase in the cerebrospinal fluid (CSF). Other protein markers associated with AD are Aβ42, resistin, and thrombospondin-1 [18]. Mitochondrial dysfunction with degeneration of mitochondria in neurons [19], inflammatory mechanisms, oxidative stress [20], vascular homeostasis, altered lipid metabolism [21], and antioxidant defence system are some of the targets used for the diagnosis of AD. CSF proteome of AD patients shows altered levels of α-1-antitrypsin, α-1b glycoprotein, APOA-I, APOE, retinol binding protein, vitamin D-binding protein, prostaglandin H2 D isomerase, and transthyretin (TTR) [22–27]. CSF biomarkers of inflammation that showed increased levels in AD are TNF-α [28], monocyte chemotactic protein-1 [29], interferon γ-inducible protein 10, IL-8 [30], IL-6 [31], transforming growth factor-β (TGFβ) [32], and vascular endothelial growth factor (VEGF) [31].

Several evidences have documented that cholesterol metabolism plays a role in AD [33]. Total serum cholesterol may be a marker of AD because high concentration of serum cholesterol is involved in tau phosphorylation and is caused due to the dysfunction of protein kinase C (PKC). The PKC function is involved in memory processes in animal models [34] and appears altered in red blood cells and lymphocytes of AD patients [35]. By inhibiting GSK3β, PKC reduces tau phosphorylation and neurofibrillary tangles formation [36] making it a potential target for drugs and the most promising marker in AD diagnosis. As many as 98 different proteins involved in oxidation reduction [37], glycolysis [38], transport [38], metabolic processes [16], protein folding [39], the response to unfolded proteins [40], and cell proliferation [40] have been reported to be associated with AD [41]. These proteins showed quantitative differences in AD and 56 of them are cytoplasmic, 28 mitochondrial, 20 nuclear, and 16 cytosolic proteins. Finally, three of them are synaptic proteins (synaptosomal-associated protein-25 (SNAP-25), synaptotagmin, and syntaxin-binding protein) which present altered expression or modification [42]. A decrease in the number of neurons, formation of amyloid plaques, and the generation of neurofibrillary tangles, which results in neuronal dysfunction, act as hallmarks of AD. Such recognition of CSF biological markers for AD gives an accurate "molecular" diagnosis and subsequent follow-up of the disease.

Biochemical biomarkers like arachidonic acid (AA) and docosahexaenoic acid (DHA), an omega-6 and omega-3 polyunsaturated fatty acid (PUFA), respectively, are very important constituents of phospholipids in cell membranes and contribute extensively to cell signalling in the brain. The CNS response to injury and to the onset (and progression) of neurodegeneration involves the release of free DHA and AA along with the synthesis of stereospecific docosanoid derivatives and prostanoids, respectively [43, 44]. Phospholipases, for example, PLA2, contribute to the conversion of AA into inflammatory molecules such as prostaglandin E2 (PGE2) by the cyclooxygenase (COX) 1 and 2 enzymes [45].

Protein biomarkers in the (CSF) such as a reduced amyloid or an elevated tau concentration have been used to diagnose early AD [38]. Lumbar puncture is an invasive procedure and may not be practically favourable for conducting large-scale studies on AD. Noninvasive neuroimaging methods such as positron emission tomography (PET) to measure amyloid in the brain or magnetic resonance imaging (MRI) to measure atrophy of medial temporal structures have also proved useful [46, 47].

However, PET is expensive and not readily available in many places, while brain atrophy, as measured by MRI, requires specialized facilities and is less specific to AD. The use of blood-based biomarkers is therefore an attractive alternative given the easy accessibility of blood [48]. Yet, there is a complex relationship between the different biomarkers. Putative biomarkers which are used in the diagnosis and prognosis of AD are positron emission tomography (PET) neuroimaging of β-amyloid (Aβ) protein deposition and magnetic resonance imaging (MRI) of hippocampal volume and other brain structures [49].

With the advent of high throughput techniques including transcriptome analysis and next generation sequencing methods, protein markers present in CSF and blood (i.e., plasma and serum) can be quantified accurately for diagnosis of AD. Extracellular plaques (Aβ42) and intracellular neurofibrillary tangles (tau) can be identified histopathologically and morphologically [50]. Aβ42, the main constituent of amyloid precursor protein (APP), is generated by sequential actions of β-secretase and γ-secretase on APP through an amyloidogenic pathway and there are several truncated Aβ isoforms in the brain [51].

Protein biomarkers involved in pathogenesis of AD are also identified by two-dimensional gel electrophoresis (2-DE) and matrix-assisted laser desorption/ionization combined with time of flight MS (MALDI-TOF-MS) and liquid chromatography combined with electrospray ionization (LC-ESIMS). In recent years, many new diagnostic tools like surface enhanced laser desorption ionization (SELDI-TOF-MS) which provides a high throughput protein expression profile analysis have evolved [52]. Isotope tagged relative and absolute quantitation (iTRAQ) [53], tandem mass tag (TMT) [54], isotope coded affinity tag (ICAT) [55], and isotope coded protein label (ICPL) [56] have been used for identification and quantification of proteins. Antibody array is another high throughput method to analyse multiple biomarkers [57].

The main tests for biomarkers classes used in the diagnosis and prognosis of AD are positron emission tomography (PET) neuroimaging of Aβ protein deposition and magnetic resonance imaging (MRI) of hippocampal volume and other brain structures [58]. These brain-imaging techniques are often used for studying the neuropathological processes and morphological and functional changes occurring in AD. Neuroimaging methods like PET and SPECT are helpful not only in the early diagnosis but also in differentiating AD from other neurodegenerative diseases.

3. Positron Emission Tomography (PET) in AD

Positron emission tomography (PET) is a nuclear medicine based molecular imaging technique that utilises a range of specially developed radiopharmaceuticals, which function as tracers. The technique is used to detect the rate of uptake of such tracers in specifically targeted cells throughout the body of the patient. The technique relies on the quantification of the radiotracer's decay, during which a positron is emitted, thereby generating a photon [7].

PET/CT thus functions as an *in vivo* imaging procedure that enables the study of systemic pathophysiological phenomenon, especially concerning neurodegenerative syndromes under its applications in the field of neurology [59]. The PET scanner detects pairs of energetic γ-rays that are indirectly emitted by the decay of the radiotracer that is administered to the patient. The radiotracer enters the brain via the blood brain barrier when administered intravenously. The radiotracer then accumulates in specific regions of the brain in accordance with the physiological condition that is being scrutinised [60]. The positrons emitted from the radiotracer transverse a few millimetres through the tissues in the vicinity of the neural vasculature transporting the radiotracer. This is accompanied with a rapid loss of kinetic energy of the traversing positrons. Further, the positrons travel slowly and interact with the electrons present in the neuronal cells to generate two 511 keV γ-rays travelling at an angle of approximately 180° to each other. This phenomenon is termed as annihilation [61]. The radiotracer utilised for the purpose of PET consists of a radiolabelled biologically active molecule that emits positrons at the time of undergoing decay [62]. The γ emissions of this radiotracer, followed by annihilation, are detected by the PET scanner, which generates three-dimensional views of the tracer localization within the patient's body (Figure 1).

The production of radiotracers utilised in PET requires the setting up of a specialised centre equipped with a significantly large cyclotron [63]. The production centre may be outsourced or on site depending on the half-life of the radiotracer being synthesised. Radiotracers that are used for PET based studies having extensive utilisation are labelled with ^{18}F ($t_{1/2}$ = 109.8 minutes), ^{11}C ($t_{1/2}$ = 20.3 minutes), or ^{15}O ($t_{1/2}$ = 2.04 minutes) [64]. The latter two must be produced at an on-site cyclotron owing to their short half-life.

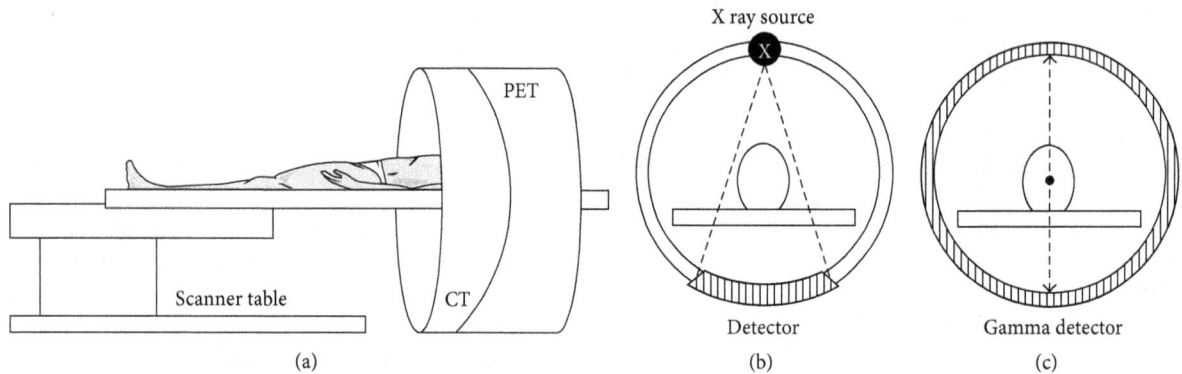

FIGURE 1: Schematic representation of (a) PET/CT scanner along with operational depiction of individual, (b) CT Module, and (c) PET Module of the scanning apparatus.

Generator based synthesis of radiotracers may also be done for labelling an active molecule with ^{68}Ga ($t_{1/2}$ = 67.83 minutes) and ^{82}Rb ($t_{1/2}$ = 1.27 minutes) [7].

Modern versions of the scanner are a hybrid between PET and CT technologies. The integration of functional imaging with structural imaging modalities plays a major role in attenuating the lacunae of anatomical acuity in the case of a simple PET based analysis. The PET/CT scanner is thus capable of generating anatomically augmented functional images of the brain [9]. By virtue of its high performance nature, PET has a wide variety of applications in the field of oncology, neurology, and cardiology [9]. The imaging modality has an extremely high sensitivity of nearly 10^{-11} to 10^{-12} mol/L and has an infinite depth of penetration [64]. The images obtained after the scan consist of PET and CT fusion images that show anatomical features along with a qualitative and quantitative distribution of the radiotracer in the brain. CT is helpful in the process of attenuation correction for accurate quantification and greater result reproducibility [65].

For the general process of image acquisition, the patient is asked to lie still in supine position on the scanner bed. The first step in image acquisition involves the initial action of performing a scout. Based on the protocol selected following the scout, a CT scan is performed which is followed by a PET scan of the defined region [66]. A brain PET/CT is performed for duration of 10 minutes without the administration of any IV contrast, which may be otherwise used in other investigations. An important pharmacological criterion that is applied in brain PET/CT based studies is that of binding potential (BP). The BP evaluates the density of neuronal receptors occupied by the radiotracer. Such an understanding aids in the characterisation of deviations in receptor localization which may further be pertinent for a particular neurological syndrome [67].

4. Single Photon Emission Computed Tomography (SPECT) in AD

Single Photon Emission Computed Tomography (SPECT) is a nuclear medicine modality that is related to PET in terms of

utilising a radioactive tracer in order to elucidate the uptake of the radiotracer in the patient. However, unlike PET, the radiotracers used in SPECT directly emit γ-rays [68].

The radiotracers used in SPECT emit a single γ-ray at the time of each decay, which is directly detected by the γ camera of the SPECT scanner. The γ camera is rotated around the patient in order to record the emitted projections [7]. Depending on the configuration of the machine, it may consist of either a single headed or a double headed γ camera.

The γ camera is fitted with collimators in order to guide the emissions towards the γ cameras of the scanner [69]. The collimator that is used is composed of lead or tungsten, which rejects any emissions that are not propagated at right angles to the reference axis as specified at the time of the scan. This is important to detect the point of origin of the emission for accurate representation in the output image [70]. The collimator used in brain SPECT imaging is a low-energy high-resolution (LEHR) collimator.

The radiotracers that are extensively used in the SPECT based investigation of neural function are labelled with ^{123}I ($t_{1/2}$ = 13.2 hours) and ^{99m}Tc ($t_{1/2}$ = 6.06 hours). The active molecule may also be labelled with ^{67}Ga ($t_{1/2}$ = 3.26 days) and ^{111}In ($t_{1/2}$ = 2.83 days) depending on the nature of analysis of the active molecule [71]. The principle of BP as discussed in PET/CT also applies to SPECT based molecular imaging. In lieu of the longer half-life of radiotracers utilised in SPECT, there is no requirement for an on-site cyclotron and a specialised radiochemistry facility. Such radiotracers are produced at a commercial scale. Owing to this, the lower expense of radiotracer generation for SPECT in comparison to PET/CT allows a wider and easily accessible utilisation of the scanning modality by patients. Brain SPECT image acquisition is performed by making the patient lie on the scanner bed in supine position. Appropriate positioning of the scanner bed and the γ cameras are done such that the collimators are in close proximity to the patient's head, while also allowing ease of movement for the γ cameras. The images obtained after the scan consist of SPECT images that show computed differential anatomical features along with a quantitative distribution of the radiotracer in the brain (Figure 2).

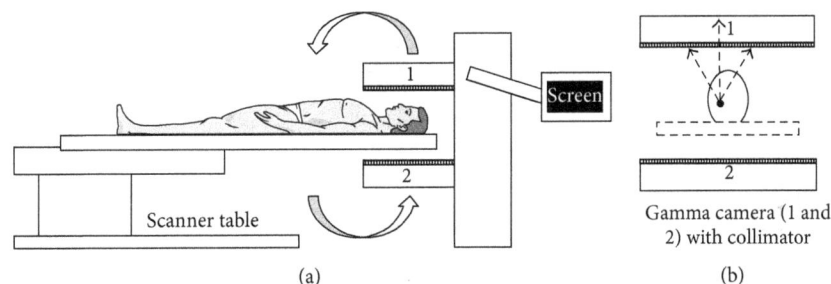

FIGURE 2: Schematic representation of (a) SPECT scanner along with depiction of (b) gamma camera placement and detection of emissions from a reference point at the time of a brain SPECT scan.

5. Radiotracers Used in PET and SPECT

A radiotracer used for neurological diagnostics must have optimal uptake, specific binding, and efficient clearance of the radiotracer [72]. The radiotracer being designed for diagnostics purposes must be of nontoxic and lipophilic nature [73]. It should have a low molecular weight so that it may easily transverse the blood brain barrier in order to enter the brain [74]. The radiotracer should be designed to reduce the incidences of nonspecific binding, should not get metabolised, and should be rapidly cleared from the blood [75]. The binding to its target must be specific and reversible in nature. The uptake of the radiotracer by the brain may further depend on a range of factors like permeability of the blood brain barrier, cerebral blood flow, plasma concentration of the radiotracer, and the noninteracting fractions of the radiotracer in the plasma and brain [74]. Furthermore, the selectivity of a particular neurological molecular imaging radiotracer is dependent on the concentration of vacant interaction site (Table 1) [73].

6. Radiotracers for Amyloid Imaging

The development of suitable radiotracers for the imaging of $A\beta$ aggregates has been taking place over the previous decades [76]. Out of the various categories of the amyloid radiotracers undergoing trial at different stages, small molecule based radiotracers have been the most successful [77] (Figure 3). In the recent years, radiotracers having high specificity have been generated using $A\beta$ antibodies and peptide fragments that have been labelled with a suitable radioactive moiety [78]. The further development of radiotracers based on stilbene, thioflavin [79], and acridine [80] aims to revolutionize $A\beta$ molecular imaging strategies. $A\beta$ specific neuroimaging radiotracers are of essential importance in the diagnosis of AD [81]. This may be attributed to the presence of moderate to severe aggregates of $A\beta$ in the form of amyloid plaques in all patients of AD [82]. The amyloid plaques are known to develop several years prior to the actual manifestation of cognitive decline and amnesia that are characteristic for AD [83].

6.1. *^{11}C-PIB*. [^{11}C]-2-[4-(Methylamino)phenyl]-1,3-benzothiazol-6-ol, also known as Pittsburgh Compound B, is the first PET based radiotracer that has been developed for specifically binding with fibrillar amyloid plaques [84] (Figure 3).

Initial studies of the radiotracer in mice showed rapid uptake in the brain upon intravenous administration. The radiotracer also showed rapid clearance from healthy neuronal tissue while showing retention in cortex of AD brain [85]. The thioflavin-T derived lipophilic structural moiety of ^{11}C-PIB is able to enter the brain via the blood brain barrier and displays sufficient specificity and high affinity to $A\beta$ aggregates found in senile plaques [86]. In studies of diseased versus healthy controls, the localization of ^{11}C-PIB after administration was found to be greater in the temporal, parietal, and frontal lobes. These findings were verified based on postmortem analysis of the same patient cohort. The areas where ^{11}C-PIB accumulated in diseased patients corresponded with areas known to have higher $A\beta$ concentrations [87]. The utilisation of ^{11}C-PIB is helpful in the differential diagnosis of AD and other types of Dementias. Comparative studies have shown that patients with Frontotemporal Dementia show normal ^{11}C-PIB uptake in a majority of clinical cases [81]. Patients that have been diagnosed with mild cognitive impairment show increased ^{11}C-PIB uptake, which is comparable to the levels of ^{11}C-PIB that have been observed in AD patients [88]. Likewise, a significant number of patients diagnosed with DLB also demonstrate an increase uptake of ^{11}C-PIB [89]. ^{11}C has a half-life of 20 minutes, limiting the utilisation of this radiotracer only in facilities that are equipped with an on-site cyclotron [90].

6.2. *^{11}C-AZD2184*. ^{11}C-AZD2184, [^{11}C]-2-[6-(methylamino)pyridin-3-yl]-1,3-benzothiazol-6-ol, is another analogue of ^{11}C-PIB, which has been synthesized by replacing the 2-phenyl moiety with a pyridine (Figure 3). The radiotracer binds to $A\beta$ aggregates in amyloid plaques with considerable affinity and demonstrates decreased levels of nonspecific binding [91]. The structure of ^{11}C-AZD2184 has a lower lipophilicity as compared to ^{11}C-PIB [92]. Such a property further decreases the chances of nonspecific interactions of the radiotracer in the white matter of the brain in contrast to ^{11}C-PIB [93].

6.3. *^{18}F-FDDNP*. 2-[1-[6-[2-[^{18}F]Fluoranylethyl(methyl)amino]naphthalen-2-yl]ethylidene]propanedinitrile (^{18}F-FDDNP) is a PET imaging radiotracer developed for the visualization of senile plaques in AD [94] (Figure 3). The radiotracer is a small molecule that has affinity to amyloid plaques as well as

TABLE 1: List of radiotracers designed for the PET as well as SPECT based analysis of AD pathophysiology.

Radiotracer	$t_{1/2}$	Emission	Modality	Specificity	Condition
[11]C-PIB	20 minutes	Positron	PET	Aβ	AD
[11]C-AZD2184	20 minutes	Positron	PET	Aβ	AD
^{18}F-FDDNP	110 minutes	Positron	PET	Aβ and Tau	AD
^{18}F-AV-45	110 minutes	Positron	PET	Aβ	AD
^{18}F-BAY94-9172	110 minutes	Positron	PET	Aβ	AD
^{18}F-GE067	110 minutes	Positron	PET	Aβ	AD
^{18}F-AZD4694	110 minutes	Positron	PET	Aβ	AD
[11]C-BF-227	20 minutes	Positron	PET	Aβ	AD
[11]C-SB-13	20 minutes	Positron	PET	Aβ	AD
^{123}I-SB-13	13.2 hours	Gamma	SPECT	Aβ	AD
^{18}F-THK523	110 minutes	Positron	PET	Tau	Tauopathies
^{18}F-THK5105	110 minutes	Positron	PET	Tau	Tauopathies
^{18}F-THK5107	110 minutes	Positron	PET	Tau	Tauopathies
[18]F-T807	110 minutes	Positron	PET	Tau	Tauopathies
[18]F-T808	110 minutes	Positron	PET	Tau	Tauopathies
[11]C-PBB3	20 minutes	Positron	PET	Tau	Tauopathies
[11]C-PK11195	20 minutes	Positron	PET	PBR-TSPO	Neuroinflammation
^{123}I-PK11195	13.2 hours	Gamma	SPECT	PBR-TSPO	Neuroinflammation
[11]C-DPA713	20 minutes	Positron	PET	PBR-TSPO	Neuroinflammation
[11]C-CLINME	20 minutes	Positron	PET	PBR-TSPO	Neuroinflammation
^{18}F-DPA714	110 minutes	Positron	PET	PBR-TSPO	Neuroinflammation
^{18}F-PBR111	110 minutes	Positron	PET	PBR-TSPO	Neuroinflammation
^{123}I-CLINDE	13.2 hours	Gamma	SPECT	PBR-TSPO	Neuroinflammation
[11]C-DED	20 minutes	Positron	PET	I_2BS	Neuroinflammation
[11]C-FTIMD	20 minutes	Positron	PET	I_2BS	Neuroinflammation
[11]C-AA	20 minutes	Positron	PET	AA analogue	Lipid metabolism
[11]C-DHA	20 minutes	Positron	PET	DHA analogue	Lipid metabolism
[11]C-Enzastaurin	20 minutes	Positron	PET	PKC	Neuroprotection
[11]C-MeDAS	20 minutes	Positron	PET	Myelin	Neuroprotection
[124]I-pQHNIG70	4.18 days	Positron	PET	HSF-1/HSP-70	Neuroprotection
[11]C-Verapamil	20 minutes	Positron	PET	P-gp	Neuroprotection

neurofibrillary tangles in patients diagnosed with AD [95]. ^{18}F-FDDNP is the first known radiotracer used in molecular imaging that has the ability to bind *in vivo* with amyloid plaques and NFTs, thereby making it possible to localize such aggregates in a noninvasive manner [96]. The first human brain PET images using ^{18}F-FDDNP were obtained in an 82-year-old female who had been clinically diagnosed with AD [97]. The examination showed relative radiotracer clearance in different regions of the brain. However, the key findings were that the radiotracer had an affinity towards regions of significant Aβ as well as hyperphosphorylated tau aggregations, which were confirmed following an autopsy of the patient [98]. Another group indicated that ^{18}F-FDDNP upon administration to AD patients in comparison to healthy controls has a higher residence time in the regions of the hippocampus, frontal lobe, parietal lobe, temporal lobe, and the occipital lobe [95]. Based on such findings it may be stated that the clearance time of ^{18}F-FDDNP in various regions

of the brain may be inversely correlated with the degree of cognitive impairment in patients that have been clinically diagnosed with AD [99].

6.4. ^{18}F-AV-45 or ^{18}F-Florbetapir. 4-[(E)-2-[6-[2-[2-(2-[^{18}F]Fluoranylethoxy)ethoxy]ethoxy]pyridin-3-yl]ethenyl]-N-methylaniline (^{18}F-AV-45 or ^{18}F-Florbetapir) is the first ^{18}F labelled PET radiotracer that has been approved by the US Food and Drug Association for the clinical evaluation of patients suspected with AD and other allied syndromes of cognitive deterioration [100] (Figure 3).

[18]F-Florbetapir applications have been able to significantly replicate imaging findings that have been examined using ^{11}C-PIB as an amyloid specific radiotracer [101, 102]. Additionally, an analysis of PET images that were obtained using ^{18}F-Florbetapir in Phase 3 clinical trials has shown a significant correlation with Aβ distributions based on post-mortem follow-ups of the trial patients [103].

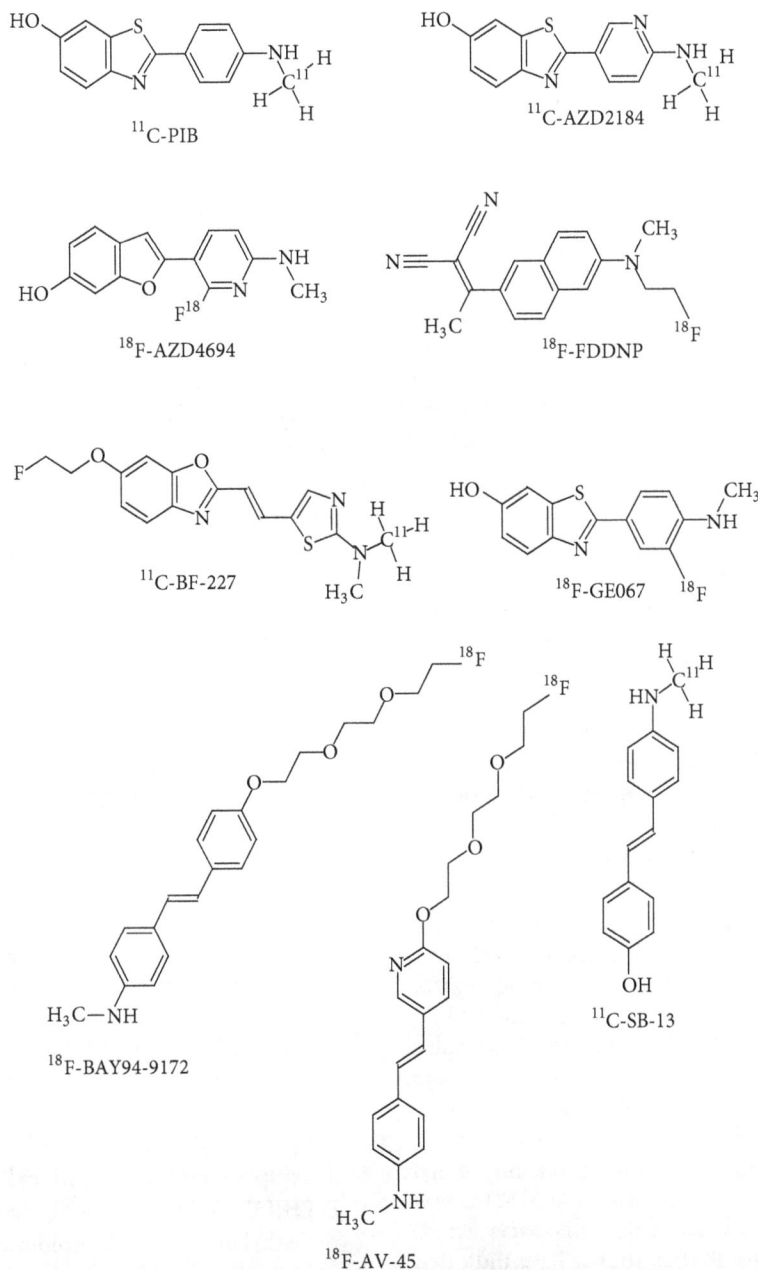

FIGURE 3: Structural representation of radiotracers for amyloid imaging.

6.5. ^{18}F-BAY94-9172 or ^{18}F-Florbetaben. 4-[(E)-2-[4-[2-[2-(2-[^{18}F]Fluoranylethoxy)ethoxy]ethoxy]phenyl]ethenyl]-N-methylaniline (^{18}F-BAY94-9172 or ^{18}F-Florbetaben) is an ^{18}F labelled radiotracer used in PET based examinations of Aβ aggregates in AD and other forms of Dementia [104] (Figure 3). The cortical distribution of ^{18}F-Florbetaben is considerably similar to that of ^{11}C-PIB [105]. In a study that has attempted to differentiate AD from Dementia with Lewy Bodies (DLB) based on ^{18}F-Florbetaben localization, the radiotracer demonstrated a lower overall retention in DLB patients in spite of a similar involvement of Aβ in the pathophysiology of DLB [83]. ^{18}F-Florbetaben thus may play a substantial role in the differential diagnosis of Frontotemporal

Dementia (FTD), Vascular Dementia (VaD), and Parkinson's disease (PD), in lieu of the absence of abnormal Aβ aggregations in such syndromes [89].

6.6. ^{18}F-GE067 or ^{18}F-Flutemetamol. 2-[3-[^{18}F]Fluoranyl-4-(methylamino)phenyl]-1,3-benzothiazol-6-ol (^{18}F-Flutemetamol) is an amyloid radiotracer that is a structural analogue of ^{11}C-PIB [91] (Figure 3). Initial studies in human subjects have shown that ^{18}F-Flutemetamol has similar neuronal uptake as well as affinity to Aβ aggregates as seen in studies using ^{11}C-PIB [106, 107]. ^{18}F labelled Aβ specific radiotracers however showcase a higher nonspecific uptake in the white matter, which may also be visualized in the PET images of healthy controls [108]. The key disadvantage of such a class of amyloid imaging radiotracers is that they generate greater levels of nonspecific background noise in comparison to ^{11}C-PIB [87].

6.7. ^{18}F-AZD4694. 2-[2-[^{18}F]Fluoro-6-(methylamino)-3-pyridinyl]-1-benzofuran-5-ol (^{18}F-AZD4694) has been developed so as to overcome the limitations of using ^{11}C-AZD2184 as an amyloid specific radiotracer. On the basis of chemical characterisation, ^{18}F-AZD4694 is an aromatic pyridinylbenzofuran that has undergone fluorosubstitution [74] (Figure 3). The uptake and distribution of ^{18}F-AZD4694 are comparable with that of ^{11}C-PIB [109]. By virtue of the shared structural similarity with ^{11}C-PIB, ^{18}F-AZD4694 thereby demonstrates similar pharmacodynamics as well as pharmacokinetics as ^{11}C-PIB while at the same time overcoming the shortcomings of using ^{11}C labelled radiotracers [110].

6.8. ^{11}C-BF-227. [^{11}C]2-(2-[2-Dimethylaminothiazol-5-yl]ethenyl)-6-(2-[fluoro]ethoxy)benzoxazole (^{11}C-BF-227) is an optimized benzoazide derivative that is being analysed as a diagnostic radiotracer for β-amyloid aggregates [111] (Figure 3). ^{11}C-BF-227 has demonstrated a good binding affinity for $A\beta$ accompanied with efficient neurological uptake [112]. ^{11}C-BF-227 localize in the frontal, temporal, lateral temporal, temporooccipital, anterior and posterior cingulate cortices, striatum, and the occipital areas of the brain where amyloid aggregates occur [111].

6.9. ^{11}C-SB-13 or ^{123}I-SB-13. [^{11}C] 4-N-Methylamino-4-hydroxystilbene (^{11}C-SB-13) is a stilbene-based derivative (Figure 3) that has selective affinity towards $A\beta$ aggregates that are as previously mentioned observed as a constituent part of senile plaques in AD [113]. The radiotracer has similar *in vivo* properties as demonstrated by ^{11}C-PIB, used for the diagnosis as well as prognosis of AD [114]. In human trials of the radiotracer initially conducted, ^{11}C-SB-13 demonstrated significant levels of localization in known regions of $A\beta$ accumulation as a part of AD pathogenesis [115]. This was possible due to efficient transport of the radiotracer across the blood brain barrier [116]. Rather, studies have indicated that the relative cortical uptake of ^{11}C-SB-13 is greater than that of ^{11}C-PIB [117]. ^{11}C-SB-13 is more likely to interact with fibrillar $A\beta$; however further studies are required to establish the same [115]. Furthermore, the shape as well as dimensions of amyloid plaques determines the degree of penetration of the radiotracer [118]. A variant of the same radiotracer has been labelled with [123]I. ^{123}I-SB-13 has demonstrated effective SPECT applications in human trials; however its use warrants further analysis [119].

7. Radiotracers for Tau Imaging

The successful molecular imaging of $A\beta$ using various developed radiotracers has given impetus to the development of tau specific radiotracers. The accumulation of hyperphosphorylated tau gives rise to neurofibrillary tangles (NFTs) [120]. However, such an aggregation occurs intracellularly among the nerve terminals [121]. This is in complete contrast to the extracellular formation of amyloid plaques [122]. In the NFTs, tau exists in the form of paired helical filaments (PHFs) [123]. The designing of tau specific radiotracers thus targets the PHF tau aggregates [124]. By virtue of the intracellular localization of PHF tau in affected neurons, it is difficult to generate tau specific radiotracers without certain affinity for $A\beta$ [125]. Such an affinity towards tau may be incorporated in the radiotracer by introducing large hydrophilic moieties that may prevent interactions with $A\beta$ [126]. A lot of initial work was focused on benzothiazole, pyrimidazole, and imadazothiazole derivatives as tau specific radiotracers [127]. Further onwards, efforts were made to characterise the use of oxindole, styryl benzimidazole, and thiohydantoin based tau radiotracers [128].

7.1. ^{18}F-THK523. 2-(4-Aminophenyl)-6-(2-([^{18}F]fluoroethoxy))quinoline (^{18}F-THK523) is a quinolone-derived radiotracer (Figure 4) used in PET based examinations of PHF tau aggregates. Studies in the tau transgenic mouse model have shown that the radiotracer is able to enter the brain via the blood brain barrier and is able to bind with PHF tau aggregates [129]. Initial *in vivo* studies in humans have indicated greater levels of interaction of the radiotracer with PHF tau in comparison to $A\beta$ [130].

In vivo examinations have demonstrated greater retention of the radiotracer in the orbitofrontal, parietal, hippocampal, lateral, and temporal regions in patients diagnosed with AD [131]. Furthermore, ^{18}F-THK523 retention is not found to be associated with that of amyloid radiotracers of the likes of ^{11}C-PIB [132]. Therefore, ^{18}F-THK523 has selective affinity to tau aggregates. However, the localization of ^{18}F-THK523 is lower in the grey matter in comparison to the white matter; this makes it difficult to examine such findings only based on visual inputs [131].

7.2. ^{18}F-THK5105 and ^{18}F-THK5117. 6-[(3-^{18}F-Fluoro-2-hydroxy)propoxy]-2-(4-dimethylaminophenyl)quinoline (^{18}F-THK5105) and 6-[(3-^{18}F-fluoro-2-hydroxy)propoxy]-2-(4-methylaminophenyl)quinoline (^{18}F-THK5117) are 2-arylquinoline derivatives that have been labelled with ^{18}F for PET based tau imaging [133] (Figure 4). These have been developed by further streamlining the binding and pharmacokinetics of ^{18}F-THK523 [134].

Autoradiography based studies using ^{18}F-THK5105 and ^{18}F-THK5117 has shown their localization in the grey matter of the temporal lobe which correlates with the localization of PHF tau aggregates in the form of NFTs [133]. Human examinations using ^{18}F-THK5105 via PET imaging have shown retention of the radiotracer in the lateral as well as mesial temporal lobes, which are otherwise known to have higher concentrations of tau aggregates in pathological cases [135]. Furthermore, the degree of retention of the radiotracer is significantly associated with the severity of Dementia and the degree of neuronal atrophy [135]. ^{18}F-THK5117 is still a newer addition to the class of tau specific radiotracers and is being thoroughly analysed at various levels of function [136].

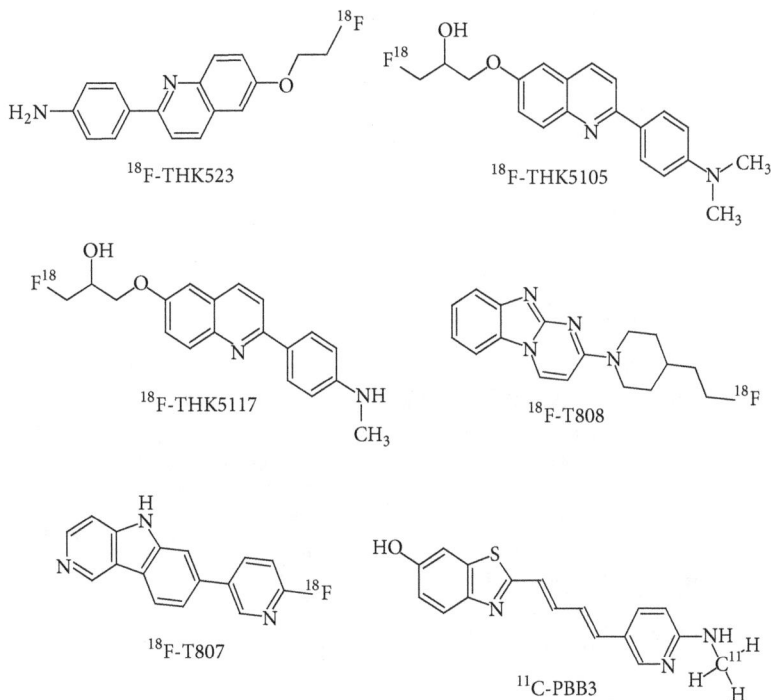

FIGURE 4: Structural representation of radiotracers for tau imaging.

7.3. *18F-T807 and* *18F-T808.* The 7-(6-[18F]Fluoropyridin-3-yl)-5H-pyrido(4,3-b)indole (18F-T807) and 2-[4-(2-[18F]fluoranylethyl)piperidin-1-yl]pyrimido[1,2-a]benzimidazole (18F-T808) radiotracers were introduced after extensive autoradiography based studies of more than 900 compounds [137] (Figure 4). These radiotracers are mainly derivatives of benzimidazole that have a high affinity to PHF tau [138]. 18F-T807 PET based studies in AD patients have shown cortical localization of the radiotracer that is consistent with the known distribution of PHF tau in the brain [139]. Such findings are significantly coherent with postmortem features that correlate PHF tau distribution with the degree of disease severity [140]. Studies using 18F-T808 have shown faster pharmacokinetics as well as delayed defluorination of the radiotracer in comparison to 18F-T807 [141].

7.4. *11C-PBB3.* The most recent member joining the ranks of other PHF tau specific radiotracers is 2-((1E,3E)-4-(6-(11C-methylamino)pyridin-3-yl)buta-1,3-dienyl)benzo[d]thiazol-6-ol (11C-PBB3), a phenyl/pyridinyl-butadienyl-benzothiazoles/benzothiazolium derivative (Figure 4). 11C-PBB3 demonstrated better visualization of tau aggregates in comparison to its predecessor 11C-PBB2 in mice models of AD, by virtue of which further work was carried out using 11C-PBB3 [142]. A human study using 11C-PBB3 demonstrated high affinity of the radiotracer to PHF tau aggregates [143]. However, significant localization of 11C-PBB3 was also noted in the venous sinuses of the subjects taking part in the same study [142]. This study also indicated that 11C-PBB3 has a low affinity to Aβ as the subjects involved in the study were also

imaged with 11C-PIB. The localization patterns of both the radiotracers were consistently different such that individual correlations could be made with the known regions of aggregation of Aβ and PHF tau [143].

8. Radiotracers for Neuroinflammation

Neuroinflammation is a well-documented ageing associated phenomenon [144]. Neuroinflammation is a key player in the progression of neurodegenerative conditions and is known to occur during the early stages of onset of such syndromes [145]. The inflammation may be correlated with the activation of microglial cells in response to neuronal degradation in conditions including AD [146]. The molecular imaging of neuroinflammation may thus contribute to the characterisation of AD while also taking into consideration specific markers of AD pathophysiology [147].

8.1. *11C-PK11195 and* *123I-Iodo-PK11195.* The most successful radiotracer for PET based neuroinflammation studies is [11C]N-butan-2-yl-1-(2-chlorophenyl)-N-methylisoquinoline-3-carboxamide (11C-PK11195) (Figure 5). 11C-PK11195 specifically binds to the 18 kDa translocator protein (TSPO) also known as the peripheral benzodiazepine receptor (PBR) [148]. In normal physiological conditions, TSPO has only a basal expression in the microglial cells [149]. However, when the microglia undergo inflammatory activation, PBR-TSPO expression is upregulated, thereby functioning as a putative biomarker for neuroinflammation [150].

As per an initial study conducted to look into the clinical validation of 11C-PK11195 as a radiotracer for neuroinflammation, there was notably high localization of the radiotracer

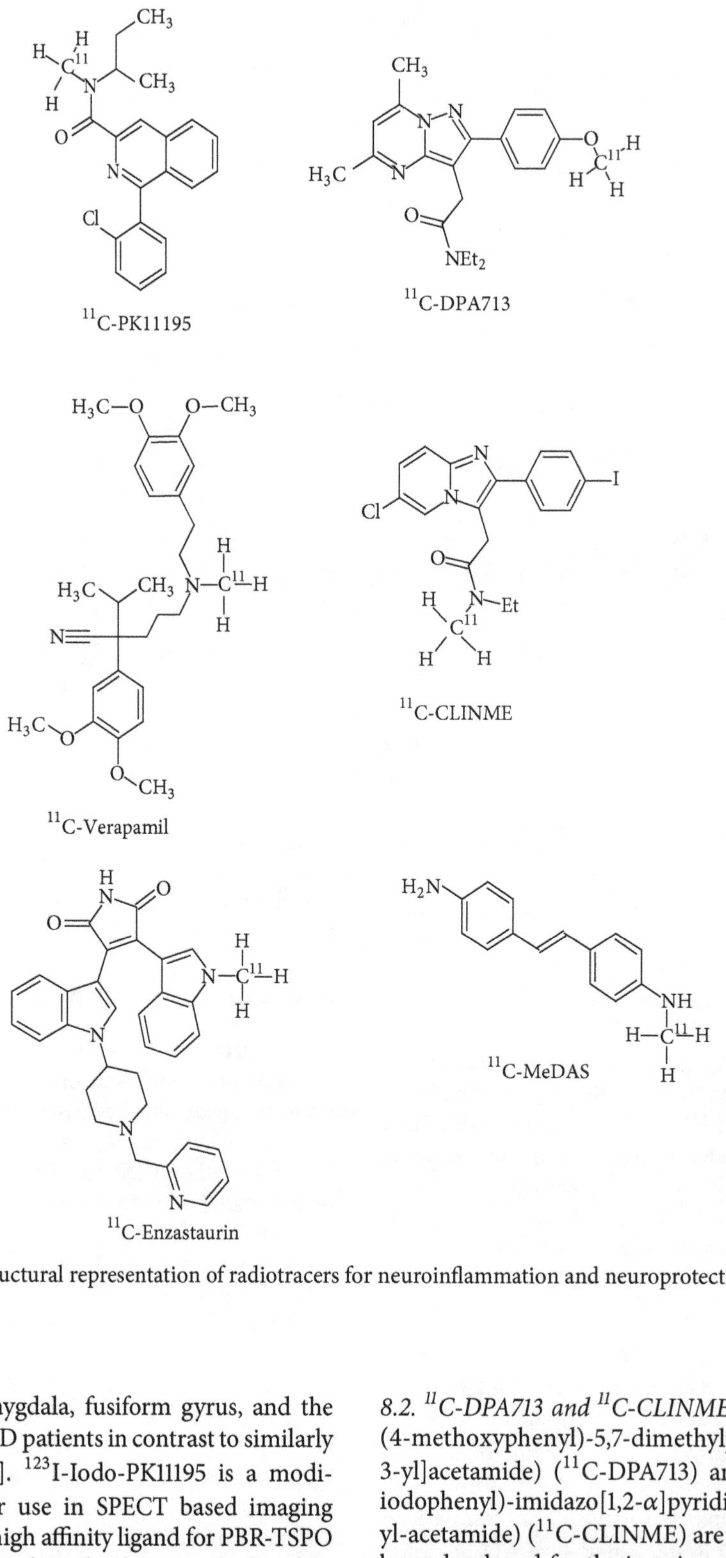

FIGURE 5: Structural representation of radiotracers for neuroinflammation and neuroprotection imaging.

in the cingulate cortex, amygdala, fusiform gyrus, and the temporoparietal cortex of AD patients in contrast to similarly aged healthy controls [151]. ^{123}I-Iodo-PK11195 is a modification of ^{11}C-PK11195 for use in SPECT based imaging protocols. It functions as a high affinity ligand for PBR-TSPO [152]. As per a SPECT based study that was undertaken using this radiotracer, an increased retention of the radiotracer was observed in the temporal, parietal, occipital, and frontal lobes, wherein such findings were in tandem with AD induced neuroinflammation [153]. However, the use of PK11195 is limited for neuroinflammation imaging due to its increased incidences of nonspecific binding and lower neuronal bioavailability [154].

8.2. ^{11}C-DPA713 and ^{11}C-CLINME. [^{11}C](N,N-Diethyl-2-[2-(4-methoxyphenyl)-5,7-dimethylpyrazolo[1,5-a]pyrimidin-3-yl]acetamide) (^{11}C-DPA713) and [^{11}C](2-[6-chloro-2-(4-iodophenyl)-imidazo[1,2-α]pyridine-3-yl]-N-ethyl-N-methyl-acetamide) (^{11}C-CLINME) are new radiotracers that have been developed for the imaging of mild neuroinflammation [155] (Figure 5). Both the radiotracers have demonstrated a lower likelihood of nonspecific neuronal interactions and are sensitive to even low levels of TSPO expression due to their high affinity to the receptor [156]. ^{11}C-DPA713 and ^{11}C-CLINME were further optimized by labelling the ligands with ^{18}F, thereby enhancing the half-life of the radiotracer. ^{18}F-DPA714 is the successor of ^{11}C-DPA713, showcasing better affinity and pharmacokinetics than PK11195 [157]. ^{18}F-PBR111 is the fluorinated analogue of ^{11}C-CLINME sharing properties that are inherent of the original radiotracer [158]. Such findings have found their basis in neuroinflammation studies that have been carried out in animal models of glioma and Multiple Sclerosis [159, 160]. ^{123}I-CLINDE is another SPECT based radiotracer that has shown promising results in the preclinical examination of neuroinflammation [161]. The radiotracer retention appreciably correlates with the variations in TSPO that are observed at the onset and progression of neuroinflammation [162]. Another prominent feature of neuroinflammation and neurodegeneration is the phenomenon of astrocytosis [163]. Astrocytosis results in increased expression of imidazoline 2 binding sites (I$_2$BS) [164]. Radiotracers that have been developed for the imaging of I$_2$BS include ^{11}C-DED and ^{11}C-FTIMD. Current studies using ^{11}C-DED in AD patients have shown increased radiotracer localization throughout the brain [165]. It has also been suggested that astrocytosis is a key feature of AD that functions as an intermediate between amyloidosis and neurodegeneration [166]. In case of ^{11}C-FTIMD, animal model based studies have demonstrated that ^{11}C-FTIMD has a high affinity to I$_2$BS and has the ability to quantitate I$_2$BS expression [167].

9. Other Molecular Radiotracers for Molecular Imaging

9.1. ^{11}C-Enzastaurin. PKC as an enzyme is one of the most important initial elements involved in the induction of the previously mentioned α-secretases, ADAM-10 and 17, which are involved in neuroprotection. A potent and selective protein kinase C (PKC) inhibitor, Enzastaurin (LY317615), was recently labelled with ^{11}C, thereby generating the radiotracer (3-(1-[^{11}C]methyl-1H-indol-3-yl)-4-[1-[1-(2-pyridinyl-methyl)-4-piperidinyl]-1H-indol-3-yl]-1H-pyrrole-2,5-dione), for PET imaging applications [168, 169] (Figure 5).

9.2. ^{11}C-MeDAS. [^{11}C]N-Methyl-4,4-diaminostilbene (^{11}C-MeDAS) is a radiotracer, which can be used as a myelin-imaging marker for the early monitoring of myelin degeneration *in vivo*, and is a potentially useful development for the investigation of neurodegeneration [170] (Figure 5).

9.3. ^{124}I-pQHNIG70. Impaired function of heat shock proteins HSP70, HSF1, and cathepsin proteins may facilitate the progression of neurodegeneration. The ^{124}I-pQHNIG70 PET reporter system for imaging specific gene includes an inducible HSP70 promoter which can be used to image and monitor the activation of the heat shock factor 1 (HSF1)/HSP70 transcription factor on exposure to drug treatment 17-allylaminodemethoxygeldanamycin [171].

9.4. ^{11}C-Verapamil. P-glycoprotein (P-gp) is a known BBB active efflux transporter involved in neuroprotection. Onset of PD and AD is characterised by its dysfunction [172].

The radiolabelled P-gp substrate 2-(3,4-dimethoxyphenyl)-5-[2-(3,4-dimethoxyphenyl)ethyl-[^{11}C]methyl-amino]-2-propan-2-yl-pentanenitrile (^{11}C-Verapamil) is used in PET studies of AD [173] (Figure 5).

9.5. ^{11}C-AA and ^{11}C-DHA. ^{11}C-Arachidonic acid (^{11}C-AA) is incorporated in brain regions with neuroinflammation [174]. ^{11}C-AA could thus be a novel marker of activated microglia to be used in studies of neurodegenerative disorders. Radiolabelled ^{11}C-docosahexaenoic acid (^{11}C-DHA) tracer is used to map the regional and global human brain DHA metabolism in relation to health and disease [175]. The quantitative imaging of DHA incorporation from plasma into the brain can be used as an *in vivo* biomarker of brain DHA metabolism and neurotransmission [176]. This may help to monitor DHA consumption *in vivo* in patients with disorders such as depression and AD, in which DHA supplementation may be helpful [177].

10. Conclusion

PET and SPECT with molecular probes are useful and reliable tools for clinical molecular neuroimaging. The methods have enabled *in vivo* assessment of molecular pathogenesis of CNS disorders. With these techniques, Aβ deposition, tau fibrillar mass, neurotransmitter turnover, and metabolism can be monitored accurately to better understand the pathological mechanisms underlying CNS diseases. In comparison to PET, SPECT is a more practical routine procedure for the detection of AD. But sensitivity, spatial resolution, and quantification of SPECT are limited. Improvements in a variety of molecular probes available for PET and SPECT will further help in identifying the biomarkers for biochemical processes underlying CNS diseases. In the forthcoming years, further advancements in imaging techniques promise to improve upon the early and accurate diagnosis, prognosis, and treatment of neurodegenerative diseases.

Conflict of Interests

The authors declare that there is no conflict of interests regarding the publication of this paper.

References

[1] D. P. Chapman, S. M. Williams, T. W. Strine, R. F. Anda, and M. J. Moore, "Dementia and its implications for public health," *Preventing Chronic Disease*, vol. 3, no. 2, article A34, 2006.

[2] D. C. Mash, D. D. Flynn, and L. T. Potter, "Loss of M2 muscarine receptors in the cerebral cortex in Alzheimer's disease and experimental cholinergic denervation," *Science*, vol. 228, no. 4703, pp. 1115–1117, 1985.

[3] J. D. Gazewood, D. R. Richards, and K. Clebak, "Parkinson disease: an update," *American Family Physician*, vol. 87, no. 4, pp. 267–273, 2013.

[4] J. Massano, "Cognitive impairment and dementia—an update," *Frontiers in Neurology*, vol. 3, article 153, 2012.

[5] V. Kljajevic, "Overestimating the effects of healthy aging," *Frontiers in Aging Neuroscience*, vol. 7, article 164, 2015.

[6] B. Frost and M. I. Diamond, "Prion-like mechanisms in neurodegenerative diseases," *Nature Reviews Neuroscience*, vol. 11, no. 3, pp. 155–159, 2010.

[7] F. M. M. Lu and Z. Yuan, "PET/SPECT molecular imaging in clinical neuroscience: recent advances in the investigation of CNS diseases," *Quantitative Imaging in Medicine and Surgery*, vol. 5, no. 3, pp. 433–447, 2015.

[8] J. F. Jiménez Bonilla and J. M. Carril Carril, "Molecular neuroimaging in degenerative dementias," *Revista Espanola de Medicina Nuclear e Imagen Molecular*, vol. 32, no. 5, pp. 301–309, 2013.

[9] P. A. Apurva, P. M. Bipin, and P. M. Kirti, "Role of PET scan in clinical practice," *Gujarat Medical Journal*, vol. 68, no. 2, pp. 19–22, 2013.

[10] R. Weissleder and U. Mahmood, "Molecular imaging," *Radiology*, vol. 219, no. 2, pp. 316–333, 2001.

[11] E. Kim, O. D. Howes, and S. Kapur, "Molecular imaging as a guide for the treatment of central nervous system disorders," *Dialogues in Clinical Neuroscience*, vol. 15, no. 3, pp. 315–328, 2013.

[12] S. P. Mueller, J. F. Polak, M. F. Kijewski, and B. L. Holman, "Collimator selection for SPECT brain imaging: the advantage of high resolution," *Journal of Nuclear Medicine*, vol. 27, no. 11, pp. 1729–1738, 1986.

[13] L. Jiang, Y. Tu, H. Shi, and Z. Cheng, "PET probes beyond ^{18}F-FDG," *Journal of Biomedical Research*, vol. 28, no. 6, pp. 435–446, 2014.

[14] W. Mier and D. Mier, "Advantages in functional imaging of the brain," *Frontiers in Human Neuroscience*, vol. 9, p. 249, 2015.

[15] T. Varghese, R. Sheelakumari, J. S. James, and P. S. Mathuranath, "A review of neuroimaging biomarkers of Alzheimer's disease," *Neurology Asia*, vol. 18, no. 3, pp. 239–248, 2013.

[16] K. Blennow, M. J. de Leon, and H. Zetterberg, "Alzheimer's disease," *The Lancet*, vol. 368, no. 9533, pp. 387–403, 2006.

[17] Alzheimer's Association, "2010 Alzheimer's disease facts and figures," *Alzheimer's and Dementia*, vol. 6, no. 2, pp. 158–194, 2010.

[18] W. T. Hu, A. Chen-Plotkin, S. E. Arnold et al., "Novel CSF biomarkers for Alzheimer's disease and mild cognitive impairment," *Acta Neuropathologica*, vol. 119, no. 6, pp. 669–678, 2010.

[19] L. Devi and H. K. Anandatheerthavarada, "Mitochondrial trafficking of APP and alpha synuclein: relevance to mitochondrial dysfunction in Alzheimer's and Parkinson's diseases," *Biochimica et Biophysica Acta (BBA)—Molecular Basis of Disease*, vol. 1802, no. 1, pp. 11–19, 2010.

[20] C. Mancuso, G. Scapagnini, D. Currò et al., "Mitochondrial dysfunction, free radical generation and cellular stress response in neurodegenerative disorders," *Frontiers in Bioscience*, vol. 12, no. 3, pp. 1107–1123, 2007.

[21] H. W. Querfurth and F. M. LaFerla, "Alzheimer's disease," *The New England Journal of Medicine*, vol. 362, no. 4, pp. 329–344, 2010.

[22] P. Davidsson, A. Westman-Brinkmalm, C. L. Nilsson et al., "Proteome analysis of cerebrospinal fluid proteins in Alzheimer patients," *NeuroReport*, vol. 13, no. 5, pp. 611–615, 2002.

[23] M. A. Korolainen, T. A. Nyman, P. Nyyssönen, E. S. Hartikainen, and T. Pirttilä, "Multiplexed proteomic analysis of oxidation and concentrations of cerebrospinal fluid proteins in Alzheimer disease," *Clinical Chemistry*, vol. 53, no. 4, pp. 657–665, 2007.

[24] H. Zetterberg, U. Rüetschi, E. Portelius et al., "Clinical proteomics in neurodegenerative disorders," *Acta Neurologica Scandinavica*, vol. 118, no. 1, pp. 1–11, 2008.

[25] C. Sihlbom, P. Davidsson, M. Sjögren, L.-O. Wahlund, and C. L. Nilsson, "Structural and quantitative comparison of cerebrospinal fluid glycoproteins in Alzheimer's disease patients and healthy individuals," *Neurochemical Research*, vol. 33, no. 7, pp. 1332–1340, 2008.

[26] M. Puchades, S. F. Hansson, C. L. Nilsson, N. Andreasen, K. Blennow, and P. Davidsson, "Proteomic studies of potential cerebrospinal fluid protein markers for Alzheimer's disease," *Molecular Brain Research*, vol. 118, no. 1-2, pp. 140–146, 2003.

[27] C. Hesse, C. L. Nilsson, K. Blennow, and P. Davidsson, "Identification of the apolipoprotein E4 isoform in cerebrospinal fluid with preparative two-dimensional electrophoresis and matrix assisted laser desorption/ionization-time of flight-mass spectrometry," *Electrophoresis*, vol. 22, no. 9, pp. 1834–1837, 2001.

[28] E. Tarkowski, K. Blennow, A. Wallin, and A. Tarkowski, "Intracerebral production of tumor necrosis factor-α, a local neuroprotective agent, in Alzheimer disease and vascular dementia," *Journal of Clinical Immunology*, vol. 19, no. 4, pp. 223–230, 1999.

[29] I. Blasko, W. Lederer, H. Oberbauer et al., "Measurement of thirteen biological markers in CSF of patients with Alzheimer's disease and other dementias," *Dementia and Geriatric Cognitive Disorders*, vol. 21, no. 1, pp. 9–15, 2005.

[30] D. Galimberti, N. Schoonenboom, P. Scheltens et al., "Intrathecal chemokine synthesis in mild cognitive impairment and Alzheimer disease," *Archives of Neurology*, vol. 63, no. 4, pp. 538–543, 2006.

[31] E. Gómez-Tortosa, I. Gonzalo, S. Fanjul et al., "Cerebrospinal fluid markers in dementia with Lewy bodies compared with Alzheimer disease," *Archives of Neurology*, vol. 60, no. 9, pp. 1218–1222, 2003.

[32] E. Rota, G. Bellone, P. Rocca, B. Bergamasco, G. Emanuelli, and P. Ferrero, "Increased intrathecal TGF-β1, but not IL-12, IFN-γ and IL-10 levels in Alzheimer's disease patients," *Neurological Sciences*, vol. 27, no. 1, pp. 33–39, 2006.

[33] R. M. Evans, S. Hui, A. Perkins, D. K. Lahiri, J. Poirier, and M. R. Farlow, "Cholesterol and APOE genotype interact to influence Alzheimer disease progression," *Neurology*, vol. 62, no. 10, pp. 1869–1871, 2004.

[34] M.-K. K. Sun, J. Hongpaisan, and D. L. Alkon, "Postischemic PKC activation rescues retrograde and anterograde long-term memory," *Proceedings of the National Academy of Sciences of the United States of America*, vol. 106, no. 34, pp. 14676–14680, 2009.

[35] J. de Barry, C. M. Liégeois, and A. Janoshazi, "Protein kinase C as a peripheral biomarker for Alzheimer's disease," *Experimental Gerontology*, vol. 45, no. 1, pp. 64–69, 2010.

[36] T. Isagawa, H. Mukai, K. Oishi et al., "Dual effects of PKNα and protein kinase C on phosphorylation of tau protein by glycogen synthase kinase-3β," *Biochemical and Biophysical Research Communications*, vol. 273, no. 1, pp. 209–212, 2000.

[37] H. Zetterberg, K. Blennow, and E. Hanse, "Amyloid β and APP as biomarkers for Alzheimer's disease," *Experimental Gerontology*, vol. 45, no. 1, pp. 23–29, 2010.

[38] H. Zetterberg, U. Andreasson, O. Hansson et al., "Elevated cerebrospinal fluid BACE1 activity in incipient alzheimer disease," *Archives of Neurology*, vol. 65, no. 8, pp. 1102–1107, 2008.

[39] J. A. Hardy and G. A. Higgins, "Alzheimer's disease: the amyloid cascade hypothesis," *Science*, vol. 256, no. 5054, pp. 184–185, 1992.

[40] T. L. Spires-Jones, W. H. Stoothoff, A. de Calignon, P. B. Jones, and B. T. Hyman, "Tau pathophysiology in neurodegeneration: a tangled issue," *Trends in Neurosciences*, vol. 32, no. 3, pp. 150–159, 2009.

[41] M. A. Korolainen, T. A. Nyman, T. Aittokallio, and T. Pirttilä, "An update on clinical proteomics in Alzheimer's research," *Journal of Neurochemistry*, vol. 112, no. 6, pp. 1386–1414, 2010.

[42] S. Davinelli, M. Intrieri, C. Russo et al., "The "Alzheimer's disease signature": potential perspectives for novel biomarkers," *Immunity and Ageing*, vol. 8, article 7, 2011.

[43] S. Dassati, A. Waldner, and R. Schweigreiter, "Apolipoprotein D takes center stage in the stress response of the aging and degenerative brain," *Neurobiology of Aging*, vol. 35, no. 7, pp. 1632–1642, 2014.

[44] S. Lorente-Cebrián, A. G. G. Costa, S. Navas-Carretero et al., "An update on the role of omega-3 fatty acids on inflammatory and degenerative diseases," *Journal of Physiology and Biochemistry*, vol. 71, no. 2, pp. 341–349, 2015.

[45] X. Li, K. S. Montine, C. D. Keene, and T. J. Montine, "Different mechanisms of apolipoprotein E isoform-dependent modulation of prostaglandin E2 production and triggering receptor expressed on myeloid cells 2 (TREM2) expression after innate immune activation of microglia," *The FASEB Journal*, vol. 29, no. 5, pp. 1754–1762, 2015.

[46] L. K. Ferreira and G. F. Busatto, "Neuroimaging in Alzheimer's disease: current role in clinical practice and potential future applications," *Clinics*, vol. 66, supplement 1, pp. 19–24, 2011.

[47] R. C. Barber, "Biomarkers for early detection of Alzheimer disease," *Journal of the American Osteopathic Association*, vol. 110, no. 9, pp. S10–S15, 2010.

[48] L. Zhang, R. C.-C. Chang, L.-W. W. Chu, and H. K.-F. Mak, "Current neuroimaging techniques in Alzheimer's disease and applications in animal models," *American Journal of Nuclear Medicine and Molecular Imaging*, vol. 2, no. 3, pp. 386–404, 2012.

[49] K. J. Anstey, R. Eramudugolla, D. E. Hosking, N. T. Lautenschlager, and R. A. Dixon, "Bridging the translation gap: from dementia risk assessment to advice on risk reduction," *Journal of Prevention of Alzheimer's Disease*, vol. 2, no. 3, pp. 189–198, 2015.

[50] T. L. Spires-Jones and B. Hyman, "The intersection of amyloid β and tau at synapses in Alzheimer's disease," *Neuron*, vol. 82, no. 4, pp. 756–771, 2014.

[51] M. Tabaton, X. Zhu, G. Perry, M. A. Smith, and L. Giliberto, "Signaling effect of amyloid-β_{42} on the processing of AβPP," *Experimental Neurology*, vol. 221, no. 1, pp. 18–25, 2010.

[52] W. Qin, L. Ho, J. Wang, E. Peskind, and G. M. Pasinetti, "S100A7, a novel Alzheimer's disease biomarker with non-amyloidogenic α-secretase activity acts via selective promotion of ADAM-10," *PLoS ONE*, vol. 4, no. 1, Article ID e4183, 2009.

[53] P. L. Ross, Y. N. Huang, J. N. Marchese et al., "Multiplexed protein quantitation in *Saccharomyces cerevisiae* using amine-reactive isobaric tagging reagents," *Molecular and Cellular Proteomics*, vol. 3, no. 12, pp. 1154–1169, 2004.

[54] A. Thompson, J. Schäfer, K. Kuhn et al., "Tandem mass tags: a novel quantification strategy for comparative analysis of complex protein mixtures by MS/MS," *Analytical Chemistry*, vol. 75, no. 8, pp. 1895–1904, 2003.

[55] S. P. Gygi, B. Rist, S. A. Gerber, F. Turecek, M. H. Gelb, and R. Aebersold, "Quantitative analysis of complex protein mixtures using isotope-coded affinity tags," *Nature Biotechnology*, vol. 17, no. 10, pp. 994–999, 1999.

[56] A. Schmidt, J. Kellermann, and F. Lottspeich, "A novel strategy for quantitative proteomics using isotope-coded protein labels," *Proteomics*, vol. 5, no. 1, pp. 4–15, 2005.

[57] C. Tian, D. Liu, W. Xiang et al., "Analyses of the similarity and difference of global gene expression profiles in cortex regions of three neurodegenerative diseases: sporadic Creutzfeldt-Jakob disease (sCJD), fatal familial insomnia (FFI), and Alzheimer's disease (AD)," *Molecular Neurobiology*, vol. 50, no. 2, pp. 473–481, 2014.

[58] G. M. McKhann, D. S. Knopman, H. Chertkow et al., "The diagnosis of dementia due to Alzheimer's disease: recommendations from the National Institute on Aging-Alzheimer's Association workgroups on diagnostic guidelines for Alzheimer's disease," *Alzheimer's & Dementia*, vol. 7, no. 3, pp. 263–269, 2011.

[59] M. Benadiba, G. Luurtsema, L. Wichert-Ana, C. A. Buchpigel, and G. B. Filho, "New molecular targets for PET and SPECT imaging in neurodegenerative diseases," *Revista Brasileira de Psiquiatria*, vol. 34, no. 2, pp. S125–S148, 2012.

[60] H. Shim, M. J. Ly, and S. K. Tighe, "Brain imaging in the differential diagnosis of young-onset dementias," *Psychiatric Clinics of North America*, vol. 38, no. 2, pp. 281–294, 2015.

[61] M. E. Phelps, "Positron emission tomography provides molecular imaging of biological processes," *Proceedings of the National Academy of Sciences of the United States of America*, vol. 97, no. 16, pp. 9226–9233, 2000.

[62] R. Dann, D. Christman, J. Fowler, B. MacGregor, and A. Wolf, "Metabolic mapping of functional activity in human subjects with the [18F] fluorodeoxyglucose technique," *Science*, vol. 212, no. 4495, pp. 678–680, 1981.

[63] K. Strijckmans, "The isochronous cyclotron: principles and recent developments," *Computerized Medical Imaging and Graphics*, vol. 25, no. 2, pp. 69–78, 2001.

[64] C. Halldin, B. Gulyás, O. Langer, and L. Farde, "Brain radioligands—state of the art and new trends," *Quarterly Journal of Nuclear Medicine*, vol. 45, no. 2, pp. 139–152, 2001.

[65] D. W. Townsend, "Dual-modality imaging: combining anatomy and function," *Journal of Nuclear Medicine*, vol. 49, no. 6, pp. 938–955, 2008.

[66] J. M. Kofler, D. D. Cody, and R. L. Morin, "CT protocol review and optimization," *Journal of the American College of Radiology*, vol. 11, no. 3, pp. 267–270, 2014.

[67] M. Laruelle, M. Slifstein, and Y. Huang, "Positron emission tomography: imaging and quantification of neurotransporter availability," *Methods*, vol. 27, no. 3, pp. 287–299, 2002.

[68] A. Baert, *Encyclopedia of Diagnostic Imaging*, Springer, Berlin, Germany, 2008.

[69] I. Buvat, S. Laffont, J. Le Cloirec, P. Bourguet, and R. Di Paola, "Importance of the choice of the collimator for the detection of small lesions in scintimammography: a phantom study," *Physics in Medicine and Biology*, vol. 46, no. 5, pp. 1343–1355, 2001.

[70] B. Palumbo, T. Buresta, S. Nuvoli et al., "SPECT and PET serve as molecular imaging techniques and *in Vivo* biomarkers for brain metastases," *International Journal of Molecular Sciences*, vol. 15, no. 6, pp. 9878–9893, 2014.

[71] S. L. Pimlott and A. Sutherland, "Molecular tracers for the PET and SPECT imaging of disease," *Chemical Society Reviews*, vol. 40, no. 1, pp. 149–162, 2011.

[72] V. L. Villemagne, M. T. Fodero-Tavoletti, K. E. Pike, R. Cappai, C. L. Masters, and C. C. Rowe, "The ART of loss: aβ imaging in the evaluation of Alzheimer's disease and other dementias," *Molecular Neurobiology*, vol. 38, no. 1, pp. 1–15, 2008.

[73] M. Laruelle, M. Slifstein, and Y. Huang, "Relationships between radiotracer properties and image quality in molecular imaging of the brain with positron emission tomography," *Molecular Imaging & Biology*, vol. 5, no. 6, pp. 363–375, 2003.

[74] V. W. Pike, "PET radiotracers: crossing the blood-brain barrier and surviving metabolism," *Trends in Pharmacological Sciences*, vol. 30, no. 8, pp. 431–440, 2009.

[75] W. M. Pardridge, "Drug and gene delivery to the brain: the vascular route," *Neuron*, vol. 36, no. 4, pp. 555–558, 2002.

[76] J. E. Maggio, E. R. Stimson, J. R. Ghilardi et al., "Reversible in vitro growth of Alzheimer disease β-amyloid plaques by deposition of labeled amyloid peptide," *Proceedings of the National Academy of Sciences of the United States of America*, vol. 89, no. 12, pp. 5462–5466, 1992.

[77] R. P. Friedland, R. E. Majocha, J. M. Reno, L. R. Lyle, and C. A. Marotta, "Development of an anti-Aβ monoclonal antibody for in vivo imaging of amyloid angiopathy in Alzheimer's disease," *Molecular Neurobiology*, vol. 9, no. 1–3, pp. 107–113, 1994.

[78] H. J. Lee, Y. Zhang, C. Zhu, K. Duff, and W. M. Pardridge, "Imaging brain amyloid of Alzheimer disease in vivo in transgenic mice with an Abeta peptide radiopharmaceutical," *Journal of Cerebral Blood Flow Metabolism*, vol. 22, no. 2, pp. 223–231, 2002.

[79] C. A. Mathis, Y. Wang, D. P. Holt, G.-F. F. Huang, M. L. Debnath, and W. E. Klunk, "Synthesis and evaluation of ^{11}C-labeled 6-substituted 2-arylbenzothiazoles as amyloid imaging agents," *Journal of Medicinal Chemistry*, vol. 46, no. 13, pp. 2740–2754, 2003.

[80] Z.-P. P. Zhuang, M.-P. P. Kung, A. Wilson et al., "Structure-activity relationship of imidazo[1,2-a]pyridines as ligands for detecting β-amyloid plaques in the brain," *Journal of Medicinal Chemistry*, vol. 46, no. 2, pp. 237–243, 2003.

[81] H. Engler, A. F. Santillo, S. X. Wang et al., "In vivo amyloid imaging with PET in frontotemporal dementia," *European Journal of Nuclear Medicine and Molecular Imaging*, vol. 35, no. 1, pp. 100–106, 2008.

[82] G. D. Rabinovici, H. J. Rosen, A. Alkalay et al., "Amyloid vs FDG-PET in the differential diagnosis of AD and FTLD," *Neurology*, vol. 77, no. 23, pp. 2034–2042, 2011.

[83] V. L. Villemagne, K. Ong, R. S. Mulligan et al., "Amyloid imaging with (18)F-florbetaben in Alzheimer disease and other dementias," *Journal of Nuclear Medicine*, vol. 52, no. 8, pp. 1210–1217, 2011.

[84] W. E. Klunk, H. Engler, A. Nordberg et al., "Imaging brain amyloid in Alzheimer's disease with Pittsburgh compound-B," *Annals of Neurology*, vol. 55, no. 3, pp. 306–319, 2004.

[85] B. J. Bacskai, G. A. Hickey, J. Skoch et al., "Four-dimensional multiphoton imaging of brain entry, amyloid binding, and clearance of an amyloid-β ligand in transgenic mice," *Proceedings of the National Academy of Sciences of the United States of America*, vol. 100, no. 21, pp. 12462–12467, 2003.

[86] C. C. Rowe, S. Ng, U. Ackermann et al., "Imaging β-amyloid burden in aging and dementia," *Neurology*, vol. 68, no. 20, pp. 1718–1725, 2007.

[87] C. C. Rowe, K. A. Ellis, M. Rimajova et al., "Amyloid imaging results from the Australian Imaging, Biomarkers and Lifestyle (AIBL) study of aging," *Neurobiology of Aging*, vol. 31, no. 8, pp. 1275–1283, 2010.

[88] A. Forsberg, H. Engler, O. Almkvist et al., "PET imaging of amyloid deposition in patients with mild cognitive impairment," *Neurobiology of Aging*, vol. 29, no. 10, pp. 1456–1465, 2008.

[89] P. Edison, C. C. Rowe, J. O. Rinne et al., "Amyloid load in Parkinson's disease dementia and Lewy body dementia measured with [^{11}C]PIB positron emission tomography," *Journal of Neurology, Neurosurgery and Psychiatry*, vol. 79, no. 12, pp. 1331–1338, 2008.

[90] M. A. Mintun, G. N. Larossa, Y. I. Sheline et al., "[11C]PIB in a nondemented population: potential antecedent marker of Alzheimer disease," *Neurology*, vol. 67, no. 3, pp. 446–452, 2006.

[91] N. S. Mason, C. A. Mathis, and W. E. Klunk, "Positron emission tomography radioligands for in vivo imaging of Aβ plaques," *Journal of Labelled Compounds and Radiopharmaceuticals*, vol. 56, no. 3-4, pp. 89–95, 2013.

[92] A. E. Johnson, F. Jeppsson, J. Sandell et al., "AZD2184: a radioligand for sensitive detection of β-amyloid deposits," *Journal of Neurochemistry*, vol. 108, no. 5, pp. 1177–1186, 2009.

[93] S. Nyberg, M. E. Jönhagen, Z. Cselényi et al., "Detection of amyloid in Alzheimer's disease with positron emission tomography using [^{11}C]AZD2184," *European Journal of Nuclear Medicine and Molecular Imaging*, vol. 36, no. 11, pp. 1859–1863, 2009.

[94] A. Nordberg, "PET imaging of amyloid in Alzheimer's disease," *The Lancet Neurology*, vol. 3, no. 9, pp. 519–527, 2004.

[95] K. Shoghi-Jadid, G. W. Small, E. D. Agdeppa et al., "Localization of neurofibrillary tangles and β-amyloid plaques in the brains of living patients with alzheimer disease," *The American Journal of Geriatric Psychiatry*, vol. 10, no. 1, pp. 24–35, 2002.

[96] P. W. Thompson, L. Ye, J. L. Morgenstern et al., "Interaction of the amyloid imaging tracer FDDNP with hallmark Alzheimer's disease pathologies," *Journal of Neurochemistry*, vol. 109, no. 2, pp. 623–630, 2009.

[97] E. D. Agdeppa, V. Kepe, K. Shoghi-Jadid et al., "In vivo and in vitro labeling of plaques and tangles in the brain of an Alzheimer's disease patient: a case study," *Journal of Nuclear Medicine*, vol. 42, no. 5, p. 65, 2001.

[98] L. M. Smid, V. Kepe, H. V. Vinters et al., "Postmortem 3-D brain hemisphere cortical tau and amyloid-β pathology mapping and quantification as a validation method of neuropathology imaging," *Journal of Alzheimer's Disease*, vol. 36, no. 2, pp. 261–274, 2013.

[99] G. W. Small, E. D. Agdeppa, V. Kepe, N. Satyamurthy, S.-C. Huang, and J. R. Barrio, "In vivo brain imaging of tangle burden in humans," *Journal of Molecular Neuroscience*, vol. 19, no. 3, pp. 321–327, 2002.

[100] H. Barthel and O. Sabri, "Florbetaben to trace amyloid-β in the Alzheimer brain by means of PET," *Journal of Alzheimer's Disease*, vol. 26, no. 3, pp. 117–121, 2011.

[101] S. R. Choi, G. Golding, Z. Zhuang et al., "Preclinical properties of 18F-AV-45: a PET agent for Abeta plaques in the brain," *Journal of Nuclear Medicine*, vol. 50, no. 11, pp. 1887–1894, 2009.

[102] D. F. Wong, P. B. Rosenberg, Y. Zhou et al., "In vivo imaging of amyloid deposition in Alzheimer disease using the radioligand ^{18}F-AV-45 (flobetapir F 18)," *Journal of Nuclear Medicine*, vol. 51, no. 6, pp. 913–920, 2010.

[103] C. M. Clark, J. A. Schneider, B. J. Bedell et al., "Use of florbetapir-PET for imaging β-amyloid pathology," *Journal of the American Medical Association*, vol. 305, no. 3, pp. 275–283, 2011.

[104] C. C. Rowe, U. Ackerman, W. Browne et al., "Imaging of amyloid β in Alzheimer's disease with 18F-BAY94-9172, a novel PET tracer: proof of mechanism," *The Lancet Neurology*, vol. 7, no. 2, pp. 129–135, 2008.

[105] S. Shokouhi, D. Claassen, and W. Riddle, "Imaging brain metabolism and pathology in Alzheimer's disease with positron emission tomography," *Journal of Alzheimer's Disease & Parkinsonism*, vol. 4, no. 2, article 143, 2014.

[106] N. Nelissen, K. Van Laere, L. Thurfjell et al., "Phase 1 study of the Pittsburgh compound B derivative ^{18}F-flutemetamol in healthy volunteers and patients with probable Alzheimer disease," *Journal of Nuclear Medicine*, vol. 50, no. 8, pp. 1251–1259, 2009.

[107] R. Vandenberghe, K. Adamczuk, P. Dupont, K. V. Laere, and G. Chételat, "Amyloid PET in clinical practice: its place in the multidimensional space of Alzheimer's disease," *NeuroImage: Clinical*, vol. 2, no. 1, pp. 497–511, 2013.

[108] C. C. Rowe and V. L. Villemagne, "Brain amyloid imaging," *Journal of Nuclear Medicine*, vol. 52, no. 11, pp. 1733–1740, 2011.

[109] Z. Cselényi, M. E. Jönhagen, A. Forsberg et al., "Clinical validation of ^{18}F-AZD4694, an amyloid-β-specific PET radioligand," *Journal of Nuclear Medicine*, vol. 53, no. 3, pp. 415–424, 2012.

[110] A. Juréus, B.-M. M. Swahn, J. Sandell et al., "Characterization of AZD4694, a novel fluorinated Aβ plaque neuroimaging PET radioligand," *Journal of Neurochemistry*, vol. 114, no. 3, pp. 784–794, 2010.

[111] Y. Kudo, N. Okamura, S. Furumoto et al., "2-(2-[2-Dimethyl-aminothiazol-5-yl]ethenyl)-6- (2-[fluoro]ethoxy)benzoxazole: a novel PET agent for in vivo detection of dense amyloid plaques in Alzheimer's disease patients," *Journal of Nuclear Medicine*, vol. 48, no. 4, pp. 553–561, 2007.

[112] Y. Kudo, "Development of amyloid imaging PET probes for an early diagnosis of Alzheimer's disease," *Minimally Invasive Therapy and Allied Technologies*, vol. 15, no. 4, pp. 209–213, 2006.

[113] M. Ono, A. Wilson, J. Nobrega et al., "^{11}C-labeled stilbene derivatives as Aβ-aggregate-specific PET imaging agents for Alzheimer's disease," *Nuclear Medicine and Biology*, vol. 30, no. 6, pp. 565–571, 2003.

[114] W. E. Klunk, H. Engler, A. Nordberg et al., "Imaging the pathology of Alzheimer's disease: amyloid-imaging with positron emission tomography," *Neuroimaging Clinics of North America*, vol. 13, no. 4, pp. 781–789, 2003.

[115] N. P. L. G. Verhoeff, A. A. Wilson, S. Takeshita et al., "In-vivo imaging of Alzheimer disease β-amyloid with [^{11}C]SB-13 PET," *American Journal of Geriatric Psychiatry*, vol. 12, no. 6, pp. 584–595, 2004.

[116] M. C. Hong, Y. K. Kim, J. Y. Choi et al., "Synthesis and evaluation of stilbene derivatives as a potential imaging agent of amyloid plaques," *Bioorganic and Medicinal Chemistry*, vol. 18, no. 22, pp. 7724–7730, 2010.

[117] K. R. Eun and X. Chen, "Development of Alzheimer's disease imaging agents for clinical studies," *Frontiers in Bioscience*, vol. 13, no. 2, pp. 777–789, 2008.

[118] C. Wu, V. W. Pike, and Y. Wang, "Amyloid imaging: from benchtop to bedside," *Current Topics in Developmental Biology*, vol. 70, pp. 171–213, 2005.

[119] M.-P. Kung, C. Hou, Z.-P. Zhuang, D. Skovronsky, and H. F. Kung, "Binding of two potential imaging agents targeting amyloid plaques in postmortem brain tissues of patients with Alzheimer's disease," *Brain Research*, vol. 1025, no. 1-2, pp. 98–105, 2004.

[120] F. Hernández and J. Avila, "Tauopathies," *Cellular and Molecular Life Sciences*, vol. 64, no. 17, pp. 2219–2233, 2007.

[121] K. Arima, "Ultrastructural characteristics of tau filaments in tauopathies: immuno-electron microscopic demonstration of tau filaments in tauopathies," *Neuropathology*, vol. 26, no. 5, pp. 475–483, 2006.

[122] P. J. Muchowski, "Protein misfolding, amyloid formation, and neurodegeneration: a critical role for molecular chaperones?" *Neuron*, vol. 35, no. 1, pp. 9–12, 2002.

[123] M. G. Spillantini and M. Goedert, "Tau pathology and neurodegeneration," *The Lancet Neurology*, vol. 12, no. 6, pp. 609–622, 2013.

[124] N. S. Honson, R. L. Johnson, W. Huang, J. Inglese, C. P. Austin, and J. Kuret, "Differentiating Alzheimer disease-associated aggregates with small molecules," *Neurobiology of Disease*, vol. 28, no. 3, pp. 251–260, 2007.

[125] K. N. Schafer, S. Kim, A. Matzavinos, and J. Kuret, "Selectivity requirements for diagnostic imaging of neurofibrillary lesions in Alzheimer's disease: a simulation study," *NeuroImage*, vol. 60, no. 3, pp. 1724–1733, 2012.

[126] A. Taghavi, S. Nasir, M. Pickhardt et al., "N^I-benzylidene-benzohydrazides as novel and selective tau-PHF ligands," *Journal of Alzheimer's Disease*, vol. 27, no. 4, pp. 835–843, 2011.

[127] S. J. Kemp, L. J. Storey, J. Storey, and J. Rickard, "Ligands for aggregated tau molecules," US Patent, 2014.

[128] V. L. Villemagne and N. Okamura, "In vivo tau imaging: obstacles and progress," *Alzheimer's & Dementia*, vol. 10, no. 3, supplement, pp. S254–S264, 2014.

[129] M. T. Fodero-Tavoletti, N. Okamura, S. Furumoto et al., "^{18}F-THK523: a novel in vivo tau imaging ligand for Alzheimer's disease," *Brain*, vol. 134, part 4, pp. 1089–1100, 2011.

[130] R. Harada, N. Okamura, S. Furumoto, T. Tago et al., "Comparison of the binding characteristics of [^{18}F] THK-523 and other amyloid imaging tracers to Alzheimer's disease pathology," *European Journal of Nuclear Medicine and Molecular Imaging*, vol. 40, no. 1, pp. 125–132, 2013.

[131] V. L. Villemagne, S. Furumoto, M. T. Fodero-Tavoletti et al., "In vivo evaluation of a novel tau imaging tracer for Alzheimer's disease," *European Journal of Nuclear Medicine and Molecular Imaging*, vol. 41, no. 5, pp. 816–826, 2014.

[132] M. T. Fodero-Tavoletti, S. Furumoto, L. Taylor et al., "Assessing THK523 selectivity for tau deposits in Alzheimer's disease and non Alzheimer's disease tauopathies," *Acta Veterinaria Scandinavica*, vol. 6, article 11, 2014.

[133] N. Okamura, S. Furumoto, R. Harada et al., "Novel 18F-labeled arylquinoline derivatives for noninvasive imaging of tau pathology in Alzheimer disease," *Journal of Nuclear Medicine*, vol. 54, no. 8, pp. 1420–1427, 2013.

[134] E. R. Zimmer, A. Leuzy, S. Gauthier, and P. Rosa-Neto, "Developments in tau PET imaging," *The Canadian Journal of Neurological Sciences*, vol. 41, no. 05, pp. 547–553, 2014.

[135] N. Okamura, S. Furumoto, M. T. Fodero-Tavoletti et al., "Non-invasive assessment of Alzheimer's disease neurofibrillary pathology using ^{18}F-THK5105 PET," *Brain*, vol. 137, no. 6, pp. 1762–1771, 2014.

[136] Y. Li, W. Tsui, H. Rusinek et al., "Cortical laminar binding of PET amyloid and tau tracers in Alzheimer disease," *Journal of Nuclear Medicine*, vol. 56, no. 2, pp. 270–273, 2015.

[137] W. Zhang, J. Arteaga, D. K. Cashion et al., "A highly selective and specific PET tracer for imaging of tau pathologies," *Journal of Alzheimer's Disease*, vol. 31, no. 3, pp. 601–612, 2012.

[138] S. Förster, T. Grimmer, I. Miederer et al., "Regional expansion of hypometabolism in Alzheimer's disease follows amyloid deposition with temporal delay," *Biological Psychiatry*, vol. 71, no. 9, pp. 792–797, 2012.

[139] D. T. Chien, S. Bahri, A. K. Szardenings et al., "Early clinical PET imaging results with the novel PHF-tau radioligand [F-18]-T807," *Journal of Alzheimer's Disease*, vol. 34, no. 2, pp. 457–468, 2013.

[140] M. Mintun, A. Schwarz, A. Joshi et al., "Exploratory analyses of regional human brain distribution of the PET tau tracer F18-labeled T807 (AV-1541) in subjects with normal cognitive function or cognitive impairment thought to be due to Alzheimer's disease," *Alzheimer's & Dementia*, vol. 9, no. 4, p. P842, 2013.

[141] D. T. Chien, A. K. Szardenings, S. Bahri et al., "Early clinical PET imaging results with the novel PHF-tau radioligand [F18]-T808," *Journal of Alzheimer's Disease*, vol. 38, no. 1, pp. 171–184, 2014.

[142] M. Maruyama, H. Shimada, T. Suhara et al., "Imaging of tau pathology in a tauopathy mouse model and in alzheimer patients compared to normal controls," *Neuron*, vol. 79, no. 6, pp. 1094–1108, 2013.

[143] G. W. Small, V. Kepe, L. M. Ercoli et al., "PET of brain amyloid and tau in mild cognitive impairment," *The New England Journal of Medicine*, vol. 355, no. 25, pp. 2652–2663, 2006.

[144] J. Stefaniak and J. O'Brien, "Imaging of neuroinflammation in dementia: a review," *Journal of Neurology, Neurosurgery & Psychiatry*, vol. 87, pp. 21–28, 2016.

[145] V. Pizza, A. Agresta, C. W. D'Acunto, M. Festa, and A. Capasso, "Neuroinflammation and ageing: current theories and an overview of the data," *Reviews on Recent Clinical Trials*, vol. 6, no. 3, pp. 189–203, 2011.

[146] R. M. Ransohoff and J. El Khoury, "Microglia in health and disease," *Cold Spring Harbor Perspectives in Biology*, 2015.

[147] D. G. Walker and L. F. F. Lue, "Immune phenotypes of microglia in human neurodegenerative disease: challenges to detecting microglial polarization in human brains," *Alzheimer's Research & Therapy*, vol. 7, no. 1, p. 56, 2015.

[148] Z. Su, F. Roncaroli, P. F. Durrenberger et al., "The 18-kDa mitochondrial translocator protein in human gliomas: an 11C-(R)PK11195 PET imaging and neuropathology study," *Journal of Nuclear Medicine*, vol. 56, no. 4, pp. 512–517, 2015.

[149] P. Gut, M. Zweckstetter, and R. B. Banati, "Lost in translocation: the functions of the 18-kD translocator protein," *Trends in Endocrinology & Metabolism*, vol. 26, no. 7, pp. 349–356, 2015.

[150] M.-K. K. Chen and T. R. R. Guilarte, "Translocator protein 18 kDa (TSPO): molecular sensor of brain injury and repair," *Pharmacology and Therapeutics*, vol. 118, no. 1, pp. 1–17, 2008.

[151] A. Cagnin, D. J. Brooks, A. M. Kennedy et al., "In-vivo measurement of activated microglia in dementia," *The Lancet*, vol. 358, no. 9280, pp. 461–467, 2001.

[152] S. Chalon, C. Pellevoisin, S. Bodard, M.-P. Vilar, J.-C. Besnard, and D. Guilloteau, "Iodinated PK 11195 as an ex vivo marker of neuronal injury in the lesioned rat brain," *Synapse*, vol. 24, no. 4, pp. 334–339, 1996.

[153] J. J. Versijpt, F. Dumont, K. J. Van Laere et al., "Assessment of neuroinflammation and microglial activation in Alzheimer's disease with radiolabelled PK11195 and single photon emission computed tomography: a pilot study," *European Neurology*, vol. 50, no. 1, pp. 39–47, 2003.

[154] S. Venneti, C. A. Wiley, and J. Kofler, "Imaging microglial activation during neuroinflammation and Alzheimer's disease," *Journal of Neuroimmune Pharmacology*, vol. 4, no. 2, pp. 227–243, 2009.

[155] A. S. C. Ching, B. Kuhnast, A. Damont, D. Roeda, B. Tavitian, and F. Dollé, "Current paradigm of the 18-kDa translocator protein (TSPO) as a molecular target for PET imaging in neuroinflammation and neurodegenerative diseases," *Insights into Imaging*, vol. 3, no. 1, pp. 111–119, 2012.

[156] H. Boutin, F. Chauveau, C. Thominiaux et al., "^{11}C-DPA-713: a novel peripheral benzodiazepine receptor PET ligand for in vivo imaging of neuroinflammation," *Journal of Nuclear Medicine*, vol. 48, no. 4, pp. 573–581, 2007.

[157] H. Boutin, C. Prenant, R. Maroy et al., "[^{18}F]DPA-714: direct comparison with [^{11}C]PK11195 in a model of cerebral ischemia in rats," *PLoS ONE*, vol. 8, no. 2, Article ID e56441, 2013.

[158] N. Van Camp, R. Boisgard, B. Kuhnast et al., "In vivo imaging of neuroinflammation: a comparative study between [^{18}F]PBR111, [^{11}C]CLINME and [^{11}C]PK11195 in an acute rodent model," *European Journal of Nuclear Medicine and Molecular Imaging*, vol. 37, no. 5, pp. 962–972, 2010.

[159] G. Abourbeh, B. Thézé, R. Maroy et al., "Imaging microglial/macrophage activation in spinal cords of experimental autoimmune encephalomyelitis rats by positron emission tomography using the mitochondrial 18 kDa translocator protein radioligand [^{18}F]DPA-714," *The Journal of Neuroscience*, vol. 32, no. 17, pp. 5728–5736, 2012.

[160] D. Tang, M. R. Hight, E. T. McKinley et al., "Quantitative preclinical imaging of TSPO expression in glioma using N,N-diethyl-2-(2-(4-(2- 18F-fluoroethoxy) phenyl)-5,7- dimethyl-pyrazolo[1,5-a]pyrimidin-3-yl)acetamide," *Journal of Nuclear Medicine*, vol. 53, no. 2, pp. 287–294, 2012.

[161] N. Arlicot, A. Katsifis, L. Garreau et al., "Evaluation of CLINDE as potent translocator protein (18 kDa) SPECT radiotracer reflecting the degree of neuroinflammation in a rat model of microglial activation," *European Journal of Nuclear Medicine and Molecular Imaging*, vol. 35, no. 12, pp. 2203–2211, 2008.

[162] F. Mattner, D. L. Bandin, M. Staykova et al., "Evaluation of [^{123}I]-CLINDE as a potent SPECT radiotracer to assess the degree of astroglia activation in cuprizone-induced neuroinflammation," *European Journal of Nuclear Medicine and Molecular Imaging*, vol. 38, no. 8, pp. 1516–1528, 2011.

[163] I. López-González, E. Aso, M. Carmona et al., "Neuroinflammatory gene regulation, mitochondrial function, oxidative stress, and brain lipid modifications with disease progression in tau P301S transgenic mice as a model of frontotemporal lobar degeneration-tau," *Journal of Neuropathology & Experimental Neurology*, vol. 74, no. 10, pp. 975–999, 2015.

[164] J. A. García-Sevilla, P. V. Escribá, and J. Guimón, "Imidazoline receptors and human brain disorders," *Annals of the New York Academy of Sciences*, vol. 881, pp. 392–409, 1999.

[165] S. F. Carter, M. Schöll, O. Almkvist et al., "Evidence for astrocytosis in prodromal Alzheimer disease provided by ^{11}C-deuterium-L-deprenyl: a multitracer PET paradigm combining ^{11}C-Pittsburgh compound B and ^{18}F-FDG," *Journal of Nuclear Medicine*, vol. 53, no. 1, pp. 37–46, 2012.

[166] A. F. Santillo, J. P. Gambini, L. Lannfelt et al., "In vivo imaging of astrocytosis in Alzheimer's disease: an 11C-L-deuteriodeprenyl and PIB PET study," *European Journal of Nuclear Medicine and Molecular Imaging*, vol. 38, no. 12, pp. 2202–2208, 2011.

[167] K. Kawamura, Y. Kimura, J. Yui et al., "PET study using [^{11}C]FTIMD with ultra-high specific activity to evaluate I$_2$-imidazoline receptors binding in rat brains," *Nuclear Medicine and Biology*, vol. 39, no. 2, pp. 199–206, 2012.

[168] M. Wang, L. Xu, M. Gao, K. D. Miller, G. W. Sledge, and Q. H. H. Zheng, "[11C]enzastaurin, the first design and radiosynthesis of a new potential PET agent for imaging of protein kinase C," *Bioorganic & Medicinal Chemistry Letters*, vol. 21, no. 6, pp. 1649–1653, 2011.

[169] M.-K. K. Sun and D. L. Alkon, "The 'memory kinases': roles of PKC isoforms in signal processing and memory formation,"

Progress in Molecular Biology and Translational Science, vol. 122, pp. 31–59, 2014.

[170] C. Wu, C. Wang, D. C. Popescu et al., "A novel PET marker for in vivo quantification of myelination," *Bioorganic & Medicinal Chemistry*, vol. 18, no. 24, pp. 8592–8599, 2010.

[171] M. Doubrovin, J. T. Che, I. Serganova et al., "Monitoring the induction of heat shock factor 1/heat shock protein 70 expression following 17-allylamino-demethoxygeldanamycin treatment by positron emission tomography and optical reporter gene imaging," *Molecular Imaging*, vol. 11, no. 1, pp. 67–76, 2012.

[172] C. Chiu, M. C. Miller, R. Monahan, D. P. Osgood, E. G. Stopa, and G. D. Silverberg, "P-glycoprotein expression and amyloid accumulation in human aging and Alzheimer's disease: preliminary observations," *Neurobiology of Aging*, vol. 36, no. 9, pp. 2475–2482, 2015.

[173] G. Luurtsema, J. Verbeek, M. Lubberink et al., "Carbon-11 labeled tracers for in vivo imaging P-glycoprotein function: kinetics, advantages and disadvantages," *Current Topics in Medicinal Chemistry*, vol. 10, no. 17, pp. 1820–1833, 2010.

[174] G. Esposito, G. Giovacchini, J.-S. S. Liow et al., "Imaging neuroinflammation in Alzheimer's disease with radiolabeled arachidonic acid and PET," *Journal of Nuclear Medicine*, vol. 49, no. 9, pp. 1414–1421, 2008.

[175] M. Singh, "Essential fatty acids, DHA and human brain," *Indian Journal of Pediatrics*, vol. 72, no. 3, pp. 239–242, 2005.

[176] S. I. Rapoport, E. Ramadan, and M. Basselin, "Docosahexaenoic acid (DHA) incorporation into the brain from plasma, as an in vivo biomarker of brain DHA metabolism and neurotransmission," *Prostaglandins& Other Lipid Mediators*, vol. 96, no. 1–4, pp. 109–113, 2011.

[177] J. A. Conquer, M. C. Tierney, J. Zecevic, W. J. Bettger, and R. H. Fisher, "Fatty acid analysis of blood plasma of patients with Alzheimer's disease, other types of dementia, and cognitive impairment," *Lipids*, vol. 35, no. 12, pp. 1305–1312, 2000.

20

Clutter Mitigation in Echocardiography Using Sparse Signal Separation

Javier S. Turek, Michael Elad, and Irad Yavneh

Department of Computer Science, Israel Institute of Technology (Technion), 3200003 Haifa, Israel

Correspondence should be addressed to Javier S. Turek; javiert@cs.technion.ac.il

Academic Editor: Michael W. Vannier

In ultrasound imaging, clutter artifacts degrade images and may cause inaccurate diagnosis. In this paper, we apply a method called Morphological Component Analysis (MCA) for sparse signal separation with the objective of reducing such clutter artifacts. The MCA approach assumes that the two signals in the additive mix have each a sparse representation under some dictionary of atoms (a matrix), and separation is achieved by finding these sparse representations. In our work, an adaptive approach is used for learning the dictionary from the echo data. MCA is compared to Singular Value Filtering (SVF), a Principal Component Analysis- (PCA-) based filtering technique, and to a high-pass Finite Impulse Response (FIR) filter. Each filter is applied to a simulated hypoechoic lesion sequence, as well as experimental cardiac ultrasound data. MCA is demonstrated in both cases to outperform the FIR filter and obtain results comparable to the SVF method in terms of contrast-to-noise ratio (CNR). Furthermore, MCA shows a lower impact on tissue sections while removing the clutter artifacts. In experimental heart data, MCA obtains in our experiments clutter mitigation with an average CNR improvement of 1.33 dB.

1. Introduction

In medical ultrasound imaging, a source of artifact called "clutter" is commonly caused by multipath reverberations or off-axis scatterers, and it materializes as a static cloud of echo signals occluding the tissue regions of interest [1, 2]. Clutter artifacts affect the contrast and the readability of images and can induce misleading functional measurements like myocardium strain in cardiac ultrasound and displacement estimation in blood flow imaging. Often, clutter artifacts degrade ultrasound images entailing the use of imaging modalities such as CT or MRI that are more expensive and involve a radiation risk to the patient.

Clutter artifacts from reverberations appear when the acoustic wave bounces back and forth between a reflective structure and the transducer surface. In echocardiography, this is a common phenomenon because the rib cage and the sternum are highly reflective structures in proximity of the path of the acoustic waves to the heart [3]. The energy of the acoustic waves decays with the distance covered and with the number of bounces, such that the effect

becomes more significant in the near-field region of the image and less visible in far-field areas. As a consequence, the myocardium is partially occluded by the artifacts, which may lead to wrong cardiac functioning diagnosis through visual inspection or tracking techniques [4, 5]. Methods that overcome the challenges imposed by reverberation echoes include interpolating data from regions of the heart where artifacts are not present [6] or inferring heart motion using probabilistic models for the challenging regions [7]. However, these techniques tend to fail in data from diseased hearts, because abnormal myocardial motion cannot be inferred using statistical assumptions or models. Therefore, a more appropriate methodology may be to separate the clutter from the signal of interest using filtering strategies, allowing motion tracking to be computed in the entire image.

Suggested filtering methods usually involve separation of the tissue and clutter echo signals by linear decomposition. Echo data is transformed to a new coordinate system in which the clutter artifacts and the signal of interest can be separated along different bases or dictionaries. Then, clutter artifacts are suppressed by reducing their respective coefficients while leaving those of the basis of the tissue signal fixed. Existing methods either use a priori orthogonal bases or learn them adaptively from the data. A priori methods use predefined bases that are orthonormal and independent of the data. Commonly used bases are the Discrete Fourier Transform (DFT), which has been used to define FIR or IIR filters for clutter mitigation in blood flow imaging [8, 9], and the wavelet transform for clutter artifact reduction [10, 11]. Also, the short-time Fourier Transform has been used to filter clutter artifacts during beamforming [12].

Although a priori bases are fast to compute, they may produce poor results when clutter and tissue characteristics overlap. Furthermore, physiological differences among patients entail space and time variability for signals characteristics. Adaptive methods have been suggested to overcome these limitations and learn a basis based on the actual data. The predominant method for determining a basis adaptively is the Principal Component Analysis (PCA) that is used to compute a basis based on the covariance characteristics of the data. Usually, adaptive techniques outperform methods that rely on choosing of bases a priori [13–16]. Some methods learn the basis from local areas of the signal [13] without exploiting the whole image information.

In the present paper, a Morphological Component Analysis (MCA) based separation algorithm [17] is introduced to mitigate clutter in ultrasound images while preserving the tissue signal. As described below, the current method learns a nonorthonormal redundant matrix (also called dictionary) from the entire data and decomposes the signal into a linear combination of a few columns (atoms) from the dictionary. Consequently, by separating the dictionary's atoms into clutter and tissue representatives, clutter filtering is achieved by selectively removing clutter atoms. The feasibility of the method is demonstrated with simulated and experimental ultrasound data. Simulation is used to quantify the performance of the method across algorithm parameters and signal motion characteristics. The suggested algorithm is also experimentally demonstrated with echocardiography images, where clutter artifacts are a significant cause of image degradation. Its performance is compared against a high-pass FIR filter and state-of-the-art Singular Value Filtering (SVF) [13].

2. Methods

2.1. Sparse Representation of a Signal. The sparse representation model [18] assumes that a signal of interest can be decomposed into a linear combination of a few vectors or "atoms" from a given matrix, also called "dictionary." The atoms that take part in the linear combination are a small subset of the dictionary, and their respective coefficients are called the sparse representation of the signal. This model is used as prior information for signals, where signal reconstruction is performed by first computing the sparse representation of the signal of interest and then by reconstructing the signal from its sparse representation and the dictionary. Selecting the dictionary is an important step in this process and it is usually dependent on the application. The objective is to find an adaptive dictionary that will enable sparse representations of relevant signals as accurately as possible.

The sparse representation principle can be illustrated by considering a signal $t \in \mathbb{C}^n$, which can be decomposed into a linear combination of atoms:

$$\mathbf{t} = \mathbf{Dx} = \sum_{i=1}^{m} x_i \mathbf{d}_i, \tag{1}$$

where vector $\mathbf{x}$ is the sparse representation of the signal $\mathbf{t}$, implying that most entries x_i are zeros, and $\mathbf{d}_i$ are the atoms (columns) of the dictionary $\mathbf{D} \in \mathbb{C}^{n \times m}$. The sparse vector $\mathbf{x}$ has $\|\mathbf{x}\|_0 = k$ nonzero elements with $k < n$. The notation $\| \cdot \|_0$ represents the ℓ_0-norm (usually, the ℓ_0-norm is wrongly known as a quasi- or pseudonorm. The ℓ_0-norm satisfies only two axioms of the norms and thus it should not be considered a norm), that is, the number of nonzero elements in the vector. The set of indices of the nonzero coefficients in $\mathbf{x}$ is defined as the support $\mathcal{S}$ and the signal can be decomposed alternatively into $\mathbf{t} = \mathbf{D}_{\mathcal{S}} \mathbf{x}_{\mathcal{S}}$, with $\mathbf{D}_{\mathcal{S}}$ being the subset $\mathcal{S}$ of columns from $\mathbf{D}$ and $\mathbf{x}_{\mathcal{S}}$ the reduced vector with only the nonzero elements. When the support of a representation vector is known, the respective coefficients in $\mathbf{x}_{\mathcal{S}}$ are computed using the pseudoinverse $\mathbf{D}_{\mathcal{S}}^{\dagger}$ of the dictionary restricted to the support, $\mathbf{D}_{\mathcal{S}}$:

$$\mathbf{t} = \mathbf{D}_{\mathcal{S}} \mathbf{x}_{\mathcal{S}} \implies \mathbf{x}_{\mathcal{S}} = \left(\mathbf{D}_{\mathcal{S}}^* \mathbf{D}_{\mathcal{S}}\right)^{-1} \mathbf{D}_{\mathcal{S}}^* \mathbf{t} = \mathbf{D}_{\mathcal{S}}^{\dagger} \mathbf{t}. \tag{2}$$

The support $\mathcal{S}$ is unknown in practice and is estimated together with the nonzero coefficient values.

The sparse representation $\mathbf{x}$ is computed by finding the sparsest vector that yields $\mathbf{t}$ when multiplied by the given dictionary $\mathbf{D}$. This problem can be written as the following optimization task:

$$\min_{\mathbf{x}} \quad \|\mathbf{x}\|_0$$
$$\text{subject to} \quad \mathbf{t} = \mathbf{Dx}. \tag{3}$$

In practice, a noisy observation $\mathbf{s}$ of the signal of interest $\mathbf{t}$ is obtained. It is often assumed that the noisy signal $\mathbf{s}$ is contaminated with additive i.i.d. white Gaussian noise $\mathbf{n} \in \mathbb{C}^n$ with noise level σ; that is, $\mathbf{s} = \mathbf{t} + \mathbf{n}$. Problem (3) is then reformulated to yield a solution that is close to the observed signal in the ℓ_2-norm sense:

$$\min_{\mathbf{x}} \quad \|\mathbf{x}\|_0$$
$$\text{subject to} \quad \|\mathbf{s} - \mathbf{Dx}\|_2^2 \le \varepsilon^2, \tag{4}$$

where ε is the desired bound on the distance from the observed signal $\mathbf{s}$ and is usually proportional to the noise standard deviation σ. The notation $\|\mathbf{v}\|_2 = \sqrt{\sum_{i=1}^{n} |v_i|^2}$ represents the ℓ_2-norm of a vector $\mathbf{v}$. An alternative to (4) may be formulated where the fidelity data term is minimized and the number of nonzero elements is constrained:

$$\min_{\mathbf{x}} \quad \|\mathbf{s} - \mathbf{Dx}\|_2^2$$
$$\text{subject to} \quad \|\mathbf{x}\|_0 \le k_0, \tag{5}$$

Task. Approximate the solution to problem (4) or (5).

Input Parameters. Input parameters are dictionary $\mathbf{D}$, the signal $\mathbf{s}$, and the error threshold ε or the maximum sparsity of the solution k_0.

Initialization. Initialization is as follows:
   (i) Initialize $k = 0$.
   (ii) The initial solution $\mathbf{x}^{(0)} = 0$.
   (iii) The initial residual $\mathbf{r}^{(0)} = \mathbf{s} - \mathbf{D}\mathbf{x}^{(0)} = \mathbf{s}$.
   (iv) The initial support $\mathcal{S}^{(0)} = \emptyset$.

Main Iteration. Increment k by 1 and perform the following steps:
   (i) Sweep: compute the projection values $\mathbf{p} = \mathbf{D}^* \mathbf{r}^{(k-1)}$, where $\mathbf{D}^*$ is the conjugate transpose of matrix $\mathbf{D}$.
   (ii) Update support: find element j, the maximizer of $|\mathbf{p}|$, and update the support, $\mathcal{S}^{(k)} = \mathcal{S}^{(k-1)} \cup \{j\}$.
   (iii) Update solution: compute $\mathbf{x}^{(k)}$, the minimizer of $\|\mathbf{s} - \mathbf{D}\mathbf{x}\|_2^2$ subject to support $\mathcal{S}^{(k)}$.
   (iv) Update residual: compute $\mathbf{r}^{(k)} = \mathbf{s} - \mathbf{D}\mathbf{x}^{(k)}$.
   (v) Stopping criterion: if $\|\mathbf{r}^{(k)}\|_2 < \varepsilon$ (for problem (4)) or $k = k_0$ (for problem (5)), stop. Otherwise, continue with the next iteration.

Output. The approximated solution is $\hat{\mathbf{x}} = \mathbf{x}^{(k)}$ obtained after k iterations.

ALGORITHM 1: Orthogonal Matching Pursuit.

where k_0 is the maximum sparsity allowed in each representation. Solving problem (4) or (5) yields an approximate sparse representation $\hat{\mathbf{x}}$ and it is used to reconstruct the clean signal by multiplying with $\mathbf{D}$; that is, $\hat{\mathbf{t}} = \mathbf{D}\hat{\mathbf{x}}$. The Orthogonal Matching Pursuit (OMP) [19] is a commonly used algorithm designed to approximate solutions to problem (4) or (5), and it is presented in Algorithm 1. The OMP is a greedy pursuit algorithm that increments the support size by one nonzero element at a time. In each iteration, an atom is chosen such that it reduces the residual distance to the observed signal the most. The stopping criterion is given by the constraint of the problem to be solved: the ℓ_2 term error bound for (4) or the number of nonzeros for (5). There are other methods for approximating the solution of (4) or (5); such is the Basis Pursuit method [20] that relaxes the ℓ_0 quasinorm in problem (4) with an ℓ_1-norm (the ℓ_1-norm of a vector $\mathbf{v}$ is defined as $\|\mathbf{v}\|_1 = \sum_{i=1}^{n} |\mathbf{v}_i|$ and it is well known [18, 20] to give preference to sparse solutions) and solves a convex optimization problem.

In ultrasound imaging, sparse representations have been used widely with interesting results. Zhang et al. [21] used Gabor atoms to denoise Doppler ultrasound blood flow signals. Also, Nieblas et al. [22] used the same dictionary to detect heart pathologies in heart sound signals with high accuracy. Furthermore, Michailovich and Adam [23] separated harmonic components using Gabor frames. Deka and Bora [24] used an adaptive dictionary for despeckling of ultrasound images. Liebgott et al. [25] applied the compressed sensing technique to reconstruct RF ultrasound signals using a dictionary of wave atoms. Also, Shi et al. [26] demonstrated compressed sensing for separating transmitted echoes and improving the resolution in ultrasound flaw detection. Wagner et al. [27] and also Chernyakova and Eldar [28] demonstrated techniques to apply compressed sensing to beamforming achieving a reduction in the sampling rate. Similarly, Zhang et al. [29] proposed an adaptive beamforming approach based on compressed sensing. Zhou et al. [30] developed an asynchronous compressed beamformer that

requires low runtime complexity for computing the sparse representations, allowing the authors to use it in portable ultrasound devices. Schiffner et al. [31] used sparse representations with a curvelet dictionary for solving the inverse scattering problem in diagnostic ultrasound images. Richy et al. [32] demonstrated a method for reconstructing the Doppler signal segment by segment in blood flow estimation that is based on compressive sensing using Fourier or wave atom dictionaries. Demirli and Saniie [33, 34] showed how to sparsely decompose ultrasound echo data using envelope and instantaneous phase for identification of signal features and data partitioning. A particular example is the work of Cloutier et al. [35]. In that work, the authors proposed to use the Matching Pursuit approximation algorithm (closely related to OMP) with Gabor atoms as an a priori dictionary to reduce clutter in Doppler blood flow signals. All these works showed performance improvements by assuming sparsity as a signal prior.

The sparse representation clearly changes with selection of the dictionary $\mathbf{D}$. There are, as noted above, two ways to select a dictionary, either defined a priori or learned adaptively from the data. Dictionaries such as the Discrete Fourier Transform (DFT) [36] and various types of wavelets such as curvelets [37], countourlets [38], and Gabor wavelets [39], among others, have been suggested as a priori dictionaries for image processing. Many of these options have a fast transformation that allows for a fast computation of a matrix-vector multiplication. However, in terms of quality, these dictionaries may limit the performance of the application [40]. For example, in an application such as ultrasound clutter filtering, using the DFT for source separation may be of limited value because tissue and clutter overlap in the frequency domain. Finding an a priori dictionary for a specific application may not be a trivial task. Alternatively, an adaptive dictionary can be learned from the data and may yield improved results.

A commonly used method to learn a dictionary from data is the K-SVD [41] technique. K-SVD is an iterative method that learns the atoms in a dictionary by fitting the data with the sparsest possible representations. As a consequence, computing an adaptive dictionary with K-SVD requires multiple data samples.

Consider the following example to illustrate how a dictionary is determined with K-SVD. Let $\mathbf{S} \in \mathbb{C}^{n \times P}$ be a matrix with P data samples ordered so that each sample appears as a column. The number of data samples P is usually much bigger than the data dimension n, enabling training a dictionary where each atom is used in several representations of samples. The K-SVD method aims to find the best dictionary $\mathbf{D}$ and the sparse representations $\mathbf{X} \in \mathbb{C}^{m \times P}$ ($\mathbf{x}_i$ for each sample $\mathbf{s}_i$) by solving the optimization problem

$$\min_{\mathbf{D}, \mathbf{X}} \quad \|\mathbf{S} - \mathbf{D}\mathbf{X}\|_F^2$$

$$\text{subject to} \quad \|\mathbf{x}_i\|_0 \leq k_0, \quad 1 \leq i \leq P \qquad (6)$$

$$\|\mathbf{d}_j\|_2^2 = 1, \quad 1 \leq j \leq m,$$

where k_0 is the maximum sparsity prescribed for each sample representation. To compute a solution to the optimization task in (6), the K-SVD method iterates between two main computational steps: sparse coding and dictionary update. The sparse coding step assumes that the dictionary $\mathbf{D}$ is fixed and the sparse representations $\mathbf{X}$ are computed. For instance, this can be done using the OMP algorithm. The dictionary update step modifies each atom one at a time. Hence, the update is computed by isolating the ith atom $\mathbf{d}_i$ from the others and rewriting the Frobenius norm:

$$\|\mathbf{S} - \mathbf{D}\mathbf{X}\|_F^2 = \left\| \left[\mathbf{S} - \sum_{j \neq i} \mathbf{d}_j \left(\mathbf{x}^T \right)_j \right] - \mathbf{d}_i \left(\mathbf{x}^T \right)_i \right\|_F^2$$

$$= \left\| \mathbf{E}_i - \mathbf{d}_i \left(\mathbf{x}^T \right)_i \right\|_F^2, \qquad (7)$$

where $(\mathbf{x}^T)_i$ stands for the ith row of $\mathbf{X}$. The terms in parentheses can be considered an error matrix $\mathbf{E}_i = \mathbf{S} - \sum_{j \neq i} \mathbf{d}_j (\mathbf{x}^T)_j$, where all the elements are fixed and are independent of atom i. The optimal solution for $\mathbf{d}_i$ and $(\mathbf{x}^T)_i$ that minimizes the functional in (7) is computed by solving a rank-1 approximation of $\mathbf{E}_i$ using the Singular Value Decomposition (SVD). In general, the SVD computation yields a dense vector $(\mathbf{x}^T)_i$ which would increase the number of nonzero elements in $(\mathbf{x}^T)_i$ and make use of the updated atom $\mathbf{d}_i$ for all the samples. Therefore, the error matrix $\mathbf{E}_i$ is restricted to those columns $\mathbf{E}_i^R$ where the atom is active, that is, for the nonzeros in $(\mathbf{x}^T)_i$. In this manner, the rank-1 problem is solved by updating only the nonzero elements in $(\mathbf{x}^T)_i$ with the respective columns $\mathbf{E}_i^R$. Once all the atoms are updated, the process repeats until some stopping criterion is satisfied. The K-SVD algorithm is presented in Algorithm 2.

2.2. Sparse Signal Separation for Clutter Mitigation. A general approach to separate signals using sparse representations is called Morphological Component Analysis (MCA) [17].

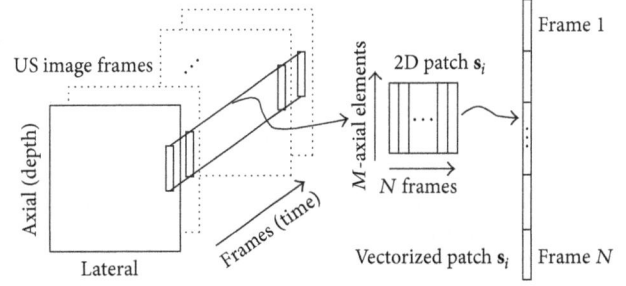

FIGURE 1: Illustration of how a patch $\mathbf{s}_i$ is extracted from a sequence of several frames of complex echo data. The small rectangles in the ultrasound image frames represent M-axial elements in each frame which are concatenated to form the patch $\mathbf{s}_i$.

In MCA, the mixed signal is decomposed into different morphological components (subdictionaries) and each source is sparse under these subdictionaries. The morphological components can be selected a priori for specific tasks and type of data [42] or can be adaptively learned [17] using some dictionary learning method such as [43, Ch. 15], [44]. Filtering a component is then applied by assigning a weight to each atom that corresponds to that component.

While MCA is a general scheme for signal separation, from now on, the discussion will concentrate on clutter artifact mitigation in the context of echocardiography ultrasound imaging. In this application, the observed signals $\mathbf{S}$ are columned versions of axial-temporal dimensional patches of real-valued raw RF or complex-valued IQ demodulated RF echo data. A signal $\mathbf{s}_i$ represents a two-dimensional patch obtained from echo data with N consecutive frames as its columns and M elements in the axial direction forming its rows (see Figure 1). (The echo data can be taken also as lateral-temporal patches. Clutter quasistatic behavior appears in the temporal dimension, while moving tissue (in any direction) appears as varying elements across the same dimension. This information is captured by such patches as well. Also, data can be taken as a three-dimensional element, by adding consecutive axial lines into every signal $\mathbf{s}_i$ and hence including adjacent A-lines in the lateral direction. This also requires us to modify the method for partitioning the atoms in the dictionary into tissue and clutter. In our experiments we found the axial-temporal patches to be slightly more effective.) In this way, every signal $\mathbf{s}_i$ contains information of the local motion characteristics in the echo data. However, the number of columns in the patch, N, dictates how much of this motion is captured. As clutter behaves quasistatically across frames, a patch with a large number of columns N may contain big motion variability making it difficult to remove clutter, whereas a small N may not contain enough tissue variability to differentiate it from the clutter artifacts. It should be noted that the amount of motion in the patch depends also on the frame rate of the acquisition. Once the data is separated, the clutter artifacts are removed, the processed signals are converted back from column vectors into two-dimensional patches, and these patches are merged

---

Task. Train a dictionary $\mathbf{D}$ to sparsely represent the data $\{\mathbf{s}_i\}_{i=1}^P$ by approximating the solution to problem (6).

Input Parameters. Input parameters include a matrix $\mathbf{S}$ containing the signals $\{\mathbf{s}_i\}_{i=1}^P$ and the maximum sparsity of the solution k_0.

Initialization. Initialization is as follows:

    (i) Initialize $k = 0$.

    (ii) Initialize $\mathbf{D}^{(0)}$ by either using m randomly chosen examples from $\mathbf{S}$ or using random entries.

    (iii) Normalize the columns of $\mathbf{D}^{(0)}$.

Main Iteration. Increment k by 1 and apply the following:

    (i) Sparse coding: obtain the sparse representations $\{\hat{\mathbf{x}}_i\}_{i=1}^P$ of each signal $\mathbf{s}_i$. Use OMP to approximate the solution of

$$\hat{\mathbf{x}}_i = \arg\min_{\mathbf{x}} \quad \left\| \mathbf{s}_i - \mathbf{D}^{(k-1)}\mathbf{x} \right\|_2^2$$
$$\text{subject to} \quad \|\mathbf{x}\|_0 \le k_0.$$

    These form the matrix $\mathbf{X}^{(k)}$.

    (ii) Dictionary update: use the following steps to update the columns of the dictionary and obtain $\mathbf{D}^{(k)}$:
    repeat for $i = 1, 2, 3, \ldots, m$.

       (a) Define the group of samples that use the atom $\mathbf{d}_i$:

$$\mathscr{G}_i = \left\{ j \mid 1 \le j \le P, \ \left(\mathbf{X}^{(k)} \right)_{i,j} \neq 0 \right\}.$$

       (b) Compute the residual matrix $\mathbf{E}_i = \mathbf{S} - \sum_{j \neq i} \mathbf{d}_j (\mathbf{x}^T)_j$, where $(\mathbf{x}^T)_j$ stands for the jth row of $\mathbf{X}^{(k)}$.

       (c) Restrict $\mathbf{E}_i$ by choosing only the columns corresponding to $\mathscr{G}_i$, and obtain $\mathbf{E}_i^R$.

       (d) Apply SVD decomposition $\mathbf{E}_i^R = \mathbf{U}\boldsymbol{\Sigma}\mathbf{V}^*$. Update the dictionary atom $\mathbf{d}_i = \mathbf{u}_1$ and the representations $(\mathbf{x}^T)_i^R = \sigma_1 \mathbf{v}_1^*$.

    (iii) Stopping rule: if the change in $\|\mathbf{S} - \mathbf{D}^{(k)}\mathbf{X}^{(k)}\|_F^2$ is small enough, stop.

Output. The desired result is the dictionary $\mathbf{D}^{(k)}$ and the sparse representations $\mathbf{X}^{(k)}$ of the signals in $\mathbf{S}$.

ALGORITHM 2: K-SVD.

to form the cleaned signal. Then, the process is repeated for the next frame.

Filtering an ultrasound sequence with MCA requires us to define the signal model and assumptions in order to construct the components in the dictionary $\mathbf{D}$. The signal model for an observed sequence of echo data $\mathbf{s}$ is assumed to be a linear superposition of the tissue $\mathbf{t}$ and clutter $\mathbf{c}$ subsignals and an additive white noise $\mathbf{n}$; that is,

$$\mathbf{s} = \mathbf{t} + \mathbf{c} + \mathbf{n}. \tag{8}$$

This assumption holds when the signal $\mathbf{s}$ is an RF or an IQ signal. On the other hand, an envelope-detected signal does not satisfy this model as the absolute value operation for computing the envelope of the signal ruins the linearity assumption.

Additionally, it is assumed that, for any patch, the corresponding $\mathbf{t}_i$ and $\mathbf{c}_i$ subsignals are sparsely generated by sparse coefficient vectors $\mathbf{x}_{t_i}$ and $\mathbf{x}_{c_i}$ multiplied by the subdictionaries $\mathbf{D}_t$ and $\mathbf{D}_c$, respectively. In other words, this assumption means that every patch can be written in the form

$$\mathbf{s}_i = \mathbf{t}_i + \mathbf{c}_i + \mathbf{n}_i = \mathbf{D}_t \mathbf{x}_{t_i} + \mathbf{D}_c \mathbf{x}_{c_i} + \mathbf{n}_i, \tag{9}$$

suggesting that clutter is separable from tissue using MCA. The second assumption is that echoes from clutter artifacts are quasistatic, meaning that the subsignal $\mathbf{c}_i$ has a quasiconstant pattern in the temporal axis, while the tissue subsignals reflect motion or variability [1].

Clutter reduction in a patch $\mathbf{s}_i$ is achieved by removing the clutter component $\mathbf{D}_c \mathbf{x}_{c_i}$ from it; that is,

$$\hat{\mathbf{s}}_i = \mathbf{s}_i - \mathbf{D}_c \mathbf{x}_{c_i}, \tag{10}$$

where $\hat{\mathbf{s}}_i$ is the resulting patch with reduced clutter. This requires computing the sparse representations $\mathbf{x}_{t_i}$ and $\mathbf{x}_{c_i}$ in (9). Note that (9) can be rewritten as follows:

$$\mathbf{s}_i = \begin{bmatrix} \mathbf{D}_t \mid \mathbf{D}_c \end{bmatrix} \begin{bmatrix} \mathbf{x}_{t_i} \\ \mathbf{x}_{c_i} \end{bmatrix} + \mathbf{n}_i = \mathbf{D}\mathbf{x}_i + \mathbf{n}_i, \tag{11}$$

where $\mathbf{D}$ is the concatenated dictionary with the tissue and clutter subdictionaries and $\mathbf{x}_i$ is the concatenation of the sparse representations of the tissue and clutter signals of the patch. Consequently, solving (4) or (5) with the concatenated dictionary $\mathbf{D}$ yields the concatenated sparse representation $\mathbf{x}_i$. The representations $\mathbf{x}_{t_i}$ and $\mathbf{x}_{c_i}$ are obtained from $\mathbf{x}_i$ relatively to the tissue or clutter atom positions in the concatenated dictionary. In this work, the Orthogonal Matching Pursuit (OMP) [19] algorithm is used to find an approximation to the sparse vector $\mathbf{x}_i$. The complete clutter reduction procedure for a patch $\mathbf{s}_i$ is illustrated in Figure 2. Additionally, for solving the problem in (4) or (5), the dictionary $\mathbf{D}$ must be known. An adaptive dictionary $\mathbf{D}$ allows the method to learn the patient's own physiological characteristics and improve the results. Hence, such a dictionary $\mathbf{D}$ is learned adaptively from the signal patches $\{\mathbf{s}_i\}_{i=1}^P$ using the K-SVD algorithm [41].

In order to separate the sparse signals in $\mathbf{x}_i$ into the tissue $\mathbf{x}_{t_i}$ and the clutter $\mathbf{x}_{c_i}$ parts, the division of $\mathbf{D}$ into the two subdictionaries, $\mathbf{D}_t$ and $\mathbf{D}_c$, needs to be known. The

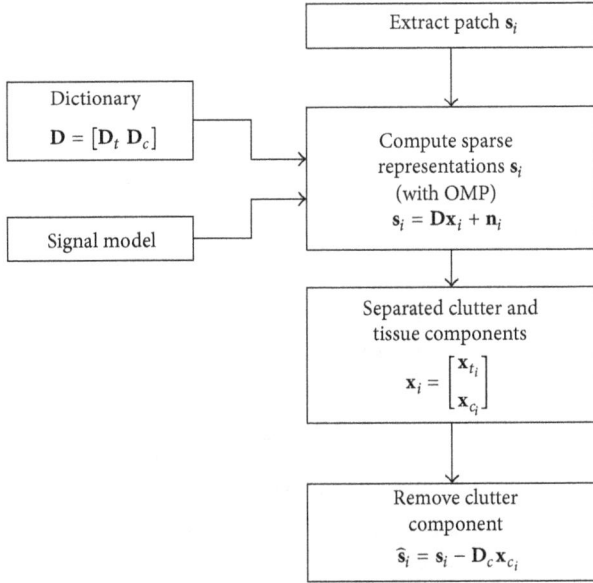

FIGURE 2: Block diagram of Morphological Component Analysis for clutter reduction for a signal patch s_i.

quality of the separation depends on dividing the dictionary obtained from the K-SVD algorithm into these two disjoint groups. For this purpose, the assumption that clutter artifact echoes are nearly static in time in comparison to the tissue echoes that move is used to differentiate between the atoms in the dictionary (a followup of the current work was recently published in [45], which presents an alternative method to train the dictionaries D_c and D_t separately). As the dictionary D is learned from columned versions of 2D (axial-temporal) patches from continuous frames of the measured signal, the learned atoms emulate the behavior of the patches in these dimensions. Therefore, an atom from D can be reshaped from a column vector into a 2D (axial-temporal) matrix with the same size of the signal patches. The quasistatic behavior of the clutter artifacts appears in a reshaped atom as a nearly constant pattern across the temporal dimension. In contrast, the atoms containing moving tissue vary in the temporal dimension. (If the tissue moves in the axial direction, the movement is captured in the axial dimension of the atom, hence varying across frames in the temporal dimension. On the other hand, a lateral movement of the tissue is translated into intermittent changes in the temporal dimension of the atom. In both cases, an atom varies across frames and has a nonconstant pattern in the temporal dimension.) An atom can be associated with one of the groups by looking at the rank behavior of its 2D matrix. A low-rank matrix means a nearly constant pattern, while a medium-to-high rank matrix suggests a moving tissue atom. Such a low-rank matrix can be revealed by a high ratio between the first singular value and the sum of all the singular values. Using a predefined cut-off value $\beta \in (0, 1)$, the atoms with the values of the above ratio greater than or equal to β are ascribed to the clutter subdictionary D_c. Note that when β is close to 1, all the atoms are assigned to the tissue subdictionary D_t and no filtering is expected to happen. Contrarily, when β tends to 0, the atoms

are assigned to the clutter subdictionary D_c and also tissue is filtered out.

3. Results

3.1. Experiments with Field II Simulator. A Field II simulation experiment [46] in MATLAB (MathWorks Inc., Natick, MA) of a hypoechoic lesion was performed to evaluate the performance of the MCA method for reducing clutter. The simulated lesion had a diameter of 5 mm and a mean scatterer amplitude ratio of −30 dB between the lesion and the background. Reconstruction of ultrasound images took place within a section of 20 mm × 10 mm where the echo data was collected.

Clutter artifact echoes were simulated from a 0.3 mm × 3.5 mm region of scatterers with reflection amplitudes 20 dB above the lesion. Scatterers for clutter artifacts were simulated separately over the same section and located in the center of the hypoechoic lesion. Scatterers outside the hypoechoic lesion were simulated several times to obtain distinct frames. These scatterers had decorrelation and axial motion across frames. Echo decorrelation between frames was achieved using the Cholesky factorization method in [47]. Clutter scatterers were assigned a small axial motion different from that of the lesion. Axial motion was achieved by oversampling echoes at 400 MHz and then downsampling at 40 MHz starting with the sample that achieves the desired subsample shift. Eventually, the hypoechoic lesion echoes were summed with the clutter artifacts echo data and with electronic noise with noise level σ (chosen for SNR of −30 dB) to obtain 19 final frames as supported by the model in (8). The default parameters used for the simulation are presented in Table 1.

The MCA method was compared against two other techniques. The first approach is a Finite Impulse Response (FIR) filter that subtracts the previous frame from the current one [48]. This is a high-pass filter applied to the echo data through time axis. The second is the Singular Value Filtering (SVF) method [13] that applies Principal Component Analysis (PCA) to every axial-temporal dimensional patch and filters clutter by soft-thresholding its normalized singular values. It uses a sigmoidal-like function with a cut-off parameter τ and a roll-off parameter α that controls the shrinkage operator. Although MCA and SVF methods work with local patches of echo data, the SVF method learns the PCA basis functions from each data patch independently.

The resulting performances of the algorithms were measured using contrast-to-noise ratio (CNR). The CNR is defined as

$$CNR = 20 \log_{10} \left(\frac{|\mu_i - \mu_o|}{\sigma_o} \right), \quad (12)$$

where μ_i and μ_o are the mean envelope-detected quantities in regions with clutter artifact and without artifacts, respectively, and σ_o is the standard deviation in the clutter-empty region. Figure 3 shows the regions of interest for computing CNR, the middle box indicating the region with clutter artifacts inside the hypoechoic lesion and the outer

TABLE 1: Default Field II simulation parameters.

Simulation parameter	Default value
Center frequency	5 MHz
Sampling frequency	40 MHz
Fractional bandwidth	50%
Tissue echo correlation	0.98
Clutter echo correlation	1.0
Tissue displacement	1 period per frame (8 pixels)
Clutter displacement	1/8 periods per frame (1 pixel)
MCA time length (N)	9 frames
MCA axial length (M)	4 periods (32 pixels)
MCA error threshold	$2.3\sigma\sqrt{2NM}$
MCA dictionary redundancy	2 : 1
MCA patch samples	84640 patches

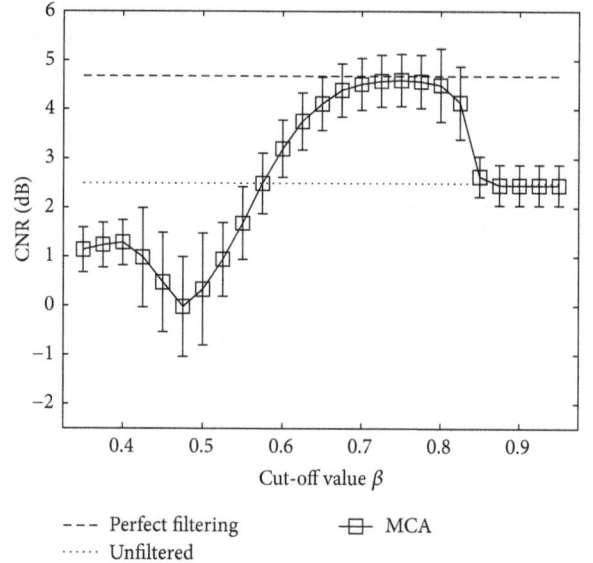

FIGURE 4: CNR measurements for MCA on complex simulated echo data for several values of the cut-off β parameter. Markers represent mean CNR and error bars the standard deviation over 100 simulations.

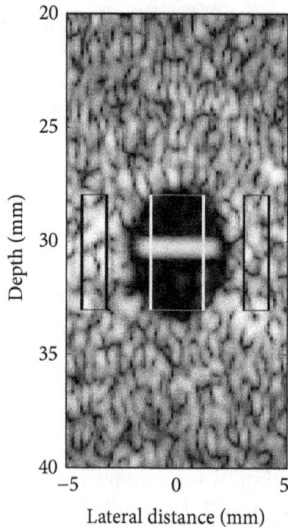

FIGURE 3: Region of interest used to compute CNR as in (12) for the simulated hypoechoic lesion. The white box corresponds to the ROI inside the lesion with clutter artifacts and the black boxes indicate the ROI outside the lesion.

boxes indicating the regions outside the lesion. The CNR performance measure may be misleading in some cases. For example, if high values of tissue speckles in the region without artifacts are being reduced, the standard deviation σ_o may decrease faster than the mean μ_o and the ratio $|\mu_o|/\sigma_o$ may increase, making the CNR higher. Subsequently, the CNR may exhibit better values than perfect filtered images. Therefore, performance was measured also using peak signal-to-noise ratio (PSNR) in a few particular cases in order to show further differences that exist between the tested methods. PSNR is computed using the following expression:

$$PSNR = 20\log_{10}\left(\frac{MAX}{\sqrt{(1/n)\,\|\mathbf{s} - \hat{\mathbf{s}}\|_2^2}}\right), \qquad (13)$$

where MAX is the maximum pixel value in the clean envelope-detected image, $\mathbf{s} \in \mathbb{R}^{\mathbf{n}}$ is the clutter-free envelope-detected signal, and $\hat{\mathbf{s}}$ is the reconstructed envelope-detected signal. PSNR measures the distance to the perfect image, penalizing for any difference from it. Thus, it is capable of measuring the remaining clutter as well as the amount of tissue removed. In contrast to CNR, PSNR requires the perfect filtered signal.

The influence of the cut-off β parameter on separation of tissue from clutter atoms in the dictionary is shown in Figure 4. Mean CNR over 100 trials was computed on complex echo data as a function of the value of the β parameter. Figure 5 presents reconstructed images after MCA for β of 0.5, 0.75, and 1. As described in Section 2.2, when β is close to one, the data remains unfiltered. In contrast, when β tends to zero, most of the data is rejected as clutter and only the noise component remains. Examples of the best reconstructions obtained from the MCA ($\beta = 0.75$) and the SVF ($\tau = 0.7, \alpha = 30$) methods are visually compared in Figures 6(a) and 6(c), respectively. The parameters for these methods were selected for the best CNR performance. Additionally, Figures 6(b) and 6(d) present the difference image between the reconstructions obtained by the algorithms and the original image. All simulation images in Figures 3, 5, and 6 are shown on a log compressed linear gray scale mapping to 0 to 30 dB. Figure 7 shows examples of (a) tissue and (b) clutter atoms in the subdictionaries obtained on one of the simulations with cut-off value β of 0.75. The atoms are shown in two-dimensional form with the same size of the patches and after envelope detection, that is, their magnitude. The axial dimension is shown in the vertical direction and the temporal dimension is in the horizontal direction.

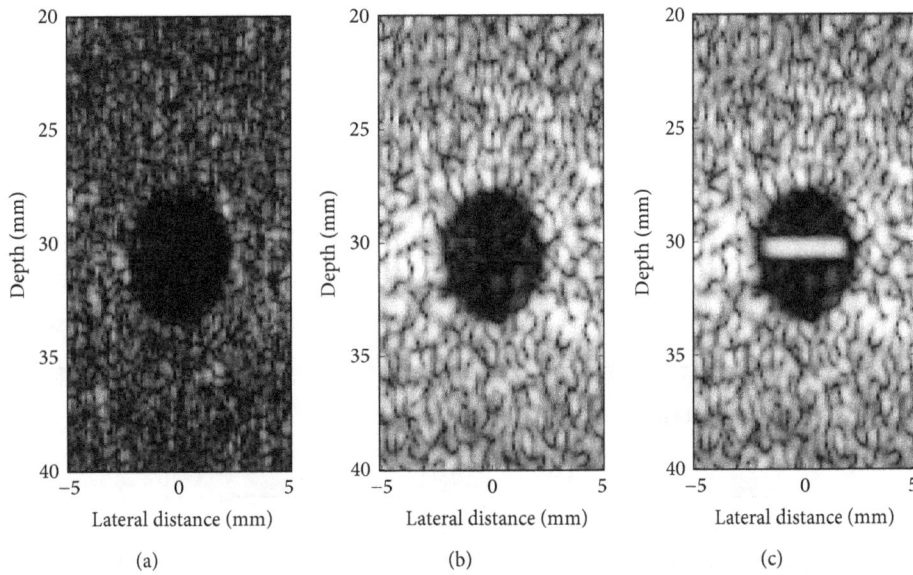

FIGURE 5: Clutter reduction using MCA on IQ data of simulation images when the cut-off β was set to (a) 0.5, (b) 0.75, and (c) 1.

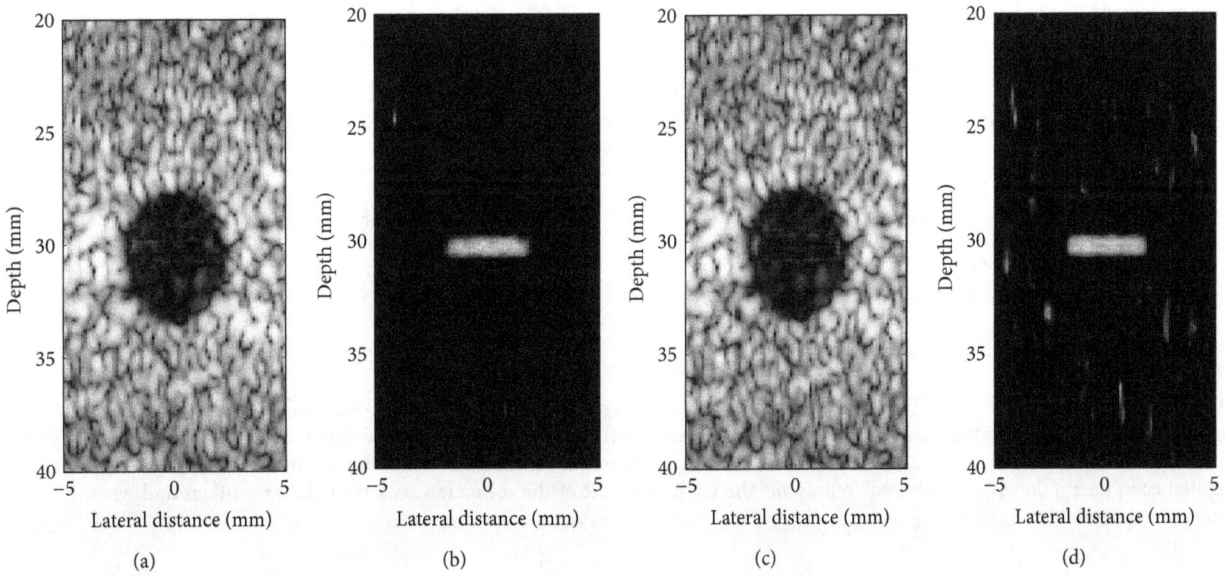

FIGURE 6: Visual comparison of clutter reduction on IQ data of simulation images obtained by (a) MCA and (c) SVF. The absolute difference between (b) the perfect filtered signal and the MCA reconstruction and (d) the perfect filtered signal and the SVF reconstruction.

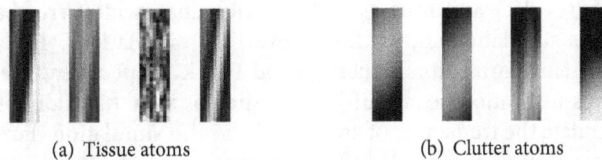

(a) Tissue atoms   (b) Clutter atoms

FIGURE 7: Example of (a) tissue atoms and (b) clutter atoms in the obtained subdictionaries from applying MCA with a cut-off value of $\beta = 0.75$. The dictionary is learned using the simulated sequence echo data. The magnitude of the atoms is presented. The atoms are shown after being transformed from vectors into 2D patches and being envelope-detected. The horizontal direction refers to the temporal dimension and the vertical direction to the axial dimension.

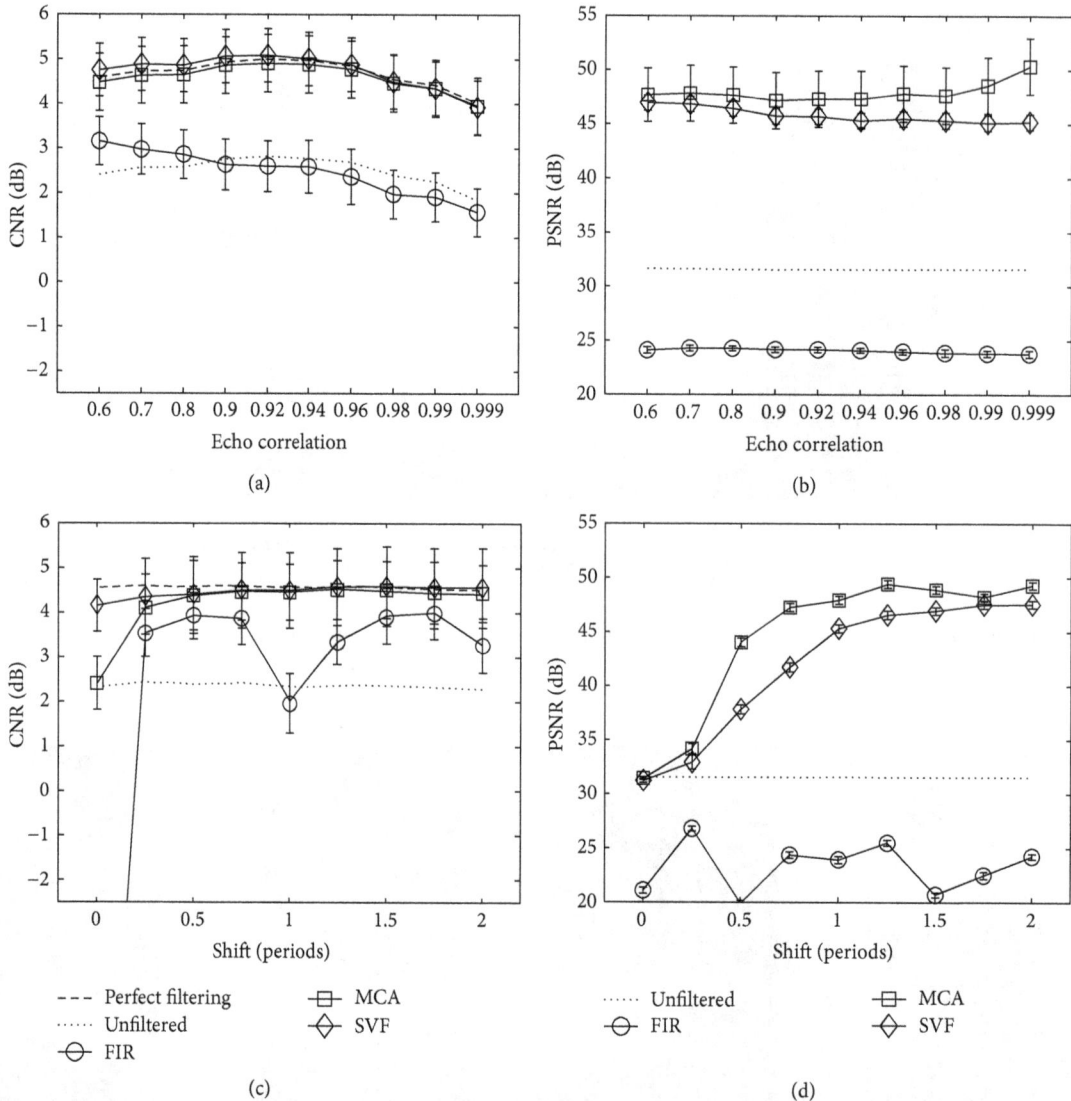

FIGURE 8: Mean CNR and mean PSNR measurements for MCA, SVF, and FIR methods for varied ((a) and (b)) echo correlation and ((c) and (d)) axial shift of the tissue scatterers. Markers represent the mean CNR and mean PSNR, respectively, and error bars the standard deviation over 100 simulations. The dashed line, labeled "perfect filtering," represents the mean CNR when the clutter artifacts are not present in the simulated echo data. Likewise, "unfiltered" represents the CNR or PSNR of the measured data with clutter artifacts and when no filtering technique is applied.

Performance of clutter reduction for the MCA, SVF, and FIR methods on IQ complex echo data measured with CNR and PSNR is presented in Figures 8(a) and 8(b) as a function of tissue echo correlation and Figures 8(c) and 8(d) as a function of tissue axial motion. This simulation shows the influence of different tissue motion and correlation values on the algorithms. The amounts of tissue motion (axial shift) and echo decorrelation serve to simulate the frame rate of an imaging device. The clutter echo correlation and axial shift were held constant at the default simulation values described in Table 1, while the tissue echo correlation and axial shift were modified for the experiment. As a reference, the dashed line labeled "perfect filtering" is included representing the mean CNR for the simulated data without the added clutter

artifacts. Additionally, the solid line with label "unfiltered" indicates the mean CNR and PSNR values when no filtering is applied. Markers in the graphs represent the mean CNR or PSNR values, while error bars represent standard deviation over 100 simulations. In Figures 9(a) and 9(b) for CNR and PSNR, respectively, the performance of the algorithms is shown as a function of the electronic signal-to-noise ratio in the simulation. Furthermore, filtering performance for several patch sizes is presented in Figure 9(c) for CNR and Figure 9(d) for PSNR as a function of the size of the temporal dimension and in Figure 9(e) for CNR and Figure 9(f) for PSNR in the axial dimension. Parameters for SVF and MCA were selected for the best performance in each case.

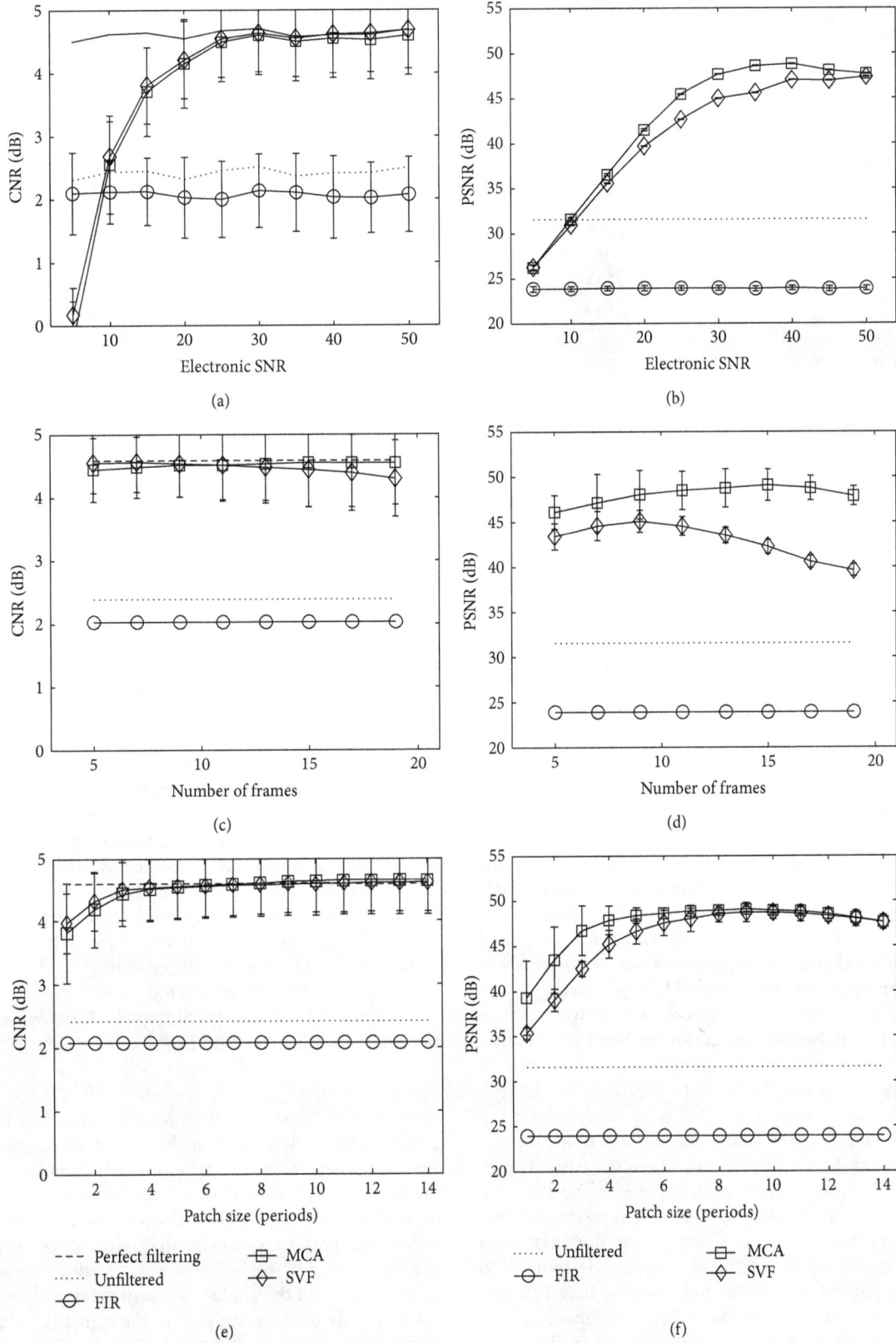

FIGURE 9: Mean CNR measurements for MCA, SVF, and FIR methods for varied (a) electronic SNR, (b) patch size in temporal dimension, and (c) patch size in axial dimension. Markers represent mean CNR and error bars the standard deviation over 100 simulations. The dashed line, labeled "perfect filtering," represents the mean CNR when the clutter artifacts are not present in the simulated echo data. Likewise, "unfiltered" represents the CNR or PSNR of the measured data with clutter artifacts and when no filtering technique is applied.

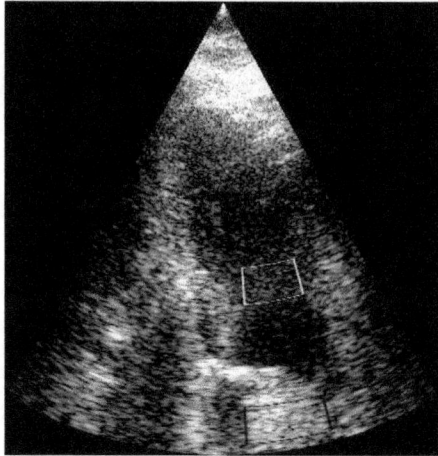

FIGURE 10: Example of ROI from an apical view of a volunteer heart view for measuring CNR. The upper white box corresponds to the artifact region and the lower black box corresponds to normal tissue.

3.2. Experiments with Human Heart Images. The MCA method was validated experimentally using frames of echo data from apical views of human hearts. The frames were acquired using a Vivid S6 (GE Medical Systems, Israel) ultrasound scanner operating at 3.3 MHz. Clutter artifact was present due to multipath reverberations mainly from the thoracic cage and sternum. Data from a full heart cycle composed of 30 to 40 frames were processed for clutter rejection. The echo sequences were acquired in in-phase and quadrature (IQ) format directly from the Vivid S6 and processed offline using MATLAB (MathWorks Inc., Natick, MA) implementation of the above mentioned three algorithms. Thirteen datasets were acquired from five male volunteers, 30–55 years old. Each dataset included different acquisitions of apical views of the heart to obtain superposed clutter artifacts that were as independent as possible between sets. The resulting performance of the algorithm was measured averaging the CNR over the sequence frames. This metric was used to compare against FIR [48] and SVF [13] methods. The parameter values of the SVF method were set to $\tau = 0.35$ and $\alpha = 25$, which were optimized for the best performance. The regions of interest (ROI) for CNR measurements of one example dataset are illustrated in Figure 10. The regions with artifacts used to measure CNR were selected with the advice from an ultrasound technician, and the tissue regions were selected in the far-field region where the tissue is predominant and clutter artifacts are not present. The electrical noise is not known for these datasets. When solving (5), the sparse representations in MCA were allowed a maximum sparsity k_0 of 20% of the patch size. The parameters used to demonstrate the MCA method and compare it to FIR and SVF techniques were a patch size of 15 axial elements and 15 frames in temporal domain with a cut-off β at 0.45. Examples of heart images from two datasets are shown in Figures 11 and 12, with the ellipses indicating regions of clutter artifacts. The filtered reconstructions using MCA and SVF are also shown in Figures 11 and 12, respectively. The arrows point to areas where tissue was incorrectly filtered. Figure 13 compares

the mean improvement CNR for the MCA, FIR, and SVF methods over the unfiltered echo data while the error bars represent standard deviation.

4. Discussion

The current study demonstrates the potential benefit of the MCA method to remove clutter artifacts that originate from multipath reverberation. The simulation and experimental results quantify the performance of the MCA method compared with a high-pass FIR method [48] and the PCA-based state-of-the-art SVF technique [13]. To our knowledge, MCA or signal separation with a sparsity prior has never been used for clutter removal in B-mode ultrasound. A sparsity prior with a priori dictionary of sinusoids was used to remove clutter in Doppler ultrasound [35].

There are two significant outcomes presented in this paper. The first outcome is the ability to separate the morphological components into clutter and tissue in the learned dictionary for complex echo data. The significance of the temporal dimension in the patches enables the atoms in the dictionary to inherit the motion characteristics of the signals. These motion properties allow us to identify and separate the tissue from the clutter sets of atoms by evaluating their temporal behavior. Because atoms in the dictionary represent the underlying data, they can be used effectively to separate (and filter) tissue and clutter components. Figure 7 depicts the morphology in the atoms of the obtained dictionary and the motion differences between the clutter atoms and the tissue ones. A separation cut-off parameter β was used to separate these morphological components. An example of the effect of this parameter β is illustrated in Figure 5. When the value of β is too low, the artifacts are filtered but part of the tissue is incorrectly identified as artifact as shown in Figure 5(a). In contrast, when β is close to 1, no visible effect is obtained (Figure 5(c)). This effect is also reflected in Figure 4, where CNR is optimized for β of 0.75 and performance tends to the CNR value of the unfiltered image as $\beta \rightarrow 1$ and to even a lower performance when $\beta \rightarrow 0$.

The second outcome is the improved performance using nonorthonormal and redundant bases for filtering. In most applications, adaptive filtering is achieved using PCA-based signal separation [2, 13–15, 49–53], which is an orthonormal basis. In this paper, we have demonstrated that separation performance is improved with a different transformation. Instead of an adaptive orthonormal basis, a redundant dictionary was shown to result in improved image quality as reflected by high CNR values and PSNR values. This redundant dictionary can effectively decompose a signal into a linear combination of a few atoms, allowing the recognition of the tissue and the clutter components in the signal. Thus, filtering only the relevant part of the signal is possible even when clutter is not much stronger than the tissue.

The simulation results show that MCA performs comparably in CNR terms and better in PSNR terms to the state-of-the-art SVF method in all the simulation tests. In Figures 8 and 9, several trends can be observed from the mean CNR and PSNR behavior of MCA as a function of the distinct

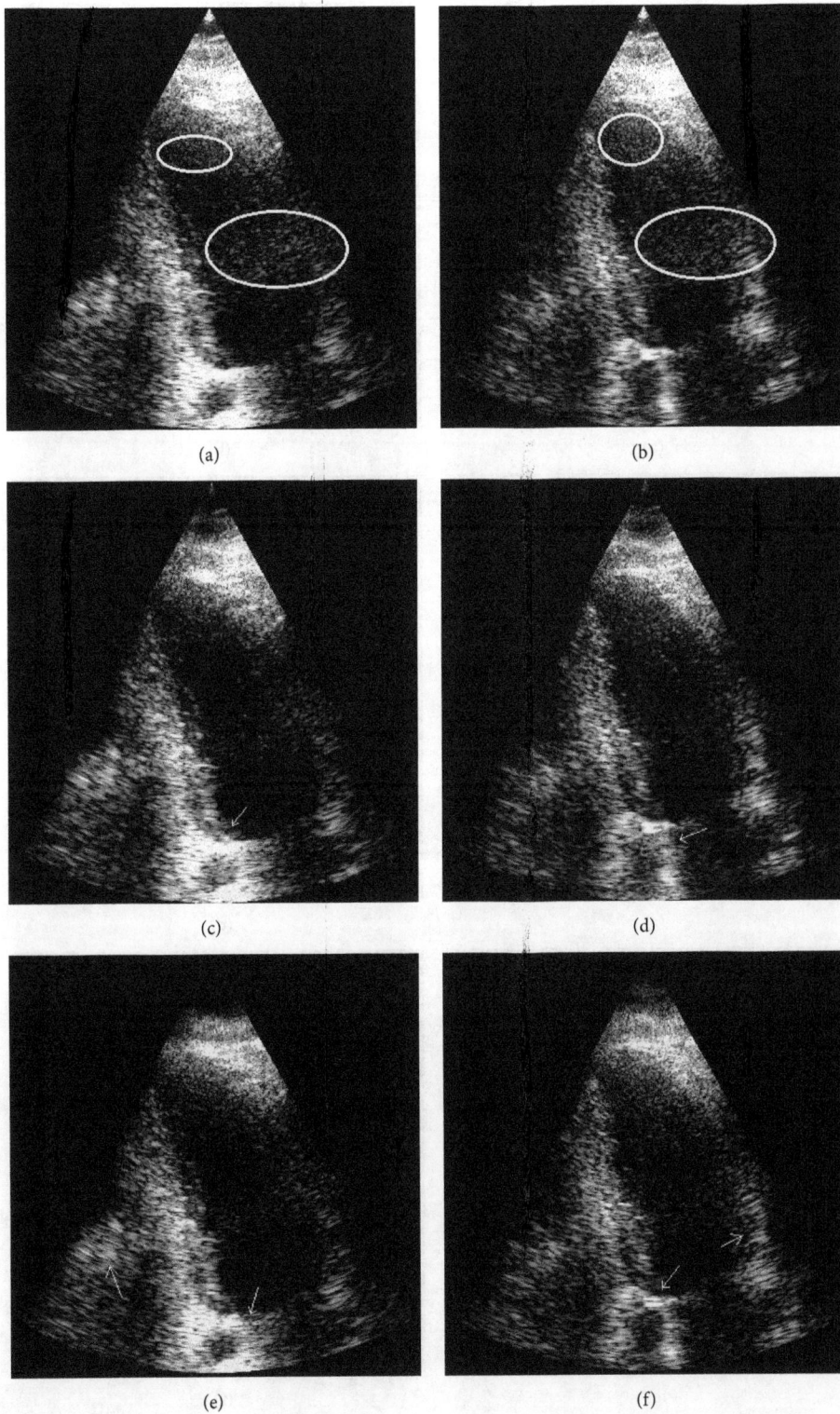

FIGURE 11: Two examples of an apical view of heart images are illustrated before clutter removal (a, b) and after clutter removal with MCA (c, d) and after applying SVF (e, f). Ellipses indicate regions of clutter artifacts due to multipath reverberations. The arrows point to regions of tissue incorrectly filtered. Images are shown on a log compressed linear gray scale mapping to 0 to 30 dB.

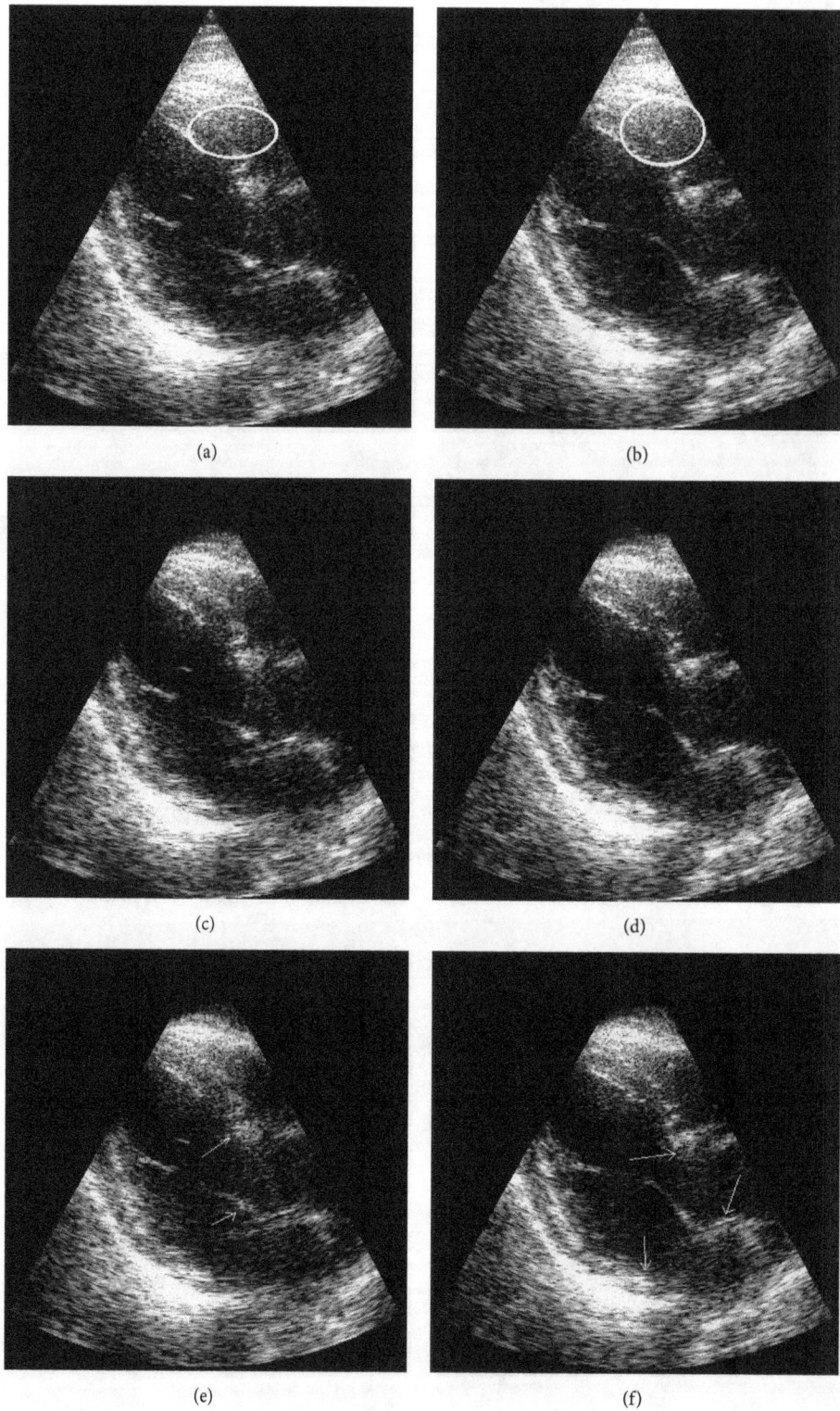

FIGURE 12: Two examples of an apical view of heart images are illustrated before filtering (a, b) and after clutter removal with MCA (c, d) and after applying SVF (e, f). Ellipses in the unfiltered images indicate regions of clutter artifacts due to multipath reverberations. The arrows point to regions of tissue incorrectly filtered. Images are shown on a log compressed linear gray scale mapping to 0 to 30 dB.

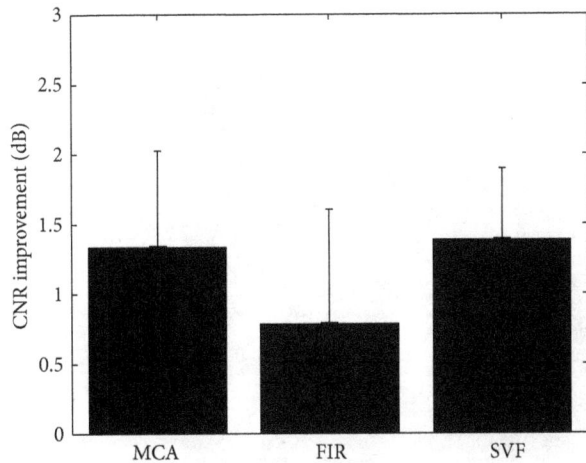

FIGURE 13: Mean improvement CNR comparison for MCA, SVF, and FIR clutter reduction methods over the unfiltered echo data. Error bars represent standard deviation over eight datasets.

simulation and algorithm parameters. First, the mean CNR and PSNR performances decrease when the tissue motion characteristics approach those of the clutter artifacts. This is clearly seen in Figures 8(c) and 8(d) when the shift motion of the tissue tends to zero and becomes close to the artifact motion. In such a case, the atoms in the learned dictionary representing tissue and clutter become similar, limiting the ability to correctly identify the atoms partitioning and hence reducing the CNR and PSNR performances. Moreover, the MCA is insensitive to the echo correlation between frames in the sequence, maintaining the same CNR gap with the perfect filtering image (Figure 8(a)). The mean PSNR performance of the MCA shown in Figure 8(b) increases when the echo correlation grows. In contrast, the PSNR performance of SVF remains steady and always below the MCA performance. Results in Figure 9 depict a performance decrease with low electronic SNR and with small patch sizes, both in axial and time dimensions. Figures 9(a) and 9(b) show that MCA and SVF have a similar reaction to low electronic SNR, with MCA having a better mean PSNR performance for middle values. In Figures 9(e) and 9(f), mean CNR and PSNR performances remain stable when the patch size in the axial dimension is at least 3 periods long (24 pixels). This occurs because local statistics are well described when a patch is large enough to include sufficient information. However, the mean PSNR performance depicts better results for MCA for small patches. When it comes to the influence of the number of frames in the patch size in Figure 9(c), the behavior of the MCA method departs from that of the SVF. The MCA method is more robust to longer patches in time because the sparsity prior assumed for the clutter signal helps separate the artifact parts that may vary slightly in time in these longer patches. On the other hand, MCA performance decreased when the size was reduced, because of the tendency to misclassify atoms when there is not enough tissue motion information. Figure 9(d) shows this behavior better and also reveals that MCA obtains PSNR values higher than those of SVF.

In Figures 8(a) and 8(c), the SVF method obtained mean CNR values that were better than the perfect filtered sequence. Such behavior can be explained by the fact that tissue is being removed, reducing the mean tissue μ_o values and their standard deviation σ_o. In particular, when "peaks" or high values in tissue are reduced, the standard deviation decreases faster than the mean, increasing the ratio $|\mu_o|/\sigma_o$ in formula (12) and thus increasing the CNR performance to higher levels than the perfect filtering. This effect may lead to misleading conclusions because in these circumstances CNR may not be a reliable indicator of contrast improvement. Such a misleading example is shown in Figure 8(d), where the PSNR performance of MCA and SVF for low axial shift is quite the same as the unfiltered image, while in Figure 8(c) SVF achieved higher CNR values than MCA (and the unfiltered data). Another example is presented in Figure 6 that visually compares the reconstructed images using MCA and SVF and the difference image of their respective reconstruction with the perfect filtered image. While the amount of artifacts removed is similar, the amount of tissue removed is higher. The PSNR measure was introduced to overcome the limitations of the CNR formula. PSNR measures the distance to the perfect filtering image, penalizing for removed tissue and for unfiltered clutter artifacts. Therefore, similar CNR values with different PSNR values suggest good clutter filtering with tissue removed for the lower PSNR result. Figures 8(b), 8(d), 9(b), 9(d), and 9(f) illustrate the experiments using the PSNR measure to show to what extent each method preserved the tissue in the overall image. In these figures, it can be seen that MCA preserved the tissue better, while both algorithms removed clutter effectively.

Unfortunately, PSNR cannot be used in real experimental data because the perfect filtered images are needed to compute it. Indeed, the CNR measure suffers from this problem and it is far from ideal to measure contrast improvements for ultrasound medical images. An alternative expression to measure contrast improvements should be developed taking into account the removed tissue and the removed clutter. How to define such a measure is an important question but it is beyond the scope of this paper.

The simulations used in this paper to obtain Figures 8 and 9 have significant limitations. The simulations do not necessarily model the physics of clutter artifacts from multipath reverberations but are used to assess the signal model given as the superposition of clutter, tissue, and noise components. Furthermore, the simulations were not intended to model the human physiology and clutter was placed at the center of the lesion for convenience. Therefore, the results of the simulations may not directly translate to human cardiac imaging. The main value of the simulation study is meant to illustrate the ability of MCA to separate clutter from the tissue component over a wide range of conditions and algorithm parameters.

The MCA technique was demonstrated in experimental human heart data with superior clutter mitigation results. In these datasets, clutter appeared mainly because of multipath reverberations from the thoracic cage. Figure 13 shows that the MCA obtained an average CNR gain of 1.33 dB, while SVF obtained 1.38 dB and FIR only 0.78 dB. The average

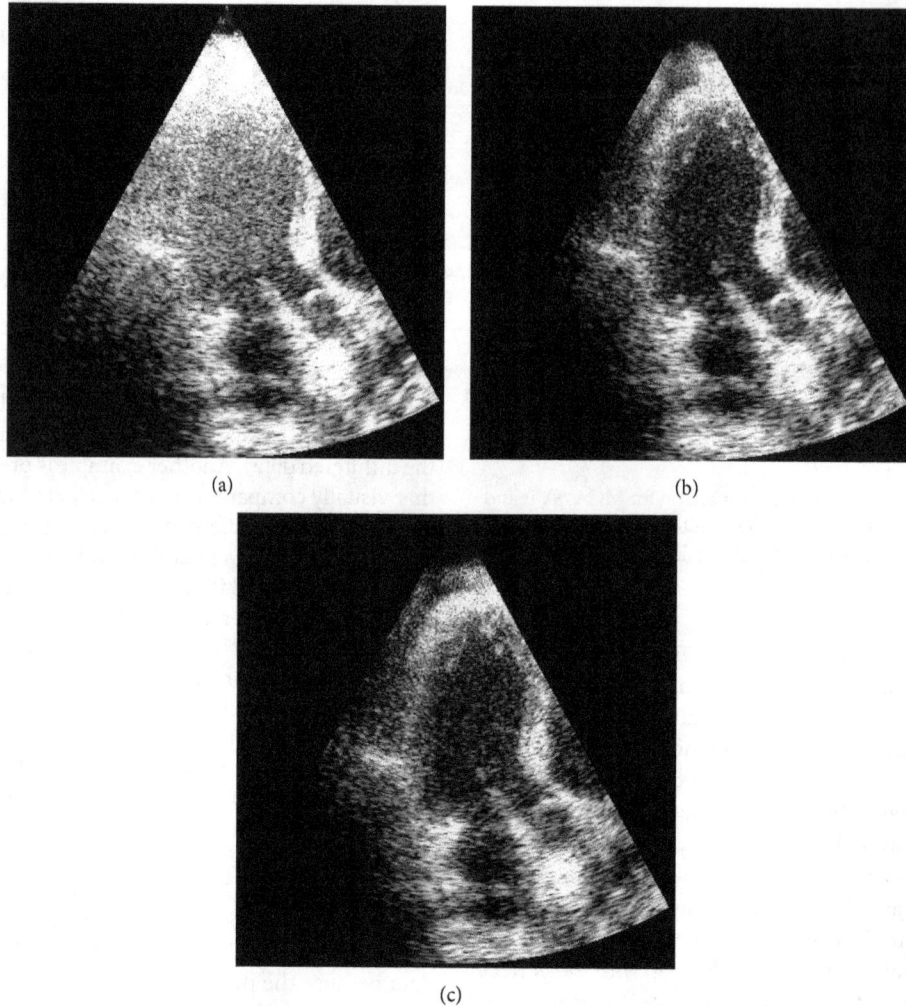

(a)

(b)

(c)

FIGURE 14: A heavily cluttered apical view of heart images illustrated before filtering (a) and after clutter removal with MCA (b) and after applying SVF (c). Images are shown on a log compressed linear gray scale mapping to 0 to 30 dB.

performance of MCA in this measure was slightly lower but still comparable to that of SVF. However, when it comes to visual comparison in Figures 11 and 12, the MCA method is seen to remove the same amounts of clutter as SVF, but less tissue than SVF. In all datasets, both MCA and SVF greatly reduced clutter artifacts independent of the clutter place in the image. In particular, better mitigation performance was obtained when the artifacts appear in the blood pool than over tissue, due to an easier recognition of the artifacts' representations. In areas where the clutter occluded the myocardium, the methods managed to reduce the artifacts without removing most or all of the tissue (see Figure 11 as an example). As an example, Figure 14 presents a frame of an additional sequence containing artifacts in the myocardium area and how the MCA (Figure 14(b)) and SVF (Figure 14(c)) methods reveal the myocardium pretty well. However, when the probe is slightly moved the method reduces its filtering performance. The reason is that clutter that moves within a few frames is confused with tissue, and OMP tends to select atoms from the tissue dictionary instead. The same undesired effect happens when applying SVF because such a patch has a higher rank due to the clutter motion. Nevertheless, this effect typically degrades the performance for a few frames, until the probe (and clutter) stops moving. An opposite effect may happen in the frames respective to diastole where the myocardium relaxes and remains quasistatic for a few frames. In this case both MCA and SVF may remove tissue. Consequently, this effect may be scaled down by taking bigger patches in the temporal domain in order to maintain information on the tissue motion before and after the relaxation period, but with performance reduction on the clutter reduction.

One of the limitations of the SVF method is that it needs to compute a singular value decomposition for every element in the echo data. On the other hand, MCA computes a singular value decomposition for every atom in the dictionary D one time for the entire sequence, which is much cheaper. However, the computational cost of MCA is dominated by sparse coding of the signals. In this case, the MCA method cost corresponds to that of the OMP method (for learning and filtering) [54]. Nevertheless, the costs can be reduced if the OMP algorithm used to solve (4) or (5) is changed by a faster approximation approach such as solving the Basis Pursuit [20] with fast convex optimization techniques. Computational runtime can be further reduced using parallel implementations, or techniques that increase speed with a small performance reduction such as a smaller patch overlapping.

It is worth mentioning that algorithm parameters for both MCA and SVF were chosen differently for the experimental data than in the simulations. Because of the differences in the characteristics in the type of data, it should be expected that such a difference exists between the experiments. One of the characteristics of the B-mode ultrasound imaging is the frame rate of the acquisition of the echo data. As the patches are taken in the time dimension, frame rate clearly affects the performance of MCA. When echo signals are acquired with a high frame rate the performance of MCA is expected to decrease because the echo correlation between frames increases and the tissue has a lower axial motion, similar to that of the clutter artifacts. In ultrafast plane wave imaging, for example, such difficulties are expected and thus additional treatment, like skipping frames, is needed for this ultrasound imaging mode. The effects of frame rate are demonstrated in the simulation results in Figure 8, where CNR and PSNR performance are quantified as a function of echo correlation and axial shift. Simulation results discussed above show that the MCA performance was stable for a wide range of these parameters and was significantly affected for small axial shift differences between the tissue and the clutter artifacts. The MCA performance deteriorated when the motion features of tissue and clutter signals became similar because of the difficulties of MCA to separate the atoms in the dictionary into the respective sets. In other words, the frame rate has a predominant influence on the optimal cut-off (β) value. As frame rate decreases, or heart rate increases, the axial motion difference grows and it is captured better in the dictionary atoms. Therefore, lower β values achieve better performance as separation becomes easier. The results in this paper show good simulation and heart dataset performances with fixed cut-off β values. Although the β value could be adaptively selected to further improve performance in every dataset separately, this was not needed to obtain good performance.

The current MCA algorithm can be extended to remove clutter in Doppler ultrasound methodologies. For example, in the blood flow application, the signal is usually assumed to be a linear superposition of a blood signal, a clutter artifact, and noise. Every echo element is measured in the temporal dimension and thus the signal or one-dimensional patches of it (as suggested in [14]) can be used to learn a dictionary. Based on the low spectrum characteristics and the intensity of the clutter and blood flow signals in Doppler [55], an approach can be suggested for detecting and partitioning a dictionary into clutter and blood flow atoms. Extending MCA to this application is being left for future work.

The appropriate separation using MCA is based on the assumption that each signal has a sparse representation and a dictionary (or "morphological component") that describes its nature. This further allows for the recognition of the clutter artifacts and tissue atoms in the dictionary based on the differences in their motion characteristics. When clutter artifacts result from multipath reverberations because of the ribs and the sternum, their exhibited motion is lower than cardiac tissue. This observation is the basis for the recognition of each group of atoms. However, the MCA algorithm as presented here is likely to be ineffective in some particular cases. In pathological cases like cardiomyopathy, in which portions of the myocardium can appear to be almost static, there is no possibility to differentiate between the tissue and the clutter artifacts. In such a case, some additional assumption on either the clutter or the tissue is required in order to detect the signal components correctly. Also, clutter may appear as an effect from the cardiac tissue or other structures in similar ultrasound applications, where the motion characteristics are very similar to those of the desirable structures. For example, the rapid movement of the heart valve leaflets may cause transient clutter to appear in Color Doppler with similar properties to those of the blood flow. Such an effect appears as a short temporal band occupying the full velocity range in the Doppler spectrogram. Applying MCA for removing transient clutter can be done by detecting this effect by analyzing the sparse representation coefficients in **x**, or even by assuming a new signal component that represents this undesirable effect.

5. Conclusions

The Morphological Component Analysis (MCA) method for signal separation has been presented for clutter mitigation in medical ultrasound. The MCA technique assumes a sparsity prior on the superposed signals. This assumption, together with a powerful dictionary learning method, such as K-SVD, allows us to translate the motion characteristics of the IQ complex echo data into the dictionary atoms. This adaptive dictionary represents an overcomplete set of directions, rather than a unique orthonormal basis as in previous works. Furthermore, it allows for a good representation of the data with its underlying statistics and for high performance filtering of the clutter artifacts. The low-rank test with the cut-off value was demonstrated to be a good separation measure for deciding whether the atoms should belong to the tissue set or to the clutter set. The MCA technique was shown to mitigate clutter artifacts in simulations of a hypoechoic lesion with mean CNR values close to the perfect filtering in a wide range of image parameters. Also, it was shown to outperform a high-pass FIR filter and to obtain results comparable to these of the state-of-the-art SVF method both on simulated and experimental data. The CNR measure was shown to be misleading in some cases, and PSNR was included to show that MCA removes less tissue than SVF. In human heart data, it was shown that a 1.33 dB gain can be obtained using MCA, comparable to that of SVF, but with improved visual results in tissue areas. In conclusion, the MCA technique is a signal separation method that allows for clutter filtering using a sparsity prior with a general and redundant basis and atoms that can be adaptively learnt from the echo data. It may be used in other medical imaging applications, given that we have shown this method to yield improved mitigation of clutter artifacts in ultrasound imaging.

Conflict of Interests

The authors declare that there is no conflict of interests regarding the publication of this paper.

Acknowledgments

The authors would like to thank F. W. Mauldin Jr. and J. A. Hossack for the simulation framework code that enabled them to run the simulations, J. Sulam for his constructive comments, and GE Medical Systems, Israel, for their kind help and technical support. This work was partially supported by MAGNETON project from the Office of the Chief Scientist (OCS) in the Israeli Ministry of Economy. The research leading to these results has received funding from the European Research Council under European Union's Seventh Framework Programme, ERC Grant Agreement no. 320649.

References

[1] M. A. Lediju, M. J. Pihl, S. J. Hsu, J. J. Dahl, C. M. Gallippi, and G. E. Trahey, "Magnitude, origins, and reduction of abdominal ultrasonic clutter," in *Proceedings of the IEEE International Ultrasonics Symposium (IUS '08)*, pp. 50–53, Beijing, China, November 2008.

[2] M. A. Lediju, M. J. Pihl, S. J. Hsu, J. J. Dahl, C. M. Gallippi, and G. E. Trahey, "A motion-based approach to abdominal clutter reduction," *IEEE Transactions on Ultrasonics, Ferroelectrics, and Frequency Control*, vol. 56, no. 11, pp. 2437–2449, 2009.

[3] G. Zwirn and S. Akselrod, "Stationary clutter rejection in echocardiography," *Ultrasound in Medicine and Biology*, vol. 32, no. 1, pp. 43–52, 2006.

[4] B. A. French, Y. Li, A. L. Klibanov, Z. Yang, and J. A. Hossack, "3D perfusion mapping in post-infarct mice using myocardial contrast echocardiography," *Ultrasound in Medicine & Biology*, vol. 32, no. 6, pp. 805–815, 2006.

[5] M. Tanabe, B. Lamia, H. Tanaka, D. Schwartzman, M. R. Pinsky, and J. Gorcsan III, "Echocar-diographic speckle tracking radial strain imaging to assess ventricular dyssynchrony in a pacing model of resynchronization therapy," *Journal of the American Society of Echocar-diography*, vol. 21, no. 12, pp. 1382–1388, 2008.

[6] Y. Li, C. D. Garson, Y. Xu, B. A. French, and J. A. Hossack, "High frequency ultra-sound imaging detects cardiac dyssynchrony in noninfarcted regions of the murine left ventricle late after reperfused myocardial infarction," *Ultrasound in Medicine & Biology*, vol. 34, no. 7, pp. 1063–1075, 2008.

[7] K. Y. E. Leung, M. G. Danilouchkine, M. van Stralen, N. de Jong, A. F. W. van der Steen, and J. G. Bosch, "Probabilistic framework for tracking in artifact-prone 3D echocardiograms," *Medical Image Analysis*, vol. 14, no. 6, pp. 750–758, 2010.

[8] S. Bjaerum, H. Torp, and K. Kristoffersen, "Clutter filter design for ultrasound color flow imaging," *IEEE Transactions on Ultrasonics, Ferroelectrics, and Frequency Control*, vol. 49, no. 2, pp. 204–216, 2002.

[9] A. P. Kadi and T. Loupas, "On the performance of regression and step-initialized IIR clutter filters for color Doppler systems in diagnostic medical ultrasound," *IEEE Transactions on Ultrasonics, Ferroelectrics, and Frequency Control*, vol. 42, no. 5, pp. 927–937, 1995.

[10] P. C. Tay, S. T. Acton, and J. A. Hossack, "A wavelet thresholding method to reduce ultrasound artifacts," *Computerized Medical Imaging and Graphics*, vol. 35, no. 1, pp. 42–50, 2011.

[11] P. C. Toy, S. T. Acton, and J. Hossack, "A transform method to remove ultrasound artifacts," in *Proceedings of the 7th IEEE Southwest Symposium on Image Analysis and Interpretation (SSIAI '06)*, pp. 110–114, March 2006.

[12] B. Byram and M. Jakovljevic, "Ultrasonic multipath and beamforming clutter reduction: a chirp model approach," *IEEE Transactions on Ultrasonics, Ferroelectrics, and Frequency Control*, vol. 61, no. 3, pp. 428–440, 2014.

[13] F. W. Mauldin Jr., D. Lin, and J. A. Hossack, "The singular value filter: a general filter design strategy for PCA-based signal separation in medical ultrasound imaging," *IEEE Transactions on Medical Imaging*, vol. 30, no. 11, pp. 1951–1964, 2011.

[14] A. C. H. Yu and L. Lovstakken, "Eigen-based clutter filter design for ultrasound color flow imaging: a review," *IEEE Transactions on Ultrasonics, Ferroelectrics, and Frequency Control*, vol. 57, no. 5, pp. 1096–1111, 2010.

[15] D. Kruse and K. Ferrara, "A new high resolution color flow system using an eigendecomposition-based adaptive filter for clutter rejection," *IEEE Transactions on Ultrasonics, Ferroelectrics, and Frequency Control*, vol. 49, no. 12, pp. 1739–1754, 2002.

[16] Z. Shen, N. Feng, Y. Shen, and C.-H. Lee, "A ridge ensemble empirical mode decomposition approach to clutter rejection for ultrasound color flow imaging," *IEEE Transactions on Biomedical Engineering*, vol. 60, no. 6, pp. 1477–1487, 2013.

[17] J.-L. Starck, M. Elad, and D. Donoho, "Redundant multiscale transforms and their application for morphological component separation," in *Advances in Imaging and Electron Physics*, vol. 132 of *Advances in Imaging and Electron Physics*, pp. 287–348, Elsevier, 2004.

[18] A. M. Bruckstein, D. L. Donoho, and M. Elad, "From sparse solutions of systems of equations to sparse modeling of signals and images," *The SIAM Review*, vol. 51, no. 1, pp. 34–81, 2009.

[19] S. G. Mallat and Z. Zhang, "Matching pursuits with time-frequency dictionaries," *IEEE Transactions on Signal Processing*, vol. 41, no. 12, pp. 3397–3415, 1993.

[20] S. S. Chen, D. L. Donoho, and M. A. Saunders, "Atomic decomposition by basis pursuit," *The SIAM Journal on Scientific Computing*, vol. 20, no. 1, pp. 33–61, 1998.

[21] Y. Zhang, L. Wang, Y. Gao, J. Chen, and X. Shi, "Automatic denoising of Doppler ultrasound signals using matching pursuit method," in *Independent Component Analysis and Blind Signal Separation*, vol. 3889 of *Lecture Notes in Computer Science*, pp. 519–526, Springer, Berlin, Germany, 2006.

[22] C. I. Nieblas, M. A. Alonso, R. Conte, and S. Villarreal, "High performance heart sound segmentation algorithm based on matching pursuit," in *Proceedings of the IEEE Digital Signal Processing and Signal Processing Education Meeting (DSP/SPE '13)*, pp. 96–100, Napa, Calif, USA, usa, August 2013.

[23] O. Michailovich and D. Adam, "A high-resolution technique for ultrasound harmonic imaging using sparse representations in gabor frames," *IEEE Transactions on Medical Imaging*, vol. 21, no. 12, pp. 1490–1503, 2002.

[24] B. Deka and P. K. Bora, "Removal of correlated speckle noise using sparse and overcomplete representations," *Biomedical Signal Processing and Control*, vol. 8, no. 6, pp. 520–533, 2013.

[25] H. Liebgott, R. Prost, and D. Friboulet, "Pre-beamformed RF signal reconstruction in medical ultrasound using compressive sensing," *Ultrasonics*, vol. 53, no. 2, pp. 525–533, 2013.

[26] G. Shi, C. Chen, J. Lin, X. Xie, and X. Chen, "Narrowband ultrasonic detection with high range resolution: separating echoes via compressed sensing and singular value decomposition," *IEEE Transactions on Ultrasonics, Ferroelectrics, and Frequency Control*, vol. 59, no. 10, pp. 2237–2252, 2012.

[27] N. Wagner, Y. C. Eldar, and Z. Friedman, "Compressed beamforming in ultrasound imaging," *IEEE Transactions on Signal Processing*, vol. 60, no. 9, pp. 4643–4657, 2012.

[28] T. Chernyakova and Y. C. Eldar, "Fourier-domain beamforming: the path to compressed ultrasound imaging," *IEEE Transactions on Ultrasonics, Ferroelectrics, and Frequency Control*, vol. 61, no. 8, pp. 1252–1267, 2014.

[29] Q. Zhang, B. Li, and M. Shen, "A measurement-domain adaptive beamforming approach for ultrasound instrument based on distributed compressed sensing: initial development," *Ultrasonics*, vol. 53, no. 1, pp. 255–264, 2013.

[30] J. Zhou, S. Hoyos, and B. Sadler, "Asynchronous compressed beamformer for portable diagnostic ultrasound systems," *IEEE Transactions on Ultrasonics, Ferroelectrics, and Frequency Control*, vol. 61, no. 11, pp. 1791–1801, 2014.

[31] M. F. Schiffner, T. Jansen, and G. Schmitz, "Compressed sensing for fast image acquisition in pulse-echo ultrasound," *Biomedical Engineering-Biomedizinische Technik*, vol. 57, no. 1, 2012.

[32] J. Richy, D. Friboulet, A. Bernard, O. Bernard, and H. Liebgott, "Blood velocity estimation using compressive sensing," *IEEE Transactions on Medical Imaging*, vol. 32, no. 11, pp. 1979–1988, 2013.

[33] R. Demirli and J. Saniie, "An efficient sparse signal decomposition technique for ultrasonic signal analysis using envelope and instantaneous phase," in *Proceedings of the IEEE International Ultrasonics Symposium (IUS '08)*, pp. 1503–1507, Beijing, China, November 2008.

[34] R. Demirli and J. Saniie, "Model-based estimation pursuit for sparse decomposition of ultrasonic echoes," *IET Signal Processing*, vol. 6, no. 4, pp. 313–325, 2012.

[35] G. Cloutier, D. Chen, and L.-G. Durand, "A new clutter rejection algorithm for Doppler ultrasound," *IEEE Transactions on Medical Imaging*, vol. 22, no. 4, pp. 530–538, 2003.

[36] M. Rudelson and R. Vershynin, "Sparse reconstruction by convex relaxation: fourier and gaussian measurements," in *Proceedings of the 40th Annual Conference on Information Sciences and Systems (CISS '06)*, pp. 207–212, March 2006.

[37] E. J. Candès and D. L. Donoho, "Recovering edges in ill-posed inverse problems: optimality of curvelet frames," *The Annals of Statistics*, vol. 30, no. 3, pp. 784–842, 2002.

[38] M. Do and M. Vetterli, "Contourlets: a new directional multiresolution image representation," in *Proceedings of the Conference Record of the 36th Asilomar Conference on Signals, Systems and Computers*, vol. 1, pp. 497–501, November 2002.

[39] S. Fischer, G. Cristóbal, and R. Redondo, "Sparse overcomplete gabor wavelet representation based on local competitions," *IEEE Transactions on Image Processing*, vol. 15, no. 2, pp. 265–272, 2006.

[40] R. Rubinstein, A. M. Bruckstein, and M. Elad, "Dictionaries for sparse representation modeling," *Proceedings of the IEEE*, vol. 98, no. 6, pp. 1045–1057, 2010.

[41] M. Aharon, M. Elad, and A. Bruckstein, "K-SVD: an algorithm for designing overcomplete dictionaries for sparse representation," *IEEE Transactions on Signal Processing*, vol. 54, no. 11, pp. 4311–4322, 2006.

[42] M. Elad, J.-L. Starck, P. Querre, and D. L. Donoho, "Simultaneous cartoon and texture image inpainting using morphological component analysis (MCA)," *Applied and Computational Harmonic Analysis*, vol. 19, no. 3, pp. 340–358, 2005.

[43] M. Elad, *Sparse and Redundant Representations: From Theory to Applications in Signal and Image Processing*, Springer, 2010.

[44] G. Peyre, J. Fadili, and J.-L. Starck, "Learning the morphological diversity," *The SIAM Journal on Imaging Sciences*, vol. 3, no. 3, pp. 646–669, 2010.

[45] J. S. Turek, M. Elad, and I. Yavneh, "Sparse signal separation with an off-line learned dictionary for clutter reduction in echocardiography," in *Proceedings of the IEEE 28th Convention of Electrical Electronics Engineers in Israel (IEEEI '14)*, pp. 1–5, December 2014.

[46] J. Jensen, "Field: a program for simulating ultrasound systems," *Medical & Biological Engineering & Computing*, vol. 4, no. 1, pp. 351–353, 1996, Proceedings of the 10th Nordic-Baltic Conference on Biomedical Imaging.

[47] F. W. Mauldin Jr., F. Viola, and W. F. Walker, "Robust motion estimation using complex principal components," in *Proceedings of the IEEE International Ultrasonics Symposium (IUS '09)*, pp. 2429–2432, Rome, Italy, September 2009.

[48] T. Hozumi, K. Yoshida, Y. Abe et al., "Visualization of clear echocardiographic images with near field noise reduction technique: experimental stud and clinical experience," *Journal of the American Society of Echocardiography*, vol. 11, no. 6, pp. 660–667, 1998.

[49] S. Bjaerum, H. Torp, and K. Kristoffersen, "Clutter filters adapted to tissue motion in ultrasound color flow imaging," *IEEE Transactions on Ultrasonics, Ferroelectrics, and Frequency Control*, vol. 49, no. 6, pp. 693–704, 2002.

[50] C. M. Gallippi and G. E. Trahey, "Adaptive clutter filtering via blind source separation for two-dimensional ultrasonic blood velocity measurement," *Ultrasonic Imaging*, vol. 24, no. 4, pp. 193–214, 2002.

[51] L. A. F. Ledoux, P. J. Brands, and A. P. G. Hoeks, "Reduction of the clutter component in Doppler ultrasound signals based on singular value decomposition: a simulation study," *Ultrasonic Imaging*, vol. 19, no. 1, pp. 1–18, 1997.

[52] A. C. H. Yu and R. S. C. Cobbold, "Single-ensemble-based eigen-processing methods for color flow imaging—part I. The Hankel-SVD filter," *IEEE Transactions on Ultrasonics, Ferroelectrics, and Frequency Control*, vol. 55, no. 3, pp. 559–572, 2008.

[53] A. C. H. Yu and R. S. C. Cobbold, "Single-ensemble-based eigen-processing methods for color flow imaging—part II. The matrix pencil estimator," *IEEE Transactions on Ultrasonics, Ferroelectrics, and Frequency Control*, vol. 55, no. 3, pp. 573–587, 2008.

[54] R. Rubinstein, M. Zibulevsky, and M. Elad, "Efficient implementation of the K-SVD algorithm using batch orthogonal matching pursuit," Tech. Rep., Technion—Israel Institute of Technology, 2009.

[55] H. Torp, "Clutter rejection filters in color flow imaging: a theoretical approach," *IEEE Transactions on Ultrasonics, Ferroelectrics, and Frequency Control*, vol. 44, no. 2, pp. 417–424, 1997.

21

Optic Disc Segmentation by Balloon Snake with Texture from Color Fundus Image

Jinyang Sun,[1] Fangjun Luan,[1] and Hanhui Wu[2]

[1]School of Information & Control Engineering, Shenyang Jianzhu University, Shenyang 110168, China
[2]Sino-Dutch Biomedical and Information Engineering School, Northeastern University, Shenyang 110819, China

Correspondence should be addressed to Fangjun Luan; luanfangjun@sjzu.edu.cn

Academic Editor: Michael W. Vannier

A well-established method for diagnosis of glaucoma is the examination of the optic nerve head based on fundus image as glaucomatous patients tend to have larger cup-to-disc ratios. The difficulty of optic segmentation is due to the fuzzy boundaries and peripapillary atrophy (PPA). In this paper a novel method for optic nerve head segmentation is proposed. It uses template matching to find the region of interest (ROI). The method of vessel erasing in the ROI is based on PDE inpainting which will make the boundary smoother. A novel optic disc segmentation approach using image texture is explored in this paper. A cluster method based on image texture is employed before the optic disc segmentation step to remove the edge noise such as cup boundary and vessels. We replace image force in the snake with image texture and the initial contour of the balloon snake is inside the optic disc to avoid the PPA. The experimental results show the superior performance of the proposed method when compared to some traditional segmentation approaches. An average segmentation dice coefficient of 94% has been obtained.

1. Introduction

Glaucoma is the second most common cause of blindness worldwide [1]. It is also the leading cause of blindness among African Americans. There will be 60.5 million people with open angle glaucoma (OAG) and angle closure glaucoma (ACG) in 2010; the number will be increasing to 79.6 million by 2020 [2]. An automatic and economic system is highly desirable for glaucoma screening for a wider range of people. The best approach to do screening is based on 2D color fundus image as it is cheap and easy to manipulate. The optic nerve head assessment based on the 2D color fundus image is the best way for glaucoma screening at the moment. But automatic glaucoma screening is based on the risk factors from the optic nerve head, so an accurate segmentation of optic nerve head is the basic and most important process in glaucoma screening.

In retinal images, the optic disc generally appears as bright, yellowish, circular or slightly oval-shaped object as shown in Figure 1.

Optic disc segmentation can be generally grouped into three categories based on the methods for extracting the optic disc boundary:

(a) template matching or Hough transform methods,

(b) deformable models like snake, level sets,

(c) supervised classification or unsupervised classification.

Shape-based template matching [3, 4] is a very easy approach to segment the disc as the optic disc is approximately circular or elliptical. But this method is not very accurate as the shape of the optic disc is not a perfect circle or ellipse due to some pathological changes and this method often fails as there is PPA near the optic disc. Mohammad et al. [5] use binary robust independent elementary features (BRIEF) and a rotation invariant BRIEF (OBRIEF) features to find approximated boundary of the optic disc. Then a pixel classification method followed by circular template matching to segment the optic disc.

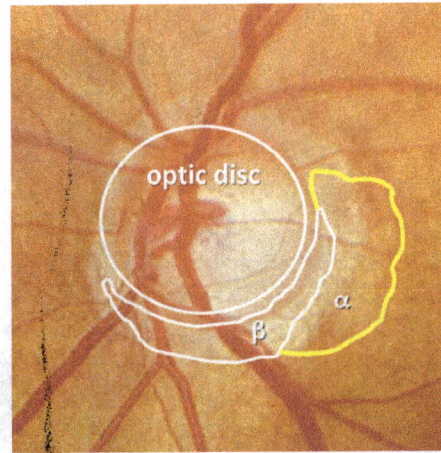

FIGURE 1: Color fundus image. The Zone alpha and beta peripapillary atrophy is near the disc.

Active contour model is one of the most promising approaches for OD segmentation as it is better in capturing irregularity disc region. GVF-snake algorithm is proposed by Osareh et al. [6] to extract the optic disc boundary. In order to remove the vessel occlusion during the deformable model, the blood vessel was first removed by morphology in the preprocessing step. Walter et al. [7] also use morphological filtering techniques to remove the blood vessels and they detect the optic disc boundary by means of watershed transformation.

Li and Chutatape [8] used principal component analysis (PCA) to locate the disc first and applied a modified active shape model (ASM) for optic disc identification. By means of shape model, this approach can handle vessel occlusion and fuzzy edges. However, the shape of the optic disc boundary may have different pathological changes. Hence, these template restrictions may reduce the accuracy of the segmentation. Lowell et al. [9] use global elliptic model to estimate the optic disc location and radius; then they apply a local deformable model with variable edge-strength dependent stiffness. This algorithm often fails where there are large numbers of white lesions, PPA, or strongly visible choroid vessel [10]. In order to solve the vessel occlusion and fuzzy contour shapes, Xu et al. [10] propose a knowledge-based clustering and smoothing update deforming model. After each deformation, the contour points are classified into two clusters by knowledge-based unsupervised learning. Then the contour is updated using both global and local information, so this method can achieve balance on contour stability and accuracy. They showed their proposed method achieves better success rate (94%) when comparing to GVF-snake (12%) and modified ASM (82%) approach. However, they also show that this method fails where there is obvious white PPA region near the disc. Dashtbozorg et al. [11] propose an automatic approach for OD segmentation using a multiresolution sliding band filter (SBF) and the OD boundary is regularized using a smoothing algorithm. This approach gets an average overlapping area of 83%, 89%, and 85% in three datasets.

All of these deformation methods are very sensitive to the initial contour. More recently, region-based active contour model is presented in [13]; this method can detect the fuzzy edge and is not sensitive to initial contour. However, the Chan-Vese model cannot handle inhomogeneous image which may lead to erroneous segmentations. Joshi et al. [14] propose a new segmentation method based on localized CV models [15] using local image information from three-dimensional feature spaces. This is a novel method by using texture feature to segment the optic disc, and they show a very nice result in their paper. But the local Chan-Vese active contour model can lead to oversegmentation as the texture of the retinal image is inhomogeneous. The selection of local neighbor radius parameter which defines the local image domain around a point of interest is very important. If the radius is too small this model is just like GVF model, while a large radius will decrease the sensitivity to small gradients and make this model be similar to the traditional Chan-Vese model and PPA region will be misclassified to optic disc region.

Another way to segment the optic disc is based on pixel classification [16, 17]. The difficulty of this approach is the shape of the classification result is often unsmooth. Moreover, it is hard to find a good texture feature to distinguish the PPA and optic disc. And this approach also needs to be trained before being applied to classification and it is very time consuming to segment the optic disc by SVM when exploiting lots of features for learning.

The difficulty in optic disc segmentation is caused by PPA as shown in Figure 1. The traditional methods often mistake PPA region as a part of optic disc. In order to solve the problem, we use the texture information from image which is robust to image inhomogeneity. This method is based on a balloon snake model, unlike other active contour models, such as snake or level set, which use gradient information to make the contour stop at the edge of disc. Thus, those methods require the initial contour to be near the true optic disc boundary. In this paper, we apply a fuzzy c means method to exclude those noises and keep the edge texture near the

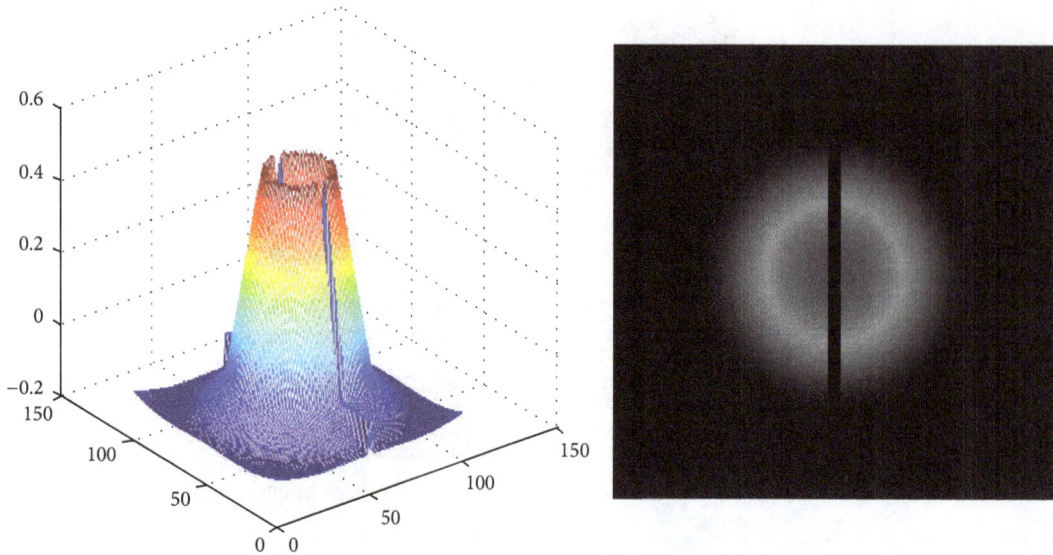

FIGURE 2: Optic disc template [12].

boundary. Then we choose the image texture rather than gradient to do segmentation, and the initial contour of the snake is a small circle in the disc region to avoid PPA region.

The organization of this paper is as follows. In Section 2, we present the methodology for OD localization and boundary segmentation. The results of our method are presented in Section 3. Comparison with results from same database by other methods can also be found in this section. Finally, Section 4 presented the conclusions of this study and future improvement.

2. Materials and Methods

The optic disc segmentation methodology of this paper can be divided into 3 main steps: (a) optic disc location, (b) vessel removal, and (c) optic nerve head segmentation.

2.1. Optic Disc Detection and ROI Selection

2.1.1. Optic Disc Detection. We use the template matching [9] to find the estimated disc region and then apply a circle Hough transform to correct the center and find an estimated disc radius. Since the appearance of the OD may vary significantly due to retinal pathologies, but the optic disc is the brightest feature of the normal fundus and shape of the optic disc is approximately vertically slightly oval (elliptical), a lot of templates have been proposed in [12] to find the optic disc. In this paper, we adopt the template from Lowell et al. [9] as shown in Figure 2. In our dataset the optic disc width is ranging from 260 to 380 pixels' length. So a template with size of 401 * 401 is used in our experiments. Then the Pearson correlation coefficient is used to measure the

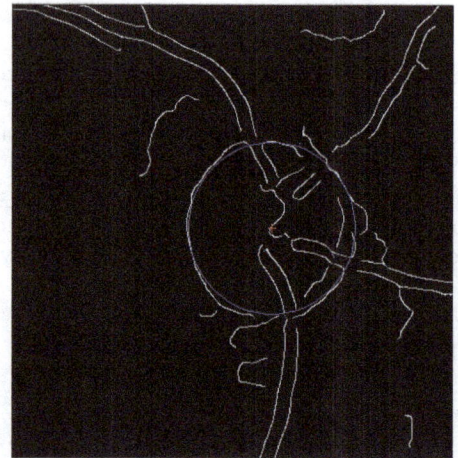

FIGURE 3: Result of circle Hough transform. The blue line is the estimated disc region.

correlation between the intensity channel from HSI color space subimage and the template in general:

$$c_{ij}$$
$$= \frac{\sum_{x,y} \left(f\left(x,y\right) - f_m \right) \left(t\left(x-i, y-j\right) - t_m \right)}{\sqrt{\left(\sum_{x,y} \left(f\left(x,y\right) - f_m \right)^2 \right) \left(\sum_{x,y} \left(t\left(x-i, y-j\right) - t_m \right)^2 \right)}},$$

(1)

where t_m is the mean intensity values of the template, which need to be calculated only once. f_m is the mean intensity values of the image region covered by the template. The location with the maximum value is selected as the optic disc location. The method is robust to small exudate and can fast

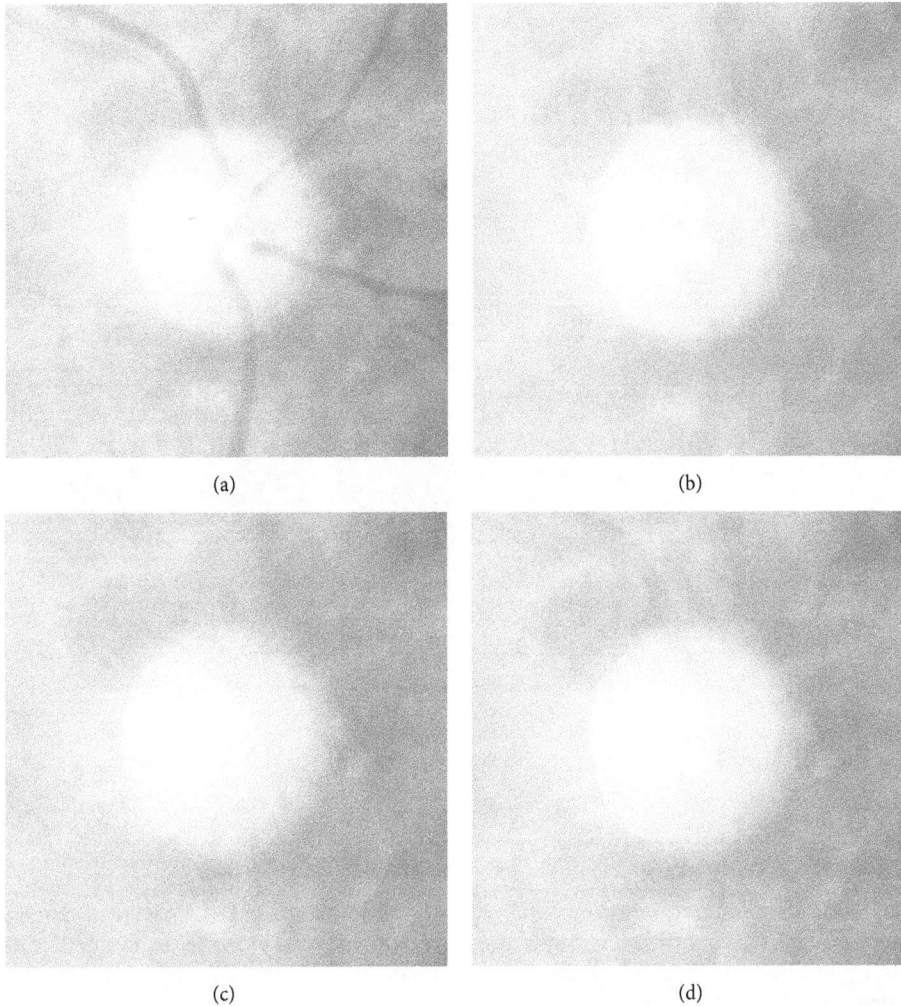

FIGURE 4: Vessel removal results. (a) Red channel image. (b) Close operation. (c) Mean pixels replacement. (d) PDE inpainting.

locate the optic disc. In the next step a circle Hough transform is used to update the center and find a disc radius.

2.1.2. ROI Selection Based on Circle Hough Transform.

Hough transform can be used to find the circular shape with fixed radius in the edge image of the fundus. An estimated disc center which is detected in the template matching step is selected as the region of interesting center. An appropriate region with size of 900 ∗ 900 is chosen as ROI. We smooth the image with a Gaussian filter to remove small noise. Canny kernel edge detection with a threshold value of 0.4 is applied to the ROI to remove weak boundaries and noises. Finally the Hough transform is applied to the edge pixels in the edge map to accumulate evidence of circles with fixed radius R in the image. In this paper, the radius is ranging from 140 to 230 with a step size of 15. The circle with the highest magnitude of evidence is chosen as the optic disc. The result is shown in Figure 3.

2.2. Vessel Removal.

Large blood vessels extending from optic disc may influence the precise edge of the optic disc. A PDE based inpainting method [18] based on the vessel mask is adopted. We also try to use morphological closing operation and mean pixels replacement method. In the morphological closing approach, a disc with radius of 15 is chosen as the structuring element, while in the mean pixels replacement approach the vessel mask pixel value is replaced by the mean value of the neighbor region.

We apply above three vessel removal methods and the results are shown in Figure 4. The advantage of morphological closing operation is that you do not need to segment the vessel first but it destroys the image texture and makes optic disc boundary become blurred. The result of image inpainting is slightly better than pixels replacement method. Moreover, it is much faster than replacement method. After the vessel removal processing, there is little information about vessel left.

2.3. Optic Nerve Head Segmentation

2.3.1. Image Texture.

In order to improve the segmentation result of the optic disc, we need to find those features which

(a)

(b)

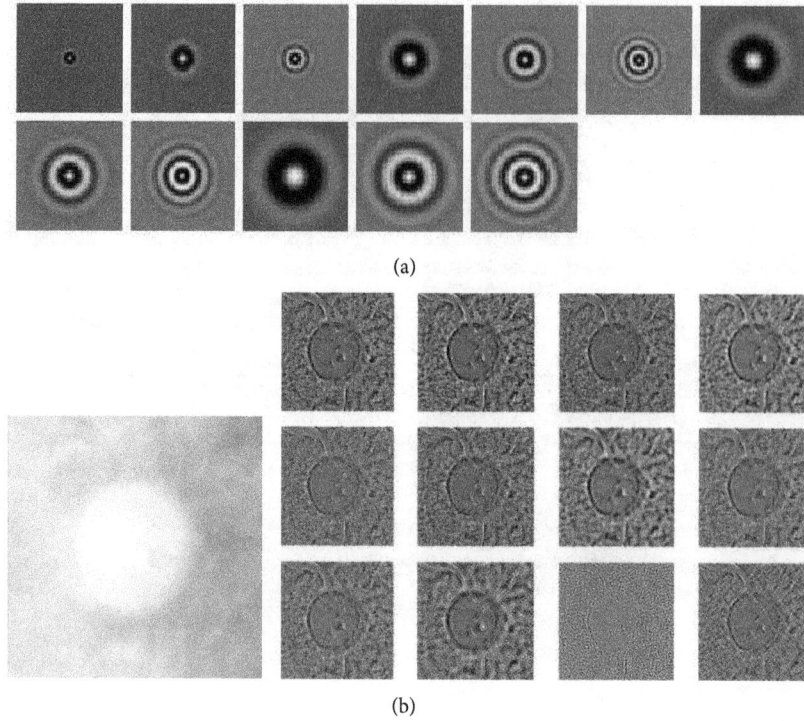

FIGURE 5: Schmid filter banks and results. (a) The Schmid filter bank. (b) The left one is the raw image. The right is the first twelve responses from Schmid.

can distinguish the optic disc region and boundary. Moreover, in consideration of the PPA region which surrounds the optic disc, we need to find those features that can also have different values between the optic disc and PPA region.

Schmid proposed texture feature filter banks which are rotationally invariant and are obtained by convolution with isotropic "Gabor-like" filters [19]. These filters combine different frequencies and scales together as follows:

$$
\begin{aligned}
F(x, y, \tau, \sigma) \\
= F_0(\tau, \sigma) + \cos\left(\frac{\sqrt{x^2 + y^2}\pi\tau}{\sigma}\right) e^{-(x^2+y^2)/2\sigma^2},
\end{aligned} \quad (2)
$$

where τ is the number of cycles of the harmonic function within the Gaussian envelope of the filters. σ represents the scale of the filter.

In this paper, several filters are generated by taking different banks parameters (σ, τ) pairs. They are taken by ranges (2,1), (4,1), (4,2), (6,1), (6,2), (6,3), (8,1), (8,2), (8,3), (10,1), (10,2), and (10,3), 12 filters in all. The filters are shown in Figure 5(a). And the responses of the image from Schmid filter bank are shown in Figure 5(b).

Another filter bank adopted is the Maximum Response Filter Banks [20]. These filters are derived from a common Root Filter Set (RFS). The RFS consists of 38 filters and is very similar to the Leung-Malik filter bank [21]. It consists of first and second derivatives of Gaussians at 6 orientations and 3 scales, 36 filters in all, and the last two filters are a

simple Gaussian and a Laplacian of Gaussian filter. To achieve rotational invariance, the authors get the Maximum Response Filter Bank from RFS by recording only the maximum filter response across all orientations for the two anisotropic filters [20]. By measuring only the maximum response across orientations, the author reduces the number of responses results from 38 to 8 (3 scales for 2 filters, plus 2 isotropic). The results of applying MR8 filter to the image are shown in Figure 6.

2.3.2. Optic Disc Segmentation with Balloon Snake

(1) The Balloon Snake. Cohen [22] added a pressure term to make the model behave like an inflatable balloon or bubble that is trapped by strong edges but expands through edges that are weak relative to the pressure and smoothing forces. The energy functional of traditional snake is changed and a pressure force is added to the formulation:

$$
\begin{aligned}
E_{\text{balloon}} = \underbrace{\frac{\alpha}{2} \oint \left|\frac{\partial \mathbf{u}}{\partial s}\right|^2 ds}_{\text{Tension}} + \underbrace{\frac{\beta}{2} \oint \left|\frac{\partial^2 \mathbf{u}}{\partial s^2}\right|^2 ds}_{\text{Stiffness}} \\
- \underbrace{\frac{\rho}{2} \oint \frac{\partial \mathbf{u}}{\partial s} \times \mathbf{u}\, ds}_{\text{Pressure}} + \underbrace{\xi \oint P(I(\mathbf{u}))\, ds}_{\text{Potential}},
\end{aligned} \quad (3)
$$

where the contour $\mathbf{u}$ depends on two parameters as below:

$$
\mathbf{u}(s, t) = (x(s, t), y(s, t)). \quad (4)
$$

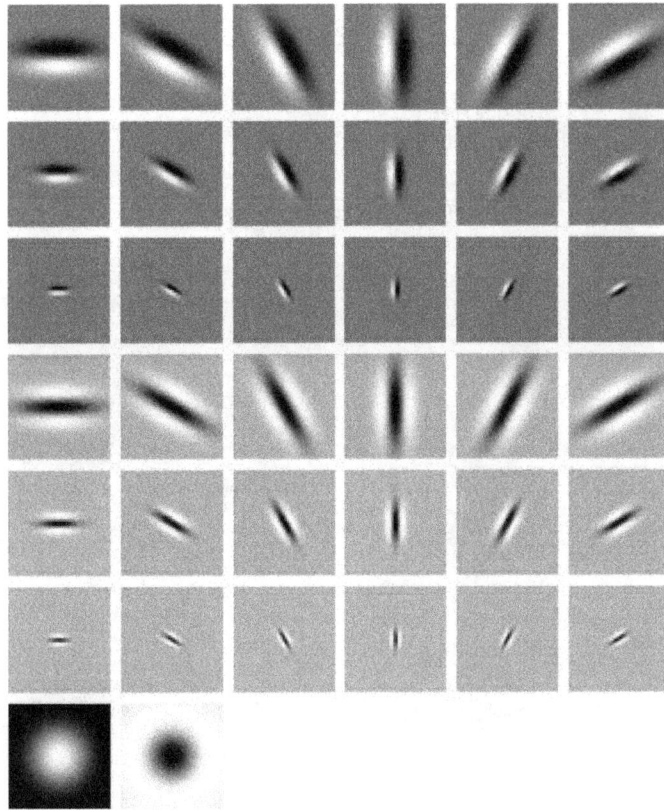

(a)

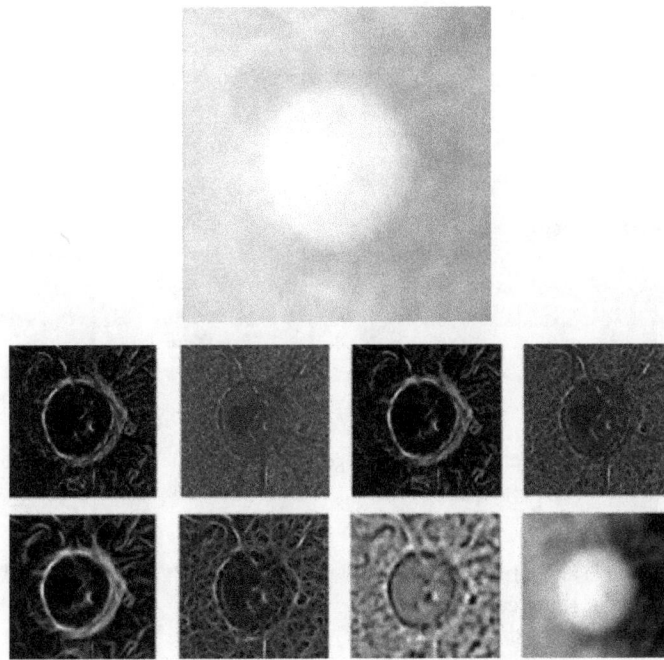

(b)

FIGURE 6: Root Filter Set and MR8 filter results. (a) Root Filter Set. (b) The upper part is the raw image. The lower part is the response result from MR8 filter.

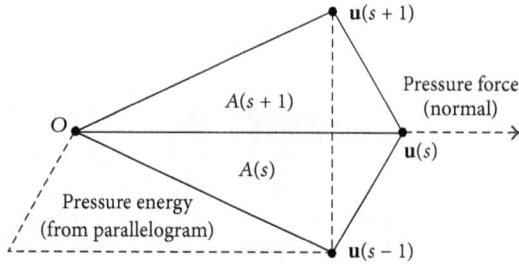

FIGURE 7: Pressure energy.

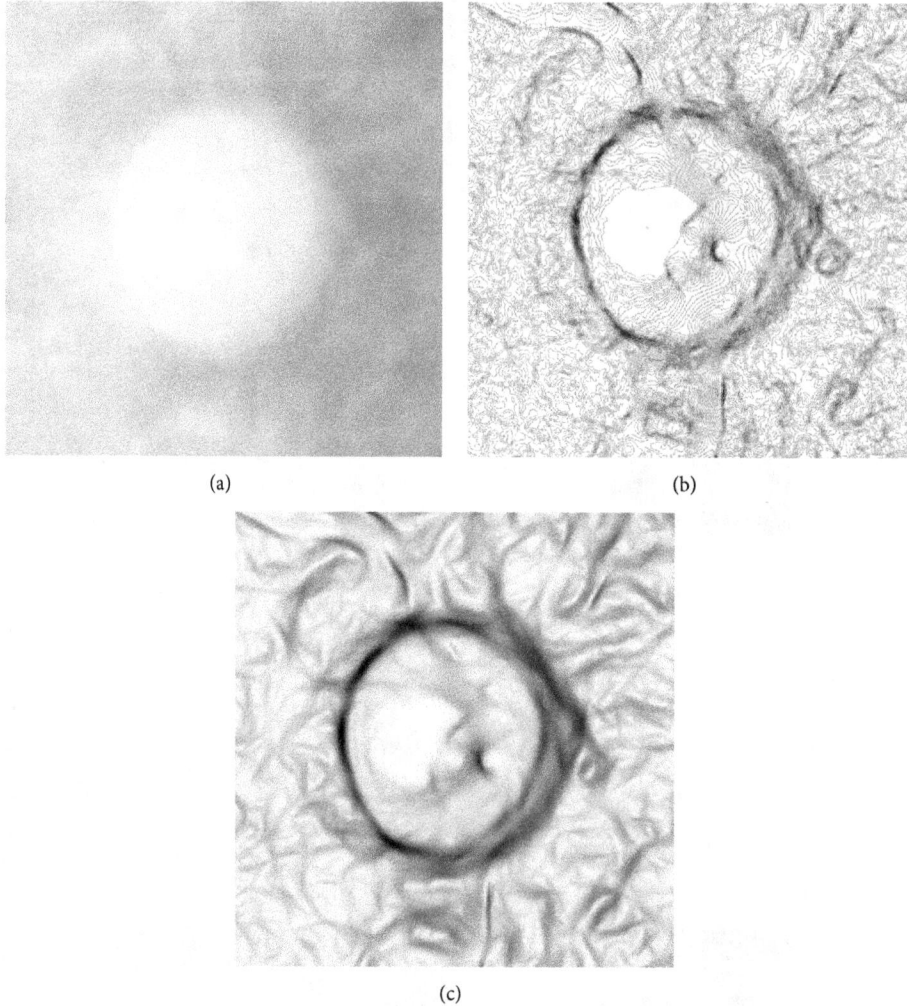

(a)

(b)

(c)

FIGURE 8: Image gradient and texture. (a) Raw image. (b) Image gradient. (c) 3rd response from MR8.

The third energy part in this equation is an isotropic pressure potential that controls the evolution of the area enclosed by the model. The energy of pressure is measured by size of the triangles region A_s in Figure 7.

The numerical solution of this equation can be found in [23]. At last we can get the total energy change of balloon snake as below:

$$\delta E = \oint \left(\frac{\partial P}{\partial \mathbf{u}} - \alpha \frac{\partial^2 \mathbf{u}}{\partial s^2} + \beta \frac{\partial^4 \mathbf{u}}{\partial s^4} + \rho \left(\frac{\partial \mathbf{u}}{\partial s} \right)^\perp \right) \cdot \delta \mathbf{u} \, ds. \quad (5)$$

At the limit of infinitesimal steps, the continuous descent equation is

$$\frac{\partial \mathbf{u}}{\partial t} = \underbrace{\alpha \frac{\partial^2 \mathbf{u}}{\partial s^2}}_{\text{Tension Force}} - \underbrace{\beta \frac{\partial^4 \mathbf{u}}{\partial s^4}}_{\text{Stiffness Force}}$$

$$- \underbrace{\rho \left(\frac{\partial \mathbf{u}}{\partial s} \right)^\perp}_{\text{Pressure Force}} - \underbrace{\frac{\partial P}{\partial \mathbf{u}}}_{\text{Image Force}}. \quad (6)$$

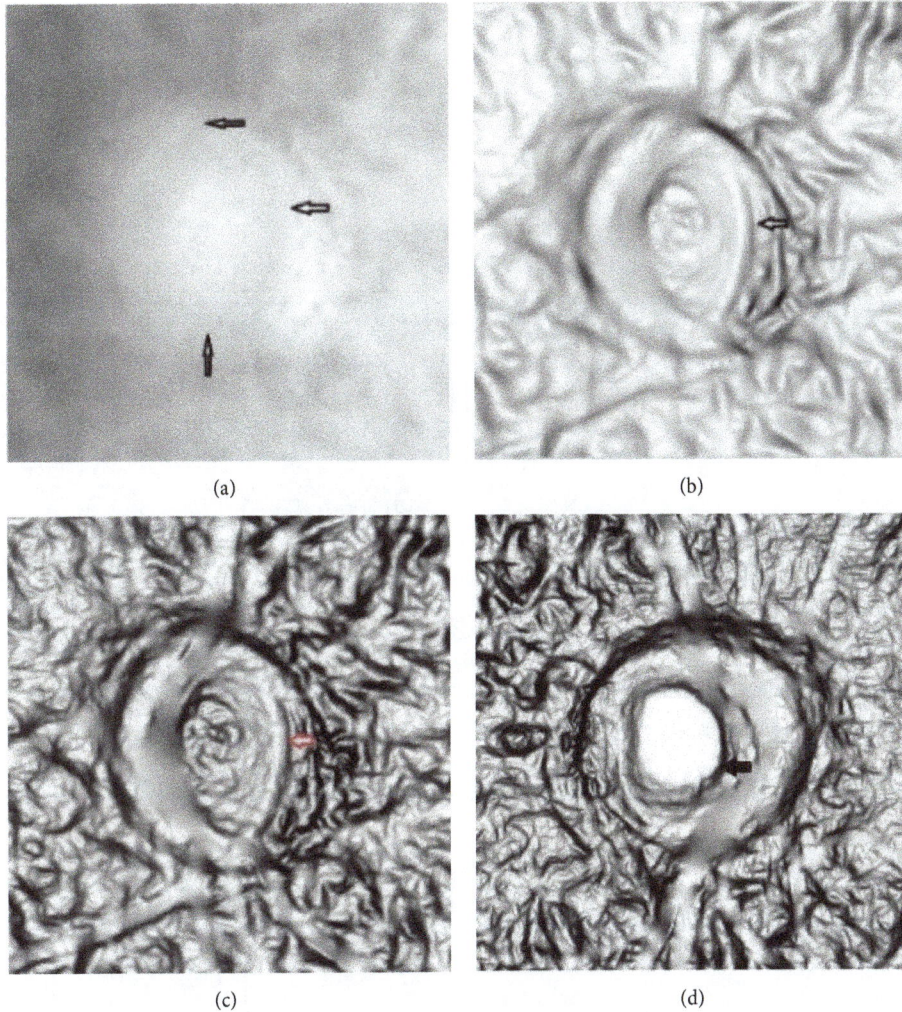

FIGURE 9: Image texture enhancement. (a) Raw image. The arrow indicates the week edges. (b) Image texture. The arrow indicates the fuzzy edge. (c) Texture enhancement. (d) Faked edges caused by enhancement.

(2) Texture Image Force. Balloon snake is difficult to use when the edges of images are weak as the image force of balloon snake is still gradient. After lots of experiments we adopt the 3rd texture response from Maximum Response Filter Bank; see Figure 8. The third texture response is good for segmentation as the boundary information is clearer than gradient and the noise texture caused by optic cup and vessel is less notable.

So the image force of balloon model is changed from gradient to texture. The energy equation of image force is as below:

$$E_{\text{image}}(x, y) = -\text{MRFilter} \odot I(x, y), \quad (7)$$

where MRFilter is the Maximum Response Filter Banks and $\odot$ means convolution.

(3) Texture Enhancement. Although this texture information is better than the image gradient for edge detection, there still remain some weak boundaries problems as shown in

Figure 9(b). We adopt the contrast-limited adaptive histogram equalization (CLAHE) to enhance the edge features. The CLAHE operation is directly applied to the image texture rather than the raw ROI image, as the CLAHE is good at enhancing small objects such as edges, and the image texture is something like small objects. The result of texture enhancement is shown in Figure 9(c).

After CLAHE enhancement, the texture becomes clearer than before. However, the noise texture which is formed by cup boundary is also clearer as shown in Figure 9(d). This will reduce the segmentation result, as the initial contour is inside the optic disc and the balloon snake may stop at the false edges formed by cup boundary or the vessel in the nasal side.

(4) Noise Textures Remove. In order to remove all noises except the disc boundary, we need to exclude those noise features and retain the texture features near the boundary. In this paper, we proposed a clustering method to find

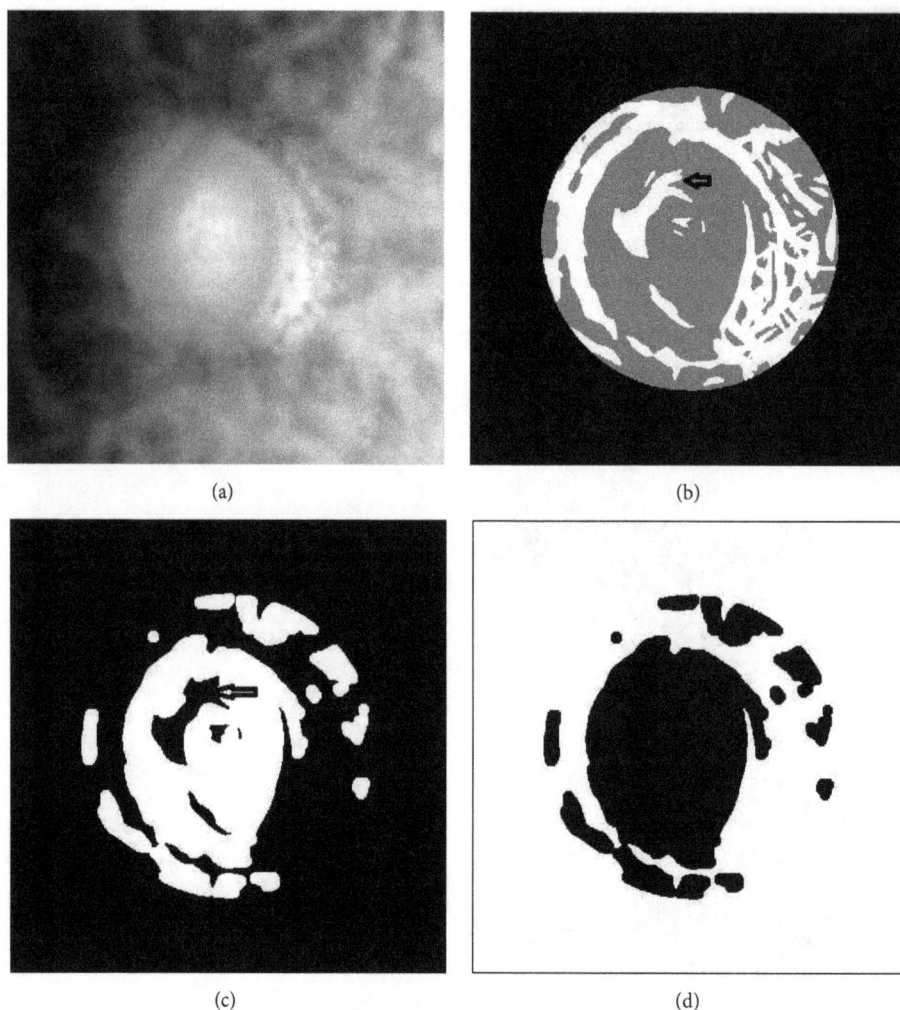

FIGURE 10: Edge region selection steps. (a) Raw image. (b) After fuzzy c means cluster. (c) After open operation. (d) Edge region.

the estimated edge region from the texture image by fuzzy c means approach. The detail of operation is as below.

(a) ROI Selection. According to estimated radius from the circle Hough transform, a larger estimated radius is selected to make sure the disc region is included in the new ROI. In this paper, we add the estimated radius by 50.

(b) Feature Selection. The feature space should have differences between the background and boundary or edge region. We give up the image intensity space as there is serious inhomogeneous intensity in fundus image which will make wrong classification. Three features are extracted from the red channel of ROI image. They are the 1st response from the Schmid filter bank and 5th and 7th response from Maximum Response (MR) Filter Bank. So every element point has three features; then they are classified into two clusters by fuzzy c means.

(c) Cluster Selection. After the classifications, the region is divided into two groups as shown in Figure 10(b). The proposed knowledge-based clustering is based on the assumption that the background region is larger than estimated

edge region. The max region is selected as the estimated background region, but there are still some holes in the background due to the cup boundary or the faked vessel edge. In order to remove the noise inside the background region, an open operation is applied to the background region as shown in Figure 10(c); this step will link the edge region; then we choose the opposite region, the estimated edge region, and select the max connect region as the estimated edge region. After this operation, small faked edge region is excluded from the edge region as shown in Figure 10(d).

(d) Noise Inpainting. After we get the edges mask, we need to remove those noises features in the optic disc. Based on the background mask from the preview step, we cannot simply assign 0 or 255 to the background region as it will produce a local maximum or minimum between background region and other regions which makes the snake contour stop. In order to make the contour smooth cross the background region, an inpainting approach [18] is employed to remove the texture noises. So in this step an inpainting operation is employed to the image again to remove the vessel edge and background region which is detected in the previous step.

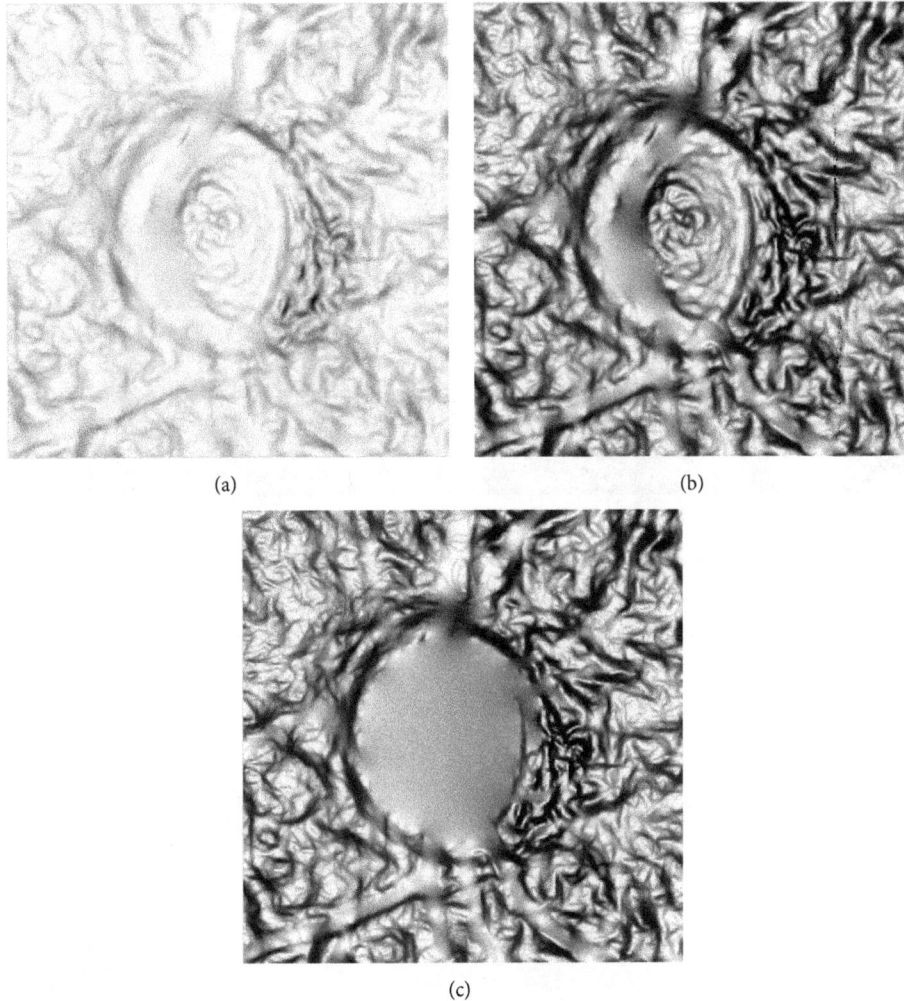

FIGURE 11: Texture noise removal. (a) Image texture. (b) After enhancement. (c) After noise inpainting.

The final result of texture enhancement and texture noises removal is shown in Figure 11.

(e) The Deformable Balloon Contour. In this paper, a circle with half of the estimated radius is adopted to make sure that the initial contour is inside the optic disc. The gradient energy is replaced by the texture energy. The contour is expanding like balloon and will stop at the texture boundary. The result of segmentation is shown in Figure 12. This segmentation method can avoid PPA as they are outside the optic disc. Moreover, if there is a PPA region near the disc, this contour will stop near the disc boundaries as long as there exists difference between the PPA and disc region.

3. Results and Discussion

3.1. Glaucoma Database. The database used in this paper is from High-Resolution Fundus (HRF) Image Database [24]. The database contains 15 images of healthy patients, 15 images of patients with diabetic retinopathy, and 15 images of glaucomatous patients at the moment. There are often some large exudates or bleeding in diabetic retinopathy images

which make it difficult to locate the disc. In this paper, we choose 15 images of healthy patients and 15 images of glaucomatous patients from this database. Binary golden standard vessel segmentation images are available for each image. The manual optic disc mask which is used as golden truth was collected by one ophthalmology expert from He Eye hospital, Shenyang.

3.2. Performance of the Algorithm. In this paper, we adopt the dice coefficient to quantify the performance of the optic disc segmentation; the dice coefficient is defined as follows:

$$DC = \frac{2 * \text{Area}(A \cap B)}{\text{Area}(A) + \text{Area}(B)}. \tag{8}$$

A represents the ground truth and *B* represents our optic disc segmentation result. A DC value of 1 indicates a perfect segmentation result with the ground truth, and a small DC value indicates a bad segmentation.

Lots of approaches have been tested to segment the disc in our experiments. The Chan-Vese [25] (CV) and an improved approach, local Gaussian distribution model [15]

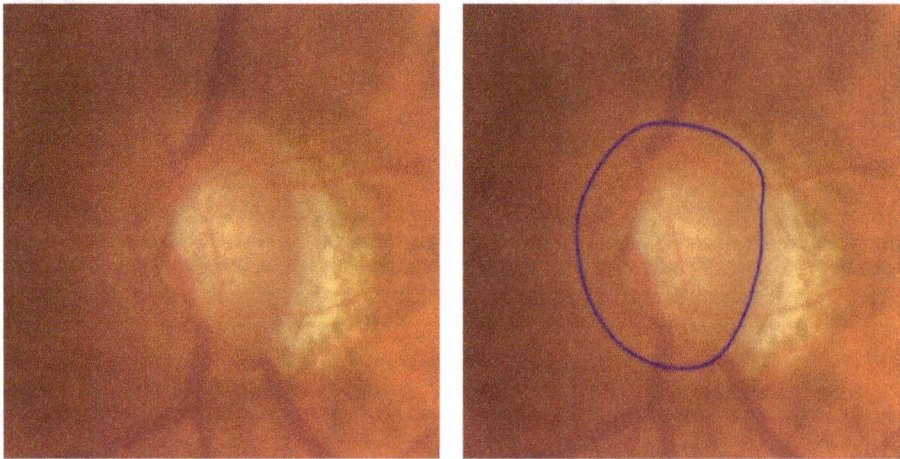

FIGURE 12: Balloon snake results.

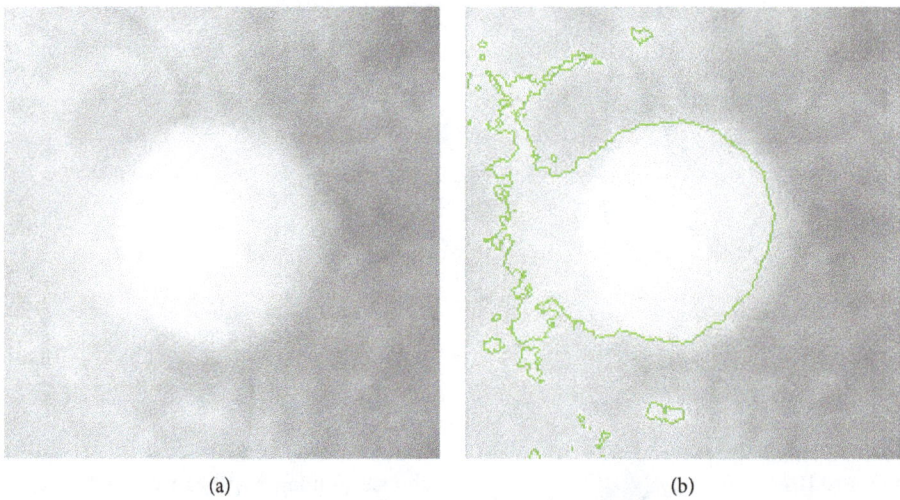

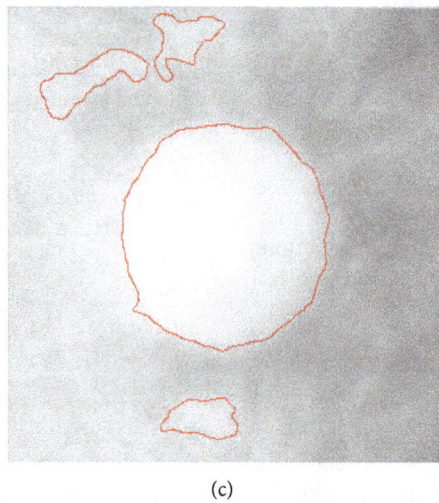

(a)

(b)

(c)

FIGURE 13: CV and local Gaussian distribution model. (a) Raw image. (b) CV model results. (c) Local Gaussian distribution model results.

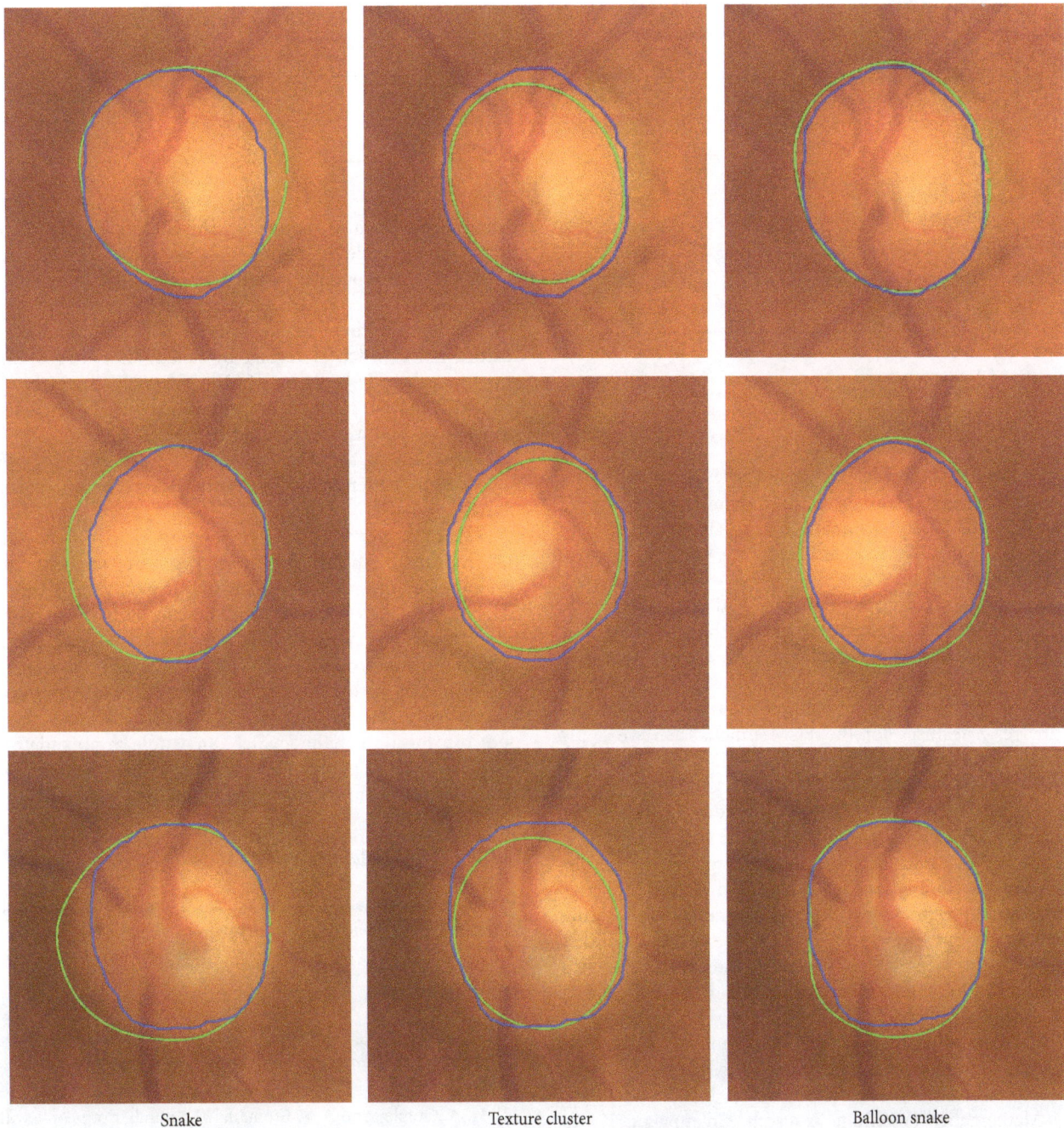

Snake   Texture cluster   Balloon snake

FIGURE 14: Three segmentation approaches. The blue is the golden mask and green is the segmentation result.

(LGD), are state-of-the-art level set segmentation methods and they are employed to segment the optic disc. Although both of them are not sensitive to the initial contour, we make the initial contour be a circle with radius smaller than the estimated disc radius from the circle Hough transform. However, we find that the CV and LGD are not suitable to do disc segmentation as shown in Figure 13. In CV model, the image intensity is used as energy to find an edge which makes the sum of inner and external energy be the minimum. This method often fails in optic disc segmentation because of inhomogeneity as shown in Figure 13(b). This image has

intensity inhomogeneity where the left part is brighter than the right part. So the CV model makes some bright region located in the left optic disc as a part of the optic disc.

While the LGD model is designed for handling image inhomogeneity problem, this method efficiently utilizes local image information rather than the global information such as CV model. We can see from Figure 13(c) that there are lots of small dark or bright regions near the optic disc which is caused by the light illumination or reflex. After we apply LGD to the ROI image, we find that it has the problem of oversegmentation as the energy minimization is achieved

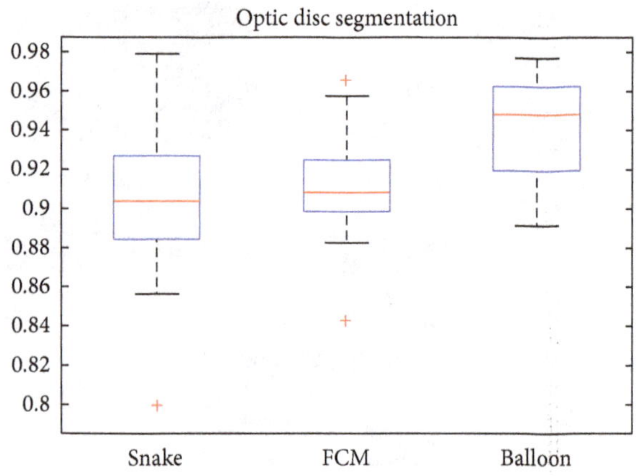

FIGURE 15: Optic disc segmentation results over 30 images.

by an interleaved level set evolution and estimation of local intensity means and variances in an iterative process. This approach will falsely segment some small regions. So we give up these two methods and regard the edge based active contour model.

We compare our proposed method with traditional snake and another texture cluster methods which is fuzzy c means cluster method. And in the texture cluster segmentation method, we adopt the 5th response from MR8 and 1st response from Schmid filter bank of the red channel values of image, 2 features for the FCM input. Then we apply morphological operation to the larger region, and an ellipse fit is applied to get this region boundary.

As shown in Figure 14, we can see from the image that the snake model often fails to detect the true edge of disc because of the fuzzy edge and PPA region. The results often include the PPA region as a part of disc. To sum up, our proposed segmentation method is more robust to the snake, as you can see from Figure 15. In the box-and-whisker figure, the proposed balloon snake is better than other two approaches, and most of segmentation dice coefficient is 94% as shown in Table 1. Although the mean dice coefficient of FCM texture cluster approach is almost the same as snake model, most of coefficient is distributed more than 90%. We utilize the Matlab (MathWorks, Inc., Natick, MA) and Mathematica (Wolfram Research, Champaign, IL) to implement our method mentioned in this paper. It costs about 2 minutes to process one image on PC (I5 Intel CPU and 4 G RAM).

4. Conclusions

In this paper, we focus on automatic segmentation of the optic disc based on 2D fundus image. Template matching and circle Hough transform are used to locate the optic disc and find an estimated circle radius. In the vessel erasing step, we use inpainting approach to remove vessel which is better than the closing operation and mean neighbor replacement.

Our proposed optic disc segmentation method is based on image texture and active contour model. We use the balloon snake model which makes the contour expand like

TABLE 1: Disc segmentation results.

	μ	δ
Snake	0.9053	0.0445
Texture cluster	0.9093	0.0311
Our method	0.9400	0.0263

balloon from the inner optic disc. This method can avoid the PPA region outside the disc boundaries and is less sensitive to the initial contour, as the initial contour of normal snake model and GVF model are recommended near the true disc boundaries. The main problem of this balloon model is the texture noise which is caused by faked vessel edges, and sometime the cup is obvious in the red channel which will make this contour mistake the cup boundary as the disc edge. So we proposed a cluster based approach to remove those texture noises in the disc. The results from our proposed approach are better than the snake model and fuzzy c means cluster approach.

The optic nerve head segmentation results show that the proposed method is able to achieve better segmentation accuracy for optic disc comparing to other existing methods. The works of this paper as a whole can be used in retina image processing system, which is highly desirable for large-scale screening programs. However, our proposed method is sensitive to optic disc location approach and vessel segmentation results; in the future we need to adopt a better optic disc location method which can handle large exudate in the diabetic retinopathy images and make our method more robust to handle inaccurate vessel segmentation results.

Conflict of Interests

The authors declare that there is no conflict of interests regarding the publication of this paper.

References

[1] S. Kingman, "Glaucoma is second leading cause of blindness globally," *Bulletin of the World Health Organization*, vol. 82, no. 11, pp. 887–888, 2004.

[2] H. A. Quigley and A. T. Broman, "The number of people with glaucoma worldwide in 2010 and 2020," *British Journal of Oph-thalmology*, vol. 90, no. 3, pp. 262–267, 2006.

[3] M. Lalonde, M. Beaulieu, and L. Gagnon, "Fast and robust optic disc detection using pyramidal decomposition and hausdorff-based template matching," *IEEE Transactions on Medical Imag-ing*, vol. 20, no. 11, pp. 1193–1200, 2001.

[4] P. M. D. S. Pallawala, W. Hsu, M. L. Lee, and K.-G. A. Eong, "Automated optic disc localization and contour detection using ellipse fitting and wavelet transform," in *Computer Vision—ECCV 2004*, vol. 3022 of *Lecture Notes in Computer Science*, pp. 139–151, Springer, Berlin, Germany, 2004.

[5] S. Mohammad, D. T. Morris, and N. Thacker, "Texture analysis for the segmentation of optic disc in retinal images," in *Proceed-ings of the IEEE International Conference on Systems, Man, and Cybernetics (SMC '13)*, pp. 4265–4270, IEEE, Manchester, UK, October 2013.

[6] A. Osareh, M. Mirmehdi, B. Thomas, and R. Markham, "Comparison of colour spaces for optic disc localisation in retinal images," in *Object Recognition Supported by User Interaction for Service Robots*, vol. 1, pp. 743–746, 2002.

[7] T. Walter, J.-C. Klein, P. Massin, and A. Erginay, "A contribution of image processing to the diagnosis of diabetic retinopathy—detection of exudates in color fundus images of the human retina," *IEEE Transactions on Medical Imaging*, vol. 21, no. 10, pp. 1236–1243, 2002.

[8] H. Li and O. Chutatape, "Boundary detection of optic disk by a modified ASM method," *Pattern Recognition*, vol. 36, no. 9, pp. 2093–2104, 2003.

[9] J. Lowell, A. Hunter, D. Steel et al., "Optic nerve head segmentation," *IEEE Transactions on Medical Imaging*, vol. 23, no. 2, pp. 256–264, 2004.

[10] J. Xu, O. Chutatape, E. Sung, C. Zheng, and P. C. T. Kuan, "Optic disk feature extraction via modified deformable model technique for glaucoma analysis," *Pattern Recognition*, vol. 40, no. 7, pp. 2063–2076, 2007.

[11] B. Dashtbozorg, A. M. Mendonça, and A. Campilho, "Optic disc segmentation using the sliding band filter," *Computers in Biology and Medicine*, vol. 56, pp. 1–12, 2015.

[12] H. Yu, E. S. Barriga, C. Agurto et al., "Fast localization and segmentation of optic disk in retinal images using directional matched filtering and level sets," *IEEE Transactions on Information Technology in Biomedicine*, vol. 16, no. 4, pp. 644–657, 2012.

[13] G. D. Joshi, J. Sivaswamy, K. Karan, and S. R. Krishnadas, "Optic disk and cup boundary detection using regional information," in *Proceedings of the 7th IEEE International Symposium on Biomedical Imaging: From Nano to Macro (ISBI '10)*, pp. 948–951, April 2010.

[14] G. D. Joshi, J. Sivaswamy, and S. R. Krishnadas, "Optic disk and cup segmentation from monocular color retinal images for glaucoma assessment," *IEEE Transactions on Medical Imaging*, vol. 30, no. 6, pp. 1192–1205, 2011.

[15] L. Wang, L. He, A. Mishra, and C. Li, "Active contours driven by local Gaussian distribution fitting energy," *Signal Processing*, vol. 89, no. 12, pp. 2435–2447, 2009.

[16] M. D. Abràmoff, W. L. M. Alward, E. C. Greenlee et al., "Automated segmentation of the optic disc from stereo color photographs using physiologically plausible features," *Investigative Ophthalmology and Visual Science*, vol. 48, no. 4, pp. 1665–1673, 2007.

[17] J. Cheng, J. Liu, Y. Xu et al., "Superpixel classification based optic disc and optic cup segmentation for glaucoma screening," *IEEE Transactions on Medical Imaging*, vol. 32, no. 6, pp. 1019–1032, 2013.

[18] M. Bertalmio, G. Sapiro, V. Caselles, and C. Ballester, "Image inpainting," in *Proceedings of the 27th annual conference on Computer graphics and interactive techniques (SIGGRAPH '00)*, pp. 417–424, July 2000.

[19] C. Schmid, "Constructing models for content-based image retrieval," in *Proceedings of the IEEE Computer Society Conference on Computer Vision and Pattern Recognition (CVPR '01)*, vol. 2, pp. II-39–II-45, December 2001.

[20] J.-M. Geusebroek, A. W. Smeulders, and J. van de Weijer, "Fast anisotropic Gauss filtering," *IEEE Transactions on Image Processing*, vol. 12, no. 8, pp. 938–943, 2003.

[21] T. Leung and J. Malik, "Representing and recognizing the visual appearance of materials using three-dimensional textons," *International Journal of Computer Vision*, vol. 43, no. 1, pp. 29–44, 2001.

[22] L. D. Cohen, "On active contour models and balloons," *CVGIP: Image Understanding*, vol. 53, no. 2, pp. 211–218, 1991.

[23] M. Kass, A. Witkin, and D. Terzopoulos, "Snakes: active contour models," *International Journal of Computer Vision*, vol. 1, no. 4, pp. 321–331, 1988.

[24] J. Odstrcilik, R. Kolar, A. Budai et al., "Retinal vessel segmentation by improved matched filtering: evaluation on a new high-resolution fundus image database," *IET Image Processing*, vol. 7, no. 4, pp. 373–383, 2013.

[25] T. F. Chan and L. A. Vese, "Active contours without edges," *IEEE Transactions on Image Processing*, vol. 10, no. 2, pp. 266–277, 2001.

22

Skin Parameter Map Retrieval from a Dedicated Multispectral Imaging System Applied to Dermatology/Cosmetology

Romuald Jolivot,[1] Yannick Benezeth,[2] and Franck Marzani[2]

[1] *National Electronic and Computer Technology Center, 112 Thailand Science Park, Phahonyothin Road, Khlong Nueng, Klong Luang, Pathumthani 12120, Thailand*

[2] *Laboratoire LE2I, UMR CNRS 6306, UFR Sciencees & Techniques, Université de Bourgogne, BP 47870, 21078 Dijon CEDEX, France*

Correspondence should be addressed to Franck Marzani; franck.marzani@u-bourgogne.fr

Academic Editor: Vincent Paquit

In vivo quantitative assessment of skin lesions is an important step in the evaluation of skin condition. An objective measurement device can help as a valuable tool for skin analysis. We propose an explorative new multispectral camera specifically developed for dermatology/cosmetology applications. The multispectral imaging system provides images of skin reflectance at different wavebands covering visible and near-infrared domain. It is coupled with a neural network-based algorithm for the reconstruction of reflectance cube of cutaneous data. This cube contains only skin optical reflectance spectrum in each pixel of the bidimensional spatial information. The reflectance cube is analyzed by an algorithm based on a Kubelka-Munk model combined with evolutionary algorithm. The technique allows quantitative measure of cutaneous tissue and retrieves five skin parameter maps: melanin concentration, epidermis/dermis thickness, haemoglobin concentration, and the oxygenated hemoglobin. The results retrieved on healthy participants by the algorithm are in good accordance with the data from the literature. The usefulness of the developed technique was proved during two experiments: a clinical study based on vitiligo and melasma skin lesions and a skin oxygenation experiment (induced ischemia) with healthy participant where normal tissues are recorded at normal state and when temporary ischemia is induced.

1. Introduction

Visual assessment of different skin pathologies is a result of ambient light that enters the skin and is scattered and diffused within it. The reemitted light carries important information about the physical and optical tissue parameters. It is a combination of selective absorption and scattering of specific light wavelengths due to the physical properties of chromophores composing the skin [1]. Well-trained dermatologists analyze the skin color and interpret the clinical pathologies based on their knowledge and experience. Dermatologists evaluate lesion conditions based on the distribution, size, shape, border, and symmetry but mostly on the color aspect. Diagnoses based on colour are subjective as colour perception depends on human visual response to light. The human eye does not have the same sensitivity for all wavelengths [2] and between individuals. Colour is sensed by the human eye over the visible wave range and is subjectively interpreted as a unique sensation while it is a combination of wavelengths. This lack of spectral discrimination means that the eye can be affected by metamerism which potentially affects the analysis.

Imaging systems for skin analysis often try to mimic the eye analysis. Nowadays, digital imaging systems are more and more available to clinicians, but imaging systems are mostly restricted to colour cameras. Such systems are limited in terms of spectral information as it is based on the trichromatic model [3]. It acquires spatially distributed information which is useful for skin lesion followup [4]. However, it does not take advantage of the skin/light interaction which occurs over the whole spectrum range.

There is a growing awareness of skin disease condition worldwide [5]. To improve the subjective assessment made on colour information, several optical acquisition systems have been developed to study the skin more objectively.

Several studies [6–8] point out the possible differentiation of skin variegation above specific wavelength values as compared to healthy skin, meaning that spectral information is an important tool of assessment. A reflectance spectrum provides precise objective physical information compared to subjective colour measurement. In vivo optical spectroscopy is based on the study of light interaction of molecules with electromagnetic radiation.

Spectroscopy measures the light intensity as a function of wavelength in form of a spectrum. This type of measurement is linked to the optical property of the skin and is a result of the absorption, scattering, and emission properties of the skin. Spectral acquisition from skin tissues returns quantitative information about its biochemical properties. This technique is proved to be potentially useful to acquire skin information [9].

Currently, there is no system that can replace the diagnosis abilities of experienced clinicians. However, the use of optical instruments increases the amount of complementary information to the dermatologist. It can potentially provide information not detectable by the human eye and can lead to objective skin chromophore quantification. This can be obtained by combining advantages of both spectrophotometer (spectral resolution) and digital camera (spatial resolution). multispectral imaging (MSI) systems overcome their respective limitations (lack of spatial variation and lack of spectral resolution).

The development of methods to assist diagnosis of skin pathology is based on objective assessment of skin characteristics. The study of skin reflectance can be correlated with its biochemical and morphological composition to reveal information about its condition. There exist two main categories to analyze human skin reflectance spectrum.

One category is based on statistical analysis. Several researches base their skin parameters retrieval by multivariate methods such as partial least squares regressions [10], support vector machine (SVM) [11], or blind source separation (BSS) [12] such as independent component analysis (ICA) [13] or principal component analysis (PCA) [14] to determine the concentration of skin chromophores. These techniques assumed that skin reflectance is a linear combination of different source component spectra weighed by their mixing quantities. The techniques are based on composition assumption. Generally, melanin and haemoglobin are assumed to be the two main components of the skin. The techniques do not have a priori information about the skin concentration and scattering. This category of analysis can be affected when the skin composition is different from the assumption. These methods are based on strong hypothesis of the skin composition and the results might be influenced when one or more hypotheses are not satisfied.

Another category refers to the analysis of reflectance spectra by means of physical models of light transportation that are based on optical skin properties. Different light propagation models have been developed such as model based on Monte Carlo simulations [15, 16], Kubelka-Munk [17, 18], and the modified Beer-Lambert law [19]. The main motivation is to retrieve skin parameters by inversing the model to match a measured reflectance spectrum.

This category of analysis is based on a priori physical knowledge of skin absorption and scattering properties and thickness. These methods tend to be more flexible regarding the skin composition and are less likely to be affected by unexpected data and to output incoherent results. A research by Shi and Dimarzio [20] presents a hyperspectral imaging system applied to foot wound care and analyzed data with two methods (Beer-Lambert law and two-layer optical model); however, the system is limited to the visible range and only three parameters (oxy/deoxyhaemoglobin concentration and epidermis thickness) are retrieved. Moncrie et al. [21] have developed a multispectral imaging system covering visible and near-infrared light combine with an algorithm retrieving five parameters (total melanin content of the epidermis and papillary dermis, collagen and haemoglobin content, and the presence of melanin in the papillary dermis) but does not consider skin layer thickness.

As a result, our development focuses on a technology combining a large amount of skin information (both spectrally and spatially) and analysis of the skin parameters quantification. We address this problem by developing an exploratory imaging system retrieving skin parameter maps dedicated to dermatology/cosmetology.

In this contribution, the development of an integrated MSI system which acquires spectral images is described. The MSI reconstructs reflectance cubes which contain only the spectral reflectance of cutaneous data by means of an artificial neural-network algorithm. Hypercubes are analyzed by using an inverse model of light propagation which retrieves skin parameter maps based on the analysis of reflectance spectra by means of a physical model of light transportation in skin. Finally, the overall system is validated on healthy and diseased skin lesions.

2. Materials and Methods

Our motivation is to provide a system for prospective study of different skin lesions. The developed multispectral imaging (MSI) system covers visible and near-infrared wave range and is suitable for dermatological and cosmetological constraints (ergonomics and fast acquisition time). The overall system is described in Figure 1.

2.1. ASCLEPIOS Multispectral Imaging System. The system presented is called ASCLEPIOS, standing for analysis of skin characteristics by light emission and processing of images of spectrum. It is an extended version of a previous multispectral camera limited to the visible [22]. An MSI is generally composed of elements similar to colour acquisition system [23]; the main difference is the increased number of channels.

2.1.1. Setup. For ergonomic purpose, the system is separated into two parts, an illumination system and a hand-held acquisition device (see Figure 2). This setting has the advantage of reducing the weight and size of the hand-held device and minimizes the number of calibration steps.

The illumination system is composed of a light source and a spectral selective device which is positioned in front

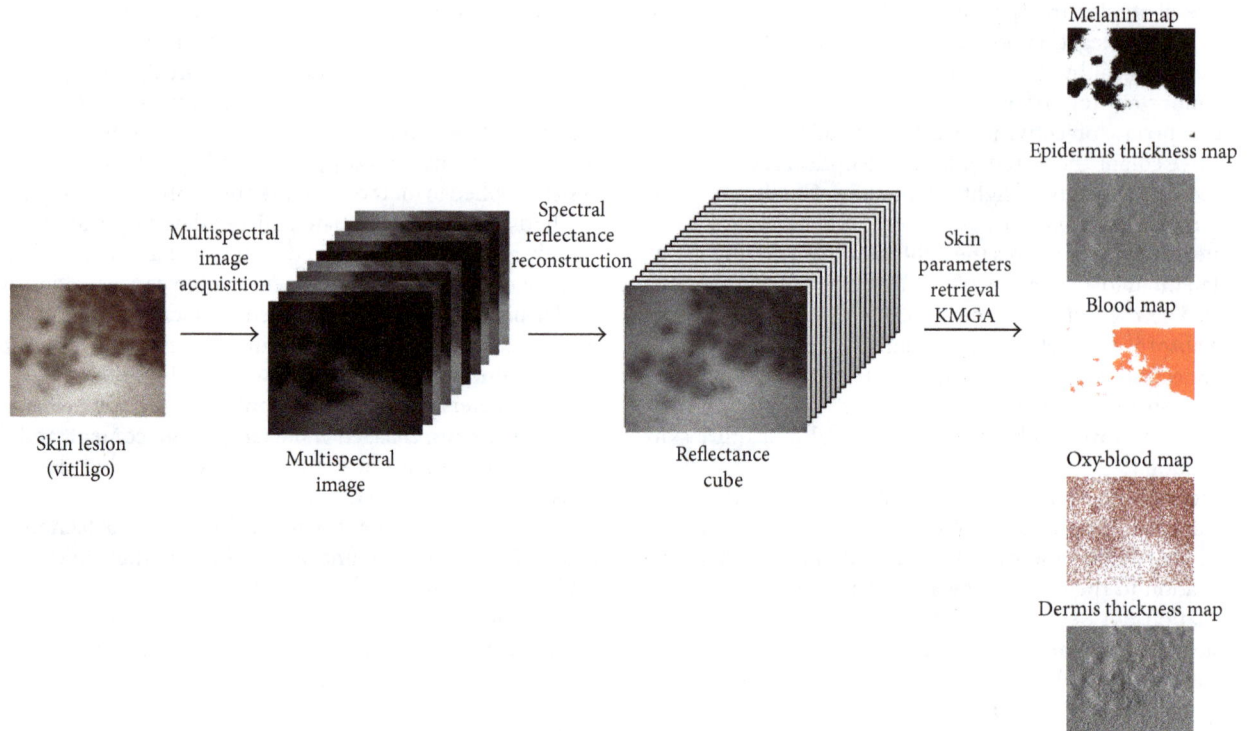

FIGURE 1: Asclepios full system: from acquisition to skin parameter map retrieval. The system is defined in three steps: (1) the acquisition of a multispectral image, (2) the reconstruction of a reflectance cube containing only skin reflectance information and finally, and (3) the retrieval of skin parameters from the analyzed reflectance cube.

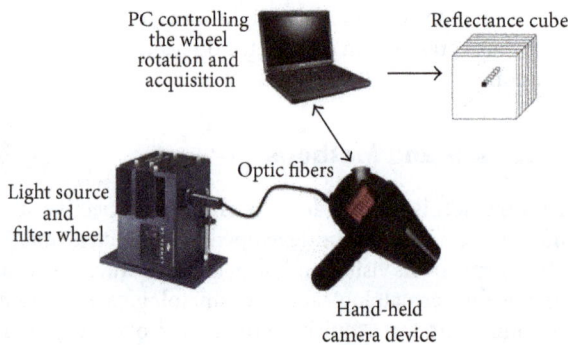

FIGURE 2: Description of the multispectral imaging system. The system is divided into two main parts: illumination device comprising of light source and filter wheel and a hand-held device with a camera. The system is controlled by a laptop and output reflectance cubes.

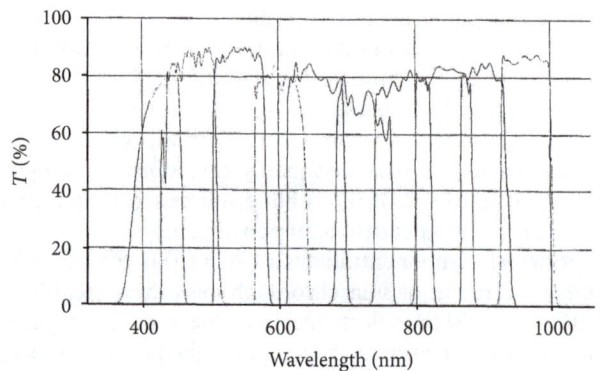

FIGURE 3: Spectral responses of the set of ten CVI Melles Griot interference filters used in the system.

of the illumination. The light source is Lambda LS Xenon Arc (Sutter Instrument, USA). It is a 175-watts light bulb with spectral range from 380 to 1000 nm. The spectral selective device is a filter wheel (Lambda 10-3, model LB10-NW, Sutter Instrument, USA) holding a set of ten interference filters (25 mm diameter) which is placed in front of the light source in the light compartment. Unlike Moncrieff et al. [24] who studied the optimal selection of spectral filters to recover human skin information in the visible range, we consider equally divided filter in both the visible and near-infrared range. The ten medium bandpass interference filters (CVI

Melles Griot, USA) have been chosen from 420 to 960 nm. The full width at half maximum of each filter is 80 nm; there are overlays between the filters to compensate the central wavelength tolerance guarantees by the manufacturer (±16 nm) (see Figure 3). The choice of interference filters for the spectral decomposition is motivated by the large commercial offer available in terms of spectral band and transmittance. The filter wheel controller is commanded by a laptop connected via a USB interface.

Light at specific waveband is transmitted from the illumination system to the back of the hand-held device by a liquid light guide.

The hand-held device is a light opaque device which protects the acquisition from external light; thus, the skin is only illuminated with light at specific wavebands. The device is composed of a wireless trigger, a camera, a lens, and liquid light guide. The extremity of the hand-held device is composed of a nozzle which sets a constant focus distance of 10 cm between the skin area and the camera. The selected camera consists of a 12 bits CMOS digital sensor (Model MV1-D1312I-160-CL, Photonfocus, Switzerland) with a resolution of 1312 × 1082 pixels and extended sensitivity in the visible and near-infrared (370 to 1100 nm). A C-mount magnifying lens (model MeVis-C, Linos, Germany) provides a useful area of 32 × 38 mm with a depth of field of 5 mm, yielding a spatial resolution of 33 pixels·mm^{-1}. After positioning the hand-held device extremity on the skin area under study, the practitioner presses a wireless remote control located in the handle. The pressure triggers the acquisition which is performed in less than two seconds. If the patient is properly installed during the acquisition process, we consider the scene completely static. The system yields ten monoband images which compose one multispectral image. The system is operated using a personal computer running on Windows XP operating system (Microsoft, Seattle, WA, USA). An in-house software, developed using Visual C++ (Microsoft, Seattle, Washington), controls the filter wheel rotation, the image acquisitions, the reflectance cube reconstruction, and the database.

2.1.2. Reflectance Reconstruction.

The interest of ASCLEPIOS system is its capacity to reconstruct reflectance cubes from acquired multispectral images. To ensure reproducibility of the reconstruction, a normalization is performed on each multispectral image [25] before the reconstruction process.

The calibration removes systematic noise introduced through the acquisition chain. Noise might cause distortion to the real reflectance property of skin. The calibration is applied to each monoband image. This specificity is linked to the different exposure time of each monoband image but also because dust or scratch might affect each filter. The corrections assume that the sensor has a linear response.

A raw monoband image can be modelled as follows:

$$[R] = [O] + [U \times S],\tag{1}$$

where $[R]$ is the raw image, $[O]$ is the offset, $[U]$ is the useful signal we want to extract, and $[S]$ is the sensor response. Using the cited modelled, it is necessary to calibrate first the offset noise and then pixel gain.

The offset corresponds to the intensity values that the camera acquires when observing a black target. The offset frame is obtained by averaging multispectral images of a Spectralon gray-scale standard target with 2% reflectance and is denoted $[O]$ in (1) (it is noted O which stands for offset frame). This process sets the zero level of the camera sensor for every monoband image.

The $[S]$ is in most cases characterized by uneven intensities in an image of a uniform surface. This effect is generally caused by nonuniform illumination, blemish on optical elements, difference of sensitivity within the sensor, and

vignetting. Flat-field correction is the technique that removes this effect. Its goal is to compensate any variation within the detector for a given amount of light. The acquisition of flat-field multispectral image is obtained by averaging multispectral image of a spectralon gray-scale standard target with 99% reflectance across the visible and is denoted F and stands for the flat-field image.

The gain correction image is composed of specific coefficient for each pixel of each monoband image. The coefficients are obtained using the following formula:

$$[S] = \frac{[F] - [O]}{\text{DR}},\tag{2}$$

where F is the flat-field monoband image and DR is the dynamic range of the camera. In the case of ASCLEPIOS, DR is equal to 4.096, corresponding to 12 bits images.

The final correction of the raw image is applied using (2):

$$[U] = \frac{[R] - [O]}{[S]}.\tag{3}$$

The cube reconstruction aims to extract only the skin reflectance spectra in each pixel of the data acquired. In order to reconstruct spectra linked to the physical properties of the skin element, the proposed method takes into account a model of light propagation in which the spectral response of all the elements involved in the acquisition process is employed (Figure 4) where $I(\lambda)$ is the spectral radiance of the illuminant, $\Phi_k(\lambda)$ is the spectral transmittance of the kth filter, $r(\lambda)$ is the spectral reflectance of the surface, $o(\lambda)$ is the spectral transmittance of the optical system, $\alpha(\lambda)$ is the spectral sensitivity of the camera and d_k is the acquired image by the kth filter. Such model aims at separating each element of the acquisition chain to only keep the reflectance information $r(\lambda)$.

There exist different methods to solve the inverse problem of spectral reflectance estimation of an object from the camera response. There are pseudoinverse calculus methods and least-squares ones; however, these methods are affected by noise amplification which is the major drawback. Another method is based on the a priori spectral reflectance information from the surface to be imaged. It is this method that we select to perform the reconstruction of reflectance cubes because this technique is robust to noise and moreover it has generalization capabilities, meaning that it can reconstruct a wide range of reflectance spectrum, even ones that it has not learnt.

The reconstruction of reflectance cube is based on an artificial neural network- (ANN) based algorithm proposed by Mansouri et al. [26]. ANN technique is a two-step process, a learning and a reconstruction part. The neural network, employed in the reflectance cube reconstruction, uses heteroassociative memories due to its modularity with regard to the different size of the input and output vectors. The learning step is based on the GretagMacBeth ColorChecker. It is made of 24 patches representing spectra of different colours. The learning step requires the acquisition of a multispectral image for the 24 patches. The ANN generates a coefficient matrix which is obtained upon association of the multispectral image of the patches with their respective known spectral values.

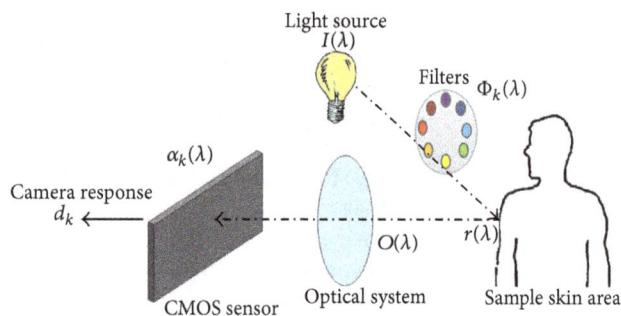

FIGURE 4: Synopsis of the spectral model of the acquisition process in a multispectral imaging system. The decomposition of the spectral model aims to retrieve only the skin reflectance spectrum $r(\lambda)$.

From Figure 4, the reflectance spectra $r(\lambda)$ of each pixel is reconstructed using the camera response $d(\lambda)$ and the result obtained from the ANN learning step (called coefficient matrix). The reconstruction requires a multispectral image as input in order to output a reflectance cube of cutaneous data. The reconstruction provides a 3-dimensional volume (x, y, λ) called a reflectance cube of cutaneous data where x and y represent the spatial dimensions and λ the spectral one [22]. The reconstruction of a reflectance cube is fast and simple as the operation is a product between the coefficient matrix and the camera response. The use of heteroassociative memory allows reconstruction with different wave ranges within the capability (420 to 780 nm) with a current step equal to ten nanometers. The limitation of the 420–780 nm window is a result of the learning protocol which is based on the Gretag MacBeth colorchart. This chart is made for visible light calibration, hence the restriction.

A study involving 150 healthy participants covering five of the six Skin PhotoTypes (SPT) (according to the Fitzpatrick scale) was performed using ASCLEPIOS [27]. Three acquisitions are performed at three different body locations, two facultative skin colour areas and a constitutive skin colour one. Constitutive skin colour is the natural, genetically determined colour of the skin whereas facultative skin colour is skin area affected by the environment (sun, hormones, etc.) resulting in modification of its original appearances over time. The reconstruction validation is performed by comparing data acquired using a commercial spectrophotometer with reflectance cube reconstructed by ASCLEPIOS. The ASCLEPIOS data used for comparison is of the same size and at similar location to that the data acquired by the spectrophotometer. The results reveal that our system reconstructs reflectance cube with an average goodness of fit coefficient (GFC) greater than of 0.997 which, according to Hernández-Andrés et al. [28], considers that the reconstruction is good if the GFC is above 0.99.

2.1.3. *Data Acquisition.* The clinical data were acquired at the Department of Dermatology of Hospital Kuala Lumpur under the supervision of Dr. R. Baba (Head of Dermatology Department) and Hospital Serdang (Malaysia) with the collaboration of Dr. N. Shamsudin during the "Skin Pigmentation Study." The data collection was performed with the collaboration of the Department of Electrical and Electronic Engineering of the University Teknologi Petronas (Malaysia). The research study was registered to the National Medical Research Register which supports the implementation of the National Institute of Health NIH guideline on the conduct of research in the Ministry of Health Malaysia (MOH). We acquired a total of 22 melasma data from 10 patients and a total of 110 vitiligo data from 32 patients.

All skin lesions were assessed by dermatologists. The acquisition process required the patient consent and all procedures were performed following the dermatology guideline.

2.2. *Skin Parameter Map Retrieval.* The interest of the previously reconstructed reflectance cube is the retrieval of skin component parameters from each spatial area by mean of spectral analysis. Analysis of reflectance cubes can provide noninvasive evaluation of skin condition through the 2D mapping of relative meaningful skin chromophore concentrations [29].

As previously mentioned, we propose to extract skin parameter maps by using spectral analysis based on a light propagation model in skin. The presentation of the method is divided into two sections, light propagation model description and genetic algorithm inversion method.

2.2.1. *Light Propagation Model Description.* The developed method for skin parameter maps by spectral analysis is based on a skin model. The structure of human skin can be seen as a three-layer medium: epidermis, dermis, and subcutaneous fat [1]. Several skin models have been developed with various number of skin parameters and different numbers of layers (2 [30], 3 [31], 5 [32], 7 [33], and even 22 layers [34]). However, regardless of the sophistication of the models, the numerous chromophores, and layers composing the skin, it is accepted that the human skin appearance, in terms of colour and reflectance spectrum in the visible domain, is mostly a result of melanin and haemoglobin concentration. Following this assessment, we selected a skin model with two layers, epidermis and dermis. The epidermis layer main component is the melanin [35] while the dermis main component is the haemoglobin. We consider the epidermal thickness to be the effective melanin layer thickness and the dermal thickness as the effective haemoglobin layer thickness. This hypothesis is considered for the entire paper. The physical and optical properties of the epidermis and dermis have been selected from the literature [1, 30, 36–39] and are summarized in Table 1. The lower value of the epidermis thickness aims to take into account the epidermis thinning related to melasma disease [39].

The light propagation model selected in this study is based on Kubelka-Munk (K-M) [40] model. It is originally based on a simple relationship between scattering and absorption coefficient of layers paint and its overall reflectance. The K-M theory describes the radiation transfer in diffuse scattering media by applying energy transport equations. It is a special case of the radiative transfer equation. K-M equations allow

TABLE 1: Five skin parameters used in the retrieval algorithm. The range of each parameter is selected from the literature. The retrieval parameters are bounded to these limits.

Skin parameter	Symbol	Range
Melanin concentration	f_{mel}	1.3 to 45%
Epidermis thickness	D_{epi}	0.01–0.15 mm
Volume fraction of haemoglobin	f_{blood}	0.2–7%
Oxygenated haemoglobin	C_{oxy}	25–90%
Dermis thickness	D_{dermis}	0.6–3 mm

quantitative studies of absorption, scattering, and luminescence in diffuse scattering media. K-M model has been extended to skin analysis by different groups [1, 17, 18, 41].

K-M model has an analytical form and it offers rapid skin optical parameters determination using inversion procedure.

We detail the principle of the Kubelka-Munk model in terms of reflectance and transmittance for a single layer. It is based on the thickness of the layer d_{layer}, the layer absorption coefficient $\mu_{a.layer}$, and the layer scattering coefficient $\mu_{s.layer}$. Both absorption and scattering coefficients are functions of the wavelength.

The equations related the melanin and haemoglobin absorption with the layer absorption coefficient $\mu_{a.layer}$ and the layer scattering coefficient $\mu_{s.layer}$ are detailed, respectively, for the epidermis and the dermis.

The epidermis absorption property is mostly due to the melanin and lightly by the baseline absorption coefficient. The melanin spectral absorption coefficient [42] is approximated by

$$\mu_{a.melanin}(\lambda) = 6.6 \times 10^{11} \lambda^{-3.33} \left[cm^{-1} \right]. \tag{4}$$

The combined absorption of the different negligible skin components (carotene, keratin, and collagen) is taken into account by Jacques which defines an equation for the baseline absorption coefficient free of the major chromophores which is similar for these two layers [42]:

$$\mu_{a.baseline}(\lambda) = 0.244 + 85.3 \exp \frac{-(\lambda - 164)}{66.2} \left[cm^{-1} \right]. \tag{5}$$

For simplification purpose, epidermis and stratum corneum are regarded as a single layer because the stratum corneum light absorption is low and transmits light uniformly in the visible wave range [43].

The optical absorption coefficient of the epidermis $\mu_{a.epidermis}$ is expressed as a function of the wavelength and depends mostly on the volume fraction of melanosome and lightly on the baseline skin absorption coefficient:

$$\mu_{a.epidermis}(\lambda) = f_{mel}\mu_{a.melanin}(\lambda) + (1 - f_{mel})\mu_{a.baseline}(\lambda) \left[cm^{-1} \right], \tag{6}$$

where λ is the wavelength in nanometres and $\mu_{a.melanin}$ is in cm^{-1}. The f_{mel} refers to the concentration of melanin in % and $\mu_{a.baseline}$ is the baseline absorption in cm^{-1}.

In the dermis, the absorption is performed by the main chromophore, the blood [42]. Within the red blood cell, the haemoglobin is a major absorber and it is decomposed into oxyhaemoglobin (HbO_2) and deoxyhaemoglobin (Hb) components. The values of absorption coefficient for the deoxy- and oxyhaemoglobin were obtained from the Oregon Medical Laser Centre website [44]. Oxyhaemoglobin absorption spectra have two absorption peaks at around 542 and 578 nm, revealing the characteristic "W" shape. For this study, blood is considered evenly distributed within the whole dermis layer.

The total haemoglobin absorption spectrum is defined as

$$\mu_{a.blood}(\lambda) = \mu_{a.oxy}(\lambda) + \mu_{a.deoxy}(\lambda) \left[cm^{-1} \right]. \tag{7}$$

The oxygenated haemoglobin can be estimated using the concentration of oxy- and deoxyhaemoglobin by the following equation:

$$R_{SO_2} = \frac{C_{HbO_2}}{C_{HbO_2} + C_{Hb}} [\%]. \tag{8}$$

The dermal absorption coefficient $\mu_{a.dermis}$ is expressed by

$$\mu_{a.dermis}(\lambda) = f_{blood}\left(C_{HbO_2}\mu_{a.oxy}(\lambda)\right)$$
$$+ f_{blood}\left(1 - C_{HbO_2}\right)\mu_{a.deoxy}(\lambda) \tag{9}$$
$$+ \left(1 - f_{blood}\right)\mu_{a.baseline}(\lambda) \left[cm^{-1} \right],$$

where λ is the wavelength in nanometres. f_{blood} is the concentration of haemoglobin in %. C_{HbO_2} is the concentration of oxyhaemoglobin in blood. $\mu_{a.oxy}$ and $\mu_{a.deoxy}$ refer, respectively, to the absorption coefficient of the oxyhaemoglobin and deoxyhaemoglobin in cm^{-1}. $\mu_{a.baseline}$ is the absorption coefficient of the skin baseline in cm^{-1}.

Subcutaneous layer is ignored because its main function is light absorption and mostly contains fat [45] and limited visible light reaches this layer.

The equations to calculate the reflectance R and transmittance T for one layer defined by Kubelka-Munk are expressed by

$$R_{layer}(\lambda) = \left(1 - \beta(\lambda)^2\right)\left(\exp\left(K(\lambda)d_{layer}\right)\right.$$
$$\left. - \exp\left(-K(\lambda)d_{layer}\right)\right)$$
$$\times \left((1 + \beta(\lambda))^2 \exp\left(K(\lambda)d_{layer}\right)\right.$$
$$\left. -(1 - \beta(\lambda))^2 \exp\left(-K(\lambda)d_{layer}\right)\right)^{-1}, \tag{10}$$

$$T_{layer}(\lambda) = 4\beta \times \left((1 + \beta)^2 \exp\left(Kd_{layer}\right)\right.$$
$$\left. -(1 - \beta)^2 \exp\left(-Kd_{layer}\right)\right)^{-1},$$

where K is the backward flux variable of one layer expressed by

$$K_{layer} = \sqrt{k_{layer}\left(k_{layer} + 2 \times s_{layer}\right)}, \tag{11}$$

and β is the forward flux variable of one layer expressed by

$$\beta_{\text{layer}} = \sqrt{\frac{k_{\text{layer}}}{k_{\text{layer}} + 2s_{\text{layer}}}}, \tag{12}$$

where k and s are expressed by

$$k_{\text{layer}} = 2 \times \mu_{a_{\text{layer}}},$$
$$s_{\text{layer}} = 2 \times \mu_{s_{\text{layer}}}. \tag{13}$$

The total reflection of a two-layer medium is defined by the following equation:

$$R_{\text{total}} = R_{\text{L1L2}} = R_1 + \frac{T_{\text{L1}}^2 R_{\text{L2}}}{1 - R_{\text{L1}} R_{\text{L2}}},$$
$$T_{\text{total}} = T_{\text{L1L2}} = \frac{T_{\text{L1}} T_{\text{L2}}}{1 - R_{\text{L1}} R_{\text{L2}}}, \tag{14}$$

where L1 and L2, respectively, refer to the epidermis layer and the dermis layer.

The model allows fast computation of the total reflectance and transmittance of a medium based on the absorption and scattering coefficient and thickness of each layer.

The five biological parameters used to simulate a reflectance spectra can be represented by an input function denoted by

$$p = \left(f_{\text{mel}}, D_{\text{epi}}, f_{\text{blood}}, C_{\text{oxy}}, D_{\text{dermis}} \right). \tag{15}$$

We presented a model of light propagation based on a two-layer skin medium using the Kubelka-Munk theory. The model generates reflectance spectra using five physiological parameters that can vary.

2.2.2. Genetic Algorithm Inversion Method.
From our research, the ASCLEPIOS system provides reflectance spectra. We need to extract information from these spectra. It requires solving an inverse problem to obtain skin parameter concentrations. This inverse problem is nonlinear due to the complex structure, in terms of scattering and absorption properties, of the two-layer skin model.

Inversion procedure aims to retrieve biochemical and optical skin properties from noninvasive measurement. The inversion means to reverse the model of light propagation in which parameters are input to generate a reflectance spectrum. The inversion of our model retrieves the five parameters by matching simulated spectra generated by the model with measured one.

Among the different existing techniques of search and optimization, our interest focused on genetic algorithm (GA) [46]. GA is a metaheuristic method that optimizes a problem through iterative improvement of a candidate solution with a quality measurement. The search of a global solution using GA is done on a population of candidates rather than a single candidate. The strengths of GA are its capacity to explore large search space (through mimic of natural evolution), and

most importantly, its strength against becoming trapped into a local minimum (by introduction of random search).

GA requires a representation of the solution space and a fitness function to evaluate the population of individuals. One individual is defined in real value of the five skin parameters of the K-M model and is bounded by its physical limit defined in Table 1 from the literature. Attempt using GA to retrieve skin parameters of a Monte Carlo for multilayered (MCML) media has been tested by Zhang et al. [47] and a hybrid version of it was developed by Choi [48]. Both prove the usefulness of the GA, but these techniques also retrieve unrealistic values mainly due to the nonconstraint of the search space. In our version, the boundary condition of each element (minimum and maximum parameter values) is restricted to their physical limit. This restriction limits the search space to realistic values. The values are not body-location-dependent to avoid user interaction. This nonrestriction aims to be applied on any data taken wherever on the body, however; this might potentially influence the results. The evolution of the population is roughly based on an iterative three-step process: selection, crossover, and mutation (see Figure 5).

The selection process is determined by a fitness function. It is probably the most important aspect of the genetic algorithm as it requires classifying the best individual which is the most similar to the measured spectrum.

Figure 6 represents the process of the fitness function. The fitness function is applied to every chromosome of the population. The genes of a chromosome are input into the forward KM model to generate a simulated spectrum. The fitness function calculates the similarity between a measured spectrum and a simulated one (using the forward KM model). The calculated fitness value is used to classify the population from the best to worst one for the selection process.

In the search of an optimal fitness function for our GA application, the following five different metric scales have been tested: the root mean squared error (RMSE), the goodness of fit coefficient (GFC), the reconstruction percentage (RecP), the modified spectral angle similarity (MSAS), and the spectral similarity value (SSV).

The first stage of the evolution process is to apply genetic operation to the population t which will generate an intermediate population t' (called mating pool). For the evolution, the population undergoes selection, crossover, and random operations. Then, most of the individuals from the intermediate population will be kept as part of the new population for the next generation. Only few individuals from the intermediate population mutate before being added to the new population.

During the next step of the evolution, the random operator selects individuals from the population and places them in the t' population. The aim of maintaining random individuals is to conserve diversity in the population.

Crossover operation consists of swapping one randomly selected parameter between two randomly chosen parents to generate two offsprings.

The mutation is applied to a low random number of children. The mutation alters randomly one parameter of

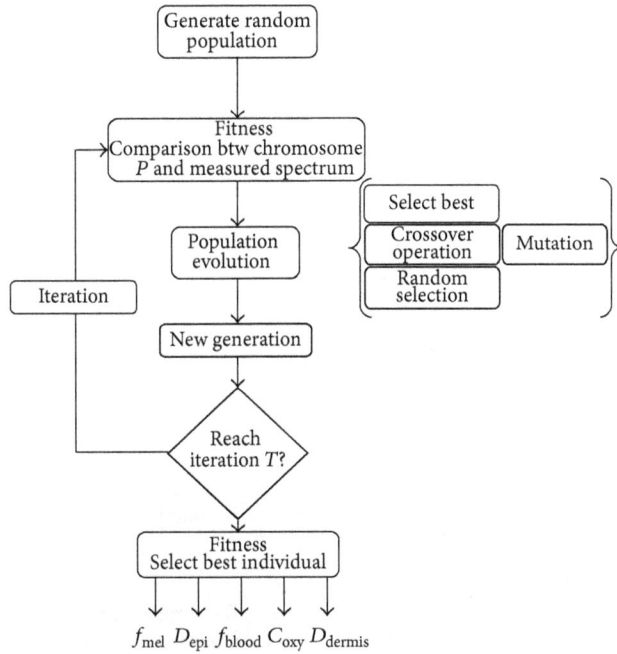

FIGURE 5: GA implementation for the inverse Kubelka-Munk model. GA is based on the evolution of a population, each step is summarized, fitness function to classify the population, population evolution to improve the solution, and parameter retrievals after T iterations.

TABLE 2: GA parameters for Kubelka-Munk inversion model.

Fitness function	RMSE
Population size	100
Termination operator	25 iterations
Best selection nb	5
Random selection nb	25
Crossing nb	30
Mutation nb	2

layer) and dermis (considered as the haemoglobin layer), and the oxygenated haemoglobin. The genetic algorithm routine and the Kubelka-Munk model have been developed on Matlab (The MathWorks, Inc., MA, USA) running on a personal computer running on Windows XP operating system (Microsoft, Seattle, WA, USA).

3. Results and Discussion

Quantitative and objective assessment of skin lesions is critical in the detection of variety of skin conditions. In order to use our method for clinically relevant skin analysis, we first validated our technique using a population of healthy participants and then applied our method to the measurement of parameters from patients with vitiligo or melasma skin lesions. The choice to study these diseases is based on the generic target of the system. These diseases are easily visually assessed by dermatologist with known parameter variation (melanin). Another experiment to validate the oxygenated haemoglobin percentage is performed on healthy participants using images of normal tissue and tissue with temporary induced ischemia.

3.1. Healthy Data Analysis. We present the results of our method based on participants from a healthy population and compare the results obtained with data from the literature.

The volume fraction of melanosome increases with the SPT type which is in accordance with the literature [33, 45, 49]. Currently, the only method to classify and compare our system is the relation between SPT and melanin concentration in skin and relation between healthy skin and skin with temporary induced ischemia.

The data for our method of skin parameters retrieval are the same as the data used for the validation of the reflectance cube reconstruction [27].

For each reflectance cube, the distribution of the skin is fairly uniform as the data were taken from healthy patient and care was taken to acquire with no visible lesions or nevus. The parameter estimation was performed on every reflectance cube. The average value of each parameter was calculated for each entire retrieved map because of low disparity within values of each map.

The aim of this test is to corroborate the skin parameter values/concentration from the literature with the parameters retrieved using our method on skin sample from various SPT.

Our results, presented by body location, show the different retrieved parameters for different SPT in Tables 3, 4, and 5.

the child chromosome by generating a new random value for the parameter.

There are different criteria to stop the evolution of the algorithm. Due to the difficulty to reach a specific fitness function value for different spectra, the termination criterion is chosen as a number of iterations. This technique has the advantage of setting a finite computation time for the algorithm and, if properly selected, one can reach optimum result. However, at the final iteration, the algorithm may not have yet converged.

As there is no golden rule to define the value of the different parameters of the GA, the selection was performed empirically through series of tests. The final parameters of our proposed genetic algorithm are detailed in Table 2. RMSE was selected because it performed better than four other metrics (reconstruction percentage, goodness of fit coefficient, modified spectral angle similarity, and spectral similarity value) tested in the optimization process of the GA.

The proposed method of combining Kubelka-Munk model (with a layered skin structure) with GA optimization can retrieve accurately simulated skin parameters as suggested by the results. The accuracy is defined by the retrieval error of two characteristic sets of parameters (one lightly and one darkly pigmented skin) with a white Gaussian noise with amplitude of ± 0.1 added to the simulated spectra. The accuracy test was performed ten times and averaged. The average root mean squared error of the fitness function is 0.25×10^{-5} with an average error of less than 1.5 percent for each parameter. This algorithm outputs the concentration of melanin, the concentration of haemoglobin, the thickness of both epidermis (considered as the melanin

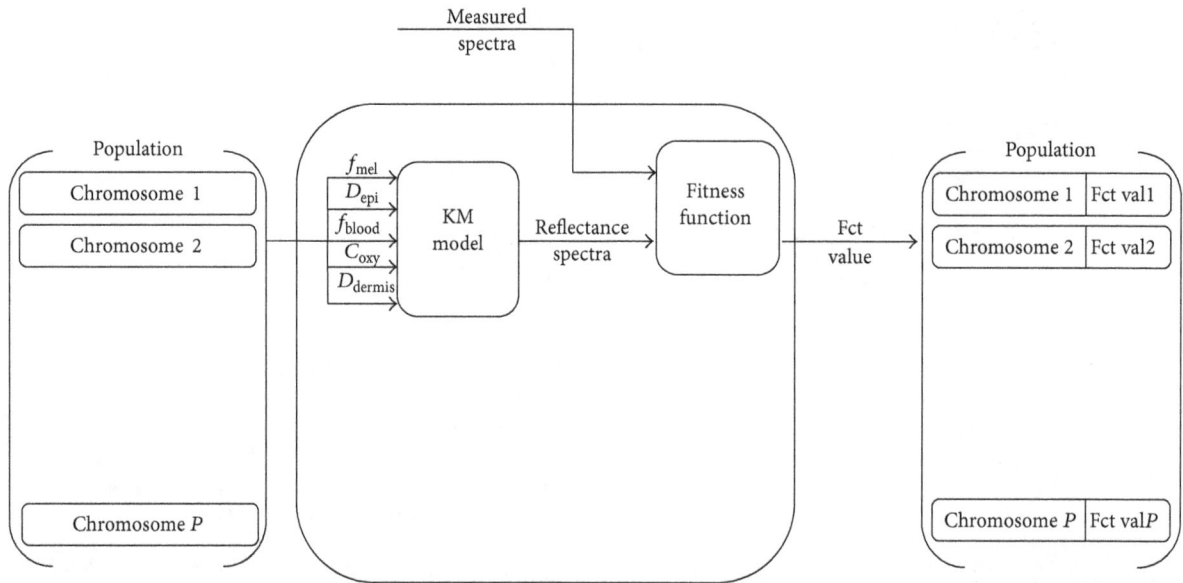

FIGURE 6: GA fitness function GA. Each chromosome of the population is used to simulate a reflectance spectrum. The simulated reflectance spectrum is compared with the measured one. The fitness function outputs a value corresponding based on the similarity between the two spectra. The fitness value is then used to classify the population.

The results are fairly consistent with the finding of Robertson and Rees [50] which reveal a thicker epidermis layer for the back of the hand which agrees with our retrieved parameters. We considered their upper back values to compare to our lower back measurement. The decrease of thickness measured by reflectance confocal microscopy (RCM) again matches the decrease of thickness calculated by our method. The major difference between the body locations is found for the melanin content of the back of the hand which is twice the one of face and lower back for SPT II, III, but the trends, while slightly lower, are similar for the remaining SPT. The oxygenated haemoglobin variation between skin types II and IV can be mostly noticed for the face and back location. This effect may be linked to the increase of melanin concentration. As the melanin concentration increases, the characteristic "W" shape of the oxygenated haemoglobin is more difficult to notice on the skin reflectance spectrum. The oxygenated haemoglobin algorithm estimation might be affected when there is a high concentration of melanin, hence the difference in the results. Also the overall values of oxygenated haemoglobin are on average 20% lower than the one reported by Zonios et al. [10] but similar to the one from Tseng et al. [51]. The difference may be a result of the interrogation depth limit of our system and requires further investigations. The volume fraction of haemoglobin is very low for SPT VI compared to other skin types; this might be a limitation of the system. It seems to be affected by the low variation of the reflectance spectrum for SPT VI. The accuracy of the method may need to be improved for this specific phototype. A possible solution to overcome this limitation is to select specific spectrum range (possibly around the characteristic "W" shape) to increase its accuracy. Further investigation is required to analyze the variation of the volume fraction of haemoglobin for the back site.

Other parameters are not significantly different between the different body locations. The model seems to be affected by the relative flat spectrum of SPT VI, especially with regard to the dermis thickness and volume fraction of haemoglobin. Further validations of the model are required. First, using ultrasound technology, the determination of the accuracy of the layer thicknesses may be verified.

3.2. Melasma and Vitiligo Data Analysis. We applied our method to quantify and compare data acquired from two populations with skin diseases that have characteristic effect on the melanin composition.

Melasma (also called chloasma) is a hyperpigmentation skin disease that is characterized by an increase level of melanin concentration released by melanocytes. The symptoms are characterized by dark, irregular, and well-demarcated skin lesions.

Vitiligo (also called leukoderma) is a common genetic autoimmune skin disease caused by the disappearance of melanocytes in the epidermis resulting in hypopigmentation. The symptom of vitiligo is the depigmentation of patches of skin with irregular shape.

All multispectral images acquired contain both healthy and hypo/hyperpigmented skin area. Every reflectance cube was analyzed using our method, generating five skin parameter maps. The average parameter values are obtained from the two different areas (healthy and diseased) which are manually selected on each map. The relative difference between healthy and hypo/hyperpigmented skin area is calculated by the following formula:

$$R_{\text{diff}} = \frac{\text{Val}_{\text{ref}}}{\text{Val}_{\text{measured}}}, \quad (16)$$

TABLE 3: Hand parameters estimation for SPT II, III, IV, V, and VI.

Hand	f_{mel}	STD	D_{epi}	STD	f_{blood}	STD	C_{oxy}	STD	D_{dermis}	STD
SPT II	10.1	0.66	0.0133	0.0002	1.1	0.04	30.2	0.17	1.06	0.018
SPT III	18.7	1.17	0.0139	0.0002	1.2	0.044	29.7	0.227	1.10	0.018
SPT IV	26.5	1.15	0.0158	0.0003	1.1	0.032	28.9	0.218	1.26	0.025
SPT V	35.8	0.98	0.0176	0.0002	1.1	0.035	28.7	0.120	1.35	0.023
SPT VI	44.7	0.26	0.0202	0.0001	0.6	0.026	31.3	0.571	2.22	0.058

STD: standard deviation. f_{mel} is the volume fraction of melanosome in %, D_{epi} is the epidermis thickness in mm, f_{blood} is the volume fraction of hemoglobin in %, C_{oxy} is the oxygenated haemoglobin in %, and D_{dermis} is the dermis thickness in mm.

TABLE 4: Face parameters estimation for SPT II, III, IV, V, and VI.

Face	f_{mel}	STD	D_{epi}	STD	f_{blood}	STD	C_{oxy}	STD	D_{dermis} (mm)	STD
SPT II	5.8	0.53	0.0116	0.0003	1.2	0.04	49.1	0.20	0.91	0.011
SPT III	7.5	0.52	0.0121	0.0001	1.3	0.046	40.9	0.167	0.10	0.002
SPT IV	15.5	0.95	0.0140	0.0002	1.4	0.054	31.1	0.689	1.08	0.029
SPT V	29.1	0.11	0.0159	0.0003	1.4	0.049	29.1	0.178	1.15	0.025
SPT VI	41.1	0.55	0.0199	0.0002	0.7	0.035	31.0	0.582	1.91	0.057

STD: standard deviation. f_{mel} is the volume fraction of melanosome in %, D_{epi} is the epidermis thickness in mm, f_{blood} is the volume fraction of haemoglobin in %, C_{oxy} is the oxygenated haemoglobin in %, and D_{dermis} is the dermis thickness in mm.

TABLE 5: Back parameters estimation for SPT II, III, IV, V, and VI.

Back	f_{mel}	STD	D_{epi}	STD	f_{blood}	STD	C_{oxy}	STD	D_{dermis}	STD
SPT II	5.3	0.06	0.0115	0.0002	0.5	0.03	46.9	0.15	0.90	0.008
SPT III	5.2	0.44	0.0118	0.0002	0.9	0.057	44.8	0.194	0.91	0.009
SPT IV	15.5	0.93	0.0138	0.0003	1.2	0.039	32.3	0.836	1.02	0.021
SPT V	33.9	0.94	0.0164	0.0003	1.2	0.046	29.6	0.269	1.13	0.022
SPT VI	43.4	0.18	0.0209	0.0001	0.7	0.031	31.0	0.430	1.87	0.058

STD: standard deviation. f_{mel} is the volume fraction of melanosome in %, D_{epi} is the epidermis thickness in mm, f_{blood} is the volume fraction of haemoglobin in %, C_{oxy} is the oxygenated haemoglobin in %, and D_{dermis} is the dermis thickness in mm.

where Val_{ref} is the retrieved healthy skin parameter value and $Val_{measured}$ is the retrieved hypo/hyperpigmented skin parameter value. The R_{diff} represents the relative change between two values. This measure is unitless.

Tables 6 and 7 summarize the difference of parameters between healthy and disease affected reflectance spectra. Melasma lesions show that the melanin volume is 2.05 higher than the healthy skin. Vitiligo lesions reveal a decrease by around four of the melanin concentration. The variation of the other parameters (epidermis and dermis thickness, haemoglobin concentration, and oxygenated haemoglobin) is not significant.

The standard deviations of the average melanin difference for both melasma and vitiligo are high. This is a result of the inclusion of all types of vitiligo (mild to severe) and all SPT types. For SPT II and III, the difference between melasma and healthy skin is very high, sometimes with a relative difference of 4, whereas for SPT V and VI, the relative difference is around 1.3 to 1.5 as the original melanin concentration is already high.

Figure 7 presents the results of the five parameters retrieved using our method on a vitiligo lesion. The melanin map is clearly affected in the area of vitiligo lesions (fair

TABLE 6: Average difference between melasma and healthy skin.

Parameter	Relative difference	STD
Melanin	2.06	0.097
Epidermis thickness	1.12	0.016
Haemoglobin concentration	1.18	0.037
Oxygenated haemoglobin	0.92	0.012
Dermis thickness	1.09	0.041

STD: standard deviation.

TABLE 7: Average difference between vitiligo and healthy skin.

Parameter	Relative difference	STD
Melanin	0.27	0.026
Epidermis thickness	0.95	0.043
Haemoglobin concentration	1.05	0.109
Oxygenated haemoglobin	1.07	0.030
Dermis thickness	1.06	0.062

STD: standard deviation.

patch on the subfigure (a)). In order to highlight the interest of the result obtained by the proposed method, the image size has been reduced to speed up the computation time.

TABLE 8: Mean parameters estimation for the data acquired on 4 healthy volunteers.

Mean 4 volunteers	f_{mel}	STD	D_{epi}	STD	f_{blood}	STD	C_{oxy}	STD	D_{dermis}	STD
Acquisition 1	13.3	0.08	0.0149	0.0001	1.6	0.004	71.9	0.15	1.02	0.018
Acquisition 2	14.2	0.08	0.0145	0.0002	2.8	0.008	55.4	0.194	1.01	0.013
Acquisition 3	13.5	0.05	0.0143	0.0002	1.7	0.005	76.7	0.836	1.01	0.022

SD: standard deviation. f_{mel} is the volume fraction of melanosome in %, D_{epi} is the epidermis thickness in mm, f_{blood} is the volume fraction of haemoglobin in %, C_{oxy} is the oxygenated hemoglobin in %, and D_{dermis} is the dermis thickness in mm.

TABLE 9: Percentage of difference between baseline acquisition (Acq1) and before occlusion release (Acq2) and one minute after release for the 5 parameters (Acq3) for the average data acquired on 4 healthy volunteers.

Percentage of difference	f_{mel}	D_{epi}	f_{blood}	C_{oxy}	D_{dermis}
Between Acq1 and Acq2	6.7	−2.6	75	−22.9	0.98
Between Acq1 and Acq3	1.5	−4.0	6.25	6.6	0.98

f_{mel} is the volume fraction of melanosome, D_{epi} is the epidermis thickness, f_{blood} is the volume fraction of haemoglobin, C_{oxy} is the oxygenated haemoglobin, and D_{dermis} is the dermis thickness.

It is to be noted that the code has not been optimized as the aim is to show the relevance of the method for skin analysis. The variation of epidermis/dermis thickness, haemoglobin concentration, and oxygenated haemoglobin parameters is only of around 10% which we do not consider to be characteristic for melasma and vitiligo diseases. This finding is consistent with the medical expectation which states that vitiligo only modifies the melanin content of the skin. As previously noted for healthy data, a difference of dermis thickness is observed between the different SPTs which does not correspond to a histological characteristic as SPT difference is due to a change of melanin concentration. The algorithm seems to retrieve dermis thickness closely related to the melanin concentration. This is particularly noticeable for a specific lesion (Figure 7) where the cross-correlation between the melanin concentration map and the dermis thickness map is 0.41. The algorithm might be affected by the limited information in the NIR to accurately retrieve dermis thickness in some case meaning a possible crosstalk in the model. This will be investigated further by adding layer to the model to try to decorrelate these parameters.

3.3. Temporary Induced Ischemia Data Analysis.
The experiment aims to induce temporary ischemia to the lower arms part of healthy volunteers. Ischemia is defined as a restriction in blood supply to tissues, leading to a decrease of oxygen (and glucose).

The protocol for this experiment involves three acquisitions and is performed as followed. The first acquisition is a baseline data acquired with the subject at rest for 5 minutes. Temporary induced ischemia is simulated by inflating a pressure cuff to the participant left upper arm. The pressure cuff blocks the blood flow and is maintained for two minutes before performing the second acquisition. This aims to record ischemia. Finally, the third acquisition is taken one minute after reperfusion (release of the cuff pressure).

The three multispectral images of the lower inner arm, acquired during the experiment, are reconstructed into reflectance cube and analyzed by the previously defined algorithm.

The data were acquired on four healthy volunteers. The data are processed by the algorithm and the average parameter values are obtained from identical areas manually selected on each map.

Table 8 presents the average retrieved skin parameters for the four healthy volunteers. The values of melanin concentration, epidermis thickness, and dermis thickness do not show significant variation between the three acquisitions. The occlusion does not have effect on these parameters, which is the result expected.

The percentage of difference between the baseline and acquisition 2 and acquisition 3 is calculated by the following formula:

$$P_{diff} = \frac{\left(Val_{Acq} - Val_{Baseline}\right)}{Val_{Baseline}}, \tag{17}$$

where Val_{Acq} is the retrieved skin parameter value for acquisition (either number 2 or 3) and $Val_{Baseline}$ is the retrieved baseline skin parameter value. The P_{diff} represents the percentage change between two values. This measure is in percentage. It aims to facilitate comparison with data from the literature.

The occlusion effect (see Table 9) shows an increase in volume fraction of haemoglobin and a decrease in oxygenated haemoglobin concentration compared to baseline. It is consistent with finding by Vogel et al. [29] and the decreased value of oxygenated haemoglobin of 22.7% is similar to the decrease reported by Zuzak et al. [52] (20.3%).

The retrieve values of both oxygenated blood concentration and volume of blood fraction for the third acquisition compared to baseline reveal only a slight increase (+6%). This potentially means that one minute after the release of the pressure cuff, the hyperemia (increase of blood flow and oxygenated haemoglobin) is nearly over and that the tissues are returning to homeostasis.

The temporary induced ischemia experiment demonstrates the potential of our system to record oxygenated haemoglobin and volume fraction of haemoglobin. Further studies might be required to fully assess the applicability

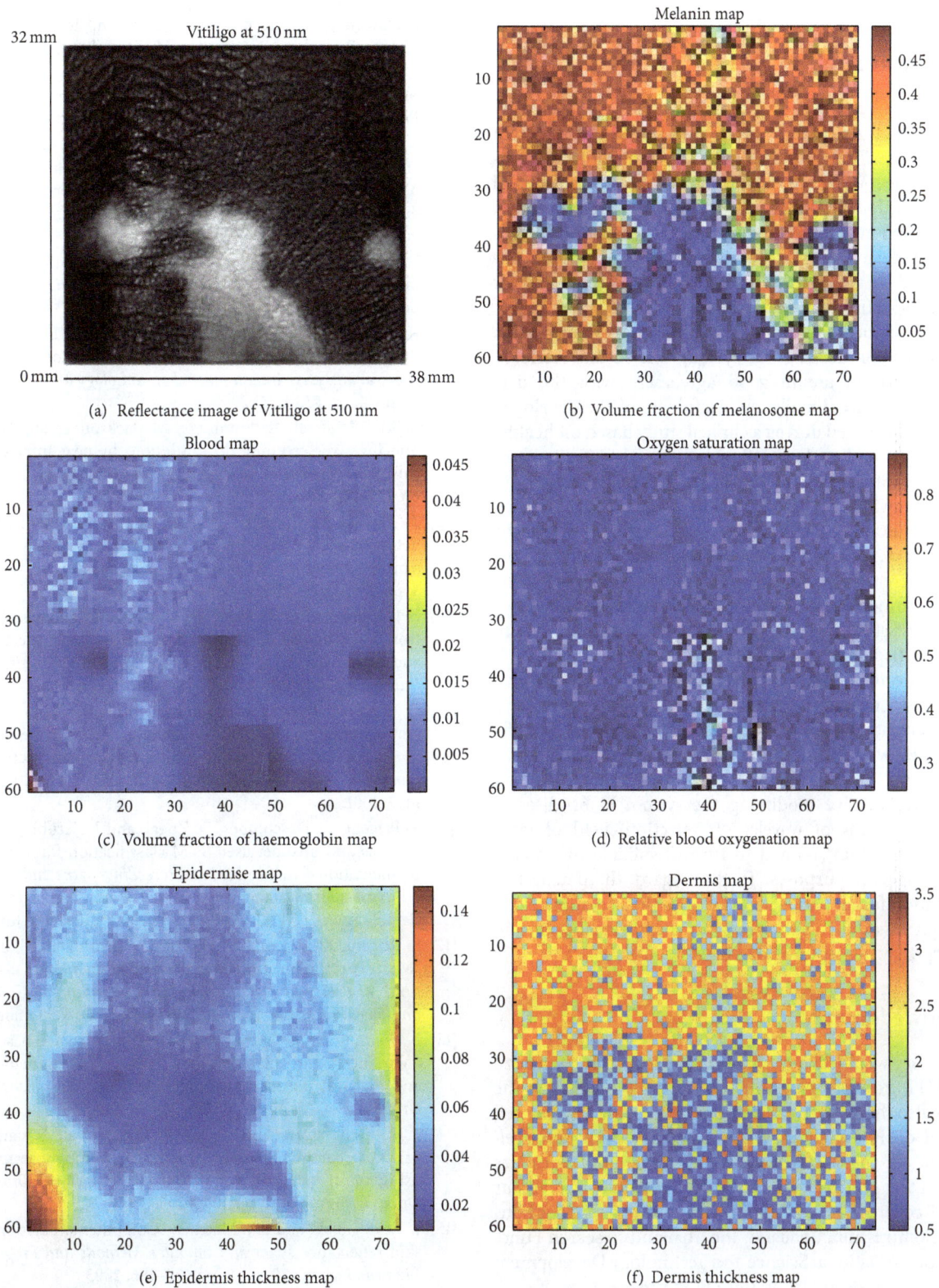

(a) Reflectance image of Vitiligo at 510 nm

(b) Volume fraction of melanosome map

(c) Volume fraction of haemoglobin map

(d) Relative blood oxygenation map

(e) Epidermis thickness map

(f) Dermis thickness map

FIGURE 7: A set of six subfigures composed of one reflectance image of vitiligo at 510 nm from the back of the left hand (a), volume fraction of melanosome map (b), volume fraction of haemoglobin map (c), oxygenated hemoglobin map (d), epidermis thickness map (e) and dermis thickness map (f). The subfigure (a) has been contrast enhanced for better viewing purpose only.

and accuracy of our system for both dermatological and cosmetological applications.

4. Conclusion

We presented a multispectral camera which has the capacity to reconstruct reflectance cubes only linked to the skin characteristics. The reflectance cube allows quantitative measure of cutaneous tissue based on a Kubelka-Munk model combined with evolutionary algorithm. Using this approach, quantification maps of five skin parameters (melanin concentration, epidermis/dermis thickness, haemoglobin concentration, and the oxygenated haemoglobin) are obtained for each multispectral image acquired.

The developed algorithm was tested on a set of healthy skin data acquired using our system. The results retrieved by the algorithm are in good agreement with the data from the literature. Finally, the usefulness of the developed technique was tested during a clinical study based on healthy skin, vitiligo, and melasma skin lesions. The results show that our research method can retrieve skin parameters in accordance with the expected skin composition for each lesion. For example, with regard to the vitiligo, where the main characteristic is a lack of melanin, the method clearly shows a decrease in melanin concentration. In the case of the melasma, some promising results are also obtained.

The first step consisting in developing a generic system for the multispectral analysis of skin data has been achieved. Because the first tests give promising results, our in vivo imaging system may be useful for prospective study for a use in dermatological and cosmetological studies. Specific pathologies with strong socioeconomic impacts could be chosen to reveal possible lesion spectral signature. The work perspectives involve modifying the system to be disease-specific (in terms of wavelength selection, field of view, contact/noncontact ...) and to further validate the system for these specific purposes. To that regard, the perspective of validation for all parameters includes the use of histology (although it is difficult to set up) or measurements of skin layer depth by ultrasound imaging system.

Acknowledgments

The authors would like to thank Professor M. H. A. Fadzil from UTP for his collaboration on this research. The authors also thank the financial support provided by Conseil Régional de Bourgogne, France, Fond Européen de Développement Régional (FEDER), France, the ministères des Affaires Étrangères (MAE) et de l'Enseignement Supérieur et de la Recherche (MESR), France, the Office of Higher Education Commission, Thailand, the Thailand Research Fund, Thailand, the National Science and Technology Development Agency, Thailand, and laboratoire Bioderma, France.

References

[1] R. Anderson, J. Hu, and J. Parrish, "Optical radiation transfer in the human skin and applications in in vivo remittance spectroscopy," in Bioengineering and the Skin, 28, MTP Press Limited, 1981.

[2] J. Dowling, "Retinal processing of vision," in Comprehensive Human Physiology, R. Greger and U. Windhorst, Eds., pp. 773–788, Springer, New York, NY, USA, 1996.

[3] M. H. Rowe, "Trichromatic color vision in primates," News in Physiological Sciences, vol. 17, no. 3, pp. 93–98, 2002.

[4] K. S. Nehal, S. A. Oliveria, A. A. Marghoob et al., "Use of and beliefs about baseline photography in the management of patients with pigmented lesions: a survey of dermatology residency programmes in the United States," Melanoma Research, vol. 12, no. 2, pp. 161–167, 2002.

[5] S. Kingman, "Growing awareness of skin disease starts flurry of initiatives," Bulletin of the World Health Organization, vol. 83, no. 12, pp. 891–892, 2005.

[6] R. Pushkarna, S. K. Bhargava, M. C. Baruah, S. Mohanty, and N. Pushkarna, "Evaluation of skin lesions with color Doppler and spectral analysis," Indian Journal of Radiology and Imaging, vol. 10, no. 4, pp. 233–236, 2000.

[7] L. M. Mcintosh, R. Summers, M. Jackson et al., "Towards non-invasive screening of skin lesions by near-infrared spectroscopy," Journal of Investigative Dermatology, vol. 116, no. 1, pp. 175–181, 2001.

[8] S. Tomatis, M. Carrara, A. Bono et al., "Automated melanoma detection with a novel multispectral imaging system: results of a prospective study," Physics in Medicine and Biology, vol. 50, no. 8, pp. 1675–1687, 2005.

[9] I. J. Bigio and J. R. Mourant, "Ultraviolet and visible spectroscopies for tissue diagnostics: fluorescence spectroscopy and elastic-scattering spectroscopy," Physics in Medicine and Biology, vol. 42, no. 5, pp. 803–814, 1997.

[10] G. Zonios, J. Bykowski, and N. Kollias, "Skin melanin, hemoglobin, and light scattering properties can be quantitatively assessed in vivo using diffuse reflectance spectroscopy," Journal of Investigative Dermatology, vol. 117, no. 6, pp. 1452–1457, 2001.

[11] S. Prigent, X. Descombes, D. Zugaj, and J. Zerubia, "Spectral analysis and unsupervised SVM classification for skin hyper-pigmentation classification," in Proceedings of the 2nd Workshop on Hyperspectral Image and Signal Processing: Evolution in Remote Sensing (WHISPERS '10), Reykjavik, Iceland, June 2010.

[12] S. Prigent, X. Descombes, D. Zugaj, P. Martel, and J. Zerubia, "Multi-spectral image analysis for skin pigmentation classification," in Proceedings of the 17th IEEE International Conference on Image Processing (ICIP '10), pp. 3641–3644, September 2010.

[13] N. Tsumura, N. Ojima, K. Sato et al., "Image-based skin color and texture analysis/synthesis by extracting hemoglobin and melanin information in the skin," ACM Transaction on Graphics, vol. 22, no. 3, pp. 770–779, 2003.

[14] J. M. Kainerstorfer, J. D. Riley, M. Ehler et al., "Quantitative principal component model for skin chromophore mapping using multi-spectral images and spatial priors," Biomedical Optics Express, vol. 2, pp. 1040–1058, 2011.

[15] I. V. Meglinski and S. J. Matcher, "Computer simulation of the skin reflectance spectra," Computer Methods and Programs in Biomedicine, vol. 70, no. 2, pp. 179–186, 2003.

[16] T. Shi and C. A. Dimarzio, "Multispectral method for skin imaging development and validation," Applied Optics, vol. 46, no. 3, pp. 8619–8626, 2007.

[17] T. Igarashi, K. Nishino, and S. K. Nayar, "The appearance of human skin: a survey," Foundations and Trends in Computer Graphics and Vision, vol. 3, no. 1, pp. 1–95, 2007.

[18] A. Krishnaswamy and G. V. G. Baranoski, "A biophysically-based spectral model of light interaction with human skin," *Computer Graphics Forum*, vol. 23, no. 3, pp. 331–340, 2004.

[19] G. N. Stamatas, B. Z. Zmudzka, N. Kollias, and J. Z. Beer, "In vivo measurement of skin erythema and pigmentation: new means of implementation of diffuse reflectance spectroscopy with a commercial instrument," *British Journal of Dermatology*, vol. 159, no. 3, pp. 683–690, 2008.

[20] D. Yudovsky, M. S. Nouvong, and L. Pilon, "Foot technology, part 2 of 2 hyperspectal imaging in diabethic foot wound care," *Journal of Diabetes Science and Technology*, vol. 4, no. 5, pp. 1099–1113, 2000.

[21] M. Moncrieff, S. Cotton, E. Claridge, and P. Hall, "Spectrophotometric intracutaneous analysis a new technique for imaging pigmented skin lesions," *British Journal of Dermatology*, vol. 146, no. 3, pp. 448–457, 2002.

[22] R. Jolivot, P. Vabres, and F. Marzani, "Reconstruction of hyperspectral cutaneous data from an artificial neural network-based multispectral imaging system," *Computerized Medical Imaging and Graphics*, vol. 35, no. 2, pp. 85–88, 2011.

[23] J. Y. Hardeberg, "Color management: principles and solutions," *NORsignalets*, vol. 3, pp. 6–12, 1999.

[24] S. J. Preece and E. Claridge, "Spectral filter optimization for the recovery of parameters which describe human skin," *IEEE Transaction on Pattern Analysis and Machine Intelligence*, vol. 26, no. 7, pp. 913–922, 2004.

[25] R. Jolivot, P. Vabres, and F. Marzani, "Calibration of multispectral imaging system applied to dermatology," in *Proceedings of the E-MEDISYS*, Fez, Morocco, January 2010.

[26] A. Mansouri, F. S. Marzani, and P. Gouton, "Neural networks in two cascade algorithms for spectral reflectance reconstruction," in *Proceedings of the IEEE International Conference on Image Processing (ICIP '05)*, pp. 718–721, September 2005.

[27] R. Jolivot, H. Nugroho, P. Vabres, M. H. Ahmad Fadzil, and F. Marzani, "Validation of a 2D multispectral camera: application to dermatology/cosmetology on a population covering five skin phototypes," in *Clinical and Biomedical Spectroscopy and Imaging*, vol. 8087 of *Proceedings of SPIE*, May 2011.

[28] J. Hernández-Andrés, J. Romero, and R. L. Lee Jr., "Colorimetric and spectroradiometric characteristics of narrow-field-of-view clear skylight in Granada, Spain," *Journal of the Optical Society of America A*, vol. 18, no. 2, pp. 412–420, 2001.

[29] A. Vogel, V. V. Chernomordik, J. D. Riley et al., "Using non-invasive multispectral imaging to quantitatively assess tissue vasculature," *Journal of Biomedical Optics*, vol. 12, no. 5, Article ID 051604, 2007.

[30] A. D. Kim and M. Moscoso, "Light transport in two-layer tissues," *Journal of Biomedical Optics*, vol. 10, no. 3, Article ID 034015, 2005.

[31] L. O. Svaasand, L. T. Norvang, E. J. Fiskerstrand, E. K. S. Stopps, M. W. Berns, and J. S. Nelson, "Tissue parameters determining the visual appearance of normal skin and port-wine stains," *Lasers in Medical Science*, vol. 10, no. 1, pp. 55–65, 1995.

[32] L. F. A. Douven and G. W. Lucassen, "Retrieval of optical properties of skin from measurement and modeling the diffuse reectance," *Laser-Tissue Interaction*, vol. 3914, no. 1, pp. 312–323, 2000.

[33] I. V. Meglinski and S. J. Matcher, "Quantitative assessment of skin layers absorption and skin reflectance spectra simulation in the visible and near-infrared spectral regions," *Physiological Measurement*, vol. 23, no. 4, pp. 741–753, 2002.

[34] C. Magnain, M. Elias, and J.-M. Frigerio, "Skin color modeling using the radiative transfer equation solved by the auxiliary function method: inverse problem," *Journal of the Optical Society of America A*, vol. 25, no. 7, pp. 1737–1743, 2008.

[35] L. T. Norvang, T. E. Milner, J. S. Nelson, M. W. Berns, and L. O. Svaasand, "Skin pigmentation characterized by visible reflectance measurements," *Lasers in Medical Science*, vol. 12, no. 2, pp. 99–112, 1997.

[36] S. L. Jacques and D. J. McAuliffe, "The melanosome: threshold temperature for explosive vaporization and internal absorption coefficient during pulsed laser irradiation," *Photochemistry and Photobiology*, vol. 53, no. 6, pp. 769–775, 1991.

[37] M. Doi and S. Tominaga, "Spectral estimation of human skin color using the Kubelka-Munk theory," in *Color Imaging VIII: Processing, Hardcopy, and Applications*, vol. 5008 of *Proceedings of SPIE*, pp. 221–228, January 2003.

[38] I. V. Meglinsky and S. J. Matcher, "Modelling the sampling volume for skin blood oxygenation measurements," *Medical and Biological Engineering and Computing*, vol. 39, no. 1, pp. 44–50, 2001.

[39] R. Hernández-Barrera, B. Torres-Alvarez, J. P. Castanedo-Cazares, C. Oros-Ovalle, and B. Moncada, "Solar elastosis and presence of mast cells as key features in the pathogenesis of melasma," *Clinical and Experimental Dermatology*, vol. 33, no. 3, pp. 305–308, 2008.

[40] P. Kubelka and F. Munk, "Ein beitrag zur optik der far-banstriche," *Zeitschrift für Technische Physik*, vol. 12, p. 543, 1931.

[41] S. Cotton, "A noninvasive skin imaging system," Tech. Rep. CSR-97-3, University of Birmingham School of Computer Science, 1997.

[42] S. L. Jacques, *Skin Optics*, Oregon Medical Laser Center News, 1998.

[43] R. R. Anderson and J. A. Parrish, "The optics of human skin," *Journal of Investigative Dermatology*, vol. 77, no. 1, pp. 13–19, 1981.

[44] S. A. Prahl, "Optical absorption of hemoglobin," 1999, http://omlc.ogi.edu/spectra/hemoglobin/.

[45] M. Shimada, Y. Yamada, M. Itoh, and T. Yatagai, "Melanin and blood concentration in a human skin model studied by multiple regression analysis: assessment by Monte Carlo simulation," *Physics in Medicine and Biology*, vol. 46, no. 9, pp. 2397–2406, 2001.

[46] J. H. Holland, *Adaptation in Natural and Artificial Systems*, University of Michigan Press, Ann Arbor, Mich, USA, 1975.

[47] R. Zhang, W. Verkruysse, B. Choi et al., "Determination of human skin optical properties from spectrophotometric measurements based on optimization by genetic algorithms," *Journal of Biomedical Optics*, vol. 10, no. 2, Article ID 024030, 2005.

[48] S. H. Choi, "Fast and robust extraction of optical and morphological properties of human skin using a hybrid stochastic-deterministic algorithm: Monte-Carlo simulation study," *Lasers in Medical Science*, vol. 25, no. 5, pp. 733–741, 2010.

[49] R. Anderson and J. Parrish, *The Science of Photomedicine, Chapter 6; Optical Properties of Human Skin*, Plenum Press, 1982.

[50] K. Robertson and J. L. Rees, "Variation in epidermal morphology in human skin at different body sites as measured by reflectance confocal microscopy," *Acta Dermato-Venereologica*, vol. 90, no. 4, pp. 368–373, 2010.

[51] S.-H. Tseng, C.-H. Hsu, and J. Yu-Yun Lee, "Noninvasive evaluation of collagen and hemoglobin contents and scattering

property of in vivo keloid scars and normal skin using diffuse reectance spectroscopy: pilot study," *Journal of Biomedical Optics*, vol. 17, no. 7, Article ID 077005, 2012.

[52] K. J. Zuzak, M. D. Schaeberle, E. N. Lewis, and I. W. Levin, "Visible reflectance hyperspectral imaging: characterization of a noninvasive, in vivo system for determining tissue perfusion," *Analytical Chemistry*, vol. 74, pp. 2021–2028, 2002.

23

Automatic Extraction of Blood Vessels in the Retinal Vascular Tree Using Multiscale Medialness

Mariem Ben Abdallah,[1] **Jihene Malek,**[1] **Ahmad Taher Azar,**[2] **Philippe Montesinos,**[3] **Hafedh Belmabrouk,**[1] **Julio Esclarín Monreal,**[4] **and Karl Krissian**[4]

[1]*Faculty of Sciences, Electronics and Microelectronics Laboratory, Monastir University, 5019 Monastir, Tunisia*
[2]*Faculty of Computers and Information, Benha University, Benha 13511, Egypt*
[3]*Institute of Mines and Ales, Laboratory of Computer and Production Engineering, 30319 Alès, France*
[4]*Imaging Technology Center (CTIM), Las Palmas-Gran Canaria University, 35017 Las Palmas de Gran Canaria, Spain*

Correspondence should be addressed to Mariem Ben Abdallah; mariembenabdallah3@gmail.com

Academic Editor: Karen Panetta

We propose an algorithm for vessel extraction in retinal images. The first step consists of applying anisotropic diffusion filtering in the initial vessel network in order to restore disconnected vessel lines and eliminate noisy lines. In the second step, a multiscale line-tracking procedure allows detecting all vessels having similar dimensions at a chosen scale. Computing the individual image maps requires different steps. First, a number of points are preselected using the eigenvalues of the Hessian matrix. These points are expected to be near to a vessel axis. Then, for each preselected point, the response map is computed from gradient information of the image at the current scale. Finally, the multiscale image map is derived after combining the individual image maps at different scales (sizes). Two publicly available datasets have been used to test the performance of the suggested method. The main dataset is the STARE project's dataset and the second one is the DRIVE dataset. The experimental results, applied on the STARE dataset, show a maximum accuracy average of around 94.02%. Also, when performed on the DRIVE database, the maximum accuracy average reaches 91.55%.

1. Introduction

For decades, retinal images are widely used by ophthalmologists for the detection and follow-up of several pathological states [1–5]. Fundus photographs, also called retinal photography, are captured using special devices called "Charged Coupled Devices" (CCD), which are cameras that show the interior surface of the eye [6–10]. These images directly provide information about the normal and abnormal features in the retina. The normal features include the optic disk, fovea, and vascular network. There are different kinds of abnormal features caused by diabetic retinopathy (DR) such as microaneurysm, hard exudate, soft exudate, hemorrhage, and neovascularization. An example of retinal images obtained by fundus photography is given in Figure 1, where two retinal images are shown. The first one does not show any DR sign (Figure 1(a)) and the second one demonstrates advanced-DR signs indicated by color arrows (Figure 1(b)). However, the manual detection of blood vessels is very difficult since the blood vessels in these images are complex and have low level contrast [11]. Also, not all the images show signs of diabetic retinopathy. Hence, a manual measurement of the information about blood vessels, such as length, width, tortuosity, and branching pattern, becomes tedious. As a result, it increases the time of diagnosis and decreases the efficiency of ophthalmologists. Therefore, automatic methods for extracting and measuring the vessels in retinal images are needed to save the workload of the ophthalmologists and to assist in characterizing the detected lesions and identifying the false positives [12].

Several works have been proposed for detecting the 2D complex vessel network, such as single scale matched

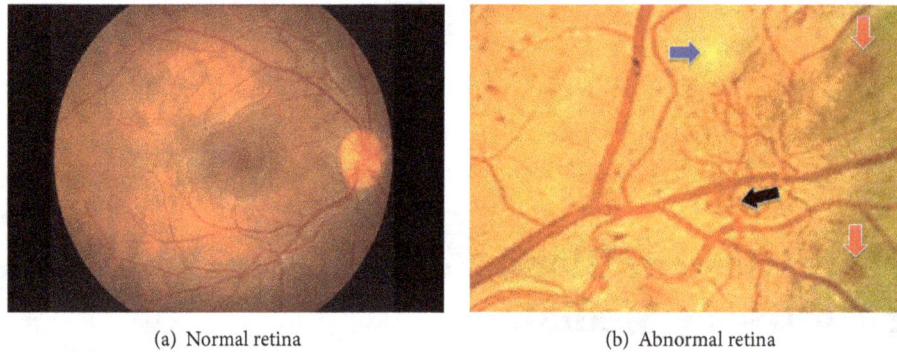

(a) Normal retina   (b) Abnormal retina

FIGURE 1: Retinal images [32].

filter [13–15], multiscale matched filter [16], adaptive local thresholding [17], single-scale Gabor filters [18], and multiscale Gabor filters [19]. Cinsdikici and Aydin [20] put forward a blood vessel segmentation based on a novel hybrid model of the matched filter and the colony algorithm, which extracts vessels perfectly but the pathological areas can affect the result. In [21–23] authors adapted another approach which applied mathematical morphological operators. The suggested method in [21] proved to be a valuable tool for the segmentation of the vascular network in retinal images, where it allowed obtaining a final image with the segmented vessels by iteratively combining the centerline image with the set of images that resulted from the vessel segments' reconstruction phase using the morphological operator. However, the inconvenience of this method is when a vessel centerline is missing, so the corresponding segmented vessel is normally not included in the final segmentation result. In [22], the authors proved that it was possible to select vessels using shape properties and connectivity, as well as differential properties like curvature. The robustness of the algorithm has been evaluated and tested on eye fundus images and on other images. Gang et al. [24] showed that the Gaussian curve is suitable for modeling the intensity profile of the cross section of the retinal vessels in color fundus images. Based on this elaboration, they proposed the amplitude-modified second-order Gaussian filter for retinal vessel detection, which optimized the matched filter and improved the successfulness of the detection. Staal et al. [25] explained a method for an automated segmentation of vessels in two-dimensional color images. The system was based on extracting image ridges that coincide approximately with vessel centerlines, where the evaluation was done using the accuracy of hard classifications and the values of soft ones. In [26], the authors presented a hybrid method for an efficient segmentation of multiple oriented blood vessels in colour retinal images. The robustness and accuracy of the method demonstrated that it might be useful in a wide range of retinal images even with the presence of lesions in the abnormal images. Dua et al. [27] presented a method for detecting blood vessels, which employs a hierarchical decomposition based on a quad tree decomposition. The algorithm was faster than the existing approaches. In the recent years, alternative approaches for an automated vessel segmentation have used the Hessian-based

multiscale detection of curvilinear structures, which has been effective in discerning both large and small vessels [28–31].

In this paper, we propose a multiscale response to detect linear structures in 2D images. We will use the formulation, which was suggested in [36, 37]. The presented detection algorithm is divided into two steps. First, we present a flux-based anisotropic diffusion method and apply it to denoise images corrupted by an additive Gaussian noise. In order to extract only the pixels belonging to a vessel region, we use a Gaussian model of the vessels for interpreting the eigenvalues and the eigenvectors of the Hessian matrix. Then, we compute the multiscale response from responses computed at a discrete set of scales. The method has been evaluated using the images of two publicly available databases, the DRIVE database [34] and the STARE database [33]. Prior to analysing fundus images, we have used the green channel alone, since it gives the highest contrast between the vessel and the background.

2. Methodology

2.1. Preprocessing Technique. In the ocular fundus image, edges and local details between heterogeneous regions are the most interesting part for clinicians. Therefore, it is very important to preserve and enhance edges and local fine structures and simultaneously reduce the noise. To reduce the image noise, several approaches have been proposed using techniques such as linear and nonlinear filtering. In linear spatial filtering, such as Gaussian filtering, the content of a pixel is given by the value of the weighted average of its immediate neighbors. This filtering not only reduces the amplitude of noise fluctuations but also degrades sharp details such as lines or edges, so the resulting images appear blurred and diffused [24, 38]. This undesirable effect can be reduced or avoided by designing nonlinear filters. The most common technique is median filtering. With it the value of an output pixel is determined by the median of the neighborhood pixels. This filtering retains edges but results in a loss of resolution by suppressing fine details [39]. In order to perform this task, Perona and Malik (PM) [18] developed an anisotropic diffusion method, a multiscale smoothing, and the edge detection scheme, which were a powerful concept in image processing. The anisotropic diffusion was inspired from the heat diffusion equation by introducing a diffusion function, g, which depended upon the norm of the gradient of the image:

$$\frac{\partial u}{\partial t} = \operatorname{div}\big(g(|\nabla u|) \cdot \nabla u\big), \tag{1}$$

where ∇ and $u(x,t)$ denote gradient operation and image intensity, respectively, div is the divergence operator, and $|\cdot|$ denotes the magnitude. The variable x represents the spatial coordinate, while the variable t is used to enumerate iteration steps in the discrete implementation. Perona and Malik suggested the following diffusion functions:

$$g(|\nabla u|) = \frac{1}{1 + (|\nabla u|/k)^2},$$
$$g(|\nabla u|) = \exp\left[-\left(\frac{|\nabla u|}{k}\right)^2\right], \tag{2}$$

where k is a parameter of the norm gradient. In this method of anisotropic diffusion, the norm gradient is used to detect edges or frontiers in the image as a step of intensity discontinuity. To understand the relation between the parameter k and the discontinuity value $|\nabla u|$, $F(\nabla u)$ can be defined as the following product $F(\nabla u) = g \times \nabla u$, called the flow diffusion.

(i) If $|\nabla u| \gg k$, then $g(|\nabla u|) \to 0$ and we have a filter pass-all.

(ii) If $|\nabla u| \ll k$, then $g(|\nabla u|) \to 1$ and we obtain an isotropic diffusion filter (like a Gaussian filter), which is a low-pass filter that attenuates high frequencies.

The one-dimensional discrete implementation of (1) is given by

$$\frac{\partial u}{\partial t}(x,t)$$
$$= \frac{\partial}{\partial x}\big(g(x,t) \cdot \nabla(u)(x,t)\big)$$
$$\approx \frac{\partial}{\partial x}\left(g(x,t) \cdot \frac{1}{dx}\left(u\left(x + \frac{dx}{2}, t\right) - u\left(x - \frac{dx}{2}, t\right)\right)\right)$$
$$\approx \frac{1}{dx^2}\left[g\left(x + \frac{dx}{2}, t\right) \cdot (u(x + dx, t) - u(x, t))\right.$$
$$\left. -g\left(x - \frac{dx}{2}, t\right) \cdot (u(x, t) - u(x - dx, t))\right]$$
$$\approx F_{\text{right}} - F_{\text{left}} \quad \text{if } dx = 1, \tag{3}$$

where $F_{\text{right}} = F(x + (dx/2), t)$ and $F_{\text{left}} = F(x - (dx/2), t)$.

The above result is generalized in n-dimensional:

$$\frac{\partial u}{\partial t} \approx \sum_{i=1}^{n} F_{x_i^+} - F_{x_i^-} \tag{4}$$

if $\forall i, dx_i = 1$, $F_{x_i^+} = F_{x_i}(x + (dx_i/2), t)$ and $F_{x_i^-} = F_{x_i}(x - (dx_i/2), t)$.

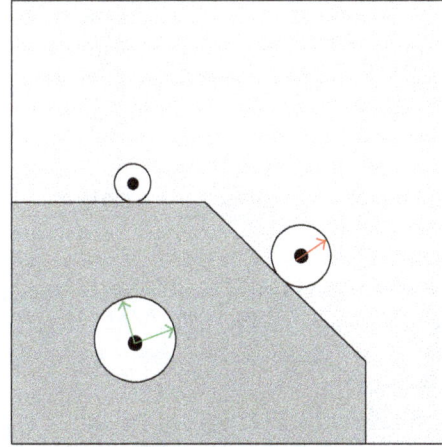

FIGURE 2: PM anisotropic diffusion.

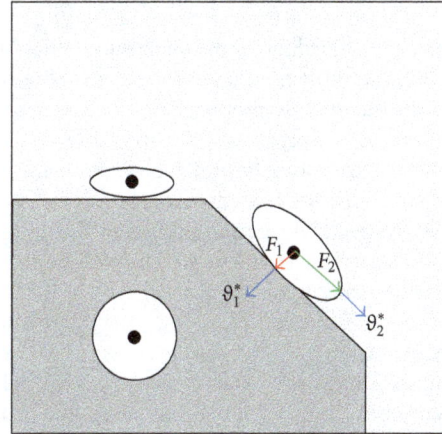

FIGURE 3: Directional anisotropic diffusion.

Up to now, the anisotropic diffusion has been defined as the case where the diffusivity is a scalar function varying with the location in the image. As described earlier, the PM diffusion (Figure 2) limits the smoothing of an image near the pixels with a high gradient magnitude (edge pixels). As the diffusion near an edge is very weak, the noise smoothing near the edge is also small. To address this, diffusions using matrices instead of scalars have been put forward [36, 40, 41], where the anisotropic diffusion allows the diffusion to be different along various directions defined by the local geometry of the structures in the image (Figure 3). Thus, the diffusion on both sides of an edge can be prevented while allowing the diffusion along the edge. This prevents the edge from being smoothed and then being removed during denoising.

The F flux of the matrix diffusion (MD) form can be written as

$$\operatorname{div}(D\nabla u), \tag{5}$$

where D is a positive definite symmetrie matrix that may be adapted to the local image structure, which can be written in

TABLE 1: Parameters and results of different filters for vessel image.

Filter	N	k	β	σ	dt	Neig.	PSNR (dB)	MSE
GF	—	—	—	2	—	9×9	37.7717	10.8620
MF	—	—	—	—	—	5×5	38.6364	8.9011
PM	13	7	—	—	0.15	—	39.6735	7.0103
DAD	**50**	**7**	**0.05**	**0.8**	**0.05**	—	**40.4337**	**5.8845**

terms of its eigenvectors v_1 and v_2 and eigenvalues λ_1 and λ_2, as follows:

$$D = \begin{bmatrix} v_1 & v_2 \end{bmatrix} \begin{bmatrix} \lambda_1 & 0 \\ 0 & \lambda_2 \end{bmatrix} \begin{bmatrix} v_1^T \\ v_2^T \end{bmatrix}. \tag{6}$$

Subsequently, the gradient vector field can be written as

$$\nabla u = u_{v_1} v_1 + u_{v_2} v_2. \tag{7}$$

Following the eigenvalues and eigenvectors that we have chosen, different matrix diffusions can be obtained [36, 41]. The diffusion matrix proposed by Weickert et al. [41] had the same eigenvectors as the structure tensor, with eigenvalues that are a function of the norm of the gradient [41, 42]. In our work, we have used a 2D basis (v_1^*, v_2^*) which corresponds, respectively, to unit vectors in the directions of the gradient and to the minimal curvature of the regularized (or smoothed) version of the image, which is the image convolved with a Gaussian filter with a standard deviation σ. This basis is of particular interest in the context of small, elongated structures such as blood vessels, where the minimal curvature holds for the axis direction orthogonal to the gradient. These directions are obtained as two of the eigenvectors of the Hessian matrix of the smoothed image: H_σ (further details are described in Section 2.3). Therefore, the eigenvectors are defined as follows:

$$\begin{aligned} v_1^* &\parallel \nabla u_\sigma, \\ v_2^* &\perp \nabla u_\sigma, \end{aligned} \tag{8}$$

where ∇u_σ is the gradient of the image convolved with a Gaussian filter with a standard deviation σ, v_2^* gives an estimation of the vessel direction, and v_1^* is its orthogonal. Also, we have used the eigenvalues in (6) as a diffusion function associated to each vector of the basis depending on the first order derivative of the intensity in this direction, instead of the traditional norm of the smoothed gradient. Furthermore, the diffusion can be decomposed as a sum of diffusions in each direction of the orthogonal basis and the divergence term can be written as [36]

$$\text{div}(F) = \text{div}\left(\sum_{i=1}^{2} \phi_i\left(u_{v_i^*}\right) \cdot v_i^*\right) = \sum_{i=1}^{2} \text{div}\left(\phi_i\left(u_{v_i^*}\right) \cdot v_i^*\right), \tag{9}$$

where $u_{v_i^*}$ and ϕ_i indicate the first order derivative of the intensity in the direction v_i and the ith diffusion function, respectively. Also, ϕ_1 can be chosen to be any of the diffusivity functions from the traditional nonhomogeneous isotropic

diffusion equation, which depends on the first order derivative of the intensity in this direction, as $\phi_1(u_{v_1^*}) = u_{v_1^*} e^{-(u_{v_1^*}/k)^2}$ and $\phi_2(u_{v_2^*}) = \alpha \cdot u_{v_2^*}$, with $0 < \alpha < 1$, being only a diffusing function to allow smoothing in a v_2^* direction. For further details, the reader could refer to [36, 43].

As in [36], we use a data attachment term with a coefficient β which allows a better control of the extent to which the restored image differs from the original image u_0 (at $t = 0$) and of the result of the diffusion process at convergence. The anisotropic diffusion equation becomes

$$\frac{\partial u}{\partial t} = \sum_{i=1}^{2} \text{div}\left(\phi_i\left(u_{v_i^*}\right) \cdot v_i^*\right) + \beta(u - u_0). \tag{10}$$

In order to evaluate the denoising effects of the directional anisotropic diffusion (DAD), we have added a Gaussian white noise to each of the images in Figure 4. Once the diffusion method is applied to these noisy images, its effectiveness in reducing the noise is got by calculating the peak signal to noise ratio (PSNR) relative to the original image as follows:

$$\text{PSNR} = 10 \cdot \log_{10}\left(\frac{d^2}{\text{MSE}}\right), \tag{11}$$

where $d = 255$ and MSE is the mean-squared error which is written as

$$\text{MSE} = \frac{1}{NM} \sum_{i=1}^{N} \sum_{j=1}^{M} \left(I_{\text{original}}(i, j) - I_{\text{denoised}}(i, j)\right)^2, \tag{12}$$

where I_{original} refers to the original image without noise and I_{denoised} is the image after the denoising process.

The higher the PSNR is, the better the effect of the denoising is. Note that this measure does not necessarily imply that an image with a higher PSNR is also more visually gratifying. However, based on our experiments using the three test images with an additive white Gaussian noise, we can draw some observations. First, all the techniques we have tried have several parameters that must be selected carefully to obtain the best results. Since we have a "clean" original image, as well as one with noise, we can use the increment in the PSNR value to guide our choice of the parameters. These parameters and the obtained results are indicated in Tables 1, 2, and 3, where we can observe that for the images corrupted with an additive Gaussian noise, the DAD method performs better than the PM method. It gains a higher PSNR (40.4337, 20.9045, and 33.3515) and a smaller MSE (5.8845, 527.9932, and 30.0557) than the aforementioned three methods.

Figure 4 represents some of the best results for the different methods (GF, MF, PM, and DAD) on the presented three

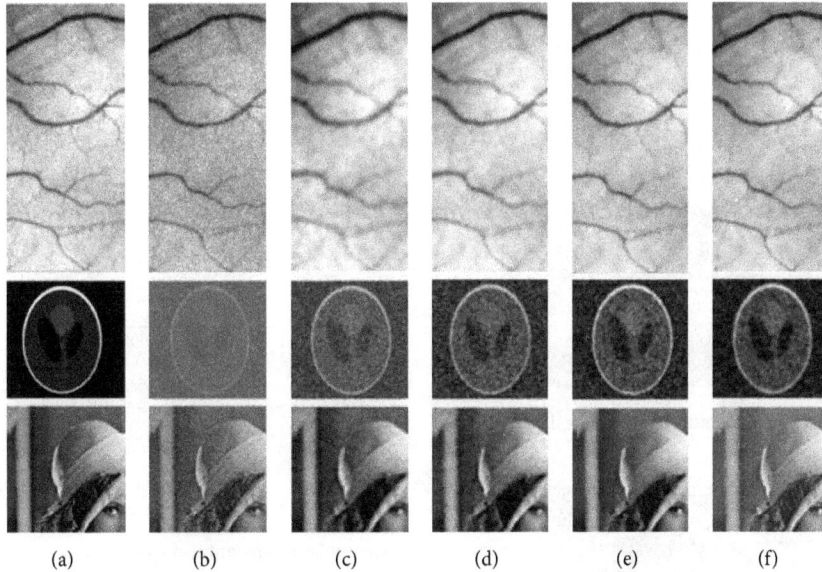

FIGURE 4: Original images (a) and the corresponding images with additive Gaussian noise (b); denoised images: best result with GF (c), best result with MF (d), best result with PM filter (e), and best result with directional anisotropic diffusion filter (f).

TABLE 2: Parameters and results of different filters for phantom image.

Filter	N	k	β	σ	dt	Neig.	PSNR (dB)	MSE
GF	—	—	—	2	—	5×5	18.8731	842.8924
MF	—	—	—	—	—	5×5	20.2437	614.7677
PM	20	3	—	—	0.15	—	20.8821	530.7294
DAD	**75**	**2**	**0.05**	**0.8**	**0.05**	—	**20.9045**	**527.9932**

TABLE 3: Parameters and results of different filters for Lena image.

Filter	N	k	β	σ	dt	Neig.	PSNR (dB)	MSE
GF	—	—	—	2	—	5×5	31.4598	46.4621
MF	—	—	—	—	—	5×5	29.14504	79.1734
PM	10	7	—	—	0.15	—	32.9911	32.6562
DAD	**20**	**7**	**0.05**	**0.8**	**0.05**	—	**33.3515**	**30.0557**

test images (Vessels, phantom, and Lena). For instance, the results recorded after applying the DAD method show that this latter improves much more the visual rendering of the image compared to other methods. As shown in the images of the first row, a DAD filter can effectively improves the quality of a noisy image and also well enhances edges and preserves more details than other filters. Indeed, the Gaussian filter smooths very strongly the planar areas which causes loss of information regarding the fine structures of the image, and it blurs the image. The Median filter, compared to the Gaussian filter, preserves edges but losses details. Comparing the results of the DAD method to those obtained by the PM diffusion in Figures 5 and 6, we can derive several observations. The denoising of PM diffusion model is sensitive to the value of the conductance parameter k, and, therefore, smoothing is performed along ridges but not across a ridge line which causes enhancing the desired ridges as well as the noise. To be compared to the DAD diffusion filter, the diffusivity

is a tensor-valued function varying with the location and orientation of edges in an image. So, when this filter is applied to a ridge line smoothing is performed along ridges as across a ridge line while preserving the details.

2.2. Multiscale Medialness. The general approach of multi-scale methods is to choose a range of scales between $t_{\min}$ and $t_{\max}$ (corresponding to $\sigma_{\min}$ and $\sigma_{\max}$), which are discretized using a logarithmic scale in order to have more accuracy for low scales and to compute a response for each scale from the initial image [36, 43, 47]. The user specifies the minimal and maximal radius of the vessels to extract. Thus, the computation of the single scale response requires different steps. First, a number of points are preselected using the eigenvalues of the Hessian matrix. These points are expected to be near a vessel axis. Then, for each preselected point, the response is computed at the current scale σ. The response function uses eigenvectors of the Hessian matrix of the image

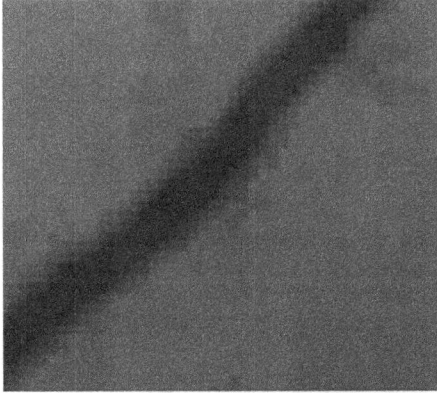

FIGURE 5: PM anisotropic diffusion ($k = 3$, $N = 100$).

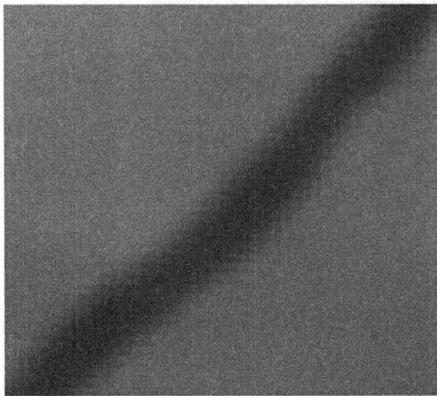

FIGURE 6: Directional anisotropic diffusion ($k = 3$, $N = 100$, $\alpha = 0.5$).

to define at each point an orientation $D(\sigma, x)$ orthogonal to the axis of a potential vessel that goes through M. From this direction, the two points located at an equal distance of M in the direction D, noted M_1 and M_2 (Figure 7). The response $R_\sigma(I)$ at M is taken as the maximum absolute value, among these two points, of the first derivative of the intensity in the D direction:

$$R_\sigma(x)$$
$$= \max\{\nabla_\sigma I(\sigma, x + \sigma \cdot d) \cdot (+d), \nabla_\sigma I(\sigma, x - \sigma \cdot d) \cdot (-d)\}, \tag{13}$$

where d is the unitary vector of the direction D, that is, $d = \vec{v_1}$, and $\nabla_\sigma I$ is the gradient of the image at the scale σ. $\nabla_\sigma I$ is obtained by the convolution with the first derivative of a Gaussian function of the standard deviation σ, where multiplying the derivatives by σ ensures the scale invariance property and allows comparing the responses obtained from different scales. The gradient vector $\nabla_\sigma I$ can be computed by a bilinear interpolation for better accuracy, which is especially needed when looking at small vessels [37, 39].

A vessel of a radius r is detected at a scale t, so we use the scales corresponding to each radius for the multiscale processing. For a fixed scale t, we calculate a response image $R_t(I)$ where I is the initial image. Then we calculate

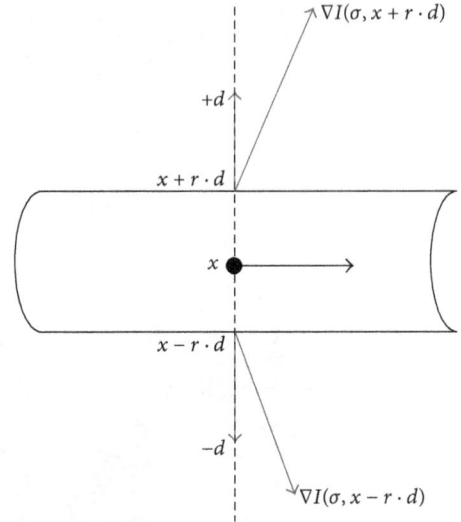

FIGURE 7: Representation of vesselness measure calculation (from the point x on the central line, d is the unit vector perpendicular to the main direction of the vessel and $r = \sigma$ is the current scale).

the multiscale response for the image $R_{\mathrm{multi}}(I)$ which is the maximum of the responses over scales: for each point $x \in I$ and a range $[t_{\min}, t_{\max}]$ of scale:

$$R_{\mathrm{multi}}(x) = \max_t\{R_t(x),\ t \in [t_{\min}, t_{\max}]\}. \tag{14}$$

This response $R_{\mathrm{multi}}(x)$ can be interpreted as an indicator that the point x belongs to the center line of a vessel, and $R_t(x)$ can be interpreted as an indicator that the point x belongs to the center line of a vessel with a radius t. Finally, this response is normalized to give a multiscale response that combines interesting features of each single scale response.

One difficulty with the multiscale approach is that we want to compare the result of a response function at different scales, whereas the intensity and its derivatives are decreasing scale functions. So far, all considerations have been made at a single scale defined by the scale parameter σ. In his work, about scale space theory, Lindeberg and Fagerström [48] showed the need for a multiscale analysis to take the varying size of objects into account. He also showed the necessity of normalizing the spatial derivatives between different scales. Thus, the normalized vesselness response is obtained by the product of the normalization term σ^γ and the final vesselness:

$$R^*(\Sigma, \gamma, x) := \max_{\sigma \in \Sigma} \sigma^\gamma \cdot R(\sigma, x) = \max_{i=1,\dots,n} \sigma_i^\gamma \cdot R(\sigma_i, x). \tag{15}$$

The parameter γ can be used to indicate the preference for a particular scale (Figure 8). If it is set to one, no scale is preferred. Besides, the multiscale response is got by selecting the maximum response over a set of different scales between $\sigma_{\min}$ and $\sigma_{\max}$.

2.3. Extraction of Local Orientations. The proposed model assumes that the intensity profile of the vessels in the cross section is Gaussian (Figure 9). This is a common assumption that it is employed in numerous algorithms [28, 35, 49].

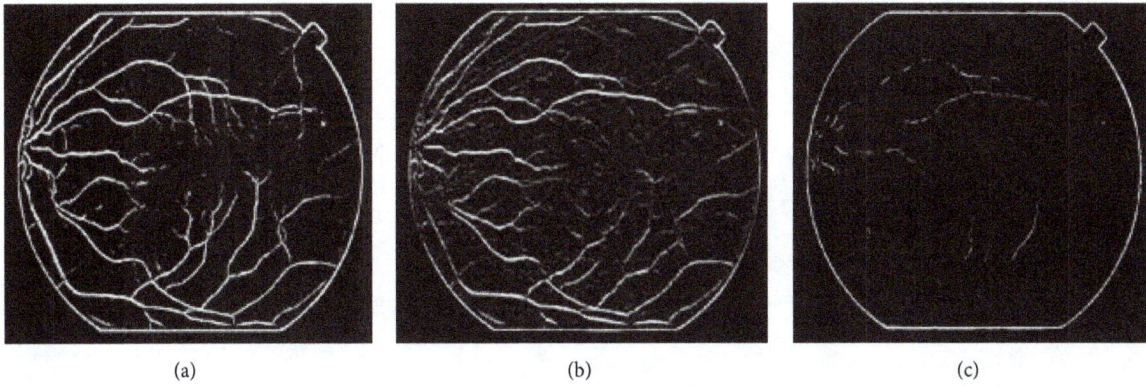

(a)   (b)   (c)

FIGURE 8: Influence of the normalization parameter γ on multiscale response; (a) $\gamma = 1$ is neutral; (b) $\gamma > 1$ favors large scales; finally, (c) $\gamma < 1$ favors small scales.

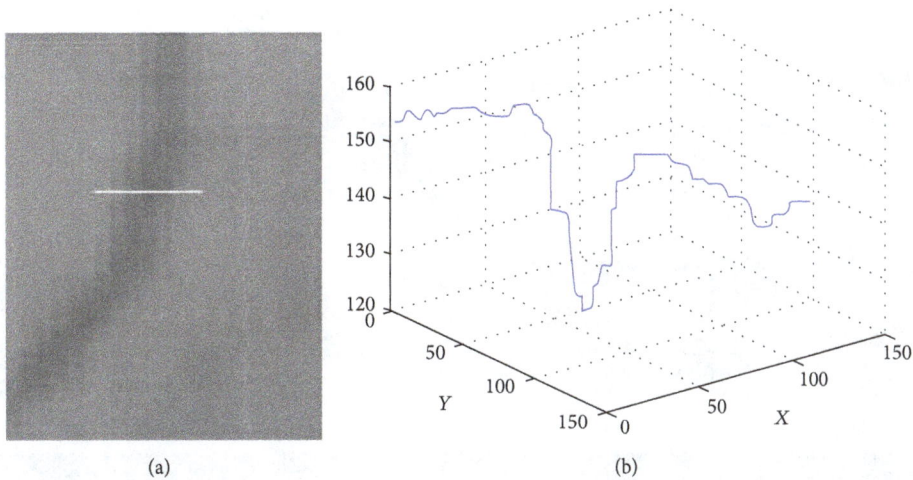

(a)   (b)

FIGURE 9: Example of cross sectional profile of blood vessel from gray scale 2D image (the gray intensities are plotted in a 3D view. The x, y axis is the position of the pixel in the 2D plane of the image, whereas the z-axis is the gray value or intensity of the pixel).

It is also commonly assumed that the intensity does not change much along vessels [49–51]. Recently, the Hessian matrix could be used to describe the local shape characteristics and orientation for elongated structures [35, 52]. The eigenvalues of this matrix, when the gradient is weak, express the local variation of the intensity in the direction of the associated eigenvectors. Subsequently, we assume that we want to characterize the dark vessels (low intensity) on a white background (high intensity).

Let us denote λ_1 and λ_2 as the eigenvalues of the Hessian matrix with $\lambda_1 \geq \lambda_2$ and $\vec{v_1}$, $\vec{v_2}$ being their associated eigenvectors (Figure 10). For a linear model with a Gaussian cross section, the vessel direction is defined by the eigenvector with the smallest eigenvalue at the center of the vessel, but it is less determined at the contours because both eigenvalues of the Hessian matrix are zero.

To summarize, for an ideal linear structure in a 2D image,

$$|\lambda_2| \approx 0,$$
$$|\lambda_1| > |\lambda_2|. \tag{16}$$

In retinal images, some large vessels may have a white line in their center and some elongated and disjoint spots (Figures 11(a), 11(b), and 11(c)); accordingly, the vessels do not invalidate the Gaussian profile assumption. So, such lines are usually lost after the preselection of vessel pixels using the Hessian eigenvalue analysis and classified as background pixels. Therefore, the responses of the gradient magnitude are a task which is of particular importance in improving the detection vessels (Figure 11). The experimental results are demonstrated in Figure 11, which shows hand labeled "truth" images, and segmented images obtained, respectively, by the Hessian eigenvalue analysis and the gradient magnitude. From these results we can deduce that responses based on the gradient magnitude can availably detect white lines as vessel pixels an removes some noise spots.

3. Results

In this section, the proposed method has been evaluated on two publicly available retinal image databases, the STARE database [33] and the DRIVE database [25]. The STARE

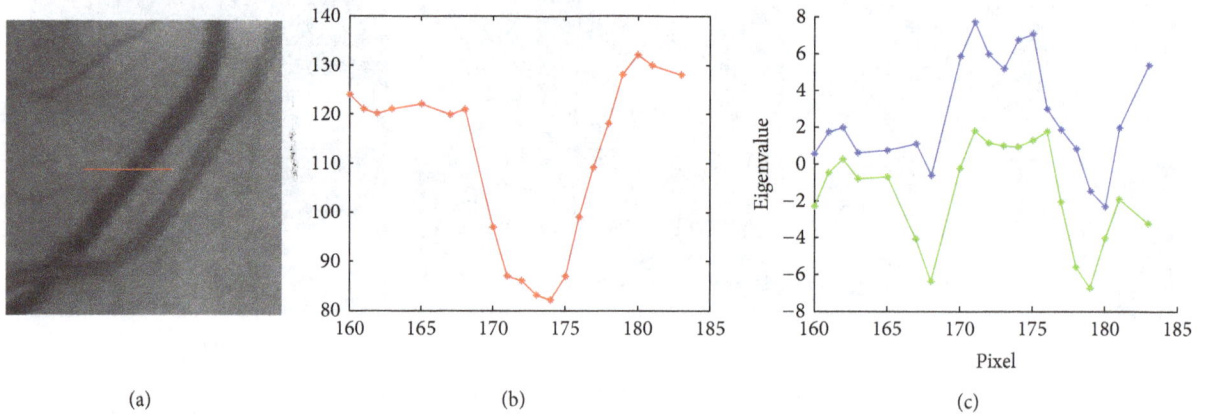

FIGURE 10: Eigenvalue analysis. (a) vessel cross section; (b) intensity distribution ($\sigma = 4.55$) vessel cross section; (c) corresponding eigenvalues.

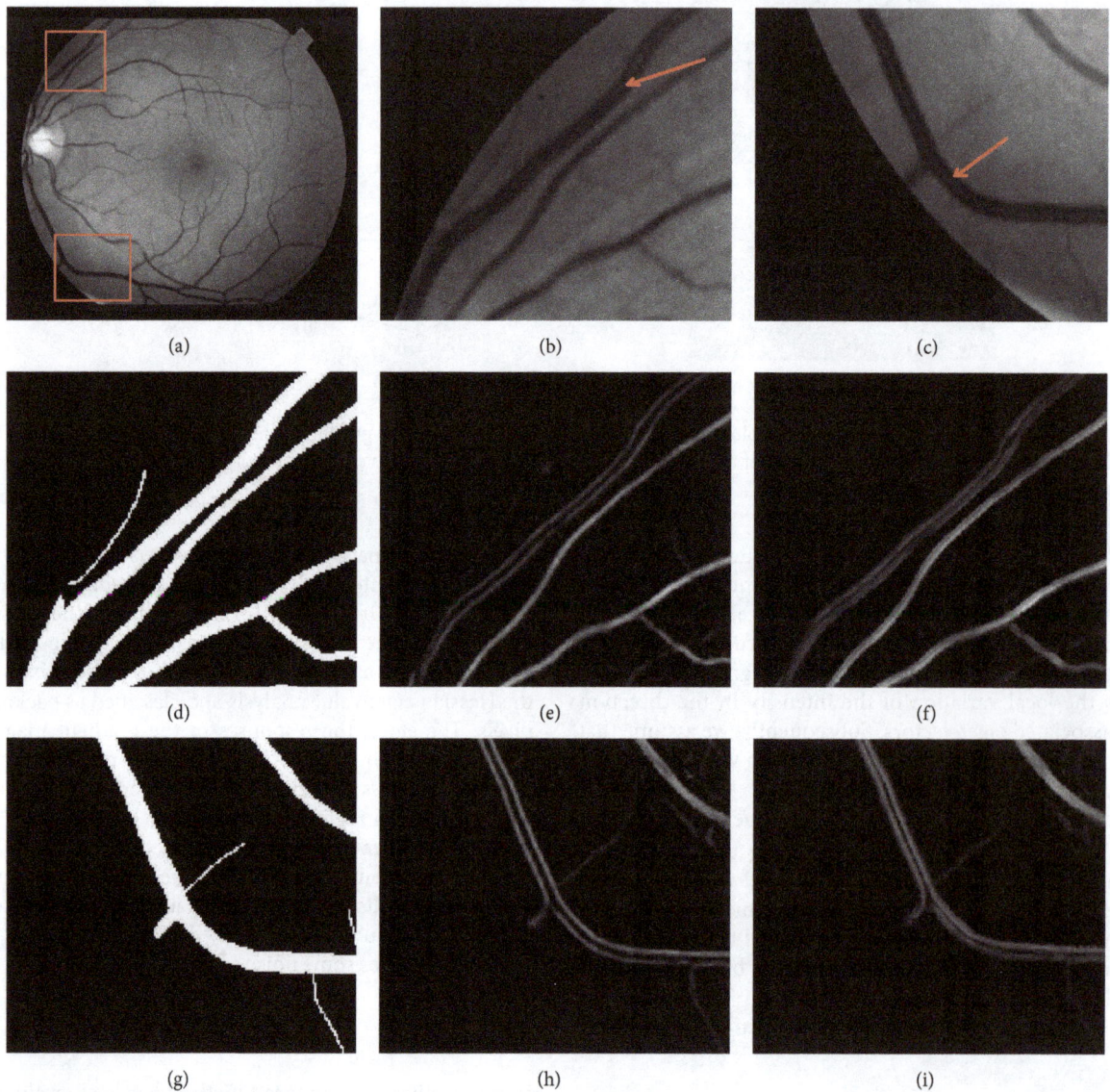

FIGURE 11: Retinal blood vessel detection. (a, b, and c) original images [33]; (d–g, e–h, and f–i) subimage of hand labeled image, vessel detection based Hessian eigenvalue analysis, and improved vessel detection with gradient magnitude.

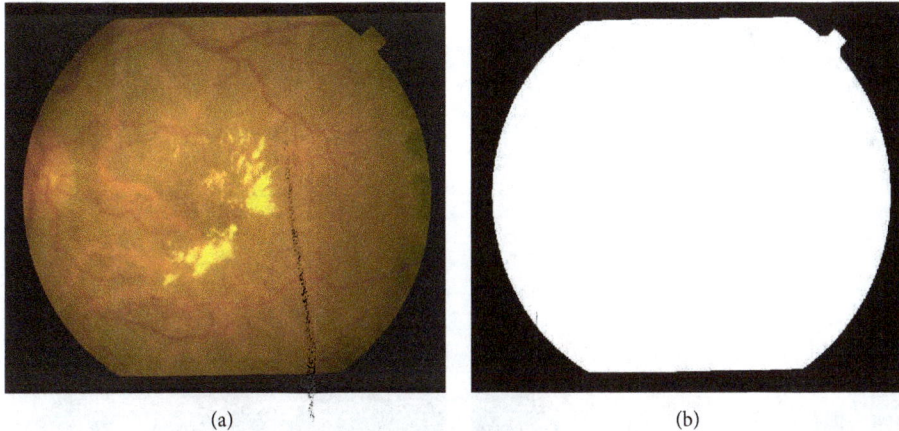

(a)   (b)

FIGURE 12: Binary mask of STARE project retinal image [33].

dataset contains twenty fundus colour retinal images, ten of which are from healthy ocular fundi and the other ten are from unhealthy ones. These images are captured by a Topcon TRV-50 fundus camera at a 35 Field Of View (FOV), which have digitized with a 24-bit gray-scale resolution and a size of 700×605 pixels. The dataset provides two sets of standard hand-labeled segmentations, which are manually segmented by two eye specialists. We create for this dataset a binary mask of the gray channel of the image using a simple threshold technique (Figure 12). We adapt the first eye specialist hand labelled as the ground truth to evaluate our vessel detection technique. The DRIVE dataset consists of 40 fundus ocular images, which have been divided into a training set and a test set by the authors of the database. These images are captured by the Canon CR5 camera at 45 FOV, which have been digitized at 24 bits with a resolution of 565×584 pixels. The dataset also gives two sets of standard hand-labeled segmentations by two human experts as a 9-ground truth.

The first expert hand labelled segmentation has been adapted as a ground truth to evaluate segmentation techniques on both STARE and DRIVE datasets. It is a common practice to evaluate the performance of retinal vessel segmentation algorithms using receiver operating characteristic (ROC) curves [25, 35]. An ROC curve plots the fraction of pixels correctly classified as vessels, namely, the true positive ra te (TPR), versus the fraction of pixels wrongly classified as vessels, namely, the false positive rate (FPR), by varying the rounding threshold T from 0 to 1 (Figure 13). The closer the curve approaches the top left corner, the better the performance of the system. In order to facilitate the comparison with other retinal vessel detection algorithms, we have selected the value of the area under the curve (AUC), which is 1 for an ideal system.

To measure the performance of the proposed enhancement filter, we ran our multiscale analysis filter with the following set of parameters:

(i) $r_{\min}$, $r_{\max}$, s, and the minimal and maximal radii used in this application are $r_{\min} = 1.25$ and $r_{\max} = 7$, discretized using $s = 4$ scales;

(ii) the parameter γ set to one to indicate no scale is preferred;

(iii) the value k is a constant threshold on the norm of gradient on the image;

(iv) N is the number of iterations for the anisotropic diffusion filter.

The computing time of our algorithm for an image of the STARE database is about 64 seconds, including anisotropic diffusion filtering, and about the same time for the DRIVE database. The implementation of the filter has been done in MATLAB, on a personal computer with a 2.13 Intel Core Duo processor and 4 GB of memory. In the first experiment, we apply a preprocessing task such as filtering data with an anisotropic diffusion version, cited above, in order to remove or at least reduce noise. The DAD filter denoises the original image by preserving edges and details. To show that the segmentation works better with anisotropic diffusion, Figure 14 presents a segmentation result before and after the application of the anisotropic diffusion scheme. In this figure, we show the improvements provided by the DAD model, which tends to remove noise effects and, unfortunately, smaller objects. So, it preserves efficiently the vessels while making the background more homogeneous.

On the other hand, for computing the response, it is possible to retain the mean of the two calculated values (the gradient of the two points located at an equal distance from the current point), like in the 3D case proposed by [36], or the minimal calculated value in the 2D case [37]. We prefer retaining the maximum of these two values. Figure 15 shows a synthetic image which consists of 100×100 pixels with an 8-bit resolution. We have chosen this image because it contains an object close to the vessel form. The latter figure shows the segmentation results by maximum, average, and minimum response functions. We note that for the case of minimum or average responses, the ring is not completely detected like in the original image, since we can see it has been missing pixels belonging to the edges, in contrast to maximum case where the extraction of the ring is complete. Table 4 presents the AUC calculated with our method for the test set of the STARE

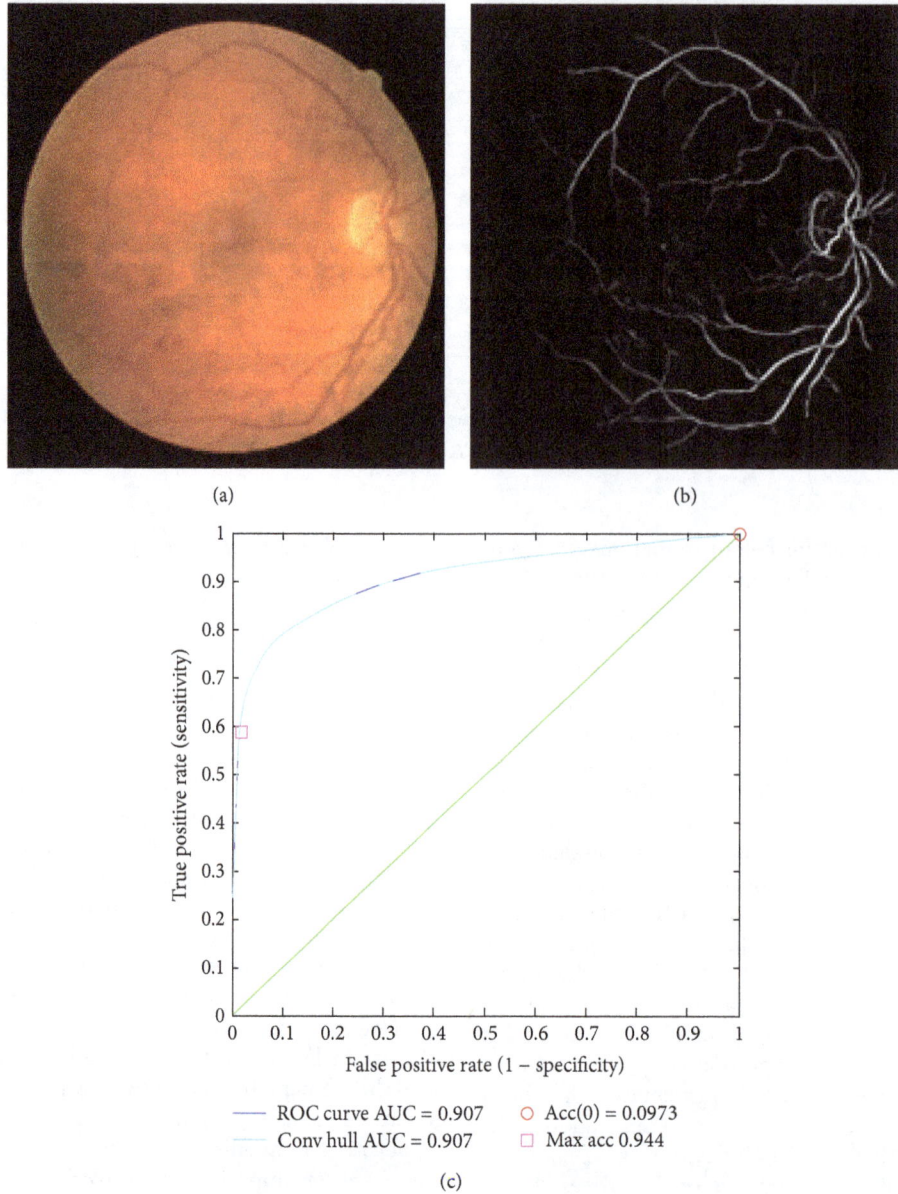

FIGURE 13: ROC curve of retinal image (06_test.tif) downloaded from DRIVE dataset [34]; (a) original image; (b) segmented image; (c) Roc curve.

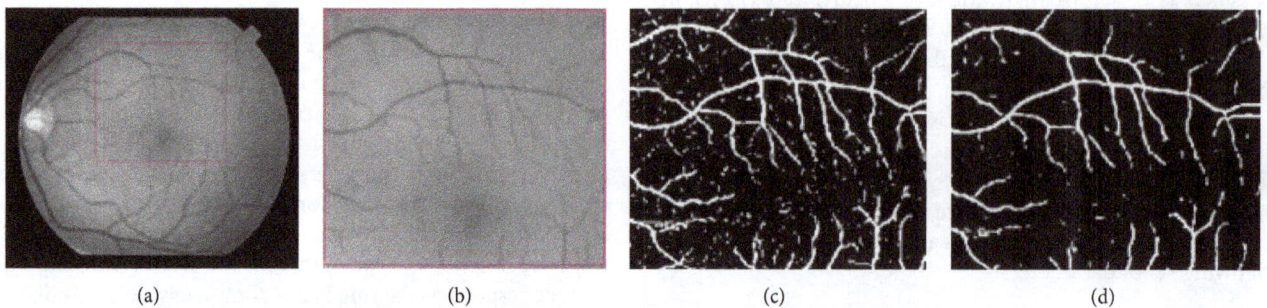

FIGURE 14: Effect of anisotropic diffusion. (a) Green channel of the original image downloaded from the STARE project dataset [33]. (b) Subimage of the original image, rescaled for better visualization, (c) segmentation without anisotropic diffusion, and (d) segmentation with anisotropic diffusion, $k = 1.25$, $\beta = 0.05$, and $N = 30$.

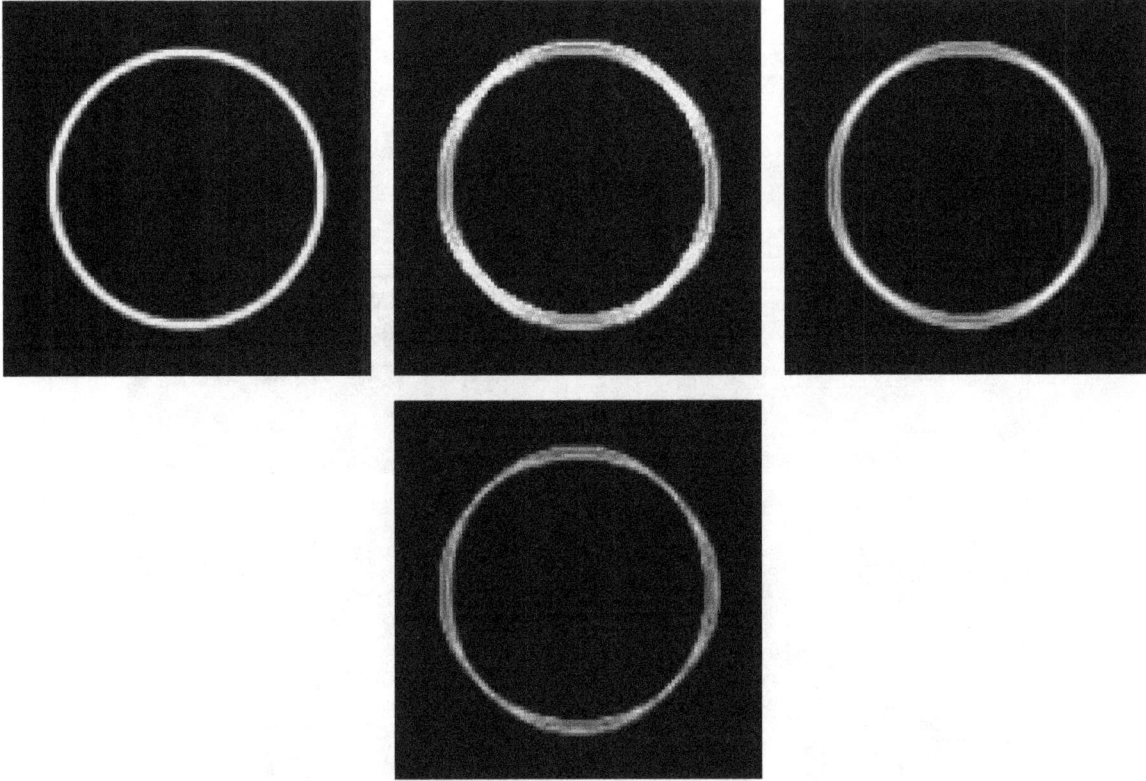

FIGURE 15: Original synthetic image, maximum response, average response, and minimum response $\sigma \in \{0.25, 0.5, 1, 2, 4\}$ (left to right-top to bottom).

TABLE 4: STARE project database [33].

	Mean	Min	Max
AUC	0.9329	0.9053	**0.9445**

TABLE 5: ROC curve analysis of STARE project database [33].

Number	MAA	TPR	FPR
1	0.9014	0.5537	0.0398
2	0.8740	0.1178	0.0045
3	0.9168	0.3819	0.0119
4	0.9286	0.5525	0.0135
5	0.9240	0.5678	0.0218
6	0.9414	0.5128	0.0139
7	0.9672	0.7626	0.0141
8	0.9683	0.7534	0.0149
9	0.9652	0.7366	0.0123
10	0.9420	0.6171	0.0182
11	0.9503	0.6379	0.0133
12	0.9655	0.7694	0.0105
13	0.9864	0.6992	0.0180
14	0.9480	0.6899	0.0162
15	0.9487	0.6882	0.0207
16	0.9226	0.6788	0.0215
17	0.9499	0.7099	0.0168
18	0.9484	0.6812	0.0102
19	0.9585	0.6058	0.0114
20	0.9345	0.6000	0.0172
	Av.MAA	Av.TPR	Av.FPR
	0.9402	0.6145	0.0162

database, using the green channel images. As given in the table, the experimental results show that the maximum model (AUC = 0.9445) performs much better than the average (AUC = 0.9329) or minimum model (AUC = 0.9053).

Figure 16 presents the obtained response image of a real retinal image, where four scales have been used for radii of vessels ranging from 1.25 to 7: $\{1.25, 2.22, 4, 7\}$. This figure shows that small and large vessels can be better distinguished in the maximum case than the minimum or average ones.

Although the contrast is not very high in the original figure (Figure 14(a)), the method detects most vessels, over a large size range. For example, in Figure 17, an image of the retinal tree vasculature is presented, where different responses recorded at increasing scales are represented. The last image shows a quite good performance of the vessel subtraction. Yet Figure 18 proves that it is possible to design a system that approaches the performance of human observers.

In order to evaluate the suggested method, experiment results of the 20-image sets of the STARE database are shown in Table 5. In Table 6, our method is compared to the most

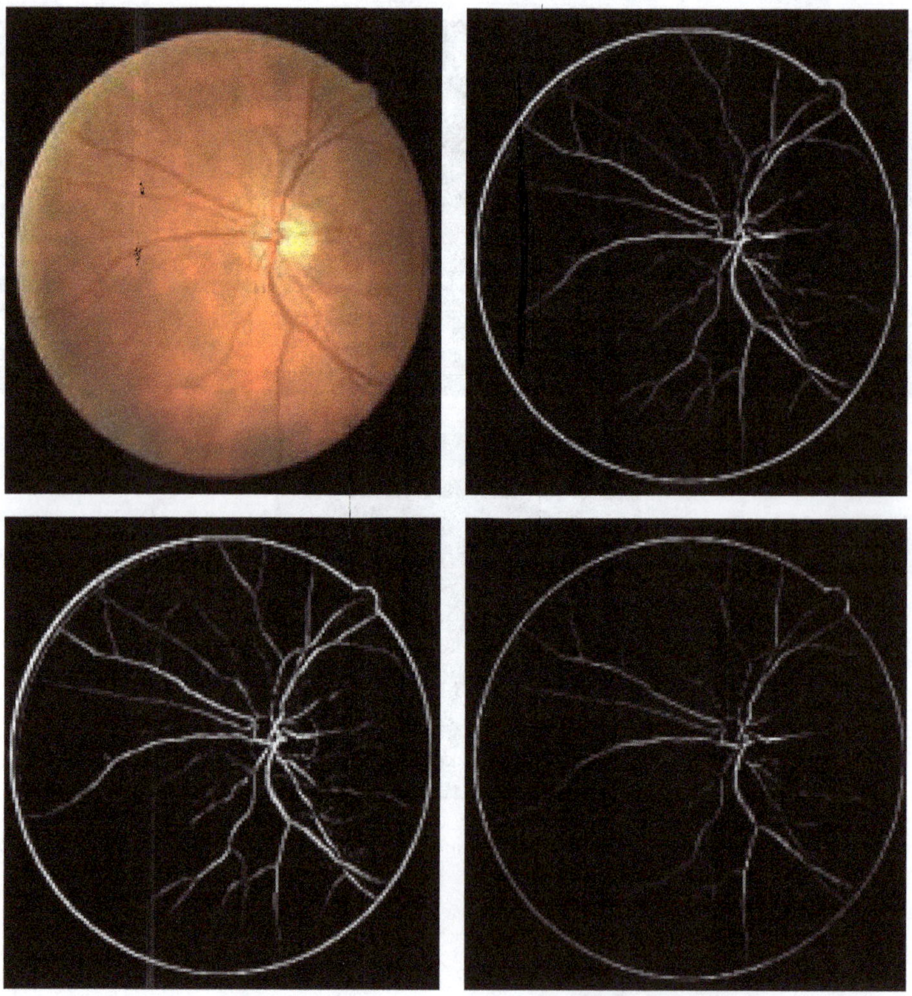

FIGURE 16: Real angiography image downloaded from DRIVE dataset [34], average response, maximum response, and minimum response (left to right-top to bottom).

TABLE 6: Comparison of vessel segmentation results on STARE project database [33].

Method	MAA	TPR	FPR
2nd human observer	0.9354	0.8949	0.0610
Hoover [33, 35]	0.9267	0.6751	0.0433
Mendonça (green) [21]	0.9440	0.6996	0.0270
Staal [25]	0.9516	0.6970	0.0190
Soares [44]	0.9480	0.7165	0.0252
Matched filter [13]	0.9384	0.6134	0.0245
Martinez-Perez [45]	0.9410	0.7506	0.0431
MF-FDOG [14]	0.9484	0.7177	0.0247
Proposed method	**0.9402**	**0.6145**	**0.0162**

recent methods in terms of TPR, FPR, and maximum accuracy average (MAA) where the maximal accuracy indicates how to extract a binary image that matches the vessel images to a high degree. The accuracy is estimated by the ratio of the sum of the number of correctly classified foreground and background pixels, divided by the total number of pixels in the image. In this latest table, the performance measures of Staal et al. [25], Zhang et al. [14], Mendonça and Campilho [21], Chaudhuri et al. [13], Martinez-Perez et al. [45], and Hoover et al. [35] have been reported by their original papers. In addition, these performance results are the average values for the whole set of 20 images, except the method of Staal [25] which used 19 out of 20 images of the STARE images, among which ten were healthy and nine were unhealthy. Table 5 presents our results on all 20 images in the STARE database, estimated using the hand-labeled images set of the first human expert designated as a ground truth. The estimated experimental results are the average TPR = 0.6145 corresponding to an FPR of around 0.0162 and a maximum average accuracy MAA = 0.9402. The results show that our method has a competitive maximum average accuracy value where it performs better than the matched filter [13] and remains close to the others.

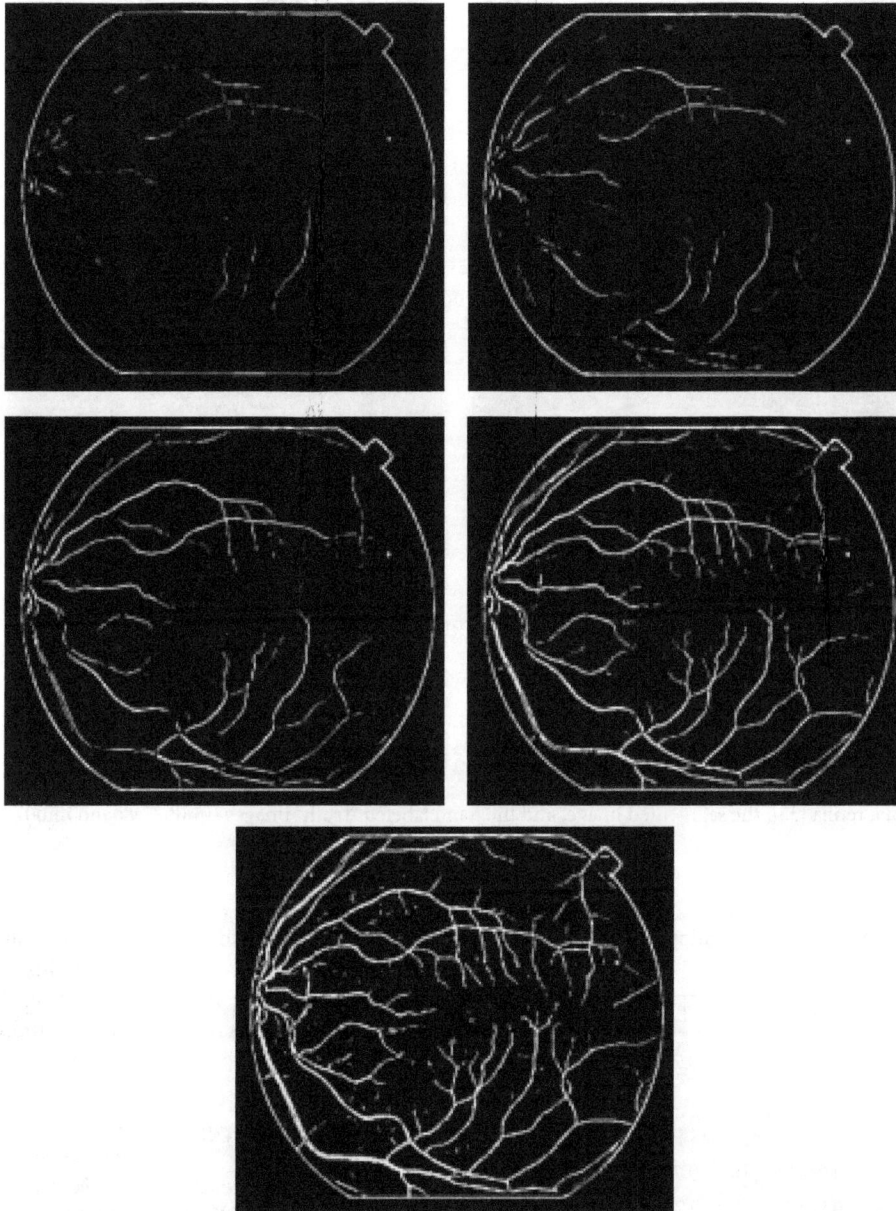

FIGURE 17: Different responses for different scales of Figure 14(a) (top to bottom); the first four images show the vesselness obtained at increasing scales. The last image is the result after the scale selection procedure (normalized image).

The results of the proposed method are also compared with those on twenty images from the DRIVE database, and the result is depicted in Table 7. The hand-labeled images by the first human expert have been used as ground truth. The experimental results show an MAA around of 0.9155. Also, we have compared the performance of the suggested technique with the sensitivities and specificities of the methods cited in Table 7. It has been found that for the DRIVE database the method has provided a sensitivity of 0.5879 and a specificity of 0.0166. We have shown that the proposed method performs well with a lower specificity even in the presence of lesions in the abnormal images.

4. Conclusion

The purpose of this work is to detect linear structures in real retinal images in order to help the interpretation of the vascular network. We put forward to combining an anisotropic diffusion filter to reduce the image noise with a multiscale response based on the eigenvectors of the Hessian matrix and on the gradient information to extract vessels from retinal images. The main advantage of this technique is its ability to extract large and fine vessels at various image resolutions. Furthermore, the directional anisotropic diffusion plays a vital role in denoising images and in decreasing

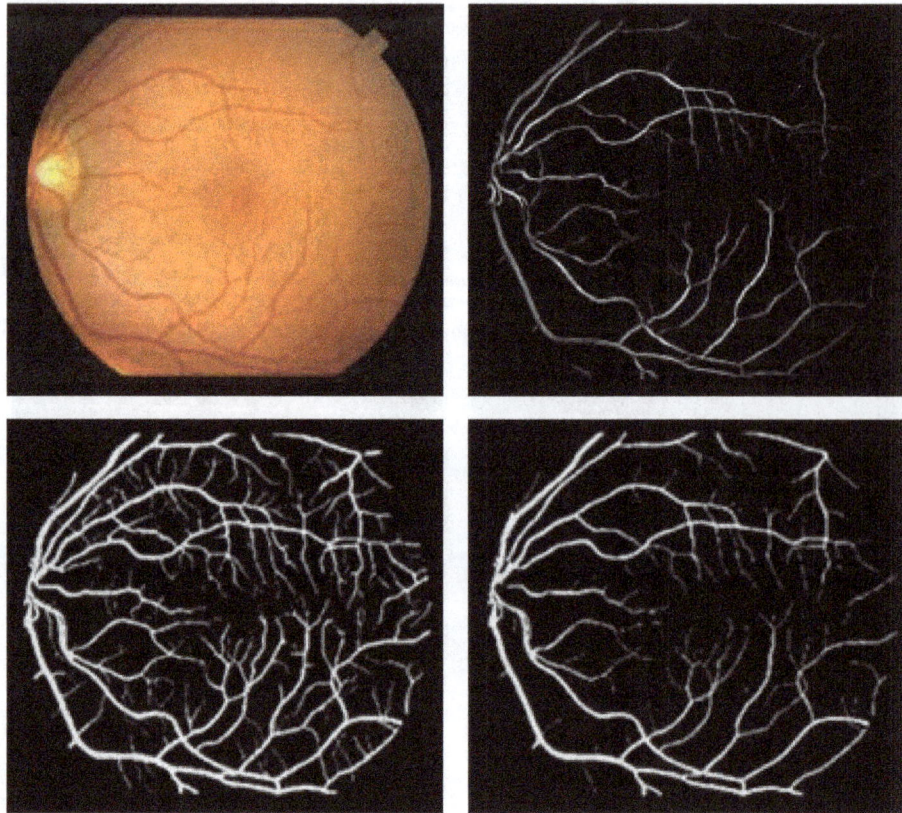

FIGURE 18: An image of a retina [35], the segmented image, and the hand labeled "truth" images (im0077.vk and im0077.ah) (left to right-top to bottom) [33].

TABLE 7: Comparison of vessel segmentation results on DRIVE database [34].

Method	MAA	TPR	FPR
2nd human observer [34]	0.9473	0.7761	0.0275
Martinez-Perez [45]	0.9344	0.7246	0.0345
Staal [25, 34]	0.9442	0.7194	0.0227
Mendonça [21]	0.9452	0.7344	0.0236
Matched filter [13]	0.9284	0.6168	0.0259
Niemeijer [34, 46]	0.9417	0.6898	0.0304
Proposed method	**0.9155**	**0.5879**	**0.0166**

the difficulty of vessel extraction especially for thin vessels. Our first results show the robustness of the method against noise as well as its applicability to detect blood vessels. The MAA is used as a performance measure, and the values achieved with our algorithm are competitive compared to the existing methods. Therefore, from the experimental results, it can be seen that the number of classified pixels has been slightly lower compared to the other methods using the same database mainly due to the weakness of blood vessels, causing missing vessels, and also because of lesions, resulting in a detection error. Also, the retinal images suffer from nonuniform illumination and have a poor contrast. Thus,

to avoid wrong classified pixels or miss classified ones, caused by an occasional false measurement, this system can very well be improved in the future with adding, for instance, some postprocessing tasks to reach more accurate measurement for blood vessels.

Conflict of Interests

The authors declare that there is no conflict of interests regarding to the publication of this paper.

References

[1] R. Williams, M. Airey, H. Baxter, J. Forrester, T. Kennedy-Martin, and A. Girach, "Epidemiology of diabetic retinopathy and macular oedema: a systematic review," *Eye*, vol. 18, no. 10, pp. 963–983, 2004.

[2] R. Gupta and P. Kumar, "Global diabetes landscape-type 2 diabetes mellitus in South Asia: epidemiology, risk factors, and control," *Insulin*, vol. 3, no. 2, pp. 78–94, 2008.

[3] J. Malek, M. Ben Abdallah, A. Mansour, and R. Tourki, "Automated optic disc detection in retinal images by applying region-based active aontour model in a variational level set formulation," in *Proceedings of the International Conference on Computer Vision in Remote Sensing (CVRS '12)*, pp. 39–44, Xiamen, China, December 2012.

[4] J. Malek and R. Tourki, "Blood vessels extraction and classification into arteries and veins in retinal images," in *Proceedings*

of the 10th International Multi-Conference on Systems, Signals & Devices (SSD '13), pp. 1–6, Hammamet, Tunisia, March 2013.

[5] J. Malek and R. Tourki, "Inertia-based vessel centerline extraction in retinal image," in *Proceedings of the International Conference on Control, Decision and Information Technologies (CoDIT '13)*, pp. 378–381, Hammamet, Tunisia, May 2013.

[6] M. Al-Rawi, M. Qutaishat, and M. Arrar, "An improved matched filter for blood vessel detection of digital retinal images," *Computers in Biology and Medicine*, vol. 37, no. 2, pp. 262–267, 2007.

[7] M. E. Tyler, L. D. Hubbard, K. Boydston, and A. J. Pugliese, "Characteristics of digital fundus camera systems affecting tonal resolution in color retinal images," *The Journal of Ophthalmic Photography*, vol. 31, no. 1, pp. 1–9, 2009.

[8] T. W. Hansen, J. Jeppesen, S. Rasmussen, H. Ibsen, and C. Torp-Pedersen, "Ambulatory blood pressure and mortality: a population-based study," *Hypertension*, vol. 45, no. 4, pp. 499–504, 2005.

[9] T. Teng, M. Lefley, and D. Claremont, "Progress towards automated diabetic ocular screening: a review of image analysis and intelligent systems for diabetic retinopathy," *Medical and Biological Engineering and Computing*, vol. 40, no. 1, pp. 2–13, 2002.

[10] M. Ben Abdallah, J. Malek, R. Tourki, J. E. Monreal, and K. Krissian, "Automatic estimation of the noise model in fundus images," in *Proceedings of the 10th International Multi-Conference on Systems, Signals & Devices (SSD '13)*, pp. 1–5, Hammamet, Tunisia, March 2013.

[11] N. Patton, T. M. Aslam, T. MacGillivray et al., "Retinal image analysis: concepts, applications and potential," in *Progress in Retinal and Eye Research*, vol. 25, pp. 99–127, 2006.

[12] T. Walter, J.-C. Klein, P. Massin, and A. Erginay, "A contribution of image processing to the diagnosis of diabetic retinopathy-detection of exudates in color fundus images of the human retina," *IEEE Transactions on Medical Imaging*, vol. 21, no. 10, pp. 1236–1243, 2002.

[13] S. Chaudhuri, S. Chatterjee, N. Katz, M. Nelson, and M. Goldbaum, "Detection of blood vessels in retinal images using two-dimensional matched filters," *IEEE Transactions on Medical Imaging*, vol. 8, no. 3, pp. 263–269, 1989.

[14] B. Zhang, L. Zhang, L. Zhang, and F. Karray, "Retinal vessel extraction by matched filter with first-order derivative of Gaussian," *Computers in Biology and Medicine*, vol. 40, pp. 438–445, 2010.

[15] J. Malek, A. T. Azar, and R. Tourki, "Impact of retinal vascular tortuosity on retinal circulation," *Neural Computing and Applications*, 2014.

[16] M. Sofka and C. V. Stewar, "Retinal vessel extraction using multiscale matched filters confidence and edge measures," Tech. Rep., Department of Computer Science, Rensselaer Polytechnic Institute, 2005.

[17] Y. Sato, S. Nakajima, N. Shiraga et al., "Three-dimensional multi-scale line filter for segmentation and visualization of curvilinear structures in medical images," *Medical Image Analysis*, vol. 2, no. 2, pp. 143–168, 1998.

[18] R. M. Rangayyan, F. Oloumi, F. Oloumi, P. Eshghzadeh-Zanjani, and F. J. Ayres, "Detection of blood vessels in the retina using Gabor filters," in *Proceedings of the 20th Canadi an Conference on Electrical and Computer Engineering (CCECE '07)*, pp. 717–720, Vancouver, Canada, April 2007.

[19] T. Pock, C. Janko, R. Beichel, and H. Bischof, "Multiscale medialness for robust segmentation of 3D tubular structures,"

in *Proceedings of the 10th Computer Vision with Workshop*, The Austrian Science Fund (FWF) under the grants P17066-N04, February 2005.

[20] M. G. Cinsdikici and D. Aydin, "Detection of blood vessels in ophthalmoscope images using MF/ant (matched filter/ant colony) algorithm," *Computer Methods and Programs in Biomedicine*, vol. 96, no. 2, pp. 85–95, 2009.

[21] A. M. Mendonça and A. Campilho, "Segmentation of retinal blood vessels by combining the detection of centerlines and morphological reconstruction," *IEEE Transactions on Medical Imaging*, vol. 25, no. 9, pp. 1200–1213, 2006.

[22] F. Zana and J.-C. Klein, "Segmentation of vessel-like patterns using mathematical morphology and curvature evaluation," *IEEE Transactions on Image Processing*, vol. 10, no. 7, pp. 1010–1019, 2001.

[23] M. M. Fraz, M. Y. Javed, and A. Basit, "Evaluation of retinal vessel segmentation methodologies based on combination of vessel centerlines and morphological processing," in *Proceedings of the 4th IEEE International Conference on Emerging Technologies (ICET '08)*, pp. 232–236, Rawalpindi, Pakistan, October 2008.

[24] L. Gang, O. Chutatape, and S. M. Krishnan, "Detection and measurement of retinal vessels in fundus images using amplitude modified second-order Gaussian filter," *IEEE Transactions on Biomedical Engineering*, vol. 49, no. 2, pp. 168–172, 2002.

[25] J. Staal, M. D. Abràmoff, M. Niemeijer, M. A. Viergever, and B. Van Ginneken, "Ridge-based vessel segmentation in color images of the retina," *IEEE Transactions on Medical Imaging*, vol. 23, no. 4, pp. 501–509, 2004.

[26] P. C. Siddalingaswamy, "Automatic detection of multiple oriented blood vessels in retinal images," *Journal of Biomedical Science and Engineering*, vol. 3, pp. 101–107, 2010.

[27] S. Dua, N. Kandiraju, and H. W. Thompson, "Design and implementation of a unique blood-vessel detection algorithm towards early diagnosis of diabetic retinopathy," in *Proceedings of the IEEE International Conference on Information Technology: Coding and Computing*, vol. 1, pp. 26–31, April 2005.

[28] A. Frangi, *Three-dimensional model -based analysis of vascular and cardiac images [Ph.D. thesis]*, Utrecht University, Utrecht, The Netherlands, 2001.

[29] C. Lorenz, I.-C. Carlsen, T. M. Buzug, C. Fassnacht, and J. Weese, "Multi scale line segmentation with automatic estimation of width, contrast and tangential direction in 2d and 3d medical images," in *Proceedings of the 1st Joint Conference Computer Vision, Virtual Reality and Robotics in Medicine and Medical Robotics and Computer-Assisted Surgery (CVRMed-MRCAS '97)*, pp. 233–242, Springer, London, UK, 1997.

[30] J. L. Federman, P. Gouras, H. Schubert et al., "Systemic diseases," in *Retina and Vitreous: Textbook of Ophthalmology*, S. M. Podos and M. Yano, Eds., vol. 9, pp. 7–24, Mosby, St. Louis, Mo, USA, 1994.

[31] W. Huang, *Automatic Detection and Quantification of Blood Vessels in the Vicinity of the Optic Disc in Digital Retinal Images*, University of Waikato, 2006.

[32] http://reference.medscape.com/features/slideshow/retina.

[33] A. Hoover, "STARE database," http://www.ces.clemson.edu/~ahoover/stare/.

[34] M. Niemeijer and B. van Ginneken, 2002, http://www.isi.uu.nl/Research/Databases/DRIVE/results.php.

[35] A. Hoover, V. Kouznetsova, and M. Goldbaum, "Locating blood vessels in retinal images by piecewise threshold probing of a matched filter response," *IEEE Transactions on Medical Imaging*, vol. 19, no. 3, pp. 203–210, 2000.

[36] K. Krissian, "Flux-based anisotropic diffusion applied to enhancement of 3-D angiogram," *IEEE Transactions on Medical Imaging*, vol. 21, no. 11, pp. 1440–1442, 2002.

[37] C. Blondel, *Modelisation 3D et 3D + t des arteres coronaires a partir de sequences rotationnelles de projections rayons X [Ph.D. thesis]*, University of Nice Sophia Antipolis, Nice, France, 2004.

[38] M. Ben Abdallah, J. Malek, R. Tourki, and K. Krissian, "Restoration of retinal images using anisotropic diffusion like algorithms," in *Proceedings of the International Conference on Computer Vision in Remote Sensing (CVRS '12)*, pp. 116–121, Xiamen, China, December 2012.

[39] K. Krissian, G. Malandain, N. Ayache, R. Vaillant, and Y. Trousset, "Model-based detection of tubular structures in 3D images," *Computer Vision and Image Understanding*, vol. 80, no. 2, pp. 130–171, 2000.

[40] G.-H. Cottet and L. Germain, "Image processing through reaction combined with nonlinear diffusion," *Mathematics of Computation*, vol. 61, no. 204, pp. 659–673, 1993.

[41] J. Weickert, "Scale-space properties of nonlinear diffusion filtering with a diffusion tensor," Tech. Rep. 110, University of Kaiserslautern, Kaiserslautern, Germany, 1994.

[42] J. Bigun, G. H. Granlund, and J. Wiklund, "Multidimensional orientation estimation with applications to texture analysis and optical flow," *IEEE Transactions on Pattern Analysis and Machine Intelligence*, vol. 13, no. 8, pp. 775–790, 1991.

[43] M. Ben Abdallah, M. Jihene, K. Krissian, and R. Tourki, "An automated vessel segmentation of retinal images using multiscale vesselness," in *Proceedings of the 8th International Multi-Conference on Systems, Signals & Devices*, IEEE, 2011.

[44] J. V. B. Soares, J. J. G. Leandro, R. M. Cesar Jr., H. F. Jelinek, and M. J. Cree, "Retinal vessel segmentation using the 2-D Gabor wavelet and supervised classification," *IEEE Transactions on Medical Imaging*, vol. 25, no. 9, pp. 1214–1222, 2006.

[45] M. E. Martinez-Perez, A. D. Hughes, S. A. Thom, A. A. Bharath, and K. H. Parker, "Segmentation of blood vessels from red-free and fluorescein retinal images," *Medical Image Analysis*, vol. 11, no. 1, pp. 47–61, 2007.

[46] M. Niemeijer, J. Staal, B. van Ginneken, M. Loog, and M. D. Abramoff, "Comparative study of retinal vessel segmentation methods on a new publicly available database," in *Proceedings of the SPIE Medical Imaging*, M. Fitzpatrick and M. Sonka, Eds., vol. 5370, pp. 648–656, 2004.

[47] X. Jiang and D. Mojon, "Adaptive local thresholding by verification-based multithreshold probing with application to vessel detection in retinal images," *IEEE Transactions on Pattern Analysis and Machine Intelligence*, vol. 25, no. 1, pp. 131–137, 2003.

[48] T. Lindeberg and D. Fagerström, "Scale-space with casual time direction," in *Proceedings of the 4th European Conference on Computer Vision (ECCV '96)*, pp. 229–240, Cambridge, UK, April 1996.

[49] W. Changhua, G. Agam, and P. Stanchev, "A general framework for vessel segmentation in retinal images," in *Proceedings of the International Symposium on Computational Intelligence in Robotics and Automation (CIRA '07)*, June 2007.

[50] X. Qian, M. P. Brennan, D. P. Dione et al., "A non-parametric vessel detection method for complex vascular structures," *Medical Image Analysis*, vol. 13, no. 1, pp. 49–61, 2008.

[51] L. Wang, A. Bhalerao, and R. Wilson, "Analysis of retinal vasculature using a multiresolution hermite model," *IEEE Transactions on Medical Imaging*, vol. 26, no. 2, pp. 137–152, 2007.

[52] A. P. Witkin, "Scale-space filtering: a new apporach to multi scale description," in *Proceedings of the IEEE International Conference on Acoustics, Speech, and Signal Processing (ICASSP '84)*, pp. 150–153, March 1984.

Permissions

List of Contributors

Seiya Tsuda, Yuji Iwahori
Department of Computer Science, Chubu University, 1200 Matsumotocho, Kasugai 487-8501, Japan

M. K. Bhuyan
Department of Electronics and Electrical Engineering, IIT Guwahati, Guwahati 781039, India

Robert J. Woodham
Department of Computer Science, University of British Columbia, Vancouver, BC, Canada V6T 1Z4

Kunio Kasugai
Department of Gastroenterology, Aichi Medical University, 1-1 Karimata, Yazako, Nagakute 480-1195, Japan

Jan Marek Marcinczak and Rolf-Rainer Grigat
Hamburg University of Technology, Schlossstraße 20, 21079 Hamburg, Germany

Marwan Abdellah, Ayman Eldeib, and Amr Sharawi
Biomedical Engineering Department, Cairo University, Giza 12613, Egypt

Eman Magdy, Nourhan Zayed and Mahmoud Fakhr
Computer and Systems Department, Electronic Research Institute, Giza 12611, Egypt

Mark W. Lenox, James Wiskin, Stephen Darrouzet, David Borup and Scott Hsieh
QT Ultrasound, LLC, Novato, CA 94949, USA

Matthew A. Lewis
Department of Radiology, University of Texas Southwestern Medical Center, Dallas, TX 75390, USA

Xiao-Quan Xu, Fei-Yun Wu, Hao Hu, Guo-Yi Su and Jie Shen
Department of Radiology, The First Affiliated Hospital of Nanjing Medical University, No. 300, Guangzhou Road, Nanjing 210029, China

Joseph Shtok, Michael Elad and Michael Zibulevsky
Computer Science Department, Technion - Israel Institute of Technology, Haifa 32000, Israel

Nourhan Zayed and Heba A. Elnemr
Computer & Systems Department, Electronics Research Institute, Cairo 12611, Egypt

Ahmad Chaddad
Department of Diagnostic Radiology, University of TexasMD Anderson Cancer Center, 1400 Pressler Street, Houston, TX 77030, USA

Joshua Kim
Tetra Imaging, 4591 Bentley Drive, Troy, MI 48098, USA
Department of Physics,Oakland University, 2200N. Squirrel Road, Rochester, MI 48309, USA

Huaiqun Guan
21st Century Oncology Inc., 4274W. Main Street, Dothan, AL 36305, USA

David Gersten
Department of Radiation Oncology, William Beaumont Hospital, 3601W.Thirteen Mile Road, Royal Oak, MI 48073, USA

Tiezhi Zhang
TetraImaging, 4591 Bentley Drive, Troy, MI 48098, USA
Department of Physics, Oakland University, 2200N. Squirrel Road, Rochester, MI 48309, USA
Department of Radiation Oncology, William Beaumont Hospital, 3601W.Thirteen Mile Road, Royal Oak, MI 48073, USA

Gurman Gill
Department of Electrical and Computer Engineering,The University of Iowa, Iowa City, IA 52242, USA
The Iowa Institute for Biomedical Imaging, The University of Iowa, Iowa City, IA 52242, USA

Reinhard R. Beichel
Department of Electrical and Computer Engineering,The University of Iowa, Iowa City, IA 52242, USA
The Iowa Institute for Biomedical Imaging, The University of Iowa, Iowa City, IA 52242, USA
Department of InternalMedicine, The University of Iowa, Iowa City, IA 52242, USA

Jimmy C. Azar, Martin Simonsson, Ewert Bengtsson and Anders Hast
Centre for Image Analysis, Department of Information Technology, Uppsala University, 75105 Uppsala, Sweden

Mohammad H. Asghari
Department of Electrical Engineering, University of California, Los Angeles, Los Angeles, CA 90095, USA

Bahram Jalali
Department of Electrical Engineering, University of California, Los Angeles, Los Angeles, CA 90095, USA
Department of Bioengineering, University of California, Los Angeles, Los Angeles, CA 90095, USA
Department of Surgery, David Geffen School of Medicine, University of California, Los Angeles, Los Angeles, CA 90095, USA

Anupama Kuruvilla
Department of BME and Center for Bioimage Informatics, Carnegie Mellon University, Pittsburgh, PA 15213, USA

Nader Shaikh, Alejandro Hoberman
Division of General Academic Pediatrics, Children's Hospital of Pittsburgh, University of Pittsburgh School of Medicine, Pittsburgh, PA 15213, USA

Jelena Kovalevi
Department of BME and Center for Bioimage Informatics, Carnegie Mellon University, Pittsburgh, PA 15213, USA
Department of ECE Carnegie Mellon University, Pittsburgh, PA 15213, USA

Anwar Abdalbari and Jing Ren
Faculty of Engineering and Applied Science, University of Ontario Institute of Technology, 2000 Simcoe Street North, Oshawa, ON, Canada L1H 7K4

Xishi Huang
Department of Medical Imaging, University of Toronto, Toronto, ON, Canada M5T 1W7

Ketil Oppedal
Department of Electrical Engineering and Computer Science, University of Stavanger, 4036 Stavanger, Norway
Centre for Age-Related Medicine, Stavanger University Hospital, Stavanger, Norway

Trygve Eftestøl, Kjersti Engan
Department of Electrical Engineering and Computer Science, University of Stavanger, 4036 Stavanger, Norway

Mona K. Beyer
Department of Radiology and Nuclear Medicine, Oslo University Hospital, Oslo, Norway
Department of Life Sciences and Health, Faculty of Health Sciences, Oslo and Akershus University College of Applied Sciences, Oslo, Norway

Dag Aarsland
Centre for Age-Related Medicine, Stavanger University Hospital, Stavanger, Norway
Alzheimer's Disease Research Centre, Karolinska Institutet (KI), Stockholm, Sweden

Alexander Heidrich
Department of Cell and Molecular Biology, Leibniz Institute for Natural Product Research and Infection Biology, Hans Kn¨oll Institute, Beutenberg Straße 11a, 07745 Jena, Germany

Jana Schmidt
Institut f¨ur Informatik/I12, Technische Universit¨at M¨unchen, Boltzmannstrraße 3, 85748 Garching bei M¨unchen, Germany

Johannes Zimmermann
Definiens AG, Bernhard-Wicki-Straße 5, 80636 M¨unchen, Germany

Hans Peter Saluz
Department of Cell and Molecular Biology, Leibniz Institute for Natural Product Research and Infection Biology, Hans Kn¨oll Institute, Beutenberg Straße 11a, 07745 Jena, Germany
Friedrich Schiller University of Jena, F¨urstengraben 1, 07743 Jena, Germany

Marco Bögel, Hannes G. Hofmann, Joachim Hornegger
Pattern Recognition Lab, Friedrich-Alexander-University Erlangen-Nuremberg, 91058 Erlangen, Germany

Rebecca Fahrig
Department of Radiology, Lucas MRS Center, Stanford University, Palo Alto, CA 94304, USA

Stefan Britzen and Andreas Maier
Siemens AG, Healthcare Sector, 91301 Forchheim, Germany

Abishek Arora
Amity Institute of Biotechnology, Amity University Uttar Pradesh, Noida 201303, India

Neeta Bhagat
Amity Institute of Biotechnology, Amity University Uttar Pradesh, Room No. 312, J3 Block, III Floor, Noida 201303, India

Javier S. Turek, Michael Elad and Irad Yavneh
Department of Computer Science, Israel Institute of Technology (Technion), 3200003 Haifa, Israel

Jinyang Sun, Fangjun Luan
School of Information & Control Engineering, Shenyang Jianzhu University, Shenyang 110168, China

Hanhui Wu
Sino-Dutch Biomedical and Information Engineering School, Northeastern University, Shenyang 110819, China

Romuald Jolivot
National Electronic and Computer Technology Center, 112Thailand Science Park, Phahonyothin Road, Khlong Nueng, Klong Luang, Pathumthani 12120,Thailand

Yannick Benezeth and Franck Marzani
Laboratoire LE2I, UMR CNRS 6306, UFR Sciencees & Techniques, Universit´e de Bourgogne, BP 47870, 21078 Dijon CEDEX, France

Mariem Ben Abdallah, Jihene Malek, Hafedh Belmabrouk
Faculty of Sciences, Electronics and Microelectronics Laboratory, Monastir University, 5019 Monastir, Tunisia

Ahmad Taher Azar
Faculty of Computers and Information, Benha University, Benha 13511, Egypt

Philippe Montesinos
Institute of Mines and Ales, Laboratory of Computer and Production Engineering, 30319 Al`es, France

Julio Esclarín Monreal and Karl Krissian
Imaging Technology Center (CTIM), Las Palmas-Gran Canaria University, 35017 Las Palmas de Gran Canaria, Spain